ULTRASOUND PHYSICS AND INSTRUMENTATION

ULTRASOUND PHYSICS AND INSTRUMENTATION

Wayne R. Hedrick, PhD
Professor, Medical Radiation Biophysics,
Northeastern Ohio Universities College of Medicine, Rootstown, Ohio
Certified Diagnostic Radiological Physicist and Medical Nuclear Physicist
American Board of Radiology,
Aultman Hospital, Canton, Ohio

David L. Hykes, PhD
Certified Radiological Physicist, American Board of Radiology,
Medical Physics Services, Inc., Canton, Ohio

Dale E. Starchman, PhD
Professor, Medical Radiation Biophysics,
Northeastern Ohio Universities College of Medicine, Rootstown, Ohio
Certified Radiological Physicist, American Board of Radiology,
Mercy Medical Center, Canton, Ohio

Fourth Edition

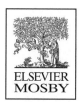

ELSEVIER
MOSBY

ELSEVIER
MOSBY

11830 Westline Industrial Drive
St. Louis, Missouri 63146

ULTRASOUND PHYSICS AND INSTRUMENTATION
Fourth Edition   0-323-03212-5
Copyright © 2005, 1995, 1992, 1985 by Mosby, Inc.

NOTICE

Ultrasound physics is an ever-changing field. Standard safety precautions must be followed, but as new research and clinical experience broaden our knowledge, changes in treatment and drug therapy may become necessary or appropriate. Readers are advised to check the most current product information provided by the manufacturer of each drug to be administered to verify the recommended dose, the method and duration of administration, and contraindications. It is the responsibility of the licensed prescriber, relying on experience and knowledge of the patient, to determine dosages and the best treatment for each individual patient. Neither the publisher nor the author assumes any liability for any injury and/or damage to persons or property arising from this publication.

The Publisher

International Standard Book Number 0-323-03212-5

Publisher: Andrew Allen
Acquisitions Editor: Jeanne Wilke
Senior Developmental Editor: Linda Woodard
Publishing Services Manager: Patricia Tannian
Project Manager: Kristine Feeherty
Designer: Jyotika Shroff

Printed in the United States of America

Last digit is the print number: 9   8   7   6   5   4   3   2   1

In memory of

Mary Mihelcic-Jones

A woman of compassion, intelligence, grace, and beauty

Reviewers

Janice Dolk, MA, RT (R), RDMS

Consultant
Owings Mills, Maryland

Thomas J. Gervaise, BS, RT, RDMS

Ultrasound Program Director
Modern Technology School
Anaheim, California

Susanna Ovel, RDMS, RVT

Senior Sonographer/Instructor
Radiological Associates of Sacramento (RAS)
Sacramento, California

Regina Swearengin, BS, RDMS

Department Chair, Sonography
Austin Community College
Austin, Texas

Preface

This new edition continues to present ultrasound physics in an easy-to-understand and comprehensive manner for diagnostic medical ultrasonography students and radiology residents. It will also benefit physicians and technologists in many medical specialties, including obstetrics, cardiology, vascular surgery, urology, general surgery, and veterinary medicine. In addition, medical physicists will find the principles of ultrasound physics and instrumentation that they need to know for clinical practice.

The field of medical diagnostic ultrasound has expanded rapidly over the past decade. Although the basic physical principles are unchanged, significant advances in instrumentation have resulted in increased clinical utilization of ultrasound in medicine. If individuals who perform and/or interpret ultrasound scans are to obtain the highest quality of diagnostic information, they must understand the underlying physical principles and instrumentation.

In the last few years the technical evolution has had an impact on computer processing techniques, PACS, Doppler imaging, tissue harmonic imaging, spatial compounding, frequency compounding, extended field of view, coded excitation, elasticity imaging, contrast agents, beam formation, broadband transducers, 1.5D and 2D transducers, and 3D ultrasound. The text has been revised and expanded to reflect these and other advances in medical diagnostic ultrasound instrumentation.

NEW CONTENT AND ORGANIZATION

Now divided into 25 chapters, the book opens with a detailed presentation of the basic physical principles of ultrasound. Chapter 1 is vitally important because the physical principles it presents form the basis for understanding all ultrasonic scanning modes. These principles are dramatically different from those that apply to diagnostic x-ray imaging. Chapter 2 discusses attenuation in tissue with some mathematical detail. Computer fundamentals are introduced in Chapter 3, followed later by digital processing techniques (Chapter 10) and computer networks (Chapter 20). Chapters 4 and 5 present single-element transducer design, pulse generation, and echo reception, which have application to multielement array transducers. Static imaging modes (A-mode, static B-mode, gated, and transmission) are discussed in Chapter 6. These instruments have been almost totally replaced with real-time scanners, which are described in Chapters 7 through 12, including separate chapters on image quality (Chapter 11) and image artifacts (Chapter 12). Hemodynamics is presented in Chapter 13 before the treatment of Doppler ultrasound (Chapters 14 through 16). Chapter 17 examines M-mode scanning. Contrast agents are discussed in Chapter 18. The usual end product of ultrasonic scanning is an image recorded on film or other media. An overview of image recording devices is presented in Chapter 19. As with other imaging techniques, ultrasound deposits energy into the body and thus has the potential for causing biological effects. Ultrasound exposure is quantified by intensity for which multiple descriptors are possible (Chapter 21). Chapter 22 reviews the literature concerning the biological effects of ultrasound. Clinical safety concerns associated with medical diagnostic ultrasound are addressed in Chapter 23. Image quality must be maintained at a high level via an appropriate quality control program as set forth in Chapter 25. Quality control has been completely revised and separated from performance testing, which is discussed in Chapter 24.

FEATURES

This text fully prepares the reader, not only by explaining the necessary principles but also by using analogies, incorporating sample problems throughout, presenting key terms, and providing review questions at the end of each chapter with answers in the back of the book. An extensive glossary of ultrasonic terms is included. Appendix A contains a comprehensive mathematics review, and Appendix B contains a short discussion of Fourier analysis, a computer processing technique in Doppler ultrasound. A separate practice exam can be found on Evolve's learning resources for students.

Problem solving is an integral part of the learning process in physics and is necessary for passing registry and certification examinations. The comprehensive examination will thoroughly test the working knowledge of readers in the physics and instrumentation of ultrasound, thus helping them prepare for examinations given by the American Registry of Diagnostic Medical Sonographers. All the learning tools integrated within this text help make comprehension easier and more successful.

EVOLVE—ONLINE COURSE MANAGEMENT

Evolve is an interactive learning environment designed to work in coordination with *Ultrasound Physics and Instru-*

mentation. Instructors may use Evolve to provide an Internet-based course component that reinforces and expands on the concepts delivered in class. Evolve may be used to publish the class syllabus, outlines, and lecture notes; set up "virtual office hours" and e-mail communication; share important dates and information through the online class calendar; and encourage student participation through chat rooms and discussion boards. Evolve allows instructors to post examinations and manage their grade book online. For more information, visit ***http://www.evolve. elsevier.com/Hedrick/ultrasound*** or contact an Elsevier sales representative.

Wayne R. Hedrick
David L. Hykes
Dale E. Starchman

Acknowledgments

As with any undertaking of this type, we are indebted to a number of people who contributed their time and expertise.

A very special thanks to Linda Metzger, RT, RDMS, RVT, for her technical assistance in the preparation of this book.

The diagnostic medical sonographers at Aultman Hospital are a resource of technical expertise who create a challenging learning environment for residents and student sonographers:

James Allman, BS, RT, RDMS, RVT
Natalie Arnold, CVT
Kelly Bourne, BA, BS
Ginger Busselman, CVT
Valerie A. Class, RT(M), RDMS
Rebecca Congon, RT, RDMS
Karen Conway, RDMS
Stephanie Davenport, RT, RDMS, RVT, RDC
Kathy Filicky, RT, RDMS
Julie Guglielmi, RT, RDMS, RVT
Christy Jones, RDMS
Karen Karlen, RT, RDMS
Thelma Lasko, RT, RDCS
Heather Massarelli, BS, RT, RDMS
Amy Mitan, BS, RT, RDMS
Lisa Montini, RT, RDMS
Sarah Poultney, SCVT
Rachael Qadri, RT, RDMS
Angela Riker, RDMS
Susan Schmidt, RT, RDMS
Charlelle Shonk, CVT
Mandy Stephens, CVT
Jennifer Stevens, RT, RDCS
Sheri Tilton, RT, RDMS, RVT

The assistance of Rob Steins, John Antol, Ken Barrett, Carol Milligan, and Kelly Beicke of Siemens Medical Solutions USA, Inc., is appreciated. We would also like to acknowledge Scott Sheldon, DO, for demonstrating clinical applications of intravascular imaging.

Discussions with medical physicists Jerry A. Thomas, MS, and Mark Rzeszotarski, PhD, have provided insight and encouragement.

We have been fortunate to work with many excellent physicians during our professional careers. Richard Albright, MD, and Mark DeGalan, MD, practice the art and science of radiology and are an inspiration to all who know them.

Contents

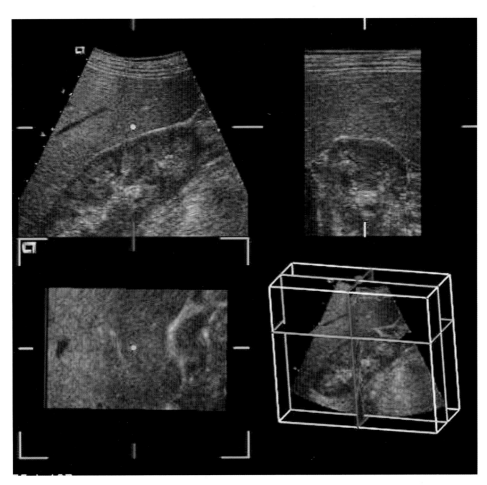

Color Plate 1 Three-dimensional multiformat. Three orthogonal planes through the kidney are displayed. The reference image denotes the orientation. (See Fig. 9-51.) (Courtesy Siemens Medical Solutions USA, Inc., Ultrasound Division, Malvern, Penn.)

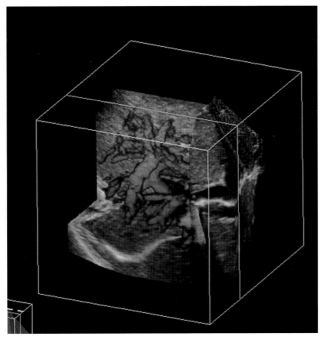

Color Plate 2 Three-dimensional polyhedron image display showing liver vasculature in a child. (See Fig. 9-52.) (Courtesy Siemens Medical Solutions USA, Inc., Ultrasound Division, Malvern, Penn.)

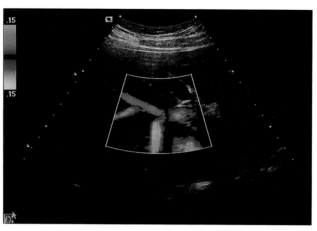

Color Plate 3 Doppler imaging of the portal vein. Flow in the anterior right portal vein and the posterior right portal vein is shown using a rainbow color map. (See Fig. 16-2.) Color Plates 4 and 5 show a color map depicting flow toward the transducer in red and blue, respectively.

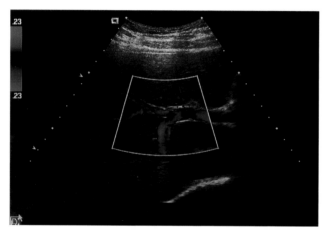

Color Plate 4 Doppler imaging of the portal vein. Flow in the anterior right portal vein and the posterior right portal vein is shown using a saturation color map. (See Fig. 16-2.) Flow toward the transducer is depicted in red.

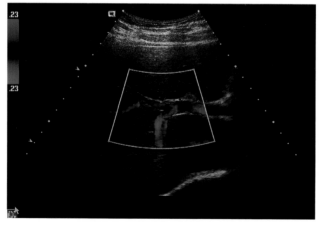

Color Plate 5 Doppler imaging of the portal vein. Flow in the anterior right portal vein and the posterior right portal vein is shown using a saturation color map. (See Fig. 16-2.) Flow toward the transducer is depicted in blue.

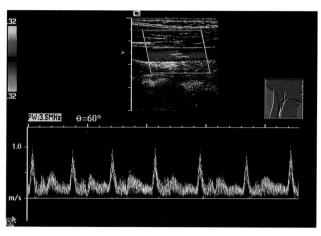

Color Plate 6 Combined Doppler mode. The color Doppler image with the sampled region identified is shown with the Doppler spectral analysis. (See Fig. 16-22.)

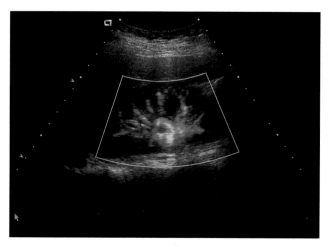

Color Plate 7 Power Doppler image of the kidney. (See Fig. 16-23.)

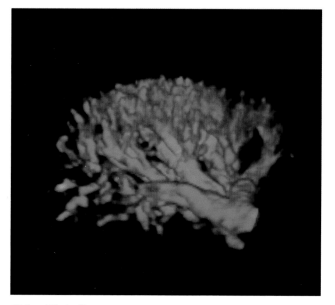

Color Plate 8 Three-dimensional power Doppler image of the kidney. (See Fig. 16-24.) (Courtesy Siemens Medical Solutions USA, Inc., Ultrasound Division, Malvern, Penn.)

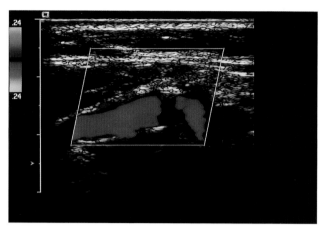

Color Plate 9 Shadowing by a calcified plaque obscures flow in the common carotid artery. (See Fig. 16-25.)

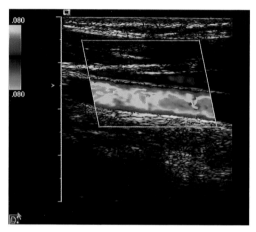

Color Plate 10 Color Doppler aliasing. Note the improper color progression—red to yellow to green to blue. If reverse flow were present, red and blue would be separated by a black region. (See Fig. 16-26.)

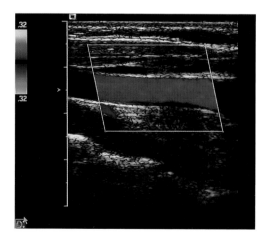

Color Plate 11 Increasing the velocity range removes the aliasing artifact in Fig. 16-26. (See Fig. 16-27.)

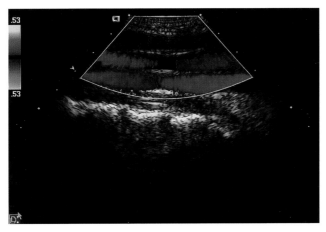

Color Plate 12 Color Doppler image of two vessels acquired with a vector transducer. (See Fig. 16-30.)

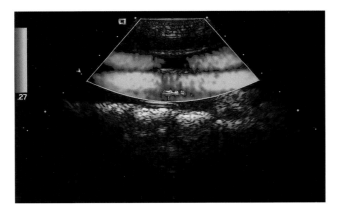

Color Plate 13 Power Doppler image of two vessels acquired with a vector transducer. (See Fig. 16-31.)

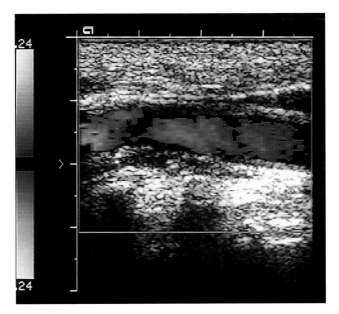

Color Plate 14 A tortuous vessel with unidirectional flow is depicted in changing colors, which suggests a reversal of flow. (See Fig. 16-32.)

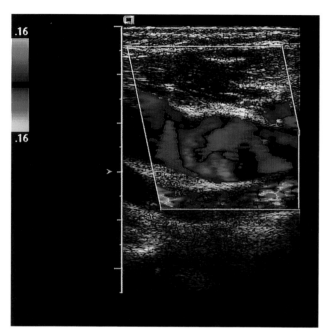

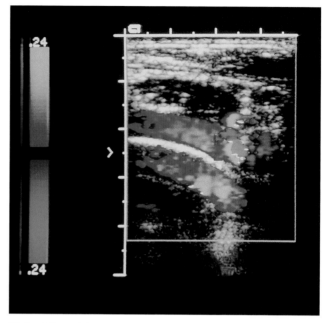

Color Plate 15 Flow reversal. (See Fig. 16-33.)

Color Plate 16 Color Doppler mirror image artifact of the subclavian artery. (See Fig. 16-34.) (Courtesy Rob Steins.)

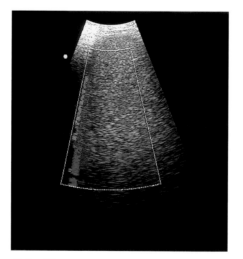

Color Plate 17 Flash artifact. Color is improperly assigned to stationary tissue (phantom material) caused by movement of the transducer. (See Fig. 16-35.)

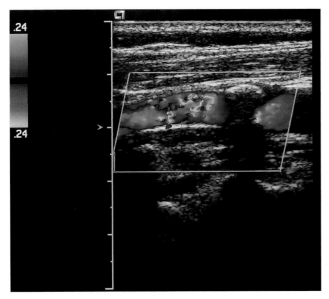

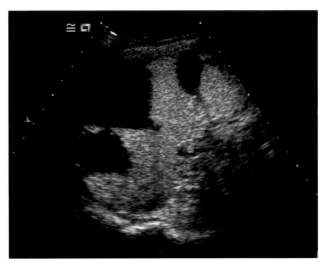

Color Plate 18 In this color flow image the internal carotid shows turbulence distal to the stenosis. (See Fig. 16-36.)

Color Plate 19 Sonogram of the liver showing the distribution of contrast agent. Three lesions that failed to accumulate contrast agent are present. (See Fig. 18-4.) (Courtesy Siemens Medical Solutions USA, Inc., Ultrasound Division, Malvern, Penn.)

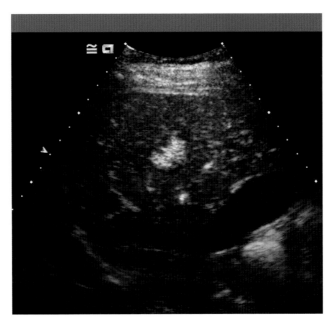

Color Plate 20 Sonogram of the liver showing the distribution of contrast agent. A mass with enhanced signal content is observed. (See Fig. 18-5.) (Courtesy Siemens Medical Solutions USA, Inc., Ultrasound Division, Malvern, Penn.)

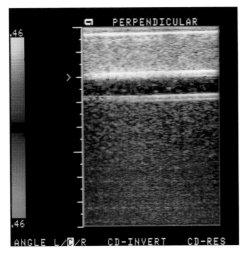

Color Plate 21 Color Doppler image of the vessel in the flow phantom obtained with a 90-degree Doppler angle. (See Fig. 24-50.)

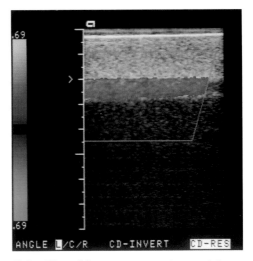

Color Plate 22 Color Doppler image of the vessel in the flow phantom obtained with a reduced Doppler angle. (See Fig. 24-51.)

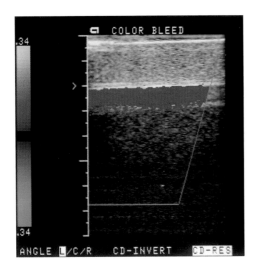

Color Plate 23 Color bleed artifact generated at high power and color gain with a Doppler flow phantom. (See Fig. 24-52.)

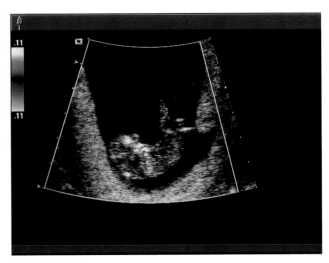

Color Plate 24 Color Doppler image of a fetus.

Basic Ultrasound Physics

SOUND WAVES

Sound is mechanical energy that is transmitted by pressure waves through a medium. Periodic changes in the pressure of the medium (air or water or iron) are created by forces acting on the molecules, causing them to oscillate about their normal, unperturbed positions. Since the motion of the molecules (particles) is repetitive, the term *cycle* is used to describe any sequence of changes in molecular motion (particle displacement, density of molecules, pressure, and particle velocity) that recurs at regular intervals.

The **frequency** of a wave is the number of vibrations (back and forth movements) that a molecule makes per second or the number of times the cycle is repeated each second. For comparative purposes, higher frequency means that the cyclic motion is executed at a faster rate and more cycles are completed in the 1-second interval than at lower frequency. Frequency is discussed in the section "Properties" later in this chapter. Sound waves are those pressure changes that the human ear can detect. They oscillate at frequencies of 20 to 20,000 cycles/second (1/s), also referred to as hertz (Hz).

Propagation

The periodic changes in pressure when vibrating molecules interact with neighboring molecules are conveyed from one location to another. The term *propagation* describes this transmittal to distant regions remote from the sound source.

Sound waves are mechanical in nature, but they are not restricted to transmission through air. Mechanical pressure waves require, however, an elastic deformable medium for propagation, which can be gas, liquid, or solid. A solid is deformable, because increased pressure applied to it causes a change in its shape. Elasticity is demonstrated by a return to the original shape when the pressure is lowered to its initial value. Electromagnetic radiation, which includes light and x-rays, consists of alternating electrical and magnetic fields that are at right angles to each other and that propagate through a vacuum at the speed of light. Sound waves are not electromagnetic radiation. Sound transmission cannot occur in a vacuum, because no molecules are available to transfer the mechanical vibrations.

Ultrasound is defined as mechanical waves with higher frequency than humans can hear: mechanical waves with frequencies of greater than 20,000 Hz, or 20 kHz (k = 10^3). Infrasound refers to mechanical waves with frequencies lower than humans can hear: less than 20 Hz. Sound, ultrasound, and infrasound have similar properties, and thus these terms are often used interchangeably in the description of physical interactions.

Wave equation. A steel ball attached to a metal spring, when pulled a small amount and released, moves back and forth, compressing and expanding the spring, displaying simple harmonic motion (Fig. 1-1). Its movement can be represented as a sinusoidal wave (Fig. 1-2). The location as a function of time can therefore be described using the wave equation

1-1

$$A = A_o \sin(2\pi ft)$$

where A is the amplitude (distance from the rest position) at time t, A_o the peak amplitude, f the frequency (cycles per second), and π a constant with the value of 3.1416. The peak amplitude is the maximum distance from the rest position.

Compression and rarefaction. Sound waves are pressure or mechanical waves that result in movement of the particles of a medium across or through their mean positions. The individual movement of each particle is described mathematically by the wave equation (Equation 1-1) and can be illustrated by looking at the movement of an audio speaker (Fig. 1-3). An electronic signal causes the mechanical movement of the speaker diaphragm. The speaker membrane mechanically vibrates or oscillates at the frequency of the sound being produced, and the sound is radiated throughout the room (Fig. 1-4).

The motion of the speaker can be visualized as a piston. When the speaker front moves forward, the air molecules immediately in front are pushed together, producing a region of increased air density, characterized by a small zone of increased pressure. The term **compression** describes the formation of the high-pressure region (Fig. 1-5). When the speaker front is pulled back, a zone of decreased molecular density results. The term **rarefaction** describes the creation of this low-pressure region.

The speaker alternately compresses the air on a forward thrust and rarefies the air on a backward thrust. The regions of compression and rarefaction are passed through the medium by molecular interactions. The originally affected molecules collide with adjacent molecules to propagate the action of the speaker. Thus the transmission of mechanical energy through the medium creates regions of varying particle density or pressure. Compression zones alternate with rarefaction zones. Between the adjacent compression zones particle density decreases to a minimum in the rarefaction zone and then increases back toward a maximum. If the action of sound propagation is frozen in time, a plot of the density of particles as a function of distance exhibits a wave pattern (Fig. 1-6, A). At a later instant the wave pattern of density variation is maintained (Fig. 1-6, B), but the compression and rarefaction zones have shifted to new locations. Molecular density is not constant at a particular position but fluctuates with a certain time dependence imposed by the frequency of the sound wave.

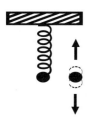

Fig. 1-1 Steel ball attached to a spring demonstrates oscillatory motion when the spring is compressed and released.

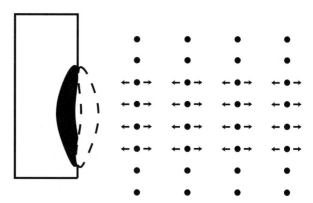

Fig. 1-3 Concept of molecular motion. Oscillation of air molecules produced by a speaker. Each molecule affected by the diaphragm movement travels back and forth over a short distance. However, the collected action of the molecules is complex.

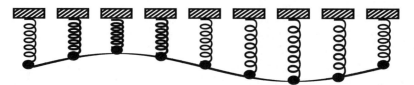

Fig. 1-2 Series of time-sequenced diagrams showing the position of the steel ball. A sinusoidal curve connects the steel ball locations with time. Maximum displacement from the position at rest is designated as the peak amplitude.

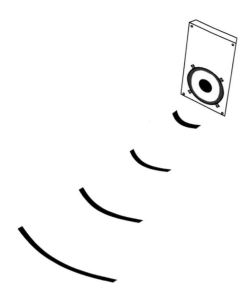

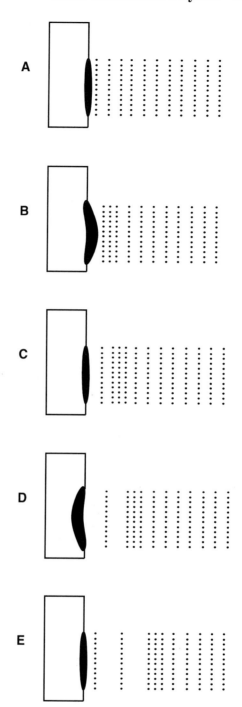

Fig. 1-4 The speaker action transfers sound throughout the room. Zones of rarefaction *(open areas)* alternate with zones of compression *(shaded areas).*

The molecules vibrate back and forth through their mean positions (a distance of only several microns) as the wave passes through the medium. A micron is equal to 10^{-6} meter. The motion of the molecules at a particular location is sinusoidal at the frequency of the sound wave (Fig. 1-7). Molecules do not travel from one end of the medium to the other; there is no flow of particles. Rather, the effect is transmitted over long distances because of neighbor-to-neighbor interactions. This molecular motion is necessary for sound transmission, which explains why sound cannot be transmitted through a vacuum.

Sound transmission is usually portrayed by showing the compression zones. A compression zone is often considered the leading portion of the sound wave and hence is called the wavefront. Wavefronts are helpful in illustrating the direction sound travels (perpendicular to the compression zone) and the region over which sound transmission takes place (the ultrasonic field).

Types of Sound Waves

Waves are divided into two basic types: longitudinal and transverse. Longitudinal waves are those in which particle motion is along the direction of the wave energy propagation; that is, the molecules vibrate back and forth in the same direction as the wave is traveling (Fig. 1-8). Sound waves in liquids and tissue are longitudinal.

Transverse waves are those in which the motion of the particles is perpendicular to the direction of propagation of the wave energy. The wave motion resulting from a stone thrown into a pool of water is an example of a transverse wave. The water molecules vibrate up and down, similar to a cork floating on the water, as the wave moves away from the point of origin across the surface of the water. An example of a transverse wave is shown in Fig. 1-9. Bone is the only biologic tissue that can cause the production of

Fig. 1-5 Influence of speaker motion on the surrounding air molecules. **A,** Undisturbed medium (no speaker motion). **B,** Speaker moving outward, compressing the medium. **C,** Speaker returning to its original position as a region of compression advances. **D,** Speaker moving inward, creating rarefaction in the medium. **E,** Speaker returning to its original position as the regions of compression and rarefaction advance.

transverse waves, which are sometimes referred to as shear waves or stress waves.

Properties of Sound Waves

Waves have certain physical characteristics that are used to describe them. Table 1-1 lists common descriptors and

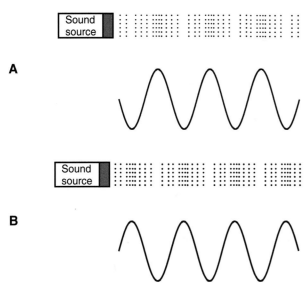

A

B

Fig. 1-6 Particle density along the path of propagation varies with time. Regions of high and low density alternate (as shown by the sinusoidal curves). **A,** Initial observation. **B,** After a short time the regions of high and low density are displaced to the right.

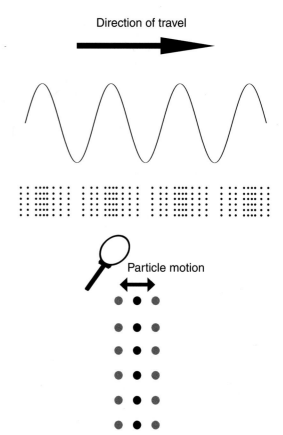

Fig. 1-8 Longitudinal wave. Molecular (particle) motion is along the direction of propagation.

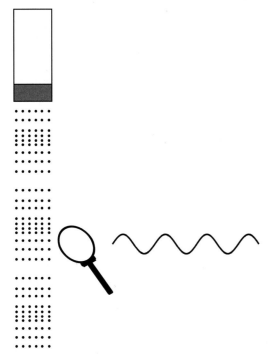

Fig. 1-7 Molecular motion as a function of time at a point within the ultrasonic field. As the sound wave propagates through the medium, individual molecules vibrate back and forth over a small distance.

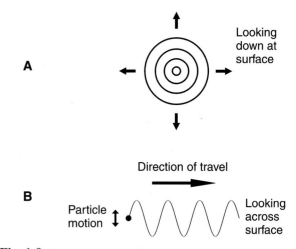

Fig. 1-9 Transverse wave. The direction of travel of the wave is radially outward from the sound source, **A,** which produces particle motion perpendicular to the direction of travel, **B.**

the corresponding symbols that are used in this text. Each descriptor is introduced and discussed in the chapter.

Physical quantities are measured in terms of a numerical value and a unit. A unit is a standard of measurement usually expressed in length, time, mass, charge, or some combination of these. Table 1-2 lists common units and the corresponding symbols that are used throughout the text.

To facilitate communication of the very large and very small numbers encountered in ultrasound physics, engineering prefixes are used. These prefixes correspond to various multiples of powers of 10, as shown in Table 1-3. When a physical parameter is expressed in scientific notation that includes some standard unit (e.g., meter, second, hertz, watt), the prefix replaces the power of 10 and becomes a modifier of the unit.

■ **Table 1-1**   List of Physical Descriptors and Symbols

Descriptor	Symbol
Absorption coefficient	α
Acoustic impedance	Z
Acoustic power	W
Acoustic pressure	p
Attenuation coefficient	a
Beam width	w
Bulk modulus	B
Compressibility	K
Density	ρ
Distance (scan depth)	z
Frequency	f
Instantaneous intensity	i
Intensity attenuation coefficient	μ
Particle displacement	s
Particle velocity	u
Percentage reflection	%R
Percentage transmission	%T
Period	τ
Reflection coefficient	α_r
Elapsed time	t
Time-averaged intensity	I
Transmission coefficient	α_t
Velocity of sound	c
Wavelength	λ

■ **Table 1-2**   List of Units and Symbols

Unit	Symbol
Meter	m
Centimeter	cm
Millimeter	mm
Micron (or micrometer)	μm
Kilogram	kg
Gram	g
Second	s
Millisecond	ms
Microsecond	μs
Hertz	Hz
Kilohertz	kHz
Megahertz	MHz
Joule	J
Watt	W
Pascal	Pa
Atmosphere	atm
Newton	Nt
Pound	lb
Volt	V
Coulomb	C
Degree Celsius	°C

■ **Table 1-3**   Unit Prefixes Representing Powers of 10

Factor	Prefix	Symbol
10^9	giga	G
10^6	mega	M
10^3	kilo	k
10^{-2}	centi	c
10^{-3}	milli	m
10^{-6}	micro	μ
10^{-9}	nano	n
10^{-12}	pico	p

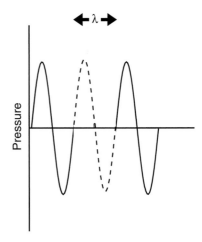

Fig. 1-10 Amplitude of particle density as a function of the distance of wave travel. The wavelength is equal to the distance between successive maxima or minima. It is also defined as the distance needed to complete one wave cycle (*dotted line*).

Wavelength.   **Wavelength** is the extent of one complete wave cycle (Fig. 1-10). A cycle is a sequence of changes in amplitude that recur at regular intervals. When particle density is plotted against distance, amplitude describes the variation in density. Wavelength is the distance between two successive equivalent density zones (i.e., two compression zones or two rarefaction zones) and is expressed in units of a meter (m), centimeter (cm), or millimeter (mm).

Amplitude.   Amplitude is the change in magnitude of a physical entity. The term can be applied to pressure in the medium or to particle density, particle displacement, or particle velocity in the medium. It has other applications, such as to characterize the size of a voltage pulse delivered to or induced within the crystal of the transducer (discussed later). When the amplitude is plotted as a function of time, the period of the wave (τ) is defined as the time necessary for one complete cycle or the time between two successive compression zones or rarefaction zones. Alternatively, the **period** is the elapsed time between compression zones as the sound wave passes through one point in the medium. The unit of the period is the second.

Frequency.   The frequency of a wave (f) is the number of cycles (pressure oscillations) occurring at a given point in one unit of time (usually 1 second). It corresponds to the inverse of the period ($1/\tau$). The unit of frequency is the hertz, which is equal to 1 cycle per second. Cycle is not a standard of measurement but is used as a descriptor to clarify the concept of frequency. Often frequency is expressed in units of inverse time only (1/s or s^{-1}).

The following equations define the relationship between period and frequency:

$$\tau = \frac{1}{f} \qquad \text{1-2}$$

and

$$f = \frac{1}{\tau} \qquad \text{1-3}$$

■ **Example 1-1**

Calculate the period of a wave whose frequency is 4,000,000 Hz or 4×10^6 cycles per second.

$$\tau = \frac{1}{f}$$

$$\tau = \frac{1}{4,000,000 \; 1/s}$$

$$\tau = 2.5 \times 10^{-7} \; s = 0.25 \; \mu s$$

■ **Example 1-2**

Calculate the frequency of a wave whose period is 5×10^{-7} second.

$$f = \frac{1}{\tau}$$

$$f = \frac{1}{5 \times 10^{-7} \; s}$$

$$f = 2 \times 10^6 \; 1/s = 2 \; MHz$$

Examples 1-1 and 1-2 illustrate the inverse relationship between frequency and period. When the period is doubled (from 2.5×10^{-7} s to 5×10^{-7} s), the frequency is halved (from 4×10^6 Hz to 2×10^6 Hz).

Acoustic velocity. The speed at which a wave propagates through the medium (rate of transfer of the mechanical vibrations) is called the **acoustic velocity** (c). In physics, velocity is usually considered a vector quantity—magnitude and direction are assigned. In ultrasound physics the term velocity traditionally refers to magnitude only (a scaler quantity). The velocity of sound is determined by the rate at which the wave energy is transmitted through the medium, which depends on the density and compressibility of the medium. Note that the acoustic velocity is not the same as the particle velocity (u), which refers to the speed at which the particles vibrate back and forth across their mean positions.

SOUND-PROPAGATION MEDIA

Properties

Elasticity. Elasticity refers to the ability of an object to return to its original shape and volume after a force is no longer acting on it. When a force is applied to the object (steel bar or soft tissue), a change in shape or volume

(distortion) is induced. The amount of this distortion depends on the strength of the force and the elastic properties of the object. The latter is determined by molecular interactions.

An ultrasound wave traveling through soft tissue causes elastic deformations by the separation and compression of neighboring molecules.

Density. Density (ρ) is the mass of a medium per unit volume. If all other physical properties of the medium are maintained unchanged, then an increase in density will impede the rate of sound propagation through the medium. As the density increases, more mass is contained within a given volume. For particles with increasingly larger mass, more force is required to produce molecular motion; and once the molecules are moving, more force is required to stop them. This is true for the rhythmic starting and stopping required to produce sound transmission. Thus on the basis of density alone, we would expect sound (ultrasound) to have a greater velocity in air (low density) than in bone (high density). However, this is not the case, and other factors must influence acoustic velocity.

Quantitatively, the velocity of sound in a medium (c) is inversely proportional to the square root of the density of the medium.

Compressibility. Another physical characteristic of a medium, **compressibility** (K), affects the velocity of sound through the medium. Compressibility indicates the fractional decrease in volume when pressure is applied to the material. The easier a medium is to reduce in volume, the higher is its compressibility.

The velocity of sound through a medium is also inversely proportional to the square root of the compressibility of the medium. However, the parameter relating the elastic properties of a medium to the velocity of sound through it is usually expressed as the reciprocal of the compressibility, termed the bulk modulus (B). Thus velocity is directly proportional to the square root of the bulk modulus.

A dense material (e.g., bone or other solid) is very difficult to reduce in volume when pressure is applied to it. This low compressibility predicts the high velocity of sound in bone. By contrast, air is easily reduced in volume, because the gas molecules are far apart and can be easily brought closer together (compressibility is high). The velocity of sound in air is low. Based on density and compressibility differences, the velocity of sound in bone is much greater than that in air.

Bulk modulus. The bulk modulus is often defined as the negative ratio of stress and strain. Stress is the force per unit area (or pressure) applied to an object. Strain is the fractional change in volume of the object. The negative sign is required since a positive pressure causes a decrease in volume. Large values for the bulk modulus indicate that a material is resistant to change in its volume when force is applied.

As the bulk modulus increases—and the compressibility decreases—the velocity of sound in the medium increases. Some authorities refer to this property as the "stiffness" of the medium.

Influences on Acoustic Velocity

Combining the compressibility (or bulk modulus) and density into one equation, we can determine the acoustic velocity for a particular medium:

1-4

$$c = \frac{1}{\sqrt{K\rho}}$$

or

$$c = \frac{\sqrt{B}}{\sqrt{\rho}}$$

If the density can be increased without affecting the compressibility, then Equation 1-4 predicts that the speed of sound will decrease. Compressibility and density of a particular substance are interdependent; a change in density is often coupled with a larger and opposing change in compressibility. Because compressibility varies more rapidly, it becomes the dominant factor in Equation 1-4. The overall effect is commonly summarized by the statement that, as density increases, the velocity of sound through a medium increases. Although exceptions can be cited, for materials of interest to the sonographer (air, lung, fat, soft tissue, plastic, bone) this statement is generally true.

As shown in Table 1-4, the velocity of sound in air is 330 meters per second (m/s) whereas in bone it is 4080 m/s. Bone is denser than air, but compressibility is the key factor in determining the relative acoustic velocities, because bone is less compressible than air.

■ **Table 1-4** Properties of Different Media

Material	Density (kg/m³)	Velocity (m/s)	Acoustic Impedance (kg/m²/s × 10⁶ or Megarayls)
Air	1.2	330	0.0004
Water (20° C)	1000	1480	1.48
Mercury	13,600	1450	20
Soft tissue			
Average*	1060	1540	1.63
Liver	1060	1550	1.64
Muscle	1080	1580	1.7
Fat	952	1459	1.38
Brain	994	1560	1.55
Kidney	1038	1560	1.62
Spleen	1045	1570	1.64
Blood	1057	1575	1.62
Bone	1912	4080	7.8
Lung	400	650	0.26
PZT	7650	3791	29
Lens	1142	1620	1.85
Aqueous humor	1000	1500	1.5
Vitreous humor	1000	1520	1.52
Lucite	1180	2680	3.16
Polystyrene	1060	2350	2.49
Castor oil	969	1477	1.43

PZT, Lead zirconate titanate.
*Average tissue (e.g., abdomen).

Density and compressibility effects can be compared by looking at two liquids. Water has a density of 1 gram per cubic centimeter (1 g/cm³) and mercury a density of 13.6 g/cm³. On the basis of density alone, water would have a velocity of sound $\sqrt{13.6}$ times greater than mercury. The compressibility of water is 13.4 times that of mercury (water is more easily compressed). Differences in compressibility and density between the two liquids cancel, so the velocities for water and mercury are similar (see Table 1-4). For liquids in general, density and compressibility offset each other, and consequently different liquids tend to transmit ultrasound at nearly the same velocity. In the transmission of sound, soft tissue behaves similarly to liquid; the acoustic velocities for various tissue types do not vary by more than a few percentage points.

In general, because their compressibility is low, more dense media (most solids) have greater velocities than do less dense media (liquids or gases). This is one of the reasons (the other will soon become evident) why, in old western movies, cowboys would put their heads to the ground or to a railroad track to hear stampeding buffalo or an approaching train. *Sound travels faster in media that are denser than air because of reduced compressibility.*

The average velocity of ultrasound in tissue is 1540 m/s or 154,000 cm/s or 1.54 mm/µs. A slight dependence on temperature of the medium and on sound frequency is exhibited; the velocity of ultrasound waves in water at 20° C is 1480 m/s but rises to 1570 m/s in water that is 37° C. For a few degrees' shift in temperature, the change in velocity through water is small. Thus room temperature fluctuations are not a problem with respect to clinical applications, because the body maintains a nearly constant temperature. Sound propagation in phantoms, however, is very dependent on temperature. To mimic tissue, a mixture of 8% ethanol and water at room temperature can be used. A change of 1° in the fluid mixture significantly alters the velocity of sound through the phantom.

The dependence of velocity or other physical parameter on frequency is called dispersion. The change in velocity with frequency is small (<0.5%) over the frequency range used in diagnostic ultrasound, which is 2 to 20 megahertz (MHz) (M = 10⁶). The velocity of sound in different materials (e.g., blood versus soft tissue) has varying frequency dependence, but these small differences have little importance in clinical imaging.

FREQUENCY, WAVELENGTH, AND VELOCITY

The velocity of sound or ultrasound remains constant for a particular medium. The velocity (c) is equal to the frequency (f) times the wavelength (λ). Stated mathematically:

1-5

$$c = f\lambda$$

This is probably the most important equation used in diagnostic ultrasound. *Because the velocity is constant for a particular medium, increasing the frequency causes the wavelength to decrease.* This phenomenon is demonstrated by Examples 1-3 and 1-4.

■ Example 1-3

Using Equation 1-5, we can determine the wavelength in tissue for a 2.5 MHz frequency ultrasound source as follows:

$$c = f \lambda$$

$$\lambda = \frac{c}{f}$$

$$\lambda = \frac{1540 \text{ m/s}}{2.5 \times 10^6 \text{ 1/s}}$$

$$\lambda = 6.2 \times 10^{-4} \text{ m}$$

$$\lambda = 0.62 \text{ mm}$$

If the frequency is increased to 5 MHz, the wavelength must decrease to half the value of 0.62 mm, because the frequency has doubled. Thus

$$\lambda = \frac{1540 \text{ m/s}}{5 \times 10^6 \text{ 1/s}}$$

$$\lambda = 3.1 \times 10^{-4} \text{ m}$$

$$\lambda = 0.31 \text{ mm}$$

When going from a medium with one acoustic velocity to a medium with another, the frequency of the sound beam remains constant. This means that a change in the wavelength of the sound beam must accompany the velocity shift, as expressed by Equation 1-5.

■ Example 1-4

The wavelength of an ultrasonic beam in tissue generated by a 2.5 MHz transducer is 0.62 mm as demonstrated in Example 1-3. If the sound beam is then transmitted into a layer of bone, the wavelength becomes

$$\lambda = \frac{4080 \text{ m/s}}{2.5 \times 10^6 \text{ 1/s}}$$

$$\lambda = 1.6 \times 10^{-3} \text{ m}$$

$$\lambda = 1.6 \text{ mm}$$

Using Equation 1-5, the wavelength of the ultrasound wave as a function of frequency can be determined for any medium for which the acoustic velocity is known. In medical imaging the medium of interest is soft tissue where an acoustic velocity of 1540 m/s is assumed. Equation 1-5 can be simplified by substituting the velocity of soft tissue:

$$\lambda \text{ (soft tissue)} = \frac{1.54 \text{ mm}}{f \text{ (MHz)}} \qquad \textbf{1-6}$$

Dividing 1.54 by the frequency expressed in megahertz yields the wavelength in millimeters.

■ Example 1-5

Using Equation 1-6, we can calculate the wavelength in tissue for a 5 MHz frequency ultrasound source as follows:

$$\lambda \text{ (soft tissue)} = \frac{1.54 \text{ mm}}{5 \text{ (MHz)}}$$

$$\lambda \text{ (soft tissue)} = 0.31 \text{ mm}$$

■ **Table 1-5** Frequency, Wavelength, and Period for Ultrasound Waves in Soft Tissue

Frequency (MHz)	Wavelength (mm)	Period (µs)
1	1.54	1
2.5	0.62	0.4
3.5	0.44	0.29
5	0.31	0.2
7.5	0.21	0.13
10	0.15	0.1
15	0.1	0.07
20	0.08	0.05

Table 1-5 lists the wavelength and period of an ultrasound wave in soft tissue as the frequency is varied.

We will see in Chapter 5 that the wavelength of ultrasound affects the axial resolution of an ultrasound system. The term *resolution* describes the ability to distinguish objects that are located close together as separate entities.

INTERACTIONS OF ULTRASOUND WITH TISSUE

In diagnostic radiography the beam of x-rays is produced outside the patient's body; the x-rays are subsequently attenuated (absorbed and scattered) as they pass through the patient's tissues. Ultimately, the transmitted photons are recorded on film. For diagnostic ultrasound the recorded image is typically based on reflected rather than transmitted energy. The single device that generates the ultrasound wave and subsequently detects the reflected energy is the transducer. An ultrasound wave is directed into the body to interact with tissues in accordance with the characteristics of the targeted tissues. The results of these interactions are recorded for diagnosis in the form of reflected ultrasound waves (echoes). The types of interactions that occur are similar to the wave behavior observed with light: reflection, refraction, scattering, diffraction, divergence, interference, and absorption. With the exception of interference, all these interactions reduce the intensity (loudness of audible sound) of the beam, termed **attenuation.** Interference may increase or decrease the intensity. In practice, reflection is often treated separately from attenuation; in other words, all interactions that decrease the intensity of the beam except for reflection are included in the attenuation process.

Reflection

The major interaction of interest for diagnostic ultrasound is **reflection.** If a sound beam is directed at right angles (called normal incidence) to a smooth interface (e.g., the boundary between different tissue types) larger than the width of the beam, it will be partially reflected toward the sound source (Fig. 1-11). These interfaces, called specular reflectors, are responsible for the major organ outlines seen in diagnostic ultrasound examinations. The diaphragm and pericardium are also examples of specular reflectors. The sonogram of

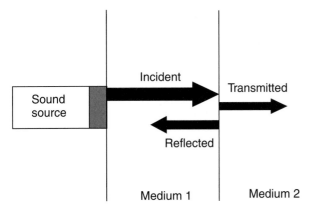

Fig. 1-11 Reflection caused by a sound wave striking a large smooth interface at normal incidence. The interface is larger than the beam width and acts as a specular reflector. The acoustic impedances of the media that compose the interface determine the relative intensities of the transmitted and reflected waves.

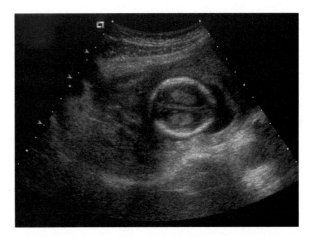

Fig. 1-12 Sonogram of the fetal head showing strong echoes from the skull.

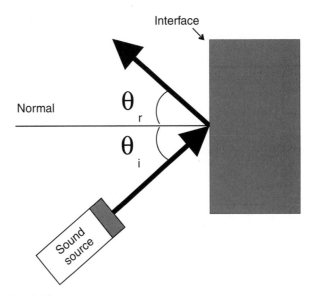

Fig. 1-13 Reflection caused by a sound wave striking a specular reflector at an angle. The resulting angle of reflection (θ_r) equals the angle of incidence (θ_i).

the fetal head in Fig. 1-12 illustrates the strong echoes obtained from the skull.

At other than normal incidence, the angle of reflection of a sound beam is equal to the angle of incidence (Fig. 1-13). These angles are defined relative to a line drawn perpendicular to the surface of the interface (normal). To obtain maximum detection of the reflected echo, we must orient the transducer (which sends and receives) so the generated sound beam will strike the interface perpendicularly, and the reflected wave travels a similar path back to the transducer.

What conditions result in a reflection of energy? A useful analogy would be throwing a baseball against a brick wall; not much energy will be transferred to the wall. Conservation of energy would permit the ball to transfer all its energy to the wall and simply stop at the surface of the wall, but conservation of momentum prevents this from occurring because of the differences in mass. Only a small portion of the energy will be transferred to the wall. Most will be retained by the baseball, which will return with almost the same velocity as when it struck the wall.

Similarly, if a Mack truck rams into a Volkswagen, very little energy will be transferred to the Volkswagen. The truck will continue at almost the same velocity as it originally had. Most of its energy will be retained, although a great deal of damage will be done to the Volkswagen. Energy cannot be transmitted readily from large objects to small ones or from small objects to large ones. If massive transfers of kinetic energy are required, collisions between objects of equal mass must occur. For example, to slow down a baseball, the maximum amount of energy transfer will result if it collides with another baseball. To transfer energy from a Mack truck by the maximum amount, it would have to collide with another Mack truck. Vibrating molecules behave in a similar manner. As long as they are transmitting energy to identically sized molecules, maximum transfer will occur. If there is a difference in the masses of the molecules, less energy will be transferred, and the energy that is not transferred will be reflected.

This analogy can be carried further by looking at the transfer of ultrasonic energy through a layer of water on top of a pool of mercury. At the water-mercury interface the small water molecules (similar to baseballs or Volkswagens) are inefficient in transferring energy to the large mercury molecules (similar to the wall or a Mack truck). They bounce off the mercury molecules, indicating that most of their energy is reflected back into themselves, with very little being transferred into the mercury. This reflection is determined by the conservation of momentum.

Acoustic impedance. In ultrasound the quantity analogous to momentum is acoustic impedance. Here we are looking not at individual molecules but at their concerted action, thereby applying the concept of mass per unit volume (density). Whereas in classical mechanics "momentum" is equal to mass times velocity, in ultrasound "density" replaces the mass and is then multiplied by the velocity. The velocity used is that of sound in the medium.

The product of density (ρ) times velocity (c) is called the **acoustic impedance** (Z):

$$Z = \rho c \tag{1-7}$$

This quantity is a measure of the resistance to sound passing through the medium. It is similar to electrical resistance, which is the degree of difficulty experienced by electrons in traversing a specific type of material. Acoustic impedance is expressed as kilograms per square meter per second ($kg/m^2/s$) and is the product of the units of density times velocity. In the international system of units (SI) this combination of $kg/m^2/s$ is given a special name, the rayl.

When a diver enters a pool, the ripple pattern expands outward and is reflected from the concrete wall of the pool. Very little wave energy is transferred from the water to the concrete wall. Now consider what would happen if the walls were made of gelatin instead of concrete. The reflected wave in the water would be less intense, and the walls would vibrate. Energy is transferred from the water to the gelatin, because the composition is similar. The acoustic impedance mismatch is less.

■ **Example 1-6**

What is the acoustic impedance of soft tissue (which has a density of $1060\ kg/m^3$)? Assume the velocity of sound in soft tissue is 1540 m/s.

$$Z = \rho c = (1060\ kg/m^3)(1540\ m/s)$$
$$Z = 1.63 \times 10^6\ kg/m^2/s\ \text{or}\ 1.63\ \text{Mrayls}$$

High-density materials give rise to high-velocity sound waves and therefore high acoustic impedances. Similarly, low-density materials such as gases have low acoustic impedances. Table 1-4 lists the acoustic impedances for several materials of interest.

Impedance mismatch. If the acoustic impedance is the same in one medium as in another, sound will be readily transmitted from one to the other. A difference in acoustic impedances causes some portion of the sound to be reflected at the interface. It is primarily the change in acoustic impedance at a biological interface (a discontinuity or an impedance mismatch) that allows visualization of soft tissue structures with an ultrasonic beam.

As mentioned earlier, watching western movies teaches that one does not listen for the train or for buffalo in a normal standing position. Every youngster learned from old westerns that you put your ear to the rail or to the ground. The late John Wayne most likely would not have said, "Put your ear to the ground, because that way you will eliminate the acoustic impedance mismatch and thus get a better sound transfer," but he should have, for that is the case.

Thus we have the second reason for placing one's ear on a solid surface. Whereas the transfer of sound from rail to air and then from air to ear is very inefficient, with direct contact the transmission from rail to air is eliminated, and vibrations pass readily across a solid–solid interface.

Another analogy that might be used, and that would be very correct, is the transmission of light. Light transmitted from one medium to another having different indices of refraction causes the major portion of the energy to be reflected rather than transmitted. This phenomenon can be observed when looking at light reflected from a shallow pool of water. The reflection occurs at the air-water boundary because of the different indices of refraction (similar to acoustic impedance). The amount of reflection is a function of the surface only. One receives the same amount of reflected light standing over a pool of water as over the deepest part of the Pacific Ocean. *Sound is reflected at the interface regardless of the thickness of the material from which it is reflected.*

Reflection coefficient. For perpendicular incidence the reflection coefficient for intensity is expressed as follows:

$$\alpha_r = \left(\frac{Z_2 - Z_1}{Z_2 + Z_1} \right)^2 \tag{1-8}$$

where α_r is the reflection coefficient, Z_2 the acoustic impedance of medium number 2 (distal to the boundary), and Z_1 the acoustic impedance of medium number 1 (proximal to the boundary). Multiplying this relation by 100 gives the percentage reflection (%R):

$$\%R = \left(\frac{Z_2 - Z_1}{Z_2 + Z_1} \right)^2 \times 100 \tag{1-9}$$

Transmission coefficient. The percentage transmission (%T) is 100 minus the percentage reflection (%R), and the transmission coefficient is 1 minus the reflection coefficient. The transmission coefficient (α_t) is calculated directly by the formula

$$\alpha_t = \frac{4Z_2Z_1}{(Z_2 + Z_1)^2} \tag{1-10}$$

Multiplying the right-hand side of Equation 1-10 by 100 gives the percentage transmission through the interface:

$$\%T = \frac{4Z_2Z_1}{(Z_2 + Z_1)^2} \times 100 \tag{1-11}$$

The equations for the transmission and reflection of ultrasound intensity are independent of frequency for specular reflection. That is, changing the transducer frequency does not alter the fraction of intensity transmitted/reflected at the interface. If the ultrasound beam strikes the interface at an angle, the angle of reflection of a sound beam is equal to the angle of incidence, but the sound wave is reflected with higher intensity compared with normal incidence. The reflection coefficient increases as the angle of incidence is increased.

Interface composition. It does not matter which impedance is the larger or smaller for two materials composing the interface—the difference between them squared gives the same number. *Thus the same percentage of reflection occurs at the interface, whether sound is going from a high acoustic impedance to a low acoustic impedance, or vice versa.* If the acoustic impedance difference is small, the magnitude of the reflected wave will be small. Because the same device transmits and receives the sound waves, maximum detection of the reflected echo occurs when the sound beam strikes the interface with normal incidence. If the acoustic impedance difference is large, such as in bone compared to soft tissue (see Example 1-7), a large fraction of sound will be reflected; little of the transmitted beam will penetrate structures behind the bone, and much will return to the detector. Consequently, for examinations involving the head, ultrasound is restricted to relatively simple noninvasive studies (echoencephalography). To visualize the liver, which is largely positioned under the ribs, one must look either through the intercostal spaces (between the ribs) or under the ribs and back up at the liver.

■ Example 1-7

Calculate the percentage reflection (%R) for a bone-tissue interface using the acoustic impedance values listed in Table 1-4:

$$\%R = \left(\frac{Z_B - Z_T}{Z_B + Z_T} \right)^2 \times 100$$

$$\%R = \left[\frac{(7.8 \times 10^6) - (1.63 \times 10^6)}{(7.8 \times 10^6) + (1.63 \times 10^6)} \right]^2 \times 100$$

$$\%R = 43\%$$

where Z_B is the acoustic impedance in bone and Z_T the acoustic impedance in tissue.

■ Example 1-8

Calculate the percentage transmission (%T) for a soft tissue–bone interface using the acoustic impedance values listed in Table 1-4:

$$\%T = \frac{4Z_2 Z_1}{(Z_2 + Z_1)^2} \times 100$$

$$\%T = \frac{4(7.8 \times 10^6)(1.63 \times 10^6)}{[(7.8 \times 10^6) + (1.63 \times 10^6)]^2} \times 100$$

$$\%T = 57\%$$

Note that the result for percentage reflection at the soft tissue–bone interface determined in Example 1-7 can be used to calculate the percentage transmission at this interface:

$$\%T = 100\% - \%R$$

$$\%T = 100\% - 43\%$$

$$\%T = 57\%$$

This is one of the reasons why bone is usually avoided during an ultrasound examination. The acoustic impedance difference is also large for an air-tissue interface, which causes most of the incident beam to be reflected.

■ Example 1-9

Calculate the percentage reflection (%R) for an air-tissue interface using the acoustic impedance values listed in Table 1-4:

$$\%R = \left(\frac{Z_T - Z_A}{Z_T + Z_A} \right)^2 \times 100$$

$$\%R = \left[\frac{(1.63 \times 10^6) - (0.0004 \times 10^6)}{(1.63 \times 10^6) + (0.0004 \times 10^6)} \right]^2 \times 100$$

$$\%R = 99.9\%$$

where Z_T is the acoustic impedance in tissue and Z_A the acoustic impedance in air.

If the acoustic impedance values are expressed in **megarayls** (Mrayls), the power of 10 can be eliminated in the calculation for percentage reflection.

■ Example 1-10

Calculate the percentage reflection (%R) for a bone-tissue interface converting the acoustic impedance values listed in Table 1-4 to Mrayls. The acoustic impedance is 1.63×10^6 rayls or 1.63 Mrayls for soft tissue and 7.8×10^6 rayls or 7.8 Mrayls for bone.

$$\%R = \left(\frac{Z_2 - Z_1}{Z_2 + Z_1} \right)^2 \times 100$$

$$\%R = \left(\frac{7.8 - 1.63}{7.8 + 1.63} \right)^2 \times 100$$

$$\%R = 43\%$$

Table 1-6 lists the percentage reflections at interfaces of varying composition. The acoustic impedances used to calculate these values were obtained from Table 1-4. Note that the thickness of the medium is not considered in the calculations; only the impedance mismatch at the interface is of concern.

Even if the air layer between a transducer and the patient is extremely thin, nearly total reflection occurs at the air-tissue interface. The ultrasound beam is not transmitted to structures distal to the air bubble, and the sonogram is void of information from this region (Fig. 1-14). During scanning, coupling gel is used to eliminate this. The gel also serves to reduce friction between the transducer and the skin.

Remember: When the heart or other thoracic structures are being studied, the lungs must be avoided because of the large amount of reflection that occurs at the multiple interfaces within them. Acoustic impedance differences at fat–soft tissue interfaces produce relatively strong echoes compared with echoes from parenchyma. Reflections from these interfaces are primarily responsible for the organ outlines seen in imaging. As an exercise, the reader should calculate the percentage reflection from a fat–soft tissue interface.

Echo-induced signals. When a device that produces and detects ultrasonic waves (i.e., a transducer) scans a patient, multiple interfaces are encountered along the path of

■ **Table 1-6** Percentage Reflection at Different Interfaces

Interface	Reflection Percent
Soft tissue–air	99.9
Soft tissue–lung	52
Soft tissue–bone	43
Aqueous humor–lens	1.1
Fat–liver	0.79
Soft tissue–fat	0.69
Soft tissue–muscle	0.04
Water–Lucite	13
Castor oil–soft tissue	0.43

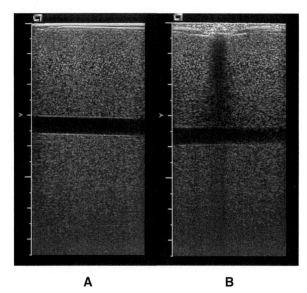

A   **B**

Fig. 1-14 Sonogram of a tissue-mimicking phantom with **(A)** and without **(B)** an air bubble present between the transducer and the phantom surface. Note that information is lost distal to the air bubble. The ultrasound energy is reflected by air-transducer interface and does not enter the phantom.

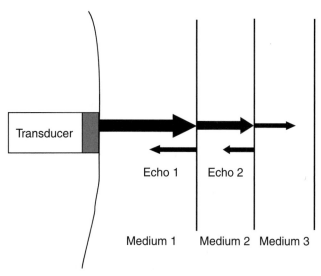

Fig. 1-15 Sound beam incident on a phantom consisting of three tissue types (or media). A fraction of the incident sound energy is reflected at each boundary between the media (labeled *Echo 1* and *Echo 2*).

travel of the ultrasound beam. A percentage of the incident beam intensity is reflected and transmitted at each interface. A series of echoes is subsequently detected (Fig. 1-15). If losses by reflection only are considered, the relative intensities of these echoes depend on the acoustic impedance mismatch at the interface that originally created the echo and on the transmission of sound energy through the interfaces along the path of travel to and from the transducer. On the return path each interface allows a fraction of the echo energy to pass through toward the transducer. *Fortunately, most of the incident intensity is transmitted across soft tissue interfaces, which enables deep-lying structures to be depicted in the ultrasound image.*

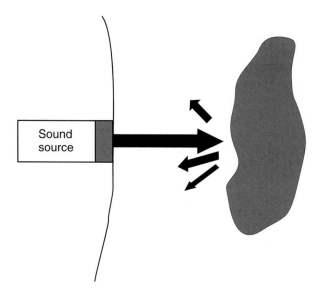

Fig. 1-16 Diffuse reflection. When a sound beam is incident on an irregular interface *(shaded area),* it is reflected in multiple directions.

Reflections occur at the transducer crystal-tissue interface, because these materials are not perfectly matched. The acoustic impedance of the crystal is usually much greater than that of tissue. Poor transmission across the crystal-tissue interface reduces the transmission of ultrasound into the body and inhibits detection of weakly reflecting interfaces. In Chapter 4 we will consider methods to decrease this effect.

Remember: In diagnostic ultrasound, reflected echoes are detected by conventional systems. Small signals are generated if the acoustic impedances are nearly the same (soft tissue to soft tissue), but strong signals occur if the difference in acoustic impedances is large (air and soft tissue). Much weaker echoes are produced by diffuse reflection and scattering.

Diffuse reflection. The large smooth surface of a specular reflector acts as a mirror to form a well-defined redirected beam (echo). A large rough-surfaced interface deflects the ultrasound beam in multiple directions (Fig. 1-16). Since the interface is not flat, the sound beam strikes the interface with various angles of incidence, which gives rise to differing angles of reflection. This is called diffuse reflection. The loss of coherence in the reflected beam weakens the echo returning to the transducer.

Before the bathroom mirror becomes fogged when you take a shower, it provides a true representation of objects placed in front of it. After you shower, the buildup of water on its surface causes it to act as a diffuse reflector, and the images of objects are less well defined. Water particles roughen its surface, reducing the coherence of reflected light.

Scattering

Another important interaction between ultrasound and tissue is **scattering,** or nonspecular reflection, which is responsible for providing the internal texture of organs in the image. The scattering occurs because the interfaces are small, with physical dimensions approximately the size of the wavelength or smaller. Each interface acts as a new separate sound source, and sound is reflected in all directions independent of the direction of the incoming sound wave (Fig. 1-17). The magnitude of scattered ultrasound intensity is much weaker than for specular reflection and depends on the number of scatterers per volume, size of the scatterers, acoustic impedance, and frequency.

Fluid regions such as cysts, urine in the bladder, and amniotic fluid lack scattering centers and produce weak ultrasound signals compared with surrounding tissue. These dark areas in the image are called hypoechoic. Areas with increased ultrasound signals compared with the surrounding tissue are called hyperechoic (Fig. 1-18).

Scattering by small particles in which the linear dimensions are much smaller than the wavelength is called Rayleigh scattering. *These nonspecular reflections have a strong frequency dependence (f^2 to f^6), which may make them useful in characterizing tissue.* Tissue characterization involves the absolute determination of tissue type via some physical measurement obtained by noninvasive means. When the frequency is changed, the altered scattering of the sound beam may provide important information for differentiating tissue types. *Specular reflectors do not exhibit a frequency dependence.*

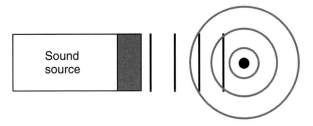

Fig. 1-17 Nonspecular reflection. The scattered wave from a small structure ($\approx\lambda$) indicated in gray is emitted in all directions, shown here in two dimensions only.

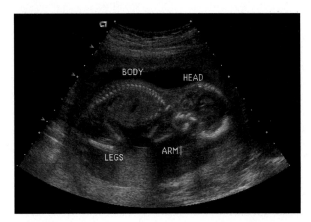

Fig. 1-18 Sonogram of a fetus. Amniotic fluid is hypoechoic and bone is hyperechoic. Soft tissue structures are intermediate shades of gray.

Reflectivity

Many factors influence the fraction of incident intensity that is reflected at an interface toward the transducer—the acoustic impedance mismatch, the angle of incidence, the size of the structure compared with the wavelength, the shape of the structure, and the texture of the surface of the interface. The combination of these factors is described by the term **reflectivity.**

Differences in reflectivity are partially responsible for the patient-to-patient variations that sonographers observe when performing a particular type of examination. Ultrasound imaging systems are capable of detecting extremely small changes in reflectivity, on the order of one in a million.

Refraction

Another interaction that occurs between ultrasound and tissue is **refraction.** If the ultrasound beam strikes an interface between two media at an angle of 90 degrees (normal incidence), a percentage will be reflected back to the first medium, and the rest will be transmitted into the second medium without a change in direction. If the beam strikes the interface at an angle other than 90 degrees, however, the transmitted part will be refracted or bent away from the straight-line path (Fig. 1-19).

Snell's law. Refraction of sound waves obeys Snell's law, which relates the angle of transmission to the relative velocities of sound in the two media. (Note that this relationship is not based on acoustic impedance.) Snell's law is given by

1-12

$$\frac{c_i}{c_t} = \frac{\sin \theta_i}{\sin \theta_t}$$

where θ_i is the incident angle, θ_t the transmitted angle, c_i the velocity of sound in the incident medium, and c_t the velocity of sound in the transmitted medium. In Snell's law the

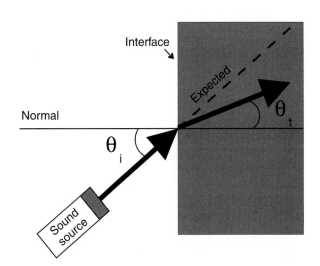

Fig. 1-19 Refraction. The velocity of a sound beam in the incident medium is greater than that in the transmitted medium, causing the beam to be bent toward the normal ($\theta_i > \theta_t$).

angles θ_i and θ_t are defined with respect to a line drawn perpendicular to the interface.

■ **Example 1-11**

Calculate the transmitted angle if an ultrasound beam is directed at an interface composed of soft tissue and fat. The angle of incidence is 10 degrees. Assume that the sound beam is moving from soft tissue into fat.

$$\frac{c_i}{c_t} = \frac{\sin \theta_i}{\sin \theta_t}$$

$$c_i = 1540 \text{ m/s}$$

$$c_t = 1459 \text{ m/s}$$

$$\theta_i = 10 \text{ degrees}$$

$$\frac{1540 \text{ m/s}}{1459 \text{ m/s}} = \frac{\sin 10°}{\sin \theta_t}$$

$$\sin \theta_t = 0.165$$

$$\theta_t = 9.5 \text{ degrees}$$

This bending occurs because the portion of the wavefront in the second medium travels at a different velocity from that in the first medium (Fig. 1-20). Note that the acoustic velocity in medium 2 is less than that in medium 1 (the spacing between successive wavefronts is smaller). The wavefront is continuous across the interface, but the portion of the wavefront in medium 2 is moving at a slower velocity than the rest and lags behind.

To illustrate this shift in wavefronts, imagine successive rows of four wheel–drive vehicles traveling through the Sahara Desert. As the vehicles cross a boundary between flat smooth terrain and sandy terrain, their velocity is reduced. If the drivers at the left who enter the sandy terrain first stubbornly maintain their alignment, the advance of this row of vehicles will be slowed compared to that of the drivers who have not yet encountered the sandy terrain. For the vehicles to continue to advance so the row remains perpendicular to their direction of travel, the drivers in the sandy terrain must turn slightly to the right. (The line of vehicles bends in the new terrain.)

Three situations regarding Snell's law should be considered:

Case 1 refraction: The velocity in the first medium is greater than that in the second medium. The angle of transmittance bends toward the normal from the expected straight-line path (see Fig. 1-19). For example, this occurs at a bone-tissue interface.

Case 2 refraction: The velocity in the first medium is less than that in the second medium. The angle of transmittance is bent away from the normal (Fig. 1-21). For example, this occurs at a tissue-bone interface.

Case 3 refraction: This is a special extension of case 2 refraction. If the velocity in the incident medium is less than that in the transmitted medium, and if the angle of incidence is beyond the so-called critical angle, the refracted beam travels along the interface, and no energy enters the second medium. This is called total reflection and occurs at an incident angle of greater than 22 degrees when the interface is composed of tissue and bone.

The critical angle (θ_c) is determined by Snell's law, in which the transmitted angle is assigned a value of 90 degrees. Since sin 90° equals 1, the critical angle for soft tissue and bone is calculated by

$$\sin \theta_c = \frac{1540 \text{ m/s}}{4080 \text{ m/s}}$$

$$\sin \theta_c = 1540 \text{ m/s} 4080 \text{ m/s}$$

$$\sin \theta_c = 0.377$$

$$\theta_c = 22.2 \text{ degrees}$$

If the velocity of sound is the same in the two media, no refraction (bending) occurs, although the acoustic impedances may be different. Nor does refraction occur at normal incidence, regardless of the relative velocities in the two media.

Transmission at nonnormal incidence. Snell's law shows that for nonnormal incidence the angle of transmission is not the same as the angle of incidence if the

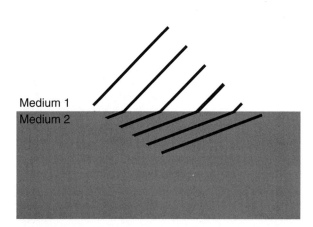

Fig. 1-20 Principle of refraction demonstrated by wavefronts striking an interface between two media having different velocities.

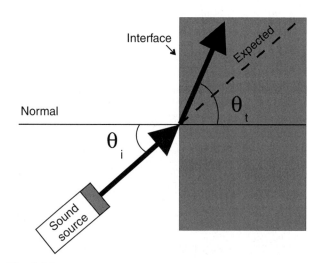

Fig. 1-21 Case 2 refraction. The velocity of a sound beam in the incident medium is less than that in the transmitted medium, causing the beam to be bent away from the normal ($\theta_i < \theta_t$).

velocities of sound in the two media are different. For non-perpendicular incidence the transmission coefficient for intensity is expressed as follows:

1-13

$$\%T = \frac{4Z_2Z_1\cos^2\theta_i}{(Z_2\cos\theta_i + Z_1\cos\theta_t)^2} \times 100$$

This equation reduces to the more familiar form of Equation 1-8, if θ_i and θ_t are equal to 90 degrees.

Misregistration. As indicated by Snell's law, the amount of deviation from the expected straight-line path changes with the angle of incidence and with the velocities in the associated media. This does not generally present any difficulty in diagnostic ultrasound, because the velocity of ultrasound in soft tissue is relatively constant (see Table 1-4). Although refraction is not a major problem in diagnostic ultrasound, under certain conditions the bending of the sound beam can cause artifacts in diagnostic images (discussed in Chapter 12). The formation of the image is predicated on the assumption that the ultrasound beam always travels in a straight line through tissue. If bending of the beam occurs along the actual path from the transducer to the object, the detected echo from an object would be placed at the wrong location in the image. The true location of the object is offset from the assumed straight-line path projected along the beam axis.

A similar effect caused by the refraction of light is seen when an object under water is viewed from above. If one reaches for the object through the water, the misregistration becomes immediately apparent. Refraction may contribute to the distortion of a curved object depicted in the image.

Diffraction

Diffraction causes the ultrasound beam to diverge or spread out as the waves move farther from the sound source (Fig. 1-22). The rate of divergence increases as the size (diameter) of the sound source decreases. Diffraction also occurs after the beam with planar wavefronts passes through a small aperture on the order of one wavelength. Because the wave is blocked everywhere but in the area of the aperture, the aperture acts as a small sound source, and the beam

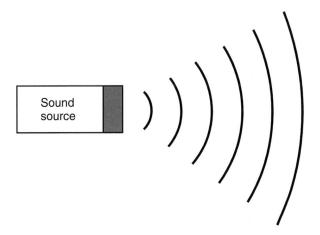

Fig. 1-22 Divergence of a sound beam from a small source.

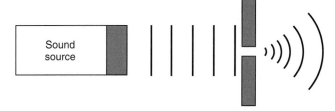

Fig. 1-23 Diffraction of a sound beam after passing through a small aperture.

diverges rapidly. This is demonstrated in Fig. 1-23. The lateral resolution of the beam and the sensitivity of the ultrasonic system are both affected by divergence.

Interference

Sound waves demonstrate interference phenomena or the superposition of waves (algebraic summation). As an example of interference, consider the ripple patterns produced in the water when three swimmers dive into a pool one after the other from three different diving boards located alongside the pool. If the entries are separated in time, then each diver will produce a characteristic ripple pattern. If all three divers reenter the water simultaneously, then the resulting complex ripple pattern consisting of large and small water disturbances is a combination of the three individual patterns.

If waves with the same frequency are *in phase*, they undergo constructive interference. Waves are in phase if crossing and inflection points are matched along the distance or time axis (Fig. 1-24). Constructive interference results in increased amplitude.

If waves with the same frequency are *out of phase*, they undergo destructive interference; that is, a decrease in amplitude results, because the peaks are not matched in the same position (Fig. 1-25). Completely destructive interference occurs when the waves are of the same frequency and amplitude and are completely out of phase (i.e., the trough of one wave corresponds to the peak of the other). The result is a wave with zero amplitude; hence, the summation wave disappears (Fig. 1-26). The effect of one wave is countered by the opposite effect of the other wave. For example, when two opposing players approach a soccer ball, the player who kicks it first controls the direction of travel. If both players kick the ball simultaneously with equal force, the forces applied will cancel each other, and the ball will not move toward either goal.

Every combination—from completely constructive to completely destructive interference—can occur, resulting in a complex wave summation. Fig. 1-27 shows the result when waves with differing frequencies create interference. This interference is important in the design of an ultrasonic transducer, because it affects the uniformity of the beam intensity throughout the ultrasonic field (see Chapter 5). Focusing of the ultrasound beam in real time imaging is based on the principle of wave interference (see Chapter 8). When combined, waves of similar frequency produce a "beat" that is used in Doppler ultrasound (see Chapter 14).

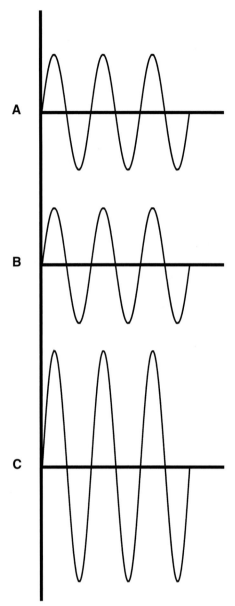

Fig. 1-24 Constructive interference or superposition (algebraic summation) of waves. The resultant wave, **C,** is the sum of waves **A** and **B.**

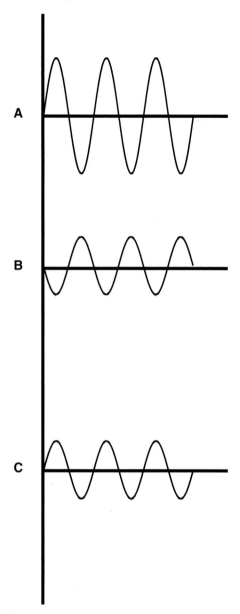

Fig. 1-25 Destructive interference. The resultant wave, **C,** is the sum of waves **A** and **B** and is reduced in amplitude, because the waves are out of phase.

Absorption

Absorption is the only process whereby sound energy is dissipated in a medium. All other modes of interactions (reflection, refraction, scattering, and divergence) decrease the ultrasonic beam intensity by redirecting the energy of the beam. **Absorption** is the process whereby ultrasonic energy is transformed into other energy forms, primarily heat. It is responsible for the medical applications of therapeutic ultrasound (physiotherapy).

Factors influencing absorption. The absorption of an ultrasonic beam is related to the beam's frequency and to the viscosity and relaxation time of the medium. The relaxation time describes the rate at which molecules return to their original positions after being displaced by a force.

If a substance has a short relaxation time, the molecules return to their original positions before the next wave compression arrives. If a substance has a long relaxation time, however, the molecules may be moving back toward their original positions as the wave crest (compression) strikes them. More energy is required to stop and then reverse the direction of the molecules, and this produces more heat (absorption).

The ability of molecules to move past one another characterizes the viscosity of a medium; high viscosity provides great resistance to molecular flow. For instance, a low-viscosity fluid (water) flows more freely than a viscous one (maple syrup). The frictional forces must be overcome by vibrating molecules, and thus more heat is produced in the maple syrup.

The frequency also affects absorption in relation to both the viscosity and the relaxation time. If the frequency is increased, the molecules must move more often, thereby

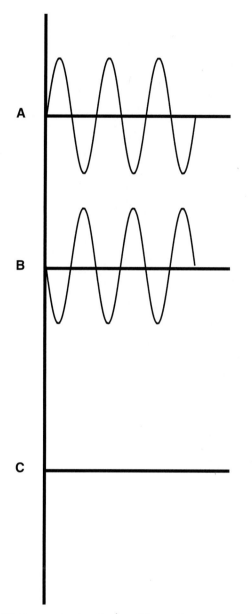

Fig. 1-26 Destructive interference. The resultant wave, **C**, is zero, because waves **A** and **B** are completely out of phase and have the same amplitude.

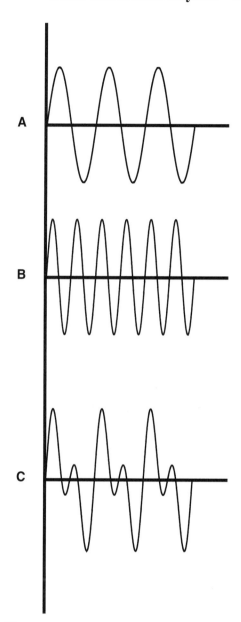

Fig. 1-27 Wave interference. Note that **B** has a slightly different frequency from **A**. Thus **C** is the summation of these two waves.

generating more heat from the drag caused by friction (viscosity). Also, as the frequency is increased, less time is available for the molecules to recover during the relaxation process. Molecules remain in motion, and more energy is necessary to stop and redirect them, again producing more absorption. *The rate of absorption is directly related to the frequency.* If the frequency doubles, the rate of absorption also doubles.

Consider the mechanical action of rubbing one's hands together. The movement produces heat. If the hands are rubbed together more rapidly (higher frequency), increased warming occurs. If lotion is placed between the palms so the resistance is decreased (lower viscosity), less heat will be generated.

The peak amplitude of acoustic pressure (mm Hg, pascals, or atmospheres), particle density (kg/m^3), particle displacement (m, cm, mm), and particle velocity (m/s, cm/s, mm/s) all decrease as the wave traverses a homogeneous medium. In Fig. 1-28 the absorption of the pulsed ultrasonic beam follows an exponential function as the pulsed wave penetrates the tissue. Absorption is enhanced if the frequency is increased (Fig. 1-29).

Attenuation

Attenuation includes the effects of both scattering and absorption in the characterization of amplitude reduction as the ultrasound wave propagates through a medium. Attenuation is also described by an exponential function dependent on the distance traveled, composition of the medium, and the frequency. As frequency is increased, the reduction of the ultrasound intensity with distance becomes more

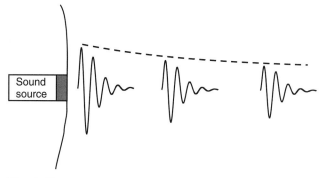

Fig. 1-28 Attenuation of acoustic pressure as a sound beam penetrates the medium. The dashed curve demonstrates an exponential decrease of the peak acoustic pressure.

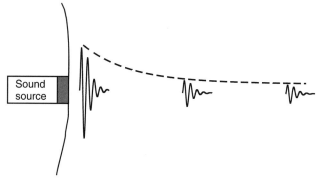

Fig. 1-29 Attenuation of acoustic pressure as a high-frequency sound beam penetrates the medium. The dashed curve demonstrates an exponential decrease of the peak acoustic pressure. Compared with Fig. 1-28 the frequency is increased, and consequently the rate of absorption is faster.

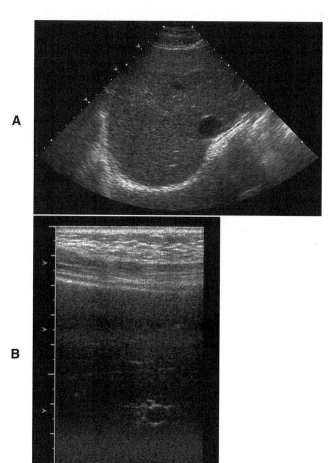

Fig. 1-30 Effect of frequency on penetration. **A,** The depth of penetration for 4 MHz transducer is 16 cm in an abdominal scan. **B,** The depth of penetration for 8 MHz transducer is 7 cm for the same patient.

pronounced. This has a practical consequence in medical imaging. The ultrasound beam and returning echoes used to form the image must travel through tissue. *The depth of penetration becomes less as frequency is increased—the ability to observe deep-lying structures is forfeited* (Fig. 1-30).

At a particular location within a continuous single-frequency ultrasonic field, the variations of pressure with time demonstrate an oscillatory behavior, the greatest deviations occurring during maximum pressure (p_o). The maximum particle velocity (u_o) and the maximum particle displacement (s_o) are related to the maximum pressure. As the maximum pressure is reduced, a corresponding decrease in particle velocity and particle displacement occurs.

INTENSITY

The **intensity** of an ultrasonic beam is the physical parameter that describes the amount of energy flowing through a cross-sectional area per second. Simply, it is the rate at which the energy is transmitted by the wave over a small area.

When characterizing audible acoustics, we use the term intensity to describe the loudness of sound. For ultrasound, increasing intensity means that the distribution of particles within the compression regions becomes more dense,

acoustic pressure is higher, length of particle oscillation increases, and maximum particle velocity is greater. The intensity of an ultrasound beam decreases as the beam propagates through tissue. The transmitted intensity and the rate of intensity loss influence the ability of a scanner to observe weakly reflecting structures. *Frequency, wavelength, and acoustic velocity of an ultrasonic beam are not affected by a change in intensity if beam propagation is linear.* For high-intensity applications such as tissue harmonic imaging, propagation is nonlinear and a change in frequency does occur (see Chapter 9).

The study of potential biologic effects is linked to intensity. Since the particle velocity and length of displacement are dictated by intensity, a high-intensity ultrasound wave is more disruptive than a low-intensity ultrasound wave is to living systems. The biological effects of ultrasound are examined in Chapter 22.

Traditionally, acoustic intensity is expressed in mixed units of watts per centimeter squared or milliwatts per centimeter squared (a combination of meter kilogram second [MKS] and centimeter gram second [CGS] system units). In other areas of physics this is considered bad form. One watt is equal to one joule per second.

Intensity Descriptors

The intensity of an ultrasound beam is proportional to the square of the pressure amplitude, particle-displacement amplitude, or particle-velocity amplitude. For example, the equation for instantaneous intensity (i) is given by

$$i = \frac{p_i^2}{\rho c}$$

1-14

where p_i is the instantaneous acoustic pressure, c the velocity of sound, and ρ the density. Acoustic pressure is expressed in pascals (Pa) in the MKS system. Pressure is the force exerted on a small area; thus a pascal is equivalent to a newton per meter squared (Nt/m^2). One atmosphere (atmospheric pressure at sea level) equals 10^5 pascals. Ultrasound instruments produce peak pressure amplitudes ranging from 0.5 to 5.5 megapascals (more than 50 times greater than atmospheric pressure).

Often the time-averaged intensity (I) is of interest. At any point through which an ultrasound beam passes, the pressure oscillates between high and low values. The greatest deviation from average pressure during a cycle is the maximum-pressure or peak-pressure amplitude (p_o). Since the pressure is fluctuating as a function of time, the instantaneous intensity is also oscillating between high and low values. By averaging the instantaneous intensity over one cycle it is possible to find the time-averaged intensity:

$$I = \frac{p_o^2}{2\rho c}$$

1-15

Power

The **power** (W) is a measure of the total energy transmitted per unit time summed over the entire cross-sectional area of the beam:

$$W = \text{Intensity} \times \text{Area}$$

1-16

The emitted power from the transducer assembly is not constant but fluctuates over the wave cycle. Ultrasonic power, averaged over a time period, is referred to as the temporal average power. The unit of power is the watt.

Decibel

Absolute values of the power and intensity of an ultrasonic beam are difficult to measure. This is particularly true of pulsed diagnostic beams, for which both temporal and spatial properties must be considered (Chapter 21).

Although no standard reference intensity for ultrasound has been established, a useful method for determining the reduced intensity of a beam is to make relative measurements that compare the value at one point with a reference intensity at another point. The following analogy may help illustrate the concept: Johnny owns 25 marbles, Tommy 50. To find out how much Johnny's marbles weigh in ounces, we place them on a scale. If we are interested only in the relative weights of the marbles, we say one batch is "half as

heavy as the other." The absolute weight in ounces is not known but can be described with respect to a standard (Tommy's marbles).

Relative measurements are usually made and given in **decibels (dB).** The intensity variation or level expressed in decibels is

$$\text{Level (dB)} = 10 \log \left(\frac{I}{I_{ref}} \right)$$

1-16

where I is the intensity at the point of interest, and I_{ref} is the initial or reference intensity.

One advantage of decibels is that they enable a wide range of intensity and power levels to be expressed in a compact form. (See "Mathematics Review" in Appendix A for further discussion.) Decibels are not restricted to the parameters of power and intensity, however. They can also be used to describe relative measurements for amplitude, noise level, percentage reflection, and many other quantities. In Equation 1-16, I_{ref} and I are replaced by the reference value and the value for the parameter of interest respectively.

Consider an ultrasonic field in which the intensity is one-half the surface intensity at 1 cm and continues to decrease to 1/10,000 of the surface intensity at a depth of 14 cm. The intensity ratio of each point to the surface requires a numerical range of 2 to 10,000. Since the decibel notation is logarithmic, a range of only –3 to –40 dB units is needed to express this same relationship. The negative sign indicates that the intensity of the beam has decreased from the reference point to the point of interest. Further examples are cited in Table 1-7.

Another advantage of the decibel notation is that decibel changes along the beam path are additive. Consider the situation illustrated in Fig. 1-31, in which the intensity at point 1 is one-tenth the original intensity, and the intensity at point 2 is half the intensity at point 1 or one twentieth the original. By using the decibel methodology, the change in decibels can be found by adding dB change from transducer to point 1 (–10 dB) with the dB change from point 1 to point 2 (–3 dB) to yield a total loss of 13 dB from the transducer to point 2. The sum of the decibel changes between points along the path is equal to the decibel change for the entire path.

The intensity of the detected echo is often compared with the intensity of the transmitted ultrasound wave. If the relative intensity of the returning echo is 60 dB less than that of the transmitted wave, Equation 1-16 demonstrates that the echo will be a small fraction (1/1,000,000) of the transmitted intensity.

Half-Value Layer

A half-value layer (HVL) or half-value thickness of material is the thickness that will reduce the intensity to half its original value. Note that a reduction in intensity by a factor of 2 results in 3 dB loss. A decrease in intensity by 3 dB indicates that one HVL of material must have been present.

■ **Table 1-7** Intensity Ratio versus Decibels

I/I_0	dB
10,000	40
1000	30
100	20
10	10
1	0
0.1	−10
0.01	−20
0.001	−30
0.0001	−40

■ **Table 1-8** Relation among Intensity Radios, Decibels, and Half-Value Layers

Percent of Sound Remaining	I/I_0	dB	Half-Value Layer
100	1	0	—
50	0.5	−3.01	1
25	0.25	−6.02	2
10	0.1	−10	3.32
5	0.05	−13.01	4.32
1	0.01	−20	6.64
0.1	0.001	−30	9.96
0.01	0.0001	−40	13.29
0.001	0.00001	−50	16.61

■ **Table 1-9** Half-Value Layers (in Centimeters) at Different Frequencies

Material	Frequency			
	1 MHz	2 MHz	5 MHz	10 MHz
Air	0.25	0.06	0.01	—
Water	1360	340	54	14
Blood	17	8.5	3	2
Bone	0.2	0.1	0.04	—
Brain	3.5	2	1	—
Fat	5	2.5	1	0.5
Liver	3	1.5	0.5	—
Muscle	1.5	0.75	0.3	0.15
Tissue (average)	4.3	2.1	0.86	0.43

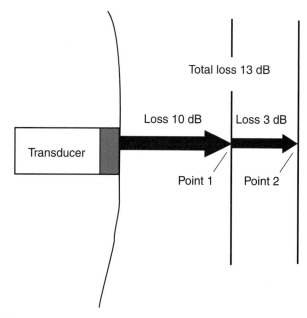

Fig. 1-31 Decibel notation. Intensity losses along the path are additive. Thus the change of intensity from the transducer to point 2 is −13 dB.

Table 1-8 shows the relation among intensity ratios, decibels, and HVLs.

Decibels and HVLs

A 9 dB reduction in intensity is expected from a thickness of material composed of 3 HVLs—that is, 9 dB divided by 3 dB/HVL equals 3 HVLs. Table 1-9 lists HVLs for various materials at different frequencies. Note that the HVLs of some materials do not vary linearly with frequency. For example, muscle exhibits a linear change in HVL with frequency, but this is not the case for water.

If the number of HVLs (n) present in an ultrasound beam is known, the reduction of intensity can be calculated from the following equation:

$$I_2 = \frac{I_1}{2^n}$$ 1-17

where I_1 is the initial intensity at point 1, and I_2 is the intensity at point 2 resulting from the attenuation of the wave through n HVLs.

The attenuation of an ultrasound beam is a measure of the decrease of power or intensity as the beam traverses a medium. All the interactions of ultrasound with tissue (reflection, refraction, scattering, divergence, and absorption) cause a decrease in beam intensity and contribute to the overall attenuation of the beam. Only absorption results in energy transfer to the tissue; all other interactions with tissue cause a redirection of ultrasonic energy.

Penetration

High-frequency sound waves are attenuated more rapidly than low-frequency sound waves. Thus the ability to penetrate tissue is reduced at higher frequencies. In addition, a reflector positioned at progressively greater depths generates progressively lower-intensity returning echoes. A method whereby the strength of the received signal is increased by amplification as a function of depth, called time gain compensation (TGC), is presented in Chapter 5. Table 1-10 shows some intensity attenuation factors for human tissues at a frequency of 1 MHz. The attenuation rate at frequencies above 1 MHz is estimated by assuming that the attenuation rate is directly proportional to the frequency. For example, the attenuation rate at 4 MHz for fat is calculated by multiplying 4 MHz times 0.6 dB/cm/MHz from Table 1-10. The result is 2.4 dB/cm for fat when the frequency is 4 MHz.

■ **Table 1-10** Attenuation of Human Tissues and Other Media at 1 MHz

Material	dB/cm
Blood	0.18
Fat	0.6
Kidney	1
Muscle (across fibers)	3.3
Muscle (along fibers)	1.2
Brain	0.85
Liver	0.9
Lung	40
Skull	20
Lens	2
Aqueous humor	0.022
Vitreous humor	0.13
Water	0.0022
Castor oil	0.95
Lucite	2

The attenuation (neglecting reflection) of an ultrasound beam propagating through soft tissue ranges from 0.5 to 1 dB/cm/MHz. As an approximation, the attenuation rate is often assumed to be 0.5 dB/cm/MHz, while the actual value is closer to 0.7 to 0.8 dB/cm/MHz. For clinical safety considerations a value of 0.5 dB/cm/MHz or less is used to calculate a conservative estimate of the intensity at depth. Signal level estimates typically apply higher values for the attenuation rate to provide system design criteria. For a 2 MHz ultrasound beam, approximately 30% of the energy is absorbed after 1 cm of travel in soft tissue. As a comparison a 7.5 MHz ultrasound beam loses more than 75% of the energy after 1 cm of travel in soft tissue. *The decrease in intensity level expressed in decibels is directly proportional to both the depth of penetration and the frequency of the ultrasound beam.*

ECHO RANGING

A system that can generate an ultrasonic pulsed wave and detect the reflected echo after a measured time permits the distance to an interface (i.e., the depth of the interface) to be determined. This technique is called **echo ranging,** a concept that formed the basis of sonar (sound navigation and ranging) developed during World War II.

In diagnostic ultrasound, reflections of the sound beam from interfaces along the ultrasonic path are of primary interest. A pulsed ultrasound wave is transmitted into the body, strikes an interface (acoustic mismatch between two media), and is partially reflected to the transducer, as determined by the percentage reflection formula. The reflected waves arising from the various acoustic impedance mismatches result in ultrasonic detection of interfaces within the body.

The distance (z) traveled by the sound beam is specified by the formula

1-18

$$z = ct$$

where *c* is the velocity, and *t* is the time of travel.

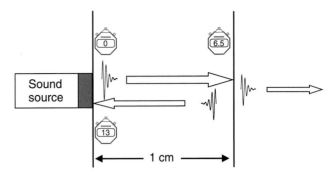

Fig. 1-32 Principle of echo ranging. The distance to the interface can be determined by measuring the time between the transmitted pulse and the received echo. A constant velocity in the medium must be assumed.

If the velocity of ultrasound in the medium and the elapsed time from the original transmitted pulse to the detection of the return echo are known, the distance to an interface is determined from Equation 1-18.

The following calculation demonstrates the time necessary to travel distances that are of clinical interest. The average velocity of ultrasound in tissue is 1540 m/s. For an interface exactly 1 cm away, the total time for the sound wave to travel out to the interface and back to the transducer is calculated by using Equation 1-18 and by solving for time (t) (Fig. 1-32). The total distance out and back is 2 cm, or 0.02 m (1 cm = 0.01 meter). Because the velocity is 1540 m/s in tissue, the elapsed time is

$$t = \frac{0.02 \text{ m}}{1540 \text{ m/s}}$$

$$t = \frac{2 \times 10^{-2} \text{ m}}{1.54 \times 10^{3} \text{ m/s}}$$

$$t = 13 \times 10^{-6} \text{ s}$$

$$t = 13 \text{ μs}$$

Only 13 μs are required for the sound beam to travel 1 cm and return 1 cm in tissue. Each centimeter of travel beam takes 6.5 μs.

■ **Example 1-12**

A pulsed ultrasound wave is transmitted through soft tissue toward an interface composed of soft tissue and bone. The elapsed time between the transmitted pulse and the detected echo is 74 μs. What is the depth of the interface?

$$z \text{ (depth)} = \frac{t}{13 \text{ μs/cm}}$$

$$z \text{ (depth)} = \frac{74 \text{ μs}}{13 \text{ μs/cm}}$$

$$z = 5.7 \text{ cm}$$

The distance to an interface is determined by the elapsed time; in other words, the time of travel to and from the interface at a constant velocity is set by the distance of travel. As the depth to the interface increases, the elapsed time increases. For an interface 10 cm away, 130 μs between the transmitted pulse and the returning echo are required.

For echo ranging to delineate the position of an interface correctly, certain conditions must hold: (1) the ultrasound wave must travel directly to the interface and back to the transducer along a straight-line path and (2) the velocity of sound must remain constant along the path of travel.

SUMMARY

An understanding of the physics of ultrasound is essential to the successful clinical application of diagnostic ultrasonographic techniques. The types and properties of sound waves and the interaction of those waves with tissues (reflection, refraction, scattering, interference, absorption, and attenuation) influence the collection and interpretation of scan data. The technique of echo ranging forms the basis of most ultrasonic scanning modes. This chapter provides a foundation for understanding the principles of all scanning modes and their associated instrumentation.

REVIEW QUESTIONS

1. The velocity of ultrasound is inversely proportional to the square root of the _____ of the medium.
2. If an ultrasound beam is directed at an interface at a 15-degree angle of incidence and the velocity in medium 1 is greater than that in medium 2, the beam will be bent (toward, away from) the normal.
3. Ultrasound waves in soft tissue are (longitudinal, transverse) waves.
4. What is the period of a wave whose frequency is 5 MHz or 5×10^6 cycles per second?
5. What is the frequency of a wave whose period is 4×10^{-7} second?
6. What is the wavelength of a 3.5 MHz sound wave in soft tissue?
7. What is the acoustic impedance of fat, whose density is 950 kg/m^3? Assume the velocity of sound in fat to be 1460 m/s.
8. What is the percentage reflection (%R) for a smooth interface composed of aqueous humor and the lens? Use the acoustic impedance values in Table 1-4 to calculate your answer.
9. What is the percentage transmission (%T) for a large smooth interface composed of fat and soft tissue? Use the acoustic impedance values listed in Table 1-4 to calculate your answer.
10. The acoustic impedance of air is 0.0004 Mrayls and that of tissue is 1.63 Mrayls. What are the percent reflection and the percent transmission at an interface composed of air and soft tissue?
11. The acoustic impedance of bone is 7.8 Mrayls, and that of tissue is 1.63 Mrayls. What are the reflection coefficient and the transmission coefficient at an interface composed of bone and soft tissue?
12. Calculate the transmitted angle if an ultrasound beam is directed at a large interface composed of soft tissue and bone. The angle of incidence is 20 degrees. Assume the sound beam to be moving from soft tissue into bone.
13. Calculate the transmitted angle if an ultrasound beam is directed at a large interface composed of fat and soft tissue. The angle of incidence is 20 degrees. Assume that the sound beam is moving from fat into soft tissue.
14. The attenuation of ultrasound propagating through soft tissue is approximately _____ dB/cm/MHz.
15. The elapsed time between the transmitted pulse and the detected echo is 39 μs. How far is the interface from the transducer?
16. The distance of a tissue interface is 2 cm from the face of the transducer. How much time elapses between the transmitted ultrasound pulse and the detected echo?
17. How far away is an interface in tissue if the elapsed time for the sound wave to travel out and back is 260 μs?
18. What is the velocity of ultrasound in a medium if the wavelength is 0.03 cm and the frequency is 5 MHz?
19. What is the wavelength of ultrasound in a medium if the velocity is 4080 m/s and the frequency is 2.5 MHz?
20. What is the frequency of ultrasound in a medium if the velocity is 333 m/s and the wavelength is 1 mm?
21. For an examination of the breast, the sonographer replaces the 5 MHz transducer with a 10 MHz transducer. The wavelength of the ultrasound wave in soft tissue will be _____ times that exhibited by the previous transducer.

BIBLIOGRAPHY

Carson PL: Physics of ultrasound propagation. In Goldman LW, Fowlkes JB, eds: *Medical CT and ultrasound: current technology and applications,* College Park, Md, 1995, American Association of Physicists in Medicine.

Carson PL: Ultrasound tissue interactions. In Goldman LW, Fowlkes JB, eds: *Categorical course in diagnostic radiology physics: CT and US cross-sectional imaging,* Oak Brook, Ill, 2000, Radiological Society of North America.

Kremkau FW: *Diagnostic ultrasound: principles and instruments,* ed 6, Philadelphia, 2002, WB Saunders.

McDicken WN: *Diagnostic ultrasonics: principles and use of instruments,* ed 3, Edinburgh, 1991, Churchill Livingstone.

Rose JL, Goldberg BB: *Basic physics in diagnostic ultrasound,* New York, 1979, John Wiley & Sons.

Wells PNT: *Physical principles of ultrasonic diagnosis,* New York, 1969, Academic Press.

Wells PNT: *Biomedical ultrasonics,* New York, 1977, Academic Press.

Zagzebski JA: *Essentials of ultrasound physics,* St Louis, 1996, Mosby-Year Book.

CHAPTER 2

Attenuation in Tissue

Absorption coefficient   Neper

Attenuation coefficient   Scattering coefficient

Absorption and scattering related to attenuation were introduced in the preceding chapter. A mathematical description of absorption and attenuation with numerous numerical examples is presented in this chapter. Calculations of attenuation and reflection losses illustrate the relatively low intensity of the received echo compared with the transmitted ultrasound beam.

ABSORPTION

At a particular location within a continuous single-frequency ultrasonic field (z), the variations of instantaneous pressure (p) with time demonstrate oscillatory behavior, in which the maximum deviation is designated as the peak amplitude pressure (p_o). The initial peak amplitude of acoustic pressure at the surface (p_{max}) decreases as the ultrasound wave moves through a homogeneous medium (Fig. 2-1). The absorption of the ultrasonic beam (reduction in acoustic pressure due to energy transfer to the medium) follows an exponential function:

2-1
$$p_o = p_{max} \exp(-\alpha z)$$

where p_o is the peak pressure amplitude of the beam at depth z, p_{max} the initial peak pressure amplitude of the beam, α the **absorption coefficient**, and z the distance traversed by the beam. *The absorption coefficient depends on the medium and frequency of the ultrasound wave.* As the ultrasound wave penetrates tissue, the peak amplitude pressure is decreased, causing smaller pressure variations at depth (Fig. 2-2). These pressure oscillations are very rapid—equal to the frequency of the ultrasound wave.

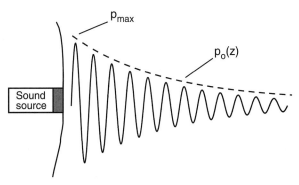

Fig. 2-1 Attenuation of acoustic pressure as a sound beam penetrates the medium. The dashed curve demonstrates an exponential decrease of the initial peak amplitude acoustic pressure (p_{max}) to peak amplitude pressure (p_o) at depth z.

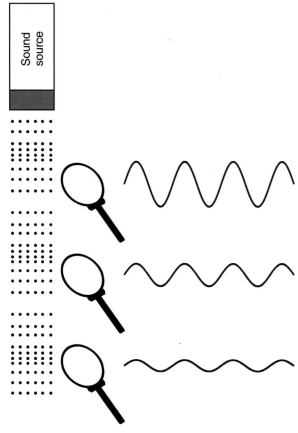

Fig. 2-2 Attenuation of the ultrasound beam causes reduced pressure oscillations as the wave penetrates tissue. The pressure change at three different depths is shown. The frequency of the pressure oscillations at each depth equals the frequency of the ultrasound wave.

ATTENUATION

Attenuation includes the effects of both scattering and absorption in the loss of pressure amplitude as the ultrasound wave propagates through a medium. Attenuation is also described by an exponential function. Thus the form of Equation 2-1 remains unchanged, but the absorption coefficient is replaced by the **attenuation coefficient** (a):

$$p_o = p_{max} \exp(-az)$$ 2-2

The attenuation coefficient (a) is given by the sum of the **scattering coefficient** (a_s) and the **absorption coefficient** (α):

$$a = a_s + \alpha$$ 2-3

The coefficients quantitate the respective fractional losses in peak amplitude pressure per unit length from absorption (α), scattering (a_s), and both processes together (a). The special unit for these coefficients is the **neper** (Np) per centimeter. The attenuation coefficients at 1 MHz for various tissue types are presented in Table 2-1. The effect of frequency must be included in any specification of attenuation coefficient. In a first approximation the attenuation coefficient

Table 2-1 Attenuation of Human Tissues at 1 MHz

Material	Np/cm
Blood	0.021
Fat	0.069
Kidney	0.115
Muscle (across fibers)	0.38
Muscle (along fibers)	0.138
Brain	0.098
Liver	0.103
Lung	4.6
Skull	2.3

increases linearly with frequency. For example, the coefficient for fat at 3.5 MHz is estimated by multiplying the value in Table 2-1 (0.069 Np/cm/MHz) by 3.5 MHz to obtain 0.24 Np/cm.

The maximum particle velocity (u_o) and the maximum particle displacement (s_o) are related to the peak amplitude pressure at that location:

$$u_o = \frac{p_o}{\rho c}$$ 2-4

and

$$s_o = \frac{p_o}{2\pi fc\rho}$$ 2-5

As the pressure is reduced, a corresponding decrease in particle velocity and particle displacement occurs.

INTENSITY

Intensity describes the amount of energy flowing through a cross-sectional area per unit of time. The units of intensity are joules/cm^2/s or watts/cm^2. Energy in this case is kinetic energy of particles as they are accelerated and decelerated by the pressure wave.

The intensity of the beam also decreases exponentially with distance from the sound source, which is given by:

$$I = I_{max} \exp(-\mu z)$$ 2-6

where *I* is the intensity at the point of interest, I_{max} the initial transmitted intensity, *z* the distance traversed by the beam, and μ the intensity attenuation coefficient. The intensity of an ultrasound beam is proportional to the square of the pressure amplitude. Thus the intensity attenuation coefficient is related to the amplitude attenuation coefficient by

$$\mu = 2a$$ 2-7

DECIBEL

Relative measurements that compare the value at one point with a reference intensity at another point are expressed in decibels (dB). The intensity change or level expressed in decibels is

2-8

$$\text{Level (dB)} = 10 \log \left(\frac{I}{I_{ref}} \right)$$

where I is the intensity at the point of interest, and I_{ref} is the reference intensity.

■ Example 2-1

Assume that the intensity at a particular point is reduced to half the transmitted intensity and that at a second point is 1/10,000 of the transmitted intensity. Convert these relative intensity measurements to decibels.

For point 1:

$$I_1 = 0.5 \, I_t$$

$$\text{Level (dB)} = 10 \log \left(\frac{0.5 \, I_t}{I_t} \right)$$

$$\text{Level (dB)} = 10 \log 0.5$$

$$\text{Level (dB)} = (10)(-0.301)$$

$$\text{Level (dB)} = -3.01$$

For point 2:

$$I_2 = 0.0001 \, I_t$$

$$\text{Level (dB)} = 10 \log \left(\frac{0.0001 \, I_t}{I_t} \right)$$

$$\text{Level (dB)} = 10 \log 0.0001$$

$$\text{Level (dB)} = 10(-4)$$

$$\text{Level (dB)} = -40$$

Note in Example 2-1 that a factor of 2 reduction in intensity corresponds to a −3 dB change. *This is the mathematical basis for the rule of thumb that each HVL results in a loss of 3 dB in intensity.*

The intensity of the detected echo is often compared with the intensity of the transmitted ultrasound wave. If the relative intensity of the returning echo is 50 dB less than that of the transmitted wave, Equation 2-8 demonstrates that the echo intensity (I_e) will be a small fraction (1/100,000) of the transmitted intensity (I_t):

$$-50 = 10 \log \left(\frac{I_e}{I_t} \right)$$

$$-5 = 10 \log \left(\frac{I_e}{I_t} \right)$$

$$\left(\frac{I_e}{I_t} \right) = \text{Antilog } (-5)$$

$$\left(\frac{I_e}{I_t} \right) = 0.00001$$

The attenuation expressed in nepers equals the attenuation coefficient times the distance traversed. The conversion to nepers for attenuation loss expressed in decibels is given as

2-9

$$\text{Attenuation loss (Np)} = 0.115 \times (\text{dB loss})$$

The conversion to decibels for attenuation loss expressed in nepers is given as

2-10

$$\text{Attenuation loss (dB)} = 8.686 \times (\text{Np loss})$$

The attenuation coefficient expressed in dB/cm or Np/cm can be converted from one unit to the other in a similar fashion.

■ Example 2-2

Find the attenuation loss in nepers and decibels for a 1 MHz ultrasound beam traversing 7 cm of liver. From Table 2-1 the attenuation coefficient for liver can be seen to be 0.103 Np/cm. A thickness of 7 cm causes a loss of 0.721 Np (0.103 Np/cm × 7 cm). The decrease in peak pressure amplitude is calculated by using Equation 2-2:

$$p_o = p_{max} \exp(-az)$$

$$p_o = p_{max} \exp(-0.721)$$

$$p_o = 0.486 \, p_{max}$$

Intensity is directly proportional to the square of the maximum pressure amplitude.

$$I = 0.236 \, I_{max}$$

The decibel loss is calculated using Equation 2-8.

$$\text{Level (dB)} = 10 \log \left(\frac{I}{I_{max}} \right)$$

$$\text{Level (dB)} = 10 \log \left(\frac{0.236 \, I_{max}}{I_{max}} \right)$$

$$\text{Level (dB)} = 10 \log (0.236)$$

$$\text{Level (dB)} = 10 \, (-0.627)$$

$$\text{Level (dB)} = -6.27$$

Note that the loss in decibels (6.27)—when multiplied by the factor 0.115 as defined by Equation 2-9—equals the loss in nepers of 0.721.

Amplitude Equation for Decibels

Equation 2-8 defines decibel using the ratio of the intensities at two different points. Another equation using the ratio of the amplitudes (usually pressure) may be employed to calculate intensity changes in decibels. Recall that the square of the amplitude is proportional to the intensity. Consequently,

2-11

$$\left(\frac{A_o}{A_{max}} \right)^2 = \frac{I}{I_{max}}$$

where A_{max} is the initial peak amplitude of the beam, and A_o is the peak amplitude at the point of interest. Substituting in Equation 2-8 for I/I_{max} using the relation in Equation 2-11:

2-12

$$\text{Level (dB)} = 10 \log \left(\frac{A_o}{A_{max}} \right)^2$$

or

$$\text{Level (dB)} = 20 \log \left(\frac{A_o}{A_{max}} \right)$$

Table 2-2 lists several examples of amplitude ratio and the corresponding decibel, calculated using Equation 2-12.

■ **Table 2-2** Amplitude Ratio versus Decibels

A/A_0	dB
100	40
20	26
10	20
2	6
1	0
0.5	−6
0.1	−20
0.05	−26
0.01	−40

A reduction in amplitude by a factor of 2 or half-amplitude ($A_o = 0.5\ A_{max}$) results in a 6 dB intensity loss. This reduction is equivalent to a reduction of intensity by a factor of 4, or 2 HVLs. One HVL corresponds to a change in amplitude by a factor of 1.414 ($A_o = 0.707\ A_{max}$). The term *half-power* describes a reduction of intensity by a factor of 2 (which corresponds to a 3 dB loss).

Decibels and HVLs

If the number of HVLs (n) for the path of the ultrasound beam is known, the reduction of intensity can be calculated from the following equation:

$$I = \frac{I_{max}}{2^n}$$

2-13

■ **Example 2-3**

Suppose a 2 MHz transducer is used to image a patient's abdomen at a depth of 15 cm. If the incident intensity is known to be 5 mW/cm^2, the intensity at 15 cm can be determined from Equation 2-13. The first step is to find the HVL for the tissue at 2 MHz, which Table 1-9 lists as 2.1 cm. In this case the number of HVLs is 7.14, because the thickness of material (15 cm) divided by the HVL (2.1 cm) equals 7.14. The intensity at 15 cm is given as

$$I = \frac{5\ mW/cm^2}{2^{7.14}}$$

$$I = \frac{5\ mW/cm^2}{141}$$

$$I = 0.035\ mW/cm^2$$

The same result could be obtained using Equation 2-8, which gives the relative intensities in decibels. The change in intensity corresponds to −21.49 dB [(7.14 HVL)(−3.01 dB/HVL)]. Substituting and solving for I gives

$$-21.49 = 10 \log \left(\frac{I}{5\ W/cm^2} \right)$$

$$-2.149 = \log \left(\frac{I}{5\ W/cm^2} \right)$$

$$\text{Antilog}\ (-2.149) = \frac{I}{5\ W/cm^2}$$

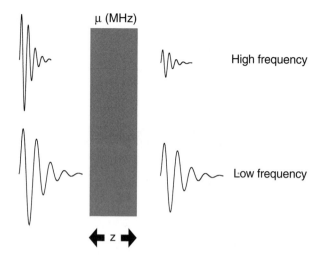

Fig. 2-3 Intensity loss depends on the tissue via the attenuation coefficient (μ), the frequency of the sound wave, and the path length (z). High frequency sound waves undergo more rapid attenuation for the same medium and path length.

$$0.007 = \frac{I}{5\ W/cm^2}$$

$$I = 0.035\ mW/cm^2$$

CALCULATION OF ATTENUATION LOSS

The intensity loss in decibels caused by attenuation as the ultrasound beam passes through a medium is calculated by the equation

2-14

$$\text{Intensity loss (dB)} = \mu f z$$

where μ is the intensity attenuation coefficient expressed in dB/cm/MHz, f is the frequency of the ultrasound wave expressed in MHz, and z is the distance traveled in the medium expressed in cm (Fig. 2-3).

A loss of intensity relative to the reference intensity (Equation 2-8) is denoted by a negative sign. The negative sign is not included in Equation 2-14, because attenuation always causes decreased intensity as the ultrasound beam penetrates a medium. The descriptor "loss" and the negative sign would be redundant. However, if the result is used in Equation 2-8 to calculate an absolute intensity expressed in W/cm^2, intensity loss by attenuation must include the negative sign. The intensity attenuation coefficient is tissue specific and accounts for differences in the attenuation rate for various tissue types. *Rapid attenuation is indicated by high values of the intensity attenuation coefficient.*

The attenuation (neglecting reflection) of an ultrasound beam propagating through soft tissue ranges from 0.5 to 1 dB/cm/MHz, but the average attenuation rate is approximated as 0.7 to 0.8 dB/cm/MHz. The decreased intensity expressed in decibels is directly proportional to both the depth of penetration and the frequency of the ultrasound beam. This can be seen more clearly by citing an example.

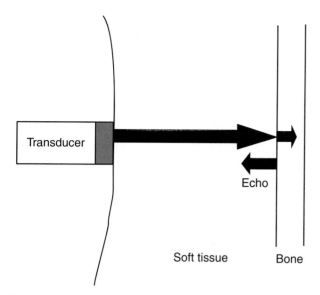

Fig. 2-4 An echo is created at an interface composed of soft tissue and bone after the sound wave penetrates 6 cm of soft tissue.

■ **Example 2-4**

Calculate the intensity loss in decibels for a 2.5 MHz ultrasound beam after traversing 6 cm of soft tissue.

$$\mu = 0.8 \text{ dB/cm/MHz}$$

$$f = 2.5 \text{ MHz}$$

$$z = 6 \text{ cm}$$

$$\text{Intensity loss (dB)} = \mu f z$$

$$\text{Intensity loss (dB)} = (0.8 \text{ dB/cm/MHz})(2.5 \text{ MHz})(6 \text{ cm})$$

$$\text{Intensity loss (dB)} = 12 \text{ dB}$$

DETERMINATION OF ECHO INTENSITY

Soft Tissue–Bone Interface

Figs. 2-4 and 2-5 depict the ultrasound beam striking an interface composed of soft tissue and bone. An echo is created at the interface that returns toward the transducer. The thickness of the soft tissue is 6 cm, and that of the bone 0.5 cm. In Fig. 2-4 the sound wave must traverse 6 cm of tissue before striking the soft tissue–bone interface. In Fig. 2-5 the order of the media is reversed: The sound wave must traverse 0.5 cm of bone before striking the interface. These figures will be used to illustrate the change in intensity of a sound beam after undergoing various interactions, specifically attenuation and reflection.

From Example 2-4, the intensity loss in decibels for a 2.5 MHz ultrasound beam after traversing 6 cm of soft tissue can be seen to be 12 dB. The intensity loss for a 2.5 MHz ultrasound beam after traversing 0.5 cm of bone is calculated in an identical manner and found to be 25 dB.

A small thickness of bone is very effective at reducing the intensity of the ultrasound beam, as indicated by the high intensity attenuation coefficient. The large reduction

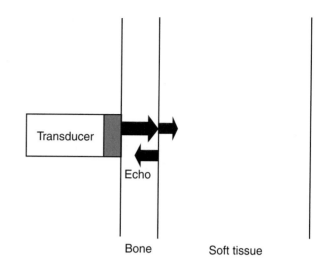

Fig. 2-5 An echo is created at an interface composed of bone and soft tissue after the sound wave penetrates 0.5 cm of bone.

attributed to attenuation in bone is the major reason why bone is generally avoided during an ultrasound examination. Additionally, there is a large amount of reflection at any soft tissue–bone interface.

In ultrasound imaging the transducer sends out a pulsed wave and subsequently detects the returning echo. Intensity loss occurs by attenuation of the transmitted wave going out to the interface and also by attenuation of the reflected wave coming back toward the transducer from the interface. The rate of attenuation depends on tissue type and wave frequency. The intensity of the detected echo from an interface is diminished by increasing the distance of travel.

■ **Example 2-5**

Calculate the relative intensity in decibels for an echo generated at a bone–soft tissue interface that is 6 cm deep in soft tissue. The transducer operates at a frequency of 2.5 MHz. Neglect the contribution of reflection at the interface.

For the transmitted wave

$$\text{Loss (dB)} = \mu f z$$

$$\text{Loss (dB)} = (0.8 \text{ dB/cm/MHz})(2.5 \text{ MHz})(6 \text{ cm})$$

$$\text{Loss (dB)} = 12 \text{ dB}$$

For the returning echo

$$\text{Loss (dB)} = 12 \text{ dB}$$

The loss as the ultrasound beam strikes the interface is the same as in Example 2-4 (i.e., 12 dB). Since the echo must repeat the path back to the transducer, the total intensity loss is twice this amount (24 dB). Remember that the dB losses along the path are additive.

Similarly, the total intensity loss of an echo returning from the bone–soft tissue interface after traveling a total distance of 1 cm in bone is 50 dB. If the frequency of the transducer is increased, the rate of attenuation between soft tissue and bone will be even more pronounced. For example, operating at a frequency of 7.5 MHz, the attenuation loss is tripled (to 72 dB and 150 dB, respectively).

Attenuation and Reflection Losses

We will now consider the combined effect of attenuation and reflection on the intensity of a detected echo. Attenuation refers to all processes (except reflection) that act to reduce ultrasound intensity. Losses from attenuation and reflection must be expressed in the same units, usually decibels. To convert percentage reflection into decibels, we modify Equation 2-8 by replacing I_{max} with 100 and I with the percentage reflection and inverting the fraction within the logarithmic function (to eliminate the negative sign):

2-15

$$Loss\ (dB) = 10\ \log\left(\frac{100}{\%R}\right)$$

The negative sign is not included, because the descriptor "loss" indicates that reflection always causes a reduction of intensity. Furthermore, losses from attenuation and reflection expressed in decibels are additive and can be easily combined. The following examples illustrate the total effect of attenuation and reflection on the intensity of the detected echo. Figs. 2-4 and 2-5 are reexamined to include the contribution of reflection.

■ **Example 2-6**

Calculate the relative intensity in decibels for an echo generated at a bone-tissue interface that is 6 cm deep in soft tissue. The transducer operates at a frequency of 2.5 MHz. Include the contribution of reflection at the interface.

For the transmitted wave

$$Loss\ (dB) = \mu fz$$
$$Loss\ (dB) = (0.8\ dB/cm/MHz)(2.5\ MHz)(6\ cm)$$
$$Loss\ (dB) = 12\ dB$$

For the returning echo

$$Loss\ (dB) = 12\ dB$$

For the reflection at this soft tissue–bone interface (i.e., the percentage reflection, 43%), which must be converted into decibels

$$Loss\ (dB) = 10\ \log\left(\frac{100}{\%R}\right)$$
$$Loss\ (dB) = 10\ \log\left(\frac{100}{43}\right)$$
$$Loss\ (dB) = 3.7\ dB$$

The total loss from attenuation and reflection

$$Loss\ (dB) = 12\ dB + 12\ dB + 3.7\ dB = 27.7\ dB$$

■ **Example 2-7**

Calculate the relative intensity in decibels for an echo generated at a bone-tissue interface that is 0.5 cm deep in bone. (The transducer operates at a frequency of 2.5 MHz.) Include the contribution of reflection at the interface.

For the transmitted wave

$$Loss\ (dB) = \mu fz$$
$$Loss\ (dB) = (20\ dB/cm/MHz)(2.5\ MHz)(0.5\ cm)$$
$$Loss\ (dB) = 25\ dB$$

For the returning echo

$$Loss\ (dB) = 25\ dB$$

For the loss from reflection at this soft tissue–bone interface (i.e., the percentage reflection, 43%), which must be converted into decibels

$$Loss\ (dB) = 10\ \log\left(\frac{100}{\%R}\right)$$
$$Loss\ (dB) = 10\ \log\left(\frac{100}{43}\right)$$
$$Loss\ (dB) = 3.7\ dB$$

The total loss from attenuation and reflection

$$Loss\ (dB) = Loss\ (going\ out) + Loss\ (returning) + Loss\ (reflection)$$
$$Loss\ (dB) = 25\ dB + 25\ dB + 3.7\ dB = 53.7\ dB$$

In general, absorption has a greater effect than reflection on the overall loss of beam intensity. This is particularly true for soft tissue interfaces in which the reflection intensity is a few percent or less. Comparing the results from the previous two examples demonstrates that the intensity of the echo at the transducer associated with a soft tissue–bone interface varies according to the attenuation along the path. *Structures with the same reflectivity are not always depicted with the same signal level.*

Calculation of Intensity

Once the total attenuation from all sources (i.e., absorption, reflection, refraction, and scattering) in decibels is found, the intensity ratio can be calculated. For a loss of 30 dB, Equation 2-8 demonstrates that the original intensity is reduced by a factor of 1000:

$$-30 = 10\ \log\left(\frac{I}{I_{max}}\right)$$
$$-3 = 10\ \log\left(\frac{I}{I_{max}}\right)$$
$$\frac{I}{I_{max}} = Antilog\ (-3)$$
$$\frac{I}{I_{max}} = 0.001$$

The intensity ratio can be used to calculate the actual intensity value for I or I_{max} if one of them is known. For example, if I_{max} is 10 mW/cm^2, the intensity at the point of interest (I) will be 0.01 mW/cm^2. An understanding of decibel notation and the various intensity parameters is essential when biologic effects of ultrasound are being discussed. (See Chapter 22.)

■ **Example 2-8**

Calculate the intensity in watts per square centimeter for the detected echo in Example 2-6. The transmitted intensity is 5 W/cm^2.

$$\text{Level (dB)} = -27.7$$
$$I_{max} = 5 \text{ W/cm}^2$$
$$I = 0.0085 \text{ W/cm}^2 \text{ or } 8.5 \text{ mW/cm}^2$$

Solid masses can be differentiated from cysts by examining the transmission of the beam through the structure. Solids attenuate the beam more rapidly than cystic (liquid-like) structures do. Liquids (blood, water, or cystic structures) are transonic or sonolucent and do not sharply attenuate. They appear in the image as hypoechoic regions. A liquid-like structure (e.g., a cyst in the breast) creates enhancement (higher signal levels) distal to the structure compared with the surrounding more attenuating tissue, as illustrated in Fig. 2-6. A solid mass in the breast exhibits little or no enhancement (Fig. 2-7). Shadowing (characterized by diminished signal levels) may occur behind sharply attenuating structures such as gallstones (Fig. 2-8).

■ **Example 2-9**

Calculate the intensity in watts per square centimeter for the detected echo in Example 2-7. The transmitted intensity is 5 W/cm^2.

$$\text{Level (dB)} = -53.7$$
$$I_{max} = 5 \text{ W/cm}^2$$
$$\text{Level (dB)} = 10 \log \left(\frac{I}{I_{max}} \right)$$
$$-53.7 = 10 \log \left(\frac{I}{5 \text{ W/cm}^2} \right)$$
$$-5.37 = \log \left(\frac{I}{5 \text{ W/cm}^2} \right)$$
$$\text{Antilog } (-5.37) = \frac{I}{5 \text{ W/cm}^2}$$
$$0.0000043 = \frac{I}{5 \text{ W/cm}^2}$$
$$I = 0.000022 \text{ W/cm}^2 \text{ or } 0.022 \text{ mW/cm}^2$$

SUMMARY

A reduction in ultrasound intensity occurs as the wave propagates through tissue. Scattering, absorption, and reflection contribute to the overall energy loss. In the absence of reflective interfaces the intensity loss is expressed mathematically as the product of the attenuation coefficient, frequency, and distance traveled in the medium. The attenuation coefficient is determined by tissue type. Lung and bone are highly attenuating, while blood and water-like fluids are weakly attenuating. The rate of energy loss

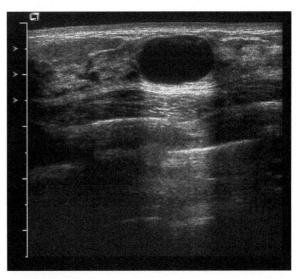

Fig. 2-6 Sonogram of a breast with a cyst. Acoustic enhancement occurs distal to the liquid-filled structure.

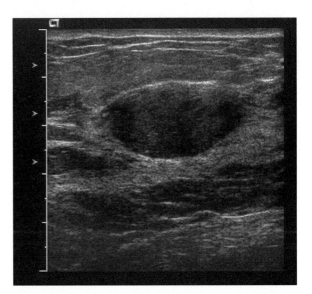

Fig. 2-7 Sonogram of a breast with a solid mass. Compare the structures distal to the mass with those distal to the cyst in Fig. 2-6.

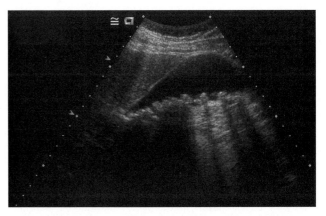

Fig. 2-8 Sonogram of a gallbladder with gallstones. Acoustic shadowing occurs distally to the strongly attenuating structures.

generally increases linearly with frequency. Intensity change is measured on a logarithmic scale in units of the decibel. Total decibel loss along the beam path composed of multiple tissue types is equal to the sum of the individual decibel losses for each path segment.

REVIEW QUESTIONS

1. Is reflection or attenuation the major cause for the loss of intensity of an ultrasound beam in soft tissue?
2. The attenuation of ultrasound propagating through soft tissue is approximately _____ dB/cm/MHz.
3. What is the attenuation loss in decibels for an ultrasound wave that penetrates 2 cm of fat? Assume the frequency to be 3 MHz, the acoustic velocity 1460 m/s, and the attenuation coefficient 0.6 dB/cm/MHz.
4. If an ultrasound beam has a transmitted intensity of 4 W/cm^2 and the detected echo has an intensity of 0.005 W/cm^2, what is the relative intensity level in decibels?
5. Calculate the relative intensity level in decibels for an echo generated at a soft tissue–bone interface that is 4 cm deep. The ultrasound beam travels through soft tissue before being reflected at the interface. The transducer frequency is 3.5 MHz.
6. Calculate the relative intensity in decibels for an echo generated at a fat–soft tissue interface that is at a depth of 2 cm. The ultrasound beam travels through fat before being reflected at the interface. The transducer frequency is 7.5 MHz.
7. Calculate the relative intensity in decibels for an echo generated at a soft tissue–lung interface that is at a depth of 5 cm. The ultrasound beam travels through soft tissue before being reflected at the interface. The transducer frequency is 5 MHz.
8. Calculate the returning echo intensity as a fraction of the transmitted intensity if the intensity of the detected echo is described as 25 dB below the transmitted intensity.
9. If intensity is decreased by a factor of 2, this corresponds to a decibel change of _____ dB.

BIBLIOGRAPHY

Carson PL: Ultrasound tissue interactions. In Goldman LW, Fowlkes JB, eds: *Categorical course in diagnostic radiology physics: CT and US cross-sectional imaging,* Oak Brook, Ill, 2000, Radiological Society of North America.

Insana MF: Sound attenuation in tissue. In Goldman LW, Fowlkes JB, eds: *Medical CT and ultrasound: current technology and applications,* College Park, Md, 1995, American Association of Physicists in Medicine.

McDicken WN: *Diagnostic ultrasonics: principles and use of instruments,* ed 3, Edinburgh, 1991, Churchill Livingstone.

NCRP Report No. 140: *Exposure criteria for medical diagnostic ultrasound: II. Criteria based on all known mechanisms,* Bethesda, Md, 2002, National Council on Radiation Protection and Measurements.

Computer Fundamentals

Analog-to-digital conversion
Binary
Bit
Buffer
Byte
Cathode ray tube (CRT)
Central processing unit (CPU)
Compact disk (CD)
Liquid crystal display (LCD)

Matrix size
Pixel
Random access memory (RAM)
Raster line
Read only memory (ROM)
Universal serial bus (USB)
Video signal
Word

During the past 15 years ultrasound instrumentation has undergone a transition from analog to digital. Digital components provide lower cost, superior performance (reliability, stability, and reproducibility), easier upgrades, flexibility of software control of scanner function, and longer life compared with their analog counterparts. The digitization of scan data provides an additional advantage: quantitative manipulation and analysis of the received echoes are possible in an expeditious fashion using current computer technology. In this chapter the binary number system, computer hardware, computer operation, analog-to-digital conversion, matrix representation of digital images, and display formats are presented. Computer techniques applied to scan data in real-time imaging are considered in Chapter 10.

BINARY REPRESENTATION

Digital computers are based on the **binary** system, in which two symbols or states are used to encode information (numbers, characters, and instructions). Similar to Morse code, in which a series of dots and dashes represents numbers and characters, the binary system employs combinations of 0s and 1s. The on-off operation of switches in the computer is ideally suited to symbolize these two possible states (the "off" position corresponding to 0 and the "on" position to 1).

The relative ease of representing 2 symbols in the binary system instead of the 10 symbols necessary in the decimal notation dictates that computers operate in binary. Furthermore, electrical circuits designed according to the Boolean principles (a mathematical treatment of logic developed by George Boole in the middle of the nineteenth century) could perform logic comparisons as well as execute complex calculations. Logic operations empower the computer to perform highly sophisticated tasks in different applications.

Bit and Byte

A single binary digit (called a **bit**) can be either 0 or 1 and thus is limited to two configurations. To increase the number of possible configurations, several bits are combined and treated as a single entity called a **word** (Fig. 3-1). Word

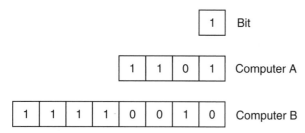

Fig. 3-1 Relationship between bit and word. Computer A has a 4-bit word, and Computer B an 8-bit word. Computer B is able to represent the detected signals with many more combinations of 0s and 1s.

length denotes the number of bits that are transferred as a group from one location in the computer to another. Word length also dictates the maximum number of bits used in computation and to encode instructions. The design of a specific computer model fixes the word length (usually 32 or 64 bits).

Another term that describes a collection of bits is **byte**. A byte is a group of 8 bits and is required to code a single character, such as one letter of the alphabet. The capacity of data storage units (e.g., magnetic disks, magnetic tape, and optical disks) is expressed in bytes or megabytes (millions of bytes). The total number of bytes indicates the total number of characters that the storage device can hold.

Binary Notation

The problem of how to represent the usual decimal numbers in this binary notation is solved as follows. In the binary system the base is 2. Each position in a multidigit binary number is denoted by a column value, which equals the base raised to a particular exponent. The integer exponent for each column increases by 1 with column position right to left. Thus, each column value increases by a factor of 2 compared with the column to the immediate right. The number 1 in a binary number signifies that the column value of the power of 2 represented by that position contributes to the overall sum. The number 0 in a binary number signifies that the column value of the power of 2 represented by that position does not contribute to the overall sum. For example:

Column value $\quad 2^3 \quad 2^2 \quad 2^1 \quad 2^0$
Binary number $\quad 0 \quad\;\; 1 \quad\;\; 0 \quad\;\; 1$

The respective value of each column right to left is 2 raised to the indicated power or 1, 2, 4, and 8. The binary digit in each column (0 or 1) indicates whether the column value contributes to the overall sum represented by the 4-bit binary number. This means that the sum of 0×8, 1×4, 0×2, and 1×1 is 5 (the corresponding decimal equivalent of the number 0101 in binary notation).

■ Example 3-1

Calculate the decimal equivalent of the binary number 1101.
Assign the value to each position.

Column value $\quad 2^3 \quad 2^2 \quad 2^1 \quad 2^0$
Binary number $\quad 1 \quad\;\; 1 \quad\;\; 0 \quad\;\; 1$

Sum the contribution from each column: $1 \times 8 + 1 \times 4 + 0 \times 2 + 1 \times 1 = 13$

The decimal equivalent of the binary number 1101 thus is 13.

Several binary numbers represented in 4 bits and the associated decimal numbers are listed in Table 3-1.

Mathematically, the number of combinations that could be denoted by a collection of bits is given by 2^n, where n is the number of bits in the binary number. A 4-bit word can represent 16 different combinations of 0s and 1s, because the base 2 raised to the fourth power equals 16. Table 3-1, which lists all unique arrangements of 4 binary digits, confirms this calculation of total possible combinations. *Obviously, a word with more bits can be configured in more combinations and can represent physical quantities with greater magnitude and/or with greater precision.* Computer B, with a bit depth of eight, corresponding to 256 combinations, is superior to computer A, which has a bit depth of four, corresponding to 16 combinations.

COMPUTER SYSTEMS

The computer system is classified into three major components: hardware, software, and documentation. Hardware is the physical equipment such as the central processing unit (CPU), memory, disk drive, printer, monitor, keyboard, mouse, trackball, and joystick. Software is the set of programs (or instructions) that tells the computer what to do. The collection of programs to perform specialized tasks is called an application package. Documentation consists of the manuals that instruct the operator how to use the computer hardware and the application package.

HARDWARE

A computer accepts information from an input device, applies some prescribed process (dictated by the software),

■ **Table 3-1** Translation of 4-bit Binary Numbers to Decimal Equivalents

Binary System	Decimal System
0000	0
0001	1
0010	2
0011	3
0100	4
0101	5
0110	6
0111	7
1000	8
1001	9
1010	10
1011	11
1100	12
1101	13
1110	14
1111	15

and communicates the results to the outside world. The input device acquires data (e.g., detector in medical imaging) and/or conveys operator instructions (e.g., keyboard or mouse). The central processing unit manipulates the data via a collection of instructions (program) and displays an image on a monitor (output device) for viewing. Both instructions and data are held in rewriteable computer memory during processing. Programs and data including patient images are retained on some type of storage device when not in active use.

Central Processing Unit

The **central processing unit (CPU)** manipulates the input data by sequentially executing programmed instructions. The components of the CPU include the arithmetic logic unit, control unit, and multiple registers, such as the program counter and accumulator. A register holds one word, which is maintained in the register until overwritten. Registers facilitate the computational process by providing information as needed within the CPU. The one word in a register could contain either datum from memory, the result of calculation, an instruction to be executed, or the address of a memory location of interest. All mathematical manipulations and logic functions are interpreted and executed by the arithmetic logic unit. The control unit coordinates all operations, including data transfers from one device to another in the system.

Since the flow of information is limited by the size of the register (number of bits contained in the register), this is the primary determinant of word length for a particular computer. The number of bits in the computer word dictates the number of different instructions that can be executed.

Memory

The **read only memory (ROM)** contains permanent instructions to be implemented by the CPU to configure the system. Usually ROM is accessed during the startup procedure, called booting. Its contents can be changed only by replacing the integrated circuit chip. **Random access memory (RAM)** is accessible by the CPU for temporary storage of data or instructions. It is erasable and can be updated with new information as required. The retrieval rate for data contained in RAM by the CPU is very fast and enables short execution times.

Input/Output Devices

Numerous input/output (I/O) devices are available that can be interfaced to the computer system. Sometimes these devices are called peripherals, because they are controlled by the CPU. A device may be designed for input only, output only, or both input and output. The output devices are used to display, list, or store the results of manipulations performed by the CPU.

Many detector systems in medicine now supply image information to the computer. Since the computer can handle only binary data, however, the analog signals coming from the detector must be translated into a digital form. This occurs at the interface, which contains an **analog-to-digital converter (ADC).**

Information in the form of alphanumerics (letters, numbers, and symbols), images, and graphs is provided to the operator. Within the computer system data communication assumes a form (e.g., magnetic fields, polarized laser light, and voltage pulse height) that is efficiently handled by the hardware devices. For example, most computers contain a keyboard. The depressed key is translated into binary code as a series of voltage pulses before being communicated to other devices.

Communication Ports

Data transfer must occur between the CPU and I/O devices. Various communication ports have been developed and standardized for ease of data transfer using equipment from different manufacturers. The most common communication ports include serial (9-pin and 25-pin), parallel, universal serial bus (USB), firewire, modem, and 10/100 Ethernet.

The serial port usually supports low-speed devices such as a mouse or joystick. The information is transferred in a series of voltage pulses, one after another in a specified time interval. Each voltage pulse codes for a 0 or 1. The RS232 standard allows transmission at rates ranging from 110 bits per second (bps) to 19.2 kilobits per second (kbps). The device must be configured for the designated rate and, once established, is fixed unless reconfigured.

The parallel port improves the data transfer rate by sending multiple bits (either 8 or 16) simultaneously. Transmission speed is increased by the number of bits in the group. The cable must contain at least as many wires as the number of bits transferred at one time. Many printers are connected to the parallel port.

The **universal serial bus (USB)** is rapidly becoming the industry standard for connection to different devices (e.g., digital cameras, printers, scanners, disk drives). The USB can support 127 devices, each with a unique 7-bit address, on a single port. A variable transfer rate from 1.5 megabits per second (Mbps) to 12 Mbps is established based on the requirements of the connected device. Version 2.0 increases the maximum transmission rate by a factor of 40. The cable has four wires (two for power and two for data transfer) and is hot swappable—no need to power down the computer to make or break the connection to the USB port.

The firewire port offers a high-speed transfer rate (100 to 400 Mbps) for applications involving large quantities of data, such as digital scanning of photographic negatives and video. Most peripherals will offer either firewire or USB connectivity.

A modem allows information to be transferred over telephone lines by converting digital data to audible tones. For analog devices such as the modem, the rate of data transmission is designated in bauds, 1 baud equaling 1 bit per second. The maximum transmission rate using the standard telephone line is 56 kbps. Frequently, transmission is slower than the maximum rate.

Computers in a local area network exchange information via the Ethernet communication system. Ethernet is a collection of hardware and operating protocols that operates at a fixed speed depending on the transmission media. The transmission rate for coaxial cable and optic cable is 10 Mbits per second and 100 Mbits per second, respectively. Each computer connected to the network has a unique address that allows routing of data to destination computers.

Buffer

Devices cannot process data as fast as the data are received. Hence, each device contains a small amount of memory (called a **buffer**) into which the data are loaded from the sending device. These data are then removed from the buffer and processed at a rate compatible with the receiving device. Since the buffer is limited in capacity, data transfer stops when the buffer is nearly full and resumes after some of the data have been removed. This technique allows devices with different processing rates to communicate with one another efficiently.

Storage Devices

Memory is relatively expensive and limited in capacity compared with storage devices. Therefore information (both program and data) is stored as files outside the memory until needed. The most common storage devices are magnetic disks (e.g., Winchester disks, removable magnetic cartridges, and floppy disks). Other storage devices such as compact disks (CD) and flash drives are increasing in popularity as a means to back up data and transfer information to another computer. The advantages of CDs are high storage capacity and low cost for the storage media. Flash drives are compact, relatively fast, and very easy to use.

Magnetic Disk

The magnetic disk consists of a base material coated with a thin layer of magnetic material, usually ferrous oxide. Data in the form of 0s and 1s are represented by small regions of magnetizations in the ferrous oxide (the magnetic field in one direction corresponding to 0 and in the opposite direction to 1).

The disk is divided into tracks and sectors, which allows a directory of the location of data on it to be generated (Fig. 3-2). Each track in a sector corresponds to one block. A block is the smallest data group that can be transferred to and from the disk. A block is usually equal to 512 bytes. If a file size is 600 bytes in memory, it requires 2 blocks on disk for storage.

The information is transferred to and from the disk via read/write heads. One read/write head is associated with each disk surface. The disk is spinning rapidly, and the read/write head moves in and out above the sensitive layer. By positioning the read/write head directly on a particular track and sector, it is possible to read or write the desired file. This is an example of random access, since the informa-

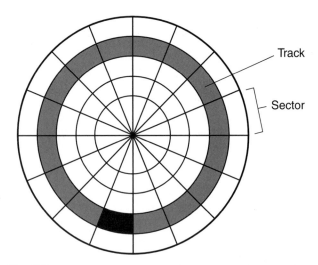

Fig. 3-2 Magnetic disk partitioned into tracks and sectors. One block of data *(black)* is contained on the track *(gray)* through one sector. The designation of track and sector of a file indicates the storage location on the disk.

tion can be transferred without examining other blocks. A particular track may contain several files, but the data making up a single file are often contiguous on the disk.

Magnetic Tape

Magnetic tape is similar to cassette audiotape. The width of the tape (1/2-inch, 8 mm, or 4 mm) is divided into nine tracks (a byte plus an error check bit) so that nine bits are written across the tape at each location along the length of the tape. The tape is contained within a cassette (two spools) or cartridge (one spool). For the cartridge the tape must be physically unwound from cartridge onto a take-up spool within the tape drive. Digital linear tape (DLT) is an example of this media package. The cassette format is less susceptible to handling problems, but holds less recording media than cartridges.

Storage capacity ranging from 4 to 110 gigabytes (GB) depends on the length of the tape and the recording density. Because sequential access provides relatively slow retrieval of data, tape storage is usually reserved for data backup. Magnetic tape provides a low-cost, removable storage option.

Optical Disk

Optical disks exist in write-once and rewriteable formats. The first type is called WORM, which means **w**rite **o**nce **r**ead **m**any. Erasable optical disks are designated MOD (magneto-optical disk). During readout a low-intensity laser light beam, less than 1 μm in diameter, scans across the reflective surface of the optical disk. At each location on the reflective surface, a value of 0 or 1 has been encoded by manipulating the reflective properties of the surface. In the WORM format a zero is represented by a pit etched into the surface by a high-intensity write laser beam to reduce the amount of light reflected by the readout laser beam. A photodetector measures the intensity of the reflected light. The presence or absence of the pit codes for a 0 or a 1 (high reflectance or low reflectance). The small physical dimensions of the laser beam allow high recording density, and thus a large storage capacity is achieved.

The erasable MOD format uses the polarization of reflected light to code for the two binary states. Polarization of the reflected light depends on the magnetization of the small region on the surface interrogated by the laser light. In the write mode an electromagnet is positioned above the disk and a laser below. The magnetization on the disk's surface is aligned in one of two directions by heating the region with the laser in the presence of a magnetic field. During readout a low-intensity laser light beam is scanned across the reflective surface of the optical disk. The polarization of the reflected light indicates a 0 or a 1 (parallel or perpendicular orientation).

WORM disks have a single platter housed in an openable or removable cartridge. Total storage for a 5.25-inch optical disk is 800 MB. Typically MODs have lower capacity than WORM disks. Optical disks generally have a much slower access time than magnetic disks. The lifetime of optical disks is 10 to 100 years.

Compact Disk

The **compact disk** is a type of optical disk that has either an erasable format (CD-RW) or a write once format (CD-R). A 120-mm diameter polycarbonate plastic disk contains a reflective aluminum layer. The CD-R encodes 0s and 1s in the same manner as the WORM optical disk. The rewriteable format has a phase-change recording layer coating the reflective surface. The optical property of the recording layer is either transparent in the crystalline form to allow light to be transmitted to the reflective surface (encodes 1) or opaque in the amorphous form to prevent light from reaching the reflective surface (encodes 0). By heating the recording layer to a particular temperature and allowing it to cool, one of the phase forms is created depending on the temperature rise. Readout is accomplished by scanning the recording layer/reflective surface with a low-intensity laser beam.

The CD contains a single track beginning at the center of the disk and spiraling outward toward the edge. A 780 nm laser burns pits along the track; each pit is 0.5 μm by 1.6 μm in size. Adjacent passes of the spiral track are separated by 1.6 μm. The high-density packing of the pits and successive spiral loops enable large information storage. A total of 333,000 sectors of 2048 bytes each compose the spiral track, yielding approximately 650 MB.

The data transfer rate established by the music industry for audio CDs is 150 kilobytes per second. The read rate for CD drives is usually expressed as a multiple of this base rate, 12x to 52x. Box 3-1 lists the characteristics of the compact disk.

Digital Video Disk

The digital video disk (DVD), also called digital versatile disk, is another type of optical disk. Although the same size

---

Box 3-1 Characteristics of the Compact Disk

Not subject to mechanical failure of read/write heads
Low cost
Industry standards
High capacity (650 MB)
Transfer rate 3 MB per second (20x)
Not affected by many environmental factors (magnetic fields, humidity)

---

as the compact disk, the DVD offers higher storage capacity by writing smaller pits with a higher packing density of the tracks. Unfortunately, no industry-wide standard has been adopted. This has resulted in several different formats such as DVD-ROM (read-only with a capacity of 4.7 to 17 GB), DVD-R (recordable with a capacity of 3.9 GB), and DVD-RAM (rewriteable with a capacity of 5.2 GB). As the technology evolves, this type of storage device will be used more often in medical applications.

Universal Serial Bus Flash Drive

The technology that enables pictures to be stored on compact flash cards in digital photography has been adapted to a compact, nonvolatile storage device, which uses the universal serial bus (USB) to transfer data. The physical size of the USB flash drive is comparable to a penlight and weighs less than an ounce. Storage capacity ranges from 32 MB to 2 GB. The flash drive contains no moving parts and is likely to be durable, but must be protected from magnetic fields.

Comparison of Storage Devices

Storage devices are characterized by size, cost, data capacity, and rate of transfer of data (Table 3-2). Each device has advantages and disadvantages (capacity, transfer rate, cost, size). The primary disadvantages of the floppy disk are its slow rate of data transfer and its limited capacity. In the past many institutions used the floppy disk as a portable storage device for the transfer of patient studies between computers. However, CDs have replaced floppy disks for this application, and as data storage requirements become even greater, the DVD will replace the CD.

Printers

Hard copy recording of text, graphics, and photographs is accomplished with a printer interfaced to the computer.

■ **Table 3-2** Characteristics of Storage Devices

Type	Storage Capacity	Transfer Rate
Floppy	0.3-3 MB	Slow
Compact disk	650 MB	Medium
Flash drive	32 MB-2 GB	Medium
Magnetic disk	10-80 GB	Fast

Often, the USB or parallel communication port is used to transfer data to the printer. Printers are usually classified as laser or inkjet. Laser printers are well suited for black and white text output: fast, high quality, and the lowest cost per page. Inkjet printers, although slower than laser printers, are more versatile and can print color photographs as well as black and white text.

Resolution is specified in the number of dots of ink that are placed on the page and is expressed as dots per inch (dpi). Higher dpi produces sharper images. Most high-quality printers can produce 600 or more dots per inch.

SOFTWARE

Software is the set of programs used to control the computer. These may be permanently stored in read-only memory (ROM), or they may be stored on magnetic disk and transferred to RAM when needed. The advantage of this storage method is that the programs can easily be rewritten with newer versions (software updates).

Software supplied by the manufacturer is designed primarily to transform the hardware into usable tools. In addition, a set of programs that allows users to create and run programs of their own design is provided. These user-generated programs are usually written in the high-level programming languages of FORTRAN, C++, JAVA, Basic, or Visual Basic, but they can also be written in assembly language.

Operating System

The **operating system** is a collection of programs that directs all the activities of the computer, including control of hardware devices and execution of application programs. Communication between the computer system and the user is essential. The computer system must offer clear and direct methods to acquire data and select processing options. The responses of the user must be converted by the operating system to forms understood by the computer. The operating system must select programs that can fulfill the request of the user. The basic approach is to separate the many functions into discrete modules, which are retrieved from the storage device and placed in memory as necessary. Each module is a program designed to do a certain task. The operating system must also maintain records of stored programs and data.

Programming Languages

Selection of a particular language to write programs depends on the application (business or scientific) and the specific hardware devices available. In all cases the program language must eventually be translated into machine code (the instruction set in 0s and 1s and equal in number to the word length for the computer). Machine code is not universal but rather is computer specific.

Assembly language programming requires every execution step by the CPU to be defined. The assembly language is converted to machine code by translation programs called assemblers. Assembly language is machine dependent. This low-level language provides for the greatest programming flexibility and speed; however, such programs often become large and complex for the general user. Operating systems are usually written in assembly language.

High-level languages are constructed so they are machine independent. This allows the software developer to write the program code once and then execute the program on any computer that has this high-level language capability. Language interpreters and translators are required to translate the program written in a high-level language to specific machine code.

Several programming languages—including Basic, Pascal, Forth, COBOL, C, and Fortran—are available. Each has a unique vocabulary of symbols, words, and letters that code for particular operations. In addition, for the computer to interpret each instruction correctly, rules of syntax must be followed exactly. Interpreters, translators, or compilers are present in the operating system so the high-level language can be converted to a machine code (instructions in binary) that is understood by the computer.

No single programming language is best for all circumstances; rather, each offers certain advantages depending on the application. For example, Fortran provides a more elaborate set of mathematical operations and a faster execution time than Basic; however, personal computer manufacturers have adopted Basic, because it is relatively easy to learn, and the difference in execution times for short simple programs is insignificant. The ease by which a Basic program can be altered, updated, and debugged also has contributed substantially to Basic's acceptance in the personal computer marketplace.

COMPUTER OPERATION

Suppose memory is represented by a group of wastepaper baskets numbered 1 through 15, as shown in Fig. 3-3. The numerical label is used to identify a particular basket. Each basket is limited—that is, it can hold only one piece of paper on which an instruction or number may be written. You are

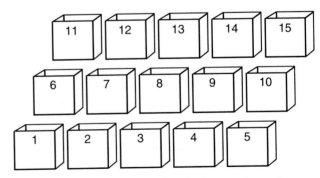

Fig. 3-3 A collection of wastepaper baskets can be used to represent computer memory. Each wastepaper basket (location in memory) has a numerical label (address) to distinguish it from the others. One instruction or multidigit binary number is held at each memory location.

■ **Table 3-3** Computer Memory Example

Location	Contents
1	Erase the pad (i.e., put number 0 on pad)
2	Add number at location 12 to contents of pad
3	Add number at location 11 to contents of pad
4	Place value on pad in wastepaper basket 10
5	Display contents at location 10 on cathode ray tube
6	Stop
7, 8, 9	0
10	8 (0000 1000)
11	5 (0000 0101)
12	3 (0000 0011)

now given a pen and a scratch pad and told to go to basket number 1, retrieve the piece of paper, and perform the instructed task. When you have completed the first assignment, move on to the next basket to retrieve your next instruction. You proceed and find the scenario outlined in Table 3-3. The result of your work is that the number 8 in binary notation with a word length of 8 (0000 1000) is stored in basket 10 and displayed on the **cathode ray tube (CRT).**

Execution of Instructions

This example illustrates how a computer works. Each location (or address) in memory, corresponding to a basket, holds one instruction or one multidigit binary number. The person represents the central processing unit (CPU), and the pad acts as the accumulator, which is a working area for calculations. A set of instructions is carried out in a carefully planned sequence (which is designated by the program). In this program the instructions are performed in order from basket 1 to basket 5. In a different program the user may be told to jump to a nonconsecutive location for the next instruction. The execution would then proceed in sequence from that point.

In the example, although you had to go to basket 12 to get some numerical information, you still came back to the next basket in sequence for the next instruction. (After completing the instruction at location 2, you went to location 3 for the next instruction.) Note that you had to be told where to start (which location in memory contained the first instruction in the program to be executed).

The program must be placed in memory before instructions are executed. This program, for example, could have been stored on a floppy disk and then transferred to computer memory before being run. The process is called "loading." Before the program was stored on the floppy, it would have to have been entered as a set of instructions line by line via the keyboard by the software developer. The data in locations 11 and 12 would also have to have been entered before the program was run or with additional programming steps that allow data input during program execution.

Memory Capacity

The total number of baskets dictates the size of the computer memory. As the number of baskets increases, more instructions and data can be held simultaneously in memory, and this results in faster execution times. The memory capacity is usually designated by the number of locations in bytes, expressed as MB. The symbol M (for mega) denotes the numerical value of 2^{20}, or 1,048,576. For example, a 64-megabyte (MB) computer would have $64 \times 1,048,576$ or 67,108,864 locations available in its memory. Memory capacity has been greatly expanded in recent years and is sometimes specified in GB or 2^{30} (1,073,700,000).

Each wastepaper basket has a numerical label to distinguish it from neighboring wastepaper baskets. This label is the unique memory address of that particular basket. The address and binary information placed in the byte are separate entities (just as the writing on the piece of paper is not the same as the numerical label of the wastepaper basket). For each 8-bit byte the information held at any memory location is coded in the form of some 8-digit combination of 0s and 1s.

Computer Speed

The clock coordinates the execution of tasks by the CPU. Each tick of the clock allows one step in the execution process to proceed. Retrieving the instruction from memory would be one step, and decoding the instruction would be another step. The repetitive ticks of the clock synchronize the movement of data and the operations applied to that data. Without the clock, each component would act independently, and all coordination would be lost. *The number of clock ticks per second, denoted in megahertz or gigahertz, describes the computer speed.* Many PCs operate at 1 GHz or higher. Clock speed is an indication of how quickly a program can be executed. Generally, higher clock speed results in shorter execution time, but this is not always true. Other descriptors also characterize computer speed.

The number (in millions) of instructions the computer can execute in 1 second, called MIPS, is another measure of computer speed. A more complex means of gauging computer speed is to note the number (in millions) of floating point operations that can be performed in 1 second (MFLOPS). These parameters establish the computer's speed on a relative scale, but other factors influence the execution time necessary for a particular program. Test programs have been used to determine the speed of different systems designed for the same application.

ANALOG-TO-DIGITAL CONVERSION

Some accuracy is sacrificed when a signal is digitized, as occurs in the translation of information from the detection system (signal amplitude and spatial location of the object) to a form that is understood by the computer. The translation process is called **analog-to-digital conversion** and is limited by the number of bits available in the digitization process. The analog signal is a continuously variable entity, whereas the digital signal is expressed in discrete steps.

Height Conversion

Imagine that there are two ways (via a staircase or a ramp) of ascending to the second floor from the first floor in a building. By using the stairs, a description of your position (height above the first floor) consists of the number of the step you are standing on multiplied by the height of a single step. You are constrained to standing on one of the steps; a position between steps is not possible. If you stand on step number 2 and each step is 2 feet high, your location is designated as 4 feet above the first floor. At step number 3 you move to a height 6 feet above the first floor. The description is limited to discrete intervals of distance established by the size of the step (in this case increments of 2 feet). However, by taking the ramp, you would reach any height above the first floor.

If we replace each step in the staircase with two smaller steps, we can now describe the height as increments of 1 foot. In Fig. 3-4, a height 5.75 feet above the first floor can be represented precisely by the ramp, but it would be approximated by step number 2 in staircase A (at a height of 4 feet) or by step number 5 in staircase B (at a height of 5 feet). An error is introduced in the quantitative description of the variable (in this case position), because discrete units are used. If we divide the discrete units into smaller and smaller steps, however, the accuracy of the conversion process is improved. In general, staircase B provides a more accurate assessment of position than does staircase A, because many more steps are used in the conversion process. The same effect is achieved by employing more bits in the digitization of analog signals.

Voltage Conversion

In medical imaging the analog signal is a voltage waveform generated by the detector. Increased signal strength is represented by an increased value of the voltage. The transformation of this analog signal to a digital format is limited to discrete steps, the size of each step being dictated by the bit depth of the analog-to-digital converter (ADC). Suppose the ADC for each of two computers is configured to digitize the received signals over a range of 0 to 5 volts. Computer A has a 2-bit ADC (or four discrete steps), and computer B a 3-bit ADC (or eight discrete steps). The corresponding step size, which is calculated by dividing the range (5 volts) by the total number of discrete steps available (either 4 or 8), is 1.25 and 0.625 V. The 2-volt peak in Fig. 3-5 is interpreted as digital step 01 (or 1×1.25 V = 1.25 V) by computer A and as digital step 011 (or 3×0.625 V = 1.875 V) by computer B. Once more, the accuracy of the conversion process is improved by increasing the bit depth, because each digital step corresponds to a smaller physical quantity.

Serial Sampling

In the previous examples one digital value was assigned to the analog signal. Other applications may require that the time dependence of the analog signal be preserved. The analog signal is repeatedly sampled during the time interval, and the instantaneous value at each sampled point is

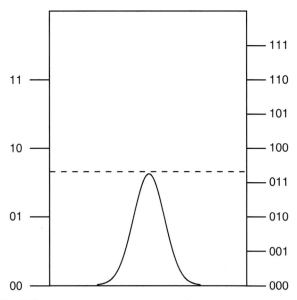

Fig. 3-5 Analog-to-digital conversion of a voltage peak. With a 2-bit scanner the voltage peak is represented as 01, but with a 3-bit scanner as 011. The smaller divisions between digitizer steps allow greater accuracy.

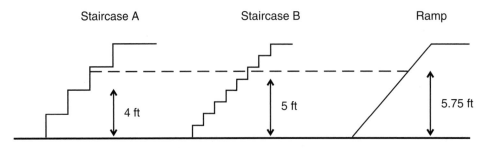

Fig. 3-4 Comparison of analog and digital representations. The 5.75-foot height above the floor *(dotted line)* can be represented exactly by the ramp but is only approximated by the staircases. Staircase A *(with large steps)* is less accurate in its representation than Staircase B. The fifth step in Staircase B is closer to the actual height than the second step of Staircase A.

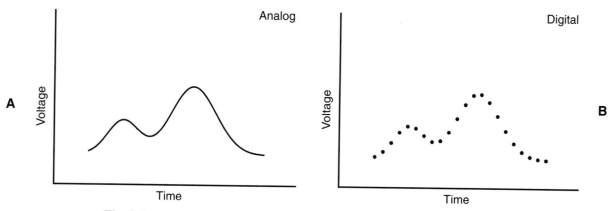

Fig. 3-6 Analog-to-digital conversion of a time-varying voltage waveform. **A,** Analog signal. **B,** Digital signal.

digitized. Fig. 3-6 illustrates the digitization of a voltage waveform varying in time. Once more, the analog-to-digital conversion process yields discrete steps (in this case, with respect both to voltage and to time).

Bit Depth

Word length sets the upper limit for the number of bits that can be used in the digitization of a signal. The actual bit depth of the ADC does not necessarily correspond to the word size. Some manufacturers use ADCs with fewer bits than the number available in a word. The prospective purchaser of imaging equipment should ascertain the bit depth maintained throughout the imaging chain, for it will ultimately affect both contrast and dynamic range.

SPATIAL REPRESENTATION

The information obtained from a scanned area is divided into small square picture elements called **pixels,** which are combined to form the image. Each pixel corresponds to a particular region, designated by spatial coordinates, and is associated with the signal strength from that region. The amplitude of the received signal is converted to a digital number (1s and 0s) by the ADC before storage in computer memory. The number of pixels available depends on the **matrix size,** which denotes the number of rows and columns in the pictorial representation. For example, a 512 × 512 matrix has 512 rows and 512 columns. The image is composed of a total of 262,144 individual pixels (the number of rows multiplied by the number of columns).

During data collection the digitized signal is stored in a particular location of memory specified by its address. Each pixel has one location reserved in memory for holding the amplitude of the signal associated with that pixel. The address is determined from the spatial coordinates of the measured parameter (e.g., the location of echo generation as illustrated in Fig. 3-7).

The digitized amplitudes for all pixels contained in computer memory must be recombined to form the image. Spatial relationships must be maintained. The image is constructed in such a manner that spatial coordinates in

the image correspond to a specific location within the area scanned. The address in memory designates the position of the pixel in the image, and the value stored at that address represents the signal amplitude of that pixel in the image. This is analogous to a jigsaw puzzle. Each piece of the puzzle is imprinted with a portion of a scene (signal amplitude) and must fit into the puzzle in a specified manner (address) to reproduce the scene.

In the digital format each piece of the puzzle is restricted to a square (which is depicted as a uniform shade of gray). Each pixel has its own shade, but only one value is stored in memory for that pixel. The same value is assumed to exist throughout the spatial extent represented by the pixel. This assumption is most appropriate for pixels with small physical dimensions. Once more, some accuracy is sacrificed by the digital representation of spatial location. As the matrix size increases, the system has the potential of presenting more spatial detail, which is demonstrated by the digitized pictures of Abraham Lincoln in varying matrix sizes (Fig. 3-8). However, computer memories with a larger capacity are then necessary to store the information. Currently, most ultrasound scanners use the 512 × 512 matrix, which is adequate for representing the spatial resolution achievable by the rest of the imaging chain. At a viewing distance of 18 inches, the individual pixel elements are not distinguished, and the image appears spatially continuous.

IMAGE DISPLAY
Cathode Ray Tube

A CRT is the simplest output device used for display purposes. It is a large evacuated (low-pressure) glass tube with a potential difference of 10,000 to 30,000 volts from back to front. This voltage difference accelerates electrons emitted from the cathode (also called electron gun or filament) at the back of the CRT toward the screen (Fig. 3-9). The glass envelope maintains the vacuum to allow the passage of electrons. A focusing cup or coil near the filament confines the electrons to a narrow beam and prevents them from spreading out over a wide area. The glass screen on the front of the CRT is covered with a phosphorescent material

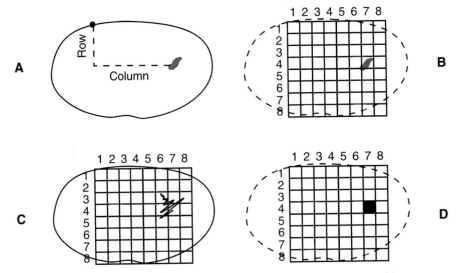

Fig. 3-7 A, The interface is located at spatial coordinates *(row, column)* with respect to a reference point (corresponding to the upper left corner of the image matrix). **B,** The position of the interface is shown in the image matrix. **C,** The echo originates at the interface. **D,** The amplitude of the detected signal is placed at the pixel location within the matrix corresponding to row 4 and column 7, designated by the spatial coordinates.

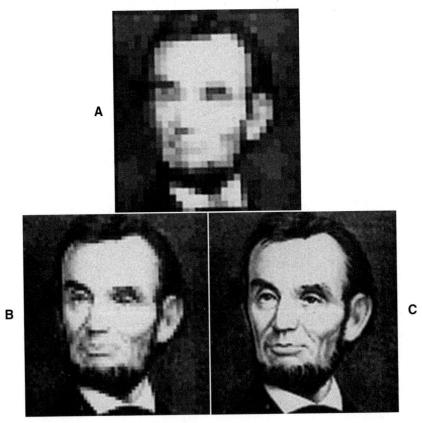

Fig. 3-8 Matrix representation of a portrait of Abraham Lincoln. **A,** 32 × 32 matrix; **B,** 64 × 64; **C,** 128 × 128.

(usually zinc sulfide, zinc sulfate, or potassium iodide) that produces light when struck with electrons. The grid near the cathode controls the number of electrons permitted to flow across the tube that ultimately strikes the phosphorescent screen.

The number of electrons striking the screen controls the brightness of the dot. The measured signal level is routed to the cathode grid. As the amplitude of the processed signal is increased, more electrons are permitted to leave the region of the cathode and strike the phosphor screen. A bright dot

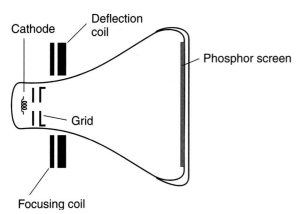

Fig. 3-9 Principal components of a cathode ray tube.

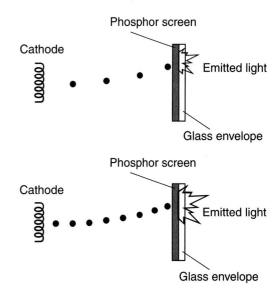

Fig. 3-10 Cathode ray tube brightness is controlled by the number of electrons striking the phosphor screen. **A,** Low beam current. **B,** High beam current.

is created by high electron beam current (Fig. 3-10). The brightness of each displayed dot (pixel) in the image matrix is adjusted independently.

Deflection plates or coils (electromagnets) within the CRT are responsible for positioning the dot in two dimensions on the screen. One pair of electrical plates (or magnetic coils) controls the position of the electron beam in the horizontal (across the screen) direction, and a second pair controls the position of the electron beam in the vertical direction. The two sets of plates, which independently control horizontal and vertical deflection, allow the beam to be positioned anywhere on the CRT screen.

Control of the electron beam placement on the phosphorescent screen is easiest to demonstrate using deflection plates. Electrical fields are produced when a voltage difference is applied to one set of plates. If no voltage is applied, no electrical field is present, and the electrons travel along a straight-line path from the filament to the center of the screen. Applying a positive voltage to one plate in the set, however, and a negative voltage to the other (i.e., creating a potential difference across the plates) deflects the beam toward the positive plate. Reversing the voltage deflects it in the opposite direction (Fig. 3-11).

Applying a linear voltage change to the plates causes the beam to move across the screen. Application of voltage to the vertical deflection plates moves it up or down, to the horizontal deflection plates moves it horizontally, and to both pairs of plates moves it diagonally (Fig. 3-12).

Liquid Crystal Display (LCD)

Solid-state flat panel monitors such as **liquid crystal displays (LCDs)** have replaced CRTs as the preferred display monitor for many applications. In the most common design the backlit LCD is composed of four functional layers—light source, polarizing filter, voltage adjust brightness control layer, and a second polarizing filter rotated 90 degrees with respect to the first filter.

The light from a uniform light source is incident on the first polarizing filter, which allows only light with a particular orientation to pass through (produces polarized light). If unchanged by the brightness control layer, then this polarized light cannot pass through the second polarizing filter, and the display is black. A voltage applied to the brightness control layer twists the light's magnetic and electric fields, changing the orientation of the light. The amount of rotation depends on the voltage. As the voltage is increased, the resulting rotation creates higher transmission through the second polarizing filter, and more light is observed. The brightness control layer is divided into small regions, pixels, similar to the image matrix. Each pixel is independently controlled for brightness level. A capacitor associated with each pixel holds charge and maintains the voltage while the remaining pixels in the LCD are displayed. Box 3-2 lists the characteristics of LCDs compared with CRTs.

Video Interface

The video interface converts the digital image to an analog format for display on a video monitor. Image data are transferred to RAM memory contained within the video interface. This allows data to be read and displayed very rapidly and essentially outside CPU control after the image(s) are sent for display. This technique enables the CPU to perform other tasks without interruptions to repeatedly direct an image for display.

Box 3-2 **Characteristics of Liquid Crystal Displays Compared with Cathode Ray Tubes**

Small physical size for the same viewing area
Less weight
Generates less heat
Lower power consumption
Smaller viewing angle
Inoperative areas on viewing surface (always black or white)
Lower luminance

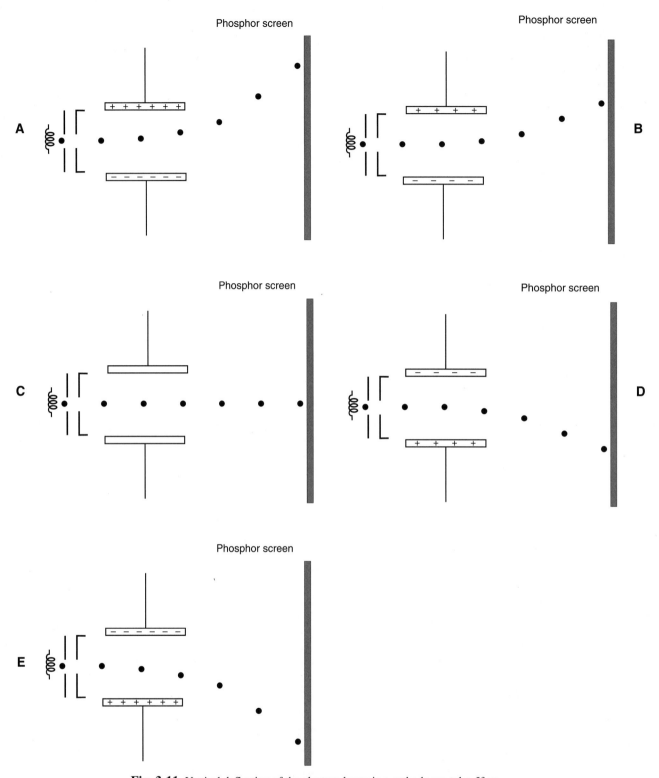

Fig. 3-11 Vertical deflection of the electron beam in a cathode ray tube. If no voltage is applied to the deflection plates, the electrons travel in a straight-line path, **C.** A voltage applied to the deflection plates alters the electron path, **A, B.** Reversing the polarity deflects the beam in the opposite direction, **D, E.** In this sequence of voltage changes to the deflection plates, five bright dots are formed along the vertical. Horizontal deflection plates (not shown) move the electron beam in and out of the page.

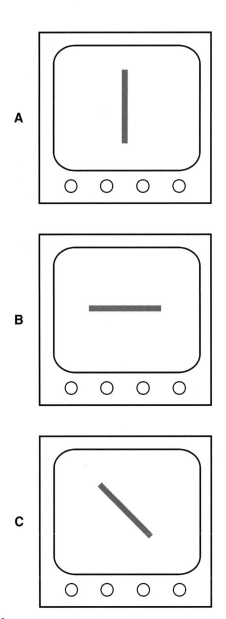

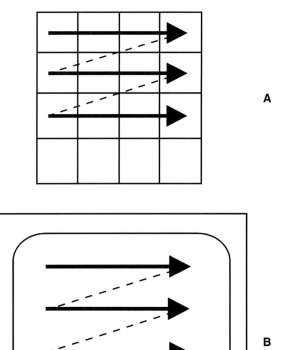

Fig. 3-13 Raster scanning. Readout of the image matrix follows a row-by-row sequence (**A**). The electron beam in the cathode ray tube is scanned across the screen in a row-by-row sequence (**B**).

Fig. 3-12 Trace of the electron beam on a cathode ray tube screen. A linear voltage applied to the vertical deflection plates moves the beam continuously upward or downward (**A**); applied to the horizontal plates moves it horizontally (**B**); and applied to both pair of plates simultaneously moves it diagonally (**C**).

Each pixel in a row of the image matrix is read sequentially left to right to form one **raster line.** After the readout for one row is completed, the pixels in the next row are then read sequentially to form another raster line. This row-by-row readout sequence continues such that a raster line is formed for each row in the image matrix. The electron beam scanning in the CRT is synchronized with the image matrix readout. That is, data obtained for a raster line in the image matrix are shown as one raster line across the screen.

In raster scanning the horizontal deflection plate voltage is changed to sweep the electron beam horizontally from left to right across the screen. The voltage to the vertical deflection plate is changed to drop the trace down one line

as the electron beam is positioned back to the left side of the display to begin the next raster line whereby the horizontal plate voltage is swept (Fig. 3-13). To avoid spurious signals, the electron beam is actually turned off during the vertical retrace. This is similar to reading a book, in which you start at the top left-hand corner and move across to the end of the line before dropping down one line to return to the left-hand side, where a new line is read.

The output, in the form of an electron beam current resulting from raster scanning of the image matrix, is connected to the cathode of the monitor and is synchronized with the raster scan of the monitor to produce the observed image (Fig. 3-14); that is, the brightness of light on the screen is dictated by the level of the input signal, and the position is governed by the raster scanning sequence. Because raster scanning of the image matrix and raster scanning of the screen are synchronized, the signal level in the image matrix—and therefore the echo measurements—is converted into a visual image.

Electronic raster scanning, invented by Philo Farnsworth in 1927, became the basis for the television industry.

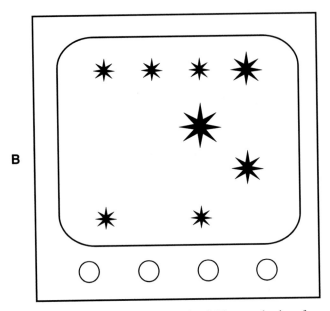

A

B

Fig. 3-14 Modulation of brightness level. The stored value of signal level at each pixel location in the image matrix (**A**) determines the brightness level for the corresponding region in the displayed image (**B**).

The screen phosphor continues to emit light for a short time after the electron beam is turned off. The decay rate of the light emission depends on the type of phosphor used. But the display of an image requires repeated raster scanning of the electron beam across the phosphor screen. The refresh rate for computer monitors is 60 to 120 times each second.

Monitor

The screen is divided into pixels similar to the matrix that holds image information. The light level or color for each screen pixel is individually controlled. Computer monitors do not comply with the information rate transfer restrictions imposed by broadcast standards. This enables an increased number of pixels in both dimensions and higher frame rates than available using a commercial TV video signal. The extended graphics array (XGA) has 1024 × 768 pixels. Other formats, which have increased resolution, are common (Table 3-4).

■ **Table 3-4** Monitor Formats

Graphics	Pixels
XGA	1024 × 768
SXGA	1280 × 1024
SXGA+	1400 × 1050
UXGA	1600 × 1200

Television Video Signal

The information obtained by raster scanning of the image matrix is assembled in a standard format called the TV **video signal**. The frame rate and number of lines that compose a frame depend on the national television industry (30 frames per second and 525 lines in the United States designated as NTSC, 25 frames per second and 625 lines in Europe designated as PAL). Odd-numbered raster lines are traced first followed by the even-numbered lines. The two sets of tracings (called fields) are interlaced to form one frame (interlaced raster scanning). The interlacing of fields doubles the refresh rate (60 fields per second) and allows flicker-free viewing, though with some sacrifice of spatial resolution. Synchronization voltage pulses are added during readout to mark horizontal (new line) and vertical (new field) positioning. This enables the displayed raster scanning on the screen to be synchronized with the readout raster scanning of the image matrix. The communication of image data between ultrasound scanner and system component (display monitor, VCR, and printer) is often accomplished by a video signal.

By repeating the raster scan of the unchanging image matrix 30 times per second, the displayed image on the monitor is continuously refreshed but appears stationary to the human eye; thus prolonged viewing of the image is now possible. If the image matrix is updated with new information (scan data) at a rate of several times per second, then the video display can show the dynamics of the acquired data.

SUMMARY

Computer technology with respect to capability, speed, and reduced cost is developing at an extremely rapid rate. For these reasons ultrasound instruments increasingly rely on digital components. Knowledge of computer fundamentals is essential for understanding the operation of present-day ultrasound scanners. The concepts of binary notation, memory capacity, analog-to-digital conversion, matrix format, image display, and storage devices were discussed. The conversion of an analog signal to the digital format often incurs a loss in accuracy. This is an inherent limitation with digital techniques, although pixel size is made relatively small so that image quality is not affected by the analog-to-digital conversion.

REVIEW QUESTIONS

1. A binary digit is called a _____.
2. Express the decimal number 14 as a binary number.
3. Express the decimal number 6 as a binary number.
4. Express the binary number 10010 as a decimal number.
5. How many locations are available in 128 MB memory?
6. Random access memory (RAM) is accessed directly, by location via a specific _____.
7. How many bits are in one byte?
8. In analog-to-digital conversion, accuracy of the digitization of the echo amplitude is improved by increasing the _____.
9. If a word contains 5 bits, what is the maximum numerical value that can be represented by this word? Assume 0 to be the lowest number represented.
10. A _____ is a small square picture element in the matrix that denotes the intensity of the reflected echo generated at an interface within the area being scanned.
11. How many pixels are used to compose an image that is displayed in a matrix 256 × 256?
12. The advantage of a 256 × 256 matrix format compared with a 64 × 64 matrix format is that greater _____ is possible.
13. Name the type of memory that can be read, but the contents cannot be changed.
14. The term _____ in conjunction with disk storage refers to a collection of words transferred in a group.
15. What are some advantages of CD storage of data?

BIBLIOGRAPHY

Bushberg JT, Siebert JA, Leidholdt Jr EM, Boone JM: *The essential physics of medical imaging,* ed 2, Baltimore, 2002, Lippincott Williams & Wilkins.

Enlander D: *Computers in medicine: an introduction,* St Louis, 1980, Mosby.

Gates SC, Becker J: *Laboratory automation using the IBM PC,* Englewood Cliffs, NJ, 1989, Prentice Hall.

Hedrick WR, Hykes DL: Computer fundamentals in diagnostic ultrasound imaging, *J Diagn Med Sonogr* 5:293, 1989.

Hunter TB: *The computer in radiology,* Rockville, Md, 1986, Aspen Systems Corporation.

Kuni CC: *Introduction to computers and digital processing in medical imaging,* Chicago, 1988, Year Book Medical Publishers.

CHAPTER 4

Single-Element Transducers: Properties

KEY TERMS

Bandwidth	Pulse repetition frequency
Duty factor (DF)	(PRF)
Fractional bandwidth	Pulse repetition period (PRP)
Matching layer	Q-value
Piezoelectric effect	Sensitivity
Pulse duration (PD)	Spatial pulse length (SPL)

Many factors have contributed to the dramatic increase in the clinical applications of medical diagnostic ultrasound: a better understanding of the design criteria for transducers; the miniaturization of electronics; the formation of computer-based signal processing; the creation of flexible microprocessor-driven instrumentation; and a lack of demonstrated adverse biologic effects. Understanding the properties of the single-element transducer discussed in this chapter is a prerequisite for understanding modifications in transducer design that are discussed in the following chapters.

The information obtained from ultrasound scanning depends in large part on the beam characteristics, which in turn are governed by transducer design. Numerous parameters are used to describe transducer performance. Physical descriptors and the corresponding symbols introduced in this chapter are listed in Table 4-1.

GENERAL REQUIREMENTS

There are three requirements for diagnostic medical ultrasound: generation of an ultrasound beam, reception of the returning echo, and processing of the signal for display. Design changes in the reception and in the processing, analysis, and display of returning echo signals differentiate one scanning mode from another. A transducer is any device that transforms one kind of energy into another (e.g., mechanical to electrical). The ultrasound transducer must convert an electrical signal into the ultrasound beam, which

Table 4-1 Physical Descriptors and Symbols

Parameter	Symbol
Bandwidth	Δf
Center frequency	f_c
Duty factor	DF
Maximum pulse repetition frequency	PRF_{max}
Number of cycles	n
Pulse duration	PD
Pulse repetition frequency	PRF
Pulse repetition period	PRP
Radiofrequency	RF
Range of scanning	R
Spatial pulse length	SPL
Mechanical coefficient	Q-value

is transmitted into the patient's body, and then convert the returning echo into an electrical signal for processing and display. The first type of transducer, which is still in use today, employed a single-element circular disk to both transmit and receive ultrasound.

FREQUENCY DETERMINATION

The first requirement of an ultrasonic scanner is that a sound wave at ultrasonic frequencies (greater than 20 kHz) be generated. The primary objectives are to produce a unidirectional beam (analogous to a flashlight beam versus a porch light) that is of uniform intensity and limited physical dimensions so that good spatial resolution is obtained. As a practical matter, the spatial variation of beam intensity can be manipulated but cannot be completely eliminated so as to produce perfect uniformity. For positional information using the echo-ranging principle, a short burst is required, and thus the sound beam must be turned on and off rapidly.

Spatial Resolution and Frequency

In echo detection, reflected mechanical vibrations from an interface are recorded. The time is measured for short pulses (which may be a single vibration) to travel from the point of sound origin to the object and back to the receiver. For example, if a Chinese gong were allowed to move only once after being struck and then were cushioned with a pillow to shorten the duration of the vibration, a single-cycle sound wave would be produced that would move out to some distant object and return toward the listener. In such circumstances, when we are listening as sound waves come back from the environment, we are actually hearing an integral number of vibrations (10 or 15 or 50) return as echoes. Since the position of any object in space can be determined only to an accuracy of about one wavelength (or a quarter wavelength if special equipment capable of measuring high-pressure or low-pressure points is used), this limitation on resolvability is imposed by wavelength. The ability to distinguish two objects separated by a small distance along the direction or propagation is called axial resolution or range resolution or depth resolution. Because frequency and wavelength are inversely related, shorter wavelengths, which produce finer resolution, correspond to higher frequencies. The question then becomes: What frequencies are needed to produce the resolution required in diagnostic ultrasound?

Wavelength of Sound Sources

The human ear can detect sound waves from approximately 20 Hz to 20 kHz. Assume that the smallest objects resolvable are one wavelength in size. A 20 Hz sound source produces a sound wave with a 77-meter (m) wavelength in tissue (the velocity of sound in tissue is 1540 m/s):

$$c = f\lambda$$
$$\lambda = \frac{c}{f}$$

$$\lambda = \frac{1540 \text{ m/s}}{20 \text{ 1/s}}$$
$$\lambda = 77 \text{ m}$$

This may be suitable for detection of aircraft carriers or submarines, but it is not appropriate for the fine resolution needed in medical diagnostic ultrasound.

In nature, bats and certain other animals (porpoises, moles, and some grasshoppers) generate ultrasound waves having frequencies of around 100 kHz. In medicine, if we had to rely on bats as a source of ultrasound, we would first need a device to contain them and then a supply of bugs to activate (or stimulate) them; then, each time a signal was needed, a new bug would be released, and the bat (if it were hungry) would generate an ultrasound wave to locate it (Fig. 4-1). Aside from the impracticality of this arrangement, there would be another problem: With a frequency of 100 kHz, the wavelength produced is 1.54 cm, which is much too long for the accurate location of small objects.

$$\lambda = \frac{c}{f}$$
$$\lambda = \frac{1540 \text{ m/s}}{100 \times 10^3 \text{ 1/s}}$$
$$\lambda = 0.0154 \text{ m} = 1.54 \text{ cm}$$

Although suitable for locating bugs and other objects in the dark, it would not be adequate for medical diagnostic ultrasound, in which objects with dimensions on the order of 1 mm (1/1000 m) or less often need to be identified.

Frequency Requirement

If one wavelength is a good approximation of the smallest detectable object, what frequency is required for a resolution of 1 mm in tissue? Using the relationship $c = f\lambda$ and solving for the frequency, we find that

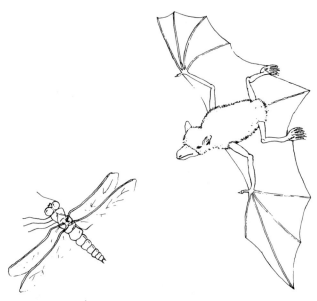

Fig. 4-1 Transducer using bat power.

$$f = \frac{c}{\lambda}$$

$$\lambda = \frac{1540 \text{ m/s}}{0.001 \text{ 1/s}}$$

$$f = 1.54 \times 10^6 \text{ 1/s} = 1.54 \text{ MHz}$$

For medical diagnostic ultrasound it is evident that megahertz frequencies are necessary.

PIEZOELECTRIC PROPERTIES

Dipole Alignment

Nothing in nature can be readily adapted to transmit ultrasonic energy in the megahertz frequency range. Consequently, the transducer must be manufactured. The construction of a high frequency transducer relies on a phenomenon first studied by Pierre Curie and his brother in the 1880s and known as the **piezoelectric (pressure electric) effect.** This effect is commonly found in crystalline materials that have dipoles (regions of positive and negative charge) on each molecule. Dipolar molecules are positive at one end and negative at the other. In the normal crystalline lattice structure these randomly arranged dipoles cannot migrate (Fig. 4-2). If the material is heated above a temperature called the Curie temperature, however, the molecules are released and can change orientation. When a pair of charged plates (one positive and one negative) is placed across the material, the negative region of each molecule points toward the positive plate, and the positive region toward the negative plate (opposite charges attract, like charges repel). The positive and negative regions of the molecules do not align directly with the electrical field produced by the plates because of thermal motion. If the material is then cooled below the Curie temperature while the charged plates are still applied, the molecules will maintain their orientations (Fig. 4-3). *Ultrasound transducers should not be autoclaved, because this destroys the piezoelectric properties of the material by raising its temperature above the Curie temperature and returning the dipoles to their random arrangement.*

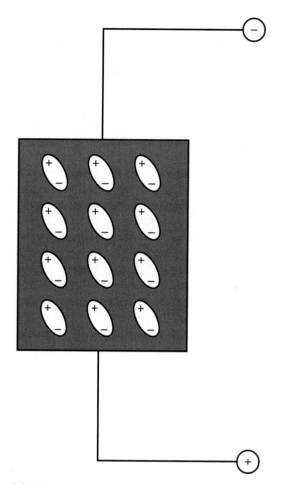

Fig. 4-3 Alignment of dipoles by applying an external electrical field during heating of the crystalline material.

Once the material is cooled below the Curie temperature, the charged plates used for alignment are removed without altering the configuration of the dipoles. The molecular arrangement of the dipolar molecules gives piezoelectric materials their unique properties. Conducting plates are placed on the opposite faces of the crystal adjacent to where the alignment electrodes were positioned (Fig. 4-4). When a voltage is applied to the conducting plates, the molecules twist to align themselves with the electrical field (positive molecules toward the negative electrode, negative molecules toward the positive electrode), thereby thickening the crystal (Fig. 4-5). If the plates are reversed in polarity, the molecules will twist back in the opposite direction, creating a decrease in the crystal thickness. The actual movement is only a few microns (10^{-6} m), although in Fig. 4-5 this change in thickness has been exaggerated for clarity. The flipping back and forth of the polarity causes expansion and contraction of the crystal, which creates mechanical vibrations. When the expanding and contracting crystal is placed on the body, sound waves (mechanical vibrations or pressure waves) are passed into the body. Thus a voltage applied across the piezoelectric material creates mechanical motion (sound waves). In the crystal this phenomenon (the converse piezoelectric effect) allows an ultrasound beam to be generated by the transducer.

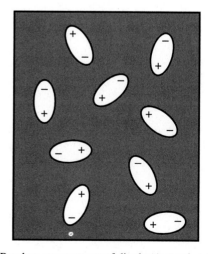

Fig. 4-2 Random arrangement of dipoles (natural state).

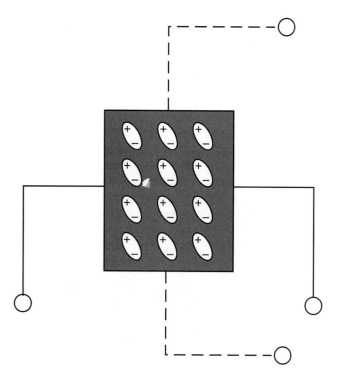

Fig. 4-4 Placement of excitation electrodes *(solid lines)* following removal of the alignment electrodes *(dashed lines).*

Alternatively, the piezoelectric effect enables the same transducer to receive an ultrasonic echo (high-frequency pressure wave). Ultrasound waves returning from interactions with interfaces in the body strike the crystal and induce electrical signals. These are processed and ultimately displayed.

Natural Vibrational Frequency

If left alone, the transducer would ring in a manner similar to a tuning fork. Note that if a tuning fork is to ring at 2000 Hz, it does not have to be struck 2000 times each second to maintain the sound (although this is a possibility, particularly for continuous wave generation). Instead, a natural vibrational frequency occurs in which the wave is transmitted back and forth (from prong to prong) at a set frequency that depends on wave interference. If a crystal suspended in air is struck with a voltage pulse, ultrasound waves are generated. Multiple wavefronts are formed: forward from the front face, backward into the crystal from the front face, into the crystal from the back face, and away from the crystal at the back face. These waves undergo constructive and destructive interference within the crystal, depending on the crystal thickness. The ultrasound moves from one face of the crystal to the other, undergoing reflection between the two crystalline surfaces. The crystal has a natural vibrational frequency (just as the tuning fork does) that is related to the distance between those two surfaces. To have constructive interference so a single wave moves back and forth across the crystal, the distance from one surface to the other must be equal to half the chosen wavelength (Fig. 4-6) so as to produce thickness mode resonance. These

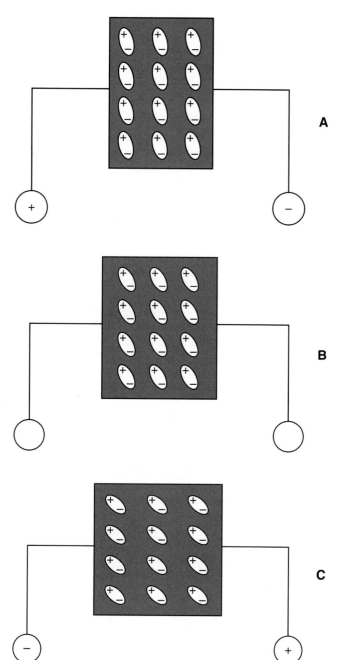

Fig. 4-5 Crystal response to voltage applied across the excitation electrodes. **A,** Contraction of the crystal caused by movement of the dipoles trying to align with an applied electrical field. **B,** Normal thickness with no applied electrical field. **C,** Expansion of the crystal caused by movement of the dipoles trying to align with an applied electrical field. The polarity is reversed from that depicted in **A.**

crystals are extremely thin. The center frequency is dictated by the crystal thickness (where crystal thickness equals $1/2\lambda$).

■ Example 4-1

What thickness of piezoelectric material is required to produce an ultrasound wave with a frequency of 1.5 MHz? (The velocity of sound in the piezoelectric material is 4350 m/s.)

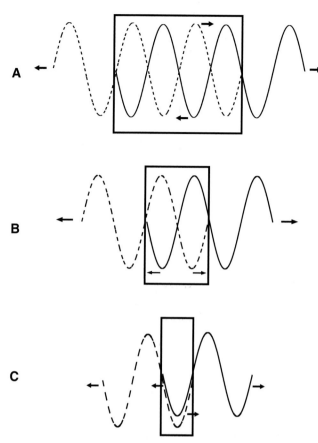

Fig. 4-6 Determination of crystal thickness using superimposition of waves. Waves generated at the back of the crystal *(dashed line)*. Waves generated from the front of the crystal *(solid line)*. Arrows indicate the direction of wave motion. **A,** Crystal thickness greater than one wavelength produces destructive interference if the thickness is not an odd-integer multiple of one half wavelength. **B,** Complete destructive interference occurs when the crystal thickness is equal to one wavelength. **C,** Complete constructive interference occurs when the crystal thickness is equal to one half wavelength or odd multiples of a half wavelength.

$$\lambda = \frac{c}{f}$$

$$\lambda = \frac{4350 \text{ m/s}}{1.5 \times 10^6 \text{ 1/s}}$$

$$\lambda = 2.9 \times 10^{-3} \text{ m} = 2.9 \text{ mm}$$

$$\text{Crystal thickness} = \frac{\lambda}{2} = 1.45 \text{ mm}$$

Note that the 1.5 MHz transducer produces an ultrasound beam having a wavelength of 1 mm in tissue.

$$\lambda = \frac{c}{f}$$

$$\lambda = \frac{1540 \text{ m/s}}{1.5 \times 10^6 \text{ 1/s}}$$

$$\lambda = 1 \times 10^{-3} \text{ m} = 1 \text{ mm}$$

Frequency does not change when the ultrasound wave enters one medium from another. The difference in wavelength between the crystal and the tissue arises from velocity differences in the two media (1540 m/s for tissue and ≈4000

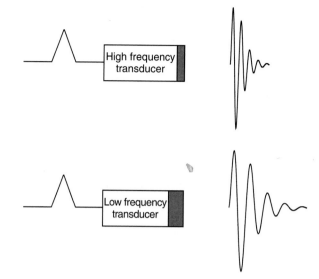

Fig. 4-7 Natural resonance frequency is controlled by crystal thickness.

m/s for the crystal). A transducer should never be dropped, because the thin crystal cracks easily.

Piezoelectric Materials

To change the frequency of a transducer often requires changing the transducer itself (with some exceptions for broadband transducers, discussed in Chapter 9). A higher-frequency transducer that produces a shorter wavelength has a thinner crystal (Fig. 4-7). For diagnostic medical applications the material almost universally used in transducers is lead zirconate titanate (PZT). PZT represents a family of piezoelectric ceramics with various additives that change the properties to match a particular application. PZT-5 is used in medical transducers, because it has the desirable properties of high electromechanical coupling coefficient, high dielectric constant, and ability to be molded in a particular size and shape. Barium lead titanate, barium lead zirconate, lead metaniobate, and lithium sulfate have also been used. Crystals of polyvinylidene fluoride have been developed with an acoustic impedance closer to that of tissue; thus the acoustic impedance mismatch at the crystal-tissue interface is less, and a higher fraction of ultrasonic energy enters the body. This material is also easy to shape. However, the low electromechanical coupling coefficient of 0.1 to 0.2 results in low sensitivity. Forming copolymers of polyvinylidene fluoride with trifluoroethylene can increase the electromechanical coupling coefficient, but this piezoelectric material is brittle and difficult to shape.

Quartz is a naturally occurring substance that can be made to have piezoelectric properties. It was the material studied by the Curies. Quartz is used in therapeutic ultrasound transducers because of its excellent transmission properties.

TRANSDUCER CONSTRUCTION

The major component of a transducer is a crystal of piezoelectric material with electrodes on opposite sides of it that create the changing polarity. The electrodes are formed by plating a thin film of gold or silver on the crystal surface. To improve the transfer of energy to and from the patient, the matching layer is located next to one of the electrodes. Crystal ringing is diminished by the introduction of the backing material that adjoins the surface electrode most distant from the point of patient contact. The entire crystal assembly, including the electrodes, matching layer, and backing material, is housed in an electrically insulating casing (usually some type of plastic). This casing also provides structural support. An acoustic insulator, made of rubber or cork, prevents the transmission of ultrasound energy into the casing. Fig. 4-8 is a cross-sectional view of a transducer.

Radiofrequency Shielding

The transducer is sensitive to electromagnetic interference, which contributes to the noise level (i.e., signals that do not correspond to physical interactions of sound waves with tissue). High noise levels prohibit the detection of weak echoes. To reduce the electromagnetic interference, a radiofrequency shield composed of a hollow metallic cylinder is placed around the crystal and backing material and electronically grounded to the front electrode surface. The acoustic insulating layer coats the inner surface of the radiofrequency shield to prevent reverberations.

Backing Material

The backing material depends on whether the transducer is designed for therapeutic purposes or diagnostic imaging. For ultrasonic therapy the objective is to deliver the maximum amount of energy in the form of heat (caused by absorption of the ultrasound) to the patient. This is achieved by a continuous output of ultrasound waves from the transducer (Fig. 4-9). Maximum output results if natural ringing (resonance) occurs in the crystal, in which case the backing material should have an acoustic impedance different from that of the crystal. Maximum reflection at the backing material–crystal interface causes the crystal to ring. Air is commonly employed as the backing material for therapy transducers. Alternatively, the crystal may be driven by an alternating voltage source of the correct frequency to induce continuous wave output. This is the typical method used for therapeutic continuous wave ultrasound transducers; this method also has applications in Doppler scanning. A crystal-producing continuous wave output cannot act as a receiver for reflected ultrasound waves.

For imaging, the transducer sends out a short burst of ultrasound (preferably one cycle, but usually two to five cycles) followed by a period of silence to listen for returning echoes (receiving mode) before another burst is generated. This is called a pulsed wave system (Fig. 4-10), and the design is based on the echo-ranging principle discussed at the end of Chapter 1.

Ideally the backing material should absorb all the energy, except for one cycle of sound produced from the front face of the transducer. *For maximum transfer of energy to occur (from crystal to backing material), the backing material must have an acoustic impedance identical to that of the crystal.* Also, the backing material should have a high absorption coefficient to prevent ultrasonic energy from reentering the crystal. An epoxy resin and tungsten powder combination is used for the backing material in diagnostic transducers to damp (shorten) the ultrasonic pulse. The rear surface of the backing material is slanted to prevent reflection of sound energy into the crystal. The **sensitivity** (ability to detect weakly reflecting interfaces) of the transducer decreases with slow damping (long pulse), because ringing lowers the instantaneous intensity of the output ultrasound wave from the transducer.

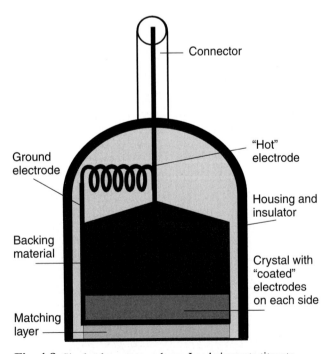

Fig. 4-8 Single-element transducer. Lead zirconate titanate (PZT) crystal, electrodes, matching layer, backing material, and acoustic insulator are shown.

Connector

"Hot" electrode

Ground electrode

Housing and insulator

Backing material

Crystal with "coated" electrodes on each side

Matching layer

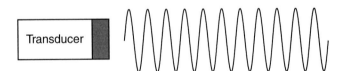

Fig. 4-9 Continuous wave output, which is used for therapeutic systems and continuous wave Doppler.

Transducer

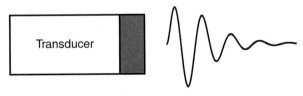

Fig. 4-10 Pulsed wave output, which is used for any scanning technique that requires depth information.

Transducer

Dynamic Damping

Dynamic damping is an electronic means to suppress ringing. A voltage pulse of opposite polarity is applied to the crystal immediately following the excitation pulse. This counteracts the expansion and contraction of the crystal stimulated by the first pulse, and ringing is inhibited.

Matching Layer

The acoustic impedance mismatch between the piezoelectric crystal and the patient causes the generated ultrasonic energy to be largely reflected at this interface. This creates a long pulse and reduces the beam intensity that enters the patient. Both effects are undesirable for imaging. *In order to shorten the pulse and improve energy transfer across the crystal-tissue interface, a material with intermediate acoustic impedance is placed between the crystal and the patient.* This material, called the **matching layer,** is mounted in the transducer on the exit side of the crystal. However, the matching layer must have low-loss properties since high attenuation would counteract the desired effect of high transmission.

PULSED WAVE OUTPUT

In echo-ranging systems the transducer must pause after transmitting the sound wave to "listen" for the returning echoes. Because the crystal cannot send and receive simultaneously, it must be pulsed for transmission after an appropriate listening time has elapsed (Fig. 4-11). The master synchronizer sends an electronic signal to a pulser or transmitter to initiate the process. The start command is, in turn, relayed to the transducer to generate a short burst

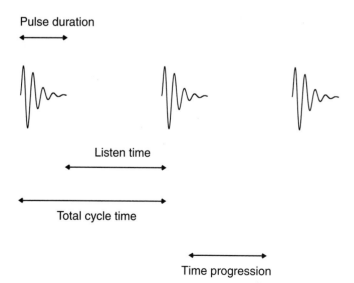

Fig. 4-11 Temporal representation of pulsed wave output. The time-dependent output from a transducer alternates between actively generating a five-cycle pulse of short duration and a longer time interval of no transmission, which allows reception of returning echoes.

of ultrasound. There are three methods by which the transmitter can work.

In the first the output from a sine-wave generator is gated to apply a rapidly alternating voltage to the crystal. If the gate is switched on for a long period, a continuous wave is produced. If it is switched on for a short period, a short pulse is created.

The second transmitter pulsing method is called shock excitation. A charged capacitor (a device that stores electrical charge) is discharged through the piezoelectric crystal, which is stimulated to vibrate at the resonance frequency as previously discussed. The capacitor is recharged while the crystal is waiting for returning echoes. The discharge time of the capacitor, in conjunction with the crystal damping and frequency, determines the pulse length (related to the number of cycles in the pulse burst). The recharge time is set to coincide with the listening time.

The excitation waveform for most modern instruments is a short, square wave burst consisting of one to three cycles with a radiowave frequency equal to the desired center frequency. The driving frequency must be within the frequency operating range of the transducer (bandwidth).

PULSE REPETITION FREQUENCY

The number of times the crystal is pulsed or electrically stimulated per second is called the **pulse repetition frequency (PRF).** Because a transducer cannot send and receive ultrasound at the same time, a limit exists with respect to the rate at which it can be pulsed. The maximum pulse repetition frequency (PRF_{max}) is limited by the maximum depth (R) to be sampled and by the velocity of ultrasound (c) in the medium, as shown in the following equation:

4-1

$$PRF_{max} = \frac{c}{2R}$$

The factor *2* accounts for the total distance traveled to the interface and back to the transducer, which is twice the scanning depth. The time (t) necessary for the wave to travel to depth R is given as

4-2

$$R = ct$$

The maximum PRF is then inversely proportional to the time of travel:

4-3

$$PRF_{max} = \frac{c}{2\,ct} = \frac{1}{2t}$$

The factor *2t* represents the down-and-back time. Because of wave transit time to the reflector and back, 13 μs (13×10^{-6} s) are required to detect an interface in tissue for each centimeter of depth that the interface is away from the face of the transducer. Thus if the maximum depth of interest in tissue is known, the transit time allows calculation of the maximum PRF from

$$\text{PRF}_{\text{max}} = \frac{1}{13 \times 10^{-6} \text{ s/cm R(cm)}}$$

4-4

Note: This equation is valid for tissue only. Equation 4-1 is valid for any medium.

Equation 4-1 illustrates that the PRF_{max} can be increased if the velocity in the medium is increased. Typically, the velocity of ultrasound in the medium does not change (being nearly constant for all types of tissue), and velocity is not adjustable by the sonographer. Equation 4-1 also indicates that the PRF_{max} can be increased if the depth of interest is decreased. Depth is the only potential parameter capable of being changed by the operator. In designing their systems, however, manufacturers often vary the PRF with the depth. The PRF set by the manufacturer is normally not a selectable parameter by the operator. These concepts are illustrated by the following three examples.

◼ **Example 4-2**

Assume that the maximum depth of interest in tissue is 10 cm. What is the maximum PRF? Express the answer using three significant figures.

$$\text{PRF}_{\text{max}} = \frac{c}{2R}$$

$$\text{PRF}_{\text{max}} = \frac{1540 \text{ m/s}}{2(0.1 \text{ m})}$$

$$\text{PRF}_{\text{max}} = 7700 \text{ 1/s}$$

or

$$\text{PRF}_{\text{max}} = \frac{1}{13 \times 10^{-6} \text{ s/cm R(cm)}}$$

$$\text{PRF}_{\text{max}} = \frac{1}{(13 \times 10^{-6} \text{ s/cm}) (10 \text{ cm})}$$

$$\text{PRF}_{\text{max}} = 7690 \text{ 1/s}$$

Note the difference in the two answers. This discrepancy occurs because the travel time is rounded off to 13 μs per centimeter (actual time, 12.987 μs) in Equation 4-4.

◼ **Example 4-3**

Assume that the maximum depth of interest in tissue is increased to 20 cm. What is the maximum PRF? Express the answer using three significant figures.

$$\text{PRF}_{\text{max}} = \frac{c}{2R}$$

$$\text{PRF}_{\text{max}} = \frac{1540 \text{ m/s}}{2(0.2 \text{ m})}$$

$$\text{PRF}_{\text{max}} = 3850 \text{ 1/s}$$

or

$$\text{PRF}_{\text{max}} = \frac{1}{13 \times 10^{-6} \text{ s/cm R(cm)}}$$

$$\text{PRF}_{\text{max}} = \frac{1}{(13 \times 10^{-6} \text{ s/cm}) (20 \text{ cm})}$$

$$\text{PRF}_{\text{max}} = 3850 \text{ 1/s}$$

For deep-lying structures to be visualized, the PRF_{max} is reduced.

◼ **Example 4-4**

Suppose that bone replaces tissue. What is the maximum PRF allowed to sample a depth of 10 cm? Express the answer using three significant figures.

$$\text{PRF}_{\text{max}} = \frac{c}{2R}$$

$$\text{PRF}_{\text{max}} = \frac{4080 \text{ m/s}}{2(0.1 \text{ m})}$$

$$\text{PRF}_{\text{max}} = 20,400 \text{ 1/s}$$

A high velocity enables the PRF_{max} to be increased dramatically. However, in this case attenuation of the ultrasound wave makes sampling impossible.

Pulse repetition frequencies range from 200 to 2000 per second for typical A-mode and static B-mode transducers. Higher PRFs (ranging from 1000 1/s to 12,000 1/s, but typically a few thousand pulses per second) are used for real-time and Doppler units. The PRF is often expressed in units of Hz or kHz (corresponding to one pulse per second or 1000 pulses per second). For example, a PRF of 5000 1/s is also described as 5000 Hz or 5 kHz.

PULSE REPETITION PERIOD

The time required to transmit a pulsed ultrasound wave plus the time devoted to listening for the returning echoes from that wave is called the **pulse repetition period (PRP).** It is equal to the reciprocal of the pulse repetition frequency:

4-5

$$\text{PRP} = \frac{1}{\text{PRF}}$$

or

$$\text{PRF} = \frac{1}{\text{PRP}}$$

◼ **Example 4-5**

What is the PRF if a pulsed sound wave is emitted every 500 μs? The time between pulses is given as 500 μs, which is equal to the PRP. Using Equation 4-5

$$\text{PRF} = \frac{1}{\text{PRP}}$$

$$\text{PRF} = \frac{1}{500 \times 10^{-6} \text{ s}}$$

$$\text{PRF} = 2000 \text{ 1/s}$$

◼ **Example 4-6**

What is the PRP if the PRF is 1 kHz?
Using Equation 4-5 and substituting a value of 1000 pulses per second for the PRF

$$\text{PRP} = \frac{1}{\text{PRF}}$$

$$\text{PRP} = \frac{1}{1000 \text{ 1/s}}$$

$$\text{PRP} = 0.001 \text{ s}$$

SPATIAL PULSE LENGTH

Ideally, for each pulse, a short packet of ultrasound energy of the appropriate frequency (i.e., 3.5 MHz for a 3.5 MHz transducer) is directed into the body. In practice, the pulse is composed of a range of different frequencies encompassing the labeled operating frequency. The operating frequency is also called the center frequency, which represents the midpoint of the frequency distribution. The length of this short-duration pulse can be estimated and is called the **spatial pulse length (SPL).** It is calculated from the wavelength (λ) associated with the center frequency and the number of cycles (n) in the pulse:

4-6
$$SPL = n \lambda$$

Assume that a transducer with a center frequency of 3 MHz produces a pulse that is three cycles in duration. The wavelength is determined from Equation 1-6:

$$\lambda = \frac{1.54 \text{ mm}}{3 \text{ (MHz)}}$$
$$\lambda = 0.513 \text{ mm}$$

With number of cycles in the pulse equal to 3, the SPL is calculated to be

$$SPL = n \lambda = (0.513 \text{ mm})(3) = 1.54 \text{ mm}$$

The SPL influences a scanner's effectiveness at depicting spatial detail. Axial resolution is the ability to distinguish as separate images two objects that are close to each other along the direction of propagation. To improve axial resolution, a pulse of short duration is desirable. To shorten the pulse spatially, the number of cycles must be reduced (Fig. 4-12), or the frequency must be increased to decrease wavelength (see Fig. 4-7). Often the pulsed wave is two to five cycles in duration.

Pulse Duration

The **pulse duration (PD),** or temporal pulse length, is the time interval for one complete pulse. It describes the actual time that the transducer is generating the ultrasonic pulse. A more formal definition is the elapsed time from initiation of the pulse to a point 20 dB below the maximum peak-to-peak pressure amplitude of the wave (Fig. 4-13). An alternative definition is the number of half cycles in which the peak amplitude is greater than 25% of the maximum peak amplitude in the pulse (6 dB). The effectiveness of the matching layer to transmit the energy into tissue and the ability of the backing material to quickly dampen the pulse are indicated by the pulse duration.

The axial resolution, and thus the ability to visualize superficial structures, depends on the pulse duration, which determines the spatial pulse length. The PD is calculated from the number of cycles in the pulse (n) and the period (τ) of the wave:

4-7
$$PD = n\tau$$

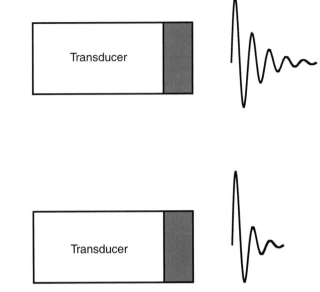

Fig. 4-12 For the same center frequency a three-cycle pulse has shorter duration than a five-cycle pulse.

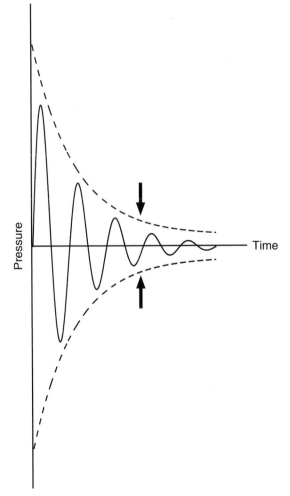

Fig. 4-13 Pulse duration or temporal pulse length. Because of damping and mechanical friction, the peak pressure amplitude decreases with time after the crystal is excited. The pulse duration is determined by the cutoff point *(arrows)* defined at 20 dB below the maximum pressure amplitude.

Consider, once more, a three-cycle pulse (at −20 dB) from a 3 MHz transducer. The following analysis can be made:

$$\tau = \frac{1}{f}$$

$$\tau = \frac{1}{3 \times 10^6 \ 1/s}$$

$$\tau = 3.3 \times 10^{-7} \ s$$

$$PD = 3 \ (3.3 \times 10^{-7} \ s)$$

$$PD = 9.9 \times 10^{-7} \ s \cong 1 \times 10^{-6} \cong 1 \ \mu s$$

The SPL varies directly with the pulse duration, the constant of proportionality being equal to the velocity in the medium:

$$SPL = (c)(PD) \qquad \textbf{4-8}$$

Given a pulse duration of 1×10^{-6} s and a velocity of 1540 m/s,

$$SPL = (1540 \ m/s)(1 \times 10^{-6} \ s) = 1.54 \times 10^{-3} \ m = 1.54 \ mm$$

which is the same answer as obtained using Equation 4-6.

Duty Factor

A typical unit with a pulse duration of 1 μs and a PRF of 1 kHz is transmitting only 0.1% of the time. By far, most of its time (99.9%) is spent in a receive mode. The **duty factor (DF)** is the fraction of time the unit is active and is calculated by obtaining the ratio of the pulse duration and the pulse repetition period:

$$DF = \frac{PD}{PRP} \qquad \textbf{4-9}$$

Both the PD and the PRP are expressed in units of time (either seconds or microseconds), but the DF has no units. It is merely the ratio of time that the pulse is on to the time between transmitted pulses. Recall that the pulse repetition period is equal to the reciprocal of the pulse repetition frequency, and thus Equation 4-9 can be expressed in the form

$$DF = (PD)(PRF) \qquad \textbf{4-10}$$

DF is important in determining some intensity parameters used to quantitate the dose response for various biologic effects.

■ Example 4-7

Calculate the DF for a 3 MHz transducer that produces three cycles per pulse. The PRF is 1500 per second.
  The pulse duration is 1 μs and the PRP 6.7×10^{-4} second (670 μs). From Equation 4-9

$$DF = \frac{PD}{PRP}$$

$$DF = \frac{1 \ \mu s}{670 \ \mu s}$$

$$DF = 0.0015$$

■ **Table 4-2** Descriptors of Transducer Performance

Transducer Factors	Function
Electromechanical coupling coefficient	Conversion from electrical energy to sound energy and vice versa
Transmission coefficient	Conversion from electrical energy to sound energy
Reception coefficient	Conversion from sound energy to electrical energy
Dielectric constant	Coupling with receiver
Acoustic impedance	Reflection at tissue interface
Mechanical coefficient (also called Q-value)	Bandwidth

TRANSDUCER FACTORS

Several parameters shown in Table 4-2 influence the overall performance of a transducer.

The electromechanical coupling coefficient describes how efficiently the transducer converts electrical stimuli from the transmitter into ultrasonic energy and converts received ultrasound energy into electrical signals. The transmission coefficient indicates the fraction of electrical energy that is converted into acoustic energy. The fraction of returning acoustic echo energy that is converted into electrical energy is given by the reception coefficient. The product of the transmission coefficient and the reception coefficient yields the electromechanical coupling coefficient.

High efficiency of energy conversion within the transducer is very desirable. This means that electrical energy used to stimulate the crystal should be radiated away as sound energy as rapidly and completely as possible, and on return the sound energy should be converted into electrical energy as rapidly and completely as possible. The result of a high electromechanical coupling coefficient is reduced oscillation time within the crystal, which allows generation of short duration pulsed waves and maximum signal amplitude on reception.

The mechanical and electrical properties of the transducer are partially characterized by the dielectric constant, which is also related to the transmission and reception coefficients. The dielectric constant describes the relative strain (movement) that the crystal undergoes when an electrical stress is applied to it and the induced voltage when it is strained. Two conditions are established to evaluate the dielectric constant: unrestricted movement and restricted (clamped) movement. This corresponds to the crystal in a free state and the crystal placed in a transducer assembly with backing and facing materials. A high dielectric constant is desirable during reception of low-megahertz frequencies, because it minimizes electronic noise from cabling and receiver amplifiers. In fact, a high dielectric constant may be more desirable than a high reception coefficient.

The acoustic impedance (Z_c) of the crystal, defined in Chapter 1 as the product of velocity times density, influences the energy transfer across the crystal-tissue interface. Matching the Z values of tissue and crystal enhances the transmission of ultrasound into the body. The mechanical coefficient (Q-value) characterizes the frequency response of the transducer. It is a major consideration when selecting a transducer for a particular application.

SENSITIVITY

Sensitivity, although not formally defined, describes the ability of an ultrasound system to distinguish low-reflectivity objects with nearly the same acoustic properties at specific locations in the medium. All the transducer factors mentioned previously influence it. Other considerations, in addition to the transducer factors, affect the overall sensitivity of an ultrasound system.

Conversion Efficiencies

Of all the transducer factors, conversion efficiencies (electrical energy to acoustic energy and vice versa) are most important in dictating the sensitivity of a transducer. To a first approximation, the product of the transmission coefficient and the reception coefficient gives transducer sensitivity. A transducer that converts 100% of the electrical energy into acoustic energy, but only 1% of the acoustic energy to electrical energy, uses 1% of the available energy. If the transmission coefficient and reception coefficient were both 0.25, then 6.25% ($0.25 \times 0.25 \times 100\%$) of the available energy would be used. The latter case permits detection of

weaker signals; a transducer with a high electromechanical coupling coefficient thus increases the sensitivity. PZT-5 has an electromechanical coupling coefficient of 0.5, which is a major determinant for the wide acceptance of this piezoelectric material for imaging.

Circuit Impedance

The electrical impedance matching of the transducer to the initiating pulser and to the receiver also affects the sensitivity. Electrical impedance mismatch at the pulser decreases the amount of electrical energy delivered to the transducer in the generator circuit, thereby creating a lower-intensity ultrasonic pulse. If there is an electrical impedance mismatch at the transducer-receiver, electrical energy is reflected into the transducer, and a smaller signal is available for processing. Again, the sensitivity of the system is reduced. The electrical impedance mismatch also causes deterioration in the axial resolution by creating a longer pulse length. Electrical impedance matching depends partially on the dielectric constant.

Backing Material

The damping characteristics (methods of reducing pulse length) of the transducer affect the sensitivity. They are partially controlled by the backing material placed next to the crystal in the transducer. In imaging systems the acoustic impedance of the backing material is made to equal the acoustic impedance of the crystal to obtain maximum transmission into the backing material and produce a short pulse (Fig. 4-14).

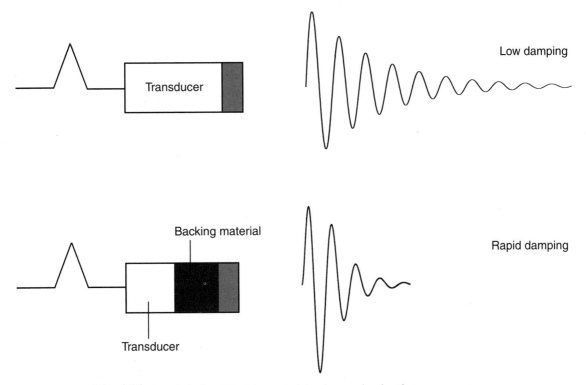

Fig. 4-14 A well-designed backing material reduces pulse duration.

Matching Layers

The acoustic impedance matching of the transducer to the object scanned is another important factor that affects sensitivity. As demonstrated in Chapter 1, an acoustic impedance mismatch at an interface causes partial reflection of the ultrasonic energy. The acoustic impedance of the crystal is large (30 Mrayls) compared with that of the tissue (1.6 Mrayls), which results in a large reflection (81%) at the crystal-tissue interface. Only 19% of the ultrasonic energy enters the tissue (percent transmission):

$$\%T = 100 - \%R$$
$$\%T = 100 - \left\{ \left[\frac{(Z_c - Z_t)}{(Z_c + Z_t)} \right]^2 \times 100 \right\}$$

where Z_c is the acoustic impedance of the crystal and Z_t the acoustic impedance of tissue.

$$\%T = 100 - \left\{ \left[\frac{(30 \text{ Mrayls} - 1.6 \text{ Mrayls})}{(30 \text{ Mrayls} + 1.6 \text{ Mrayls})} \right]^2 \times 100 \right\}$$
$$\%T = 100 - 81 = 19\%$$

The introduction of facing materials or matching layers between the crystal and the tissue partially eliminates this problem. The facing material of proper acoustic impedance provides a better match between the crystal and the tissue (i.e., reduces the acoustic impedance mismatch by interposing a material with intermediate acoustic impedance between the crystal and tissue). The transfer of sound energy from the crystal to soft tissue, and vice versa, is enhanced (Fig. 4-15). Matching layers are composed of fine particles (aluminum powder) dispersed in an epoxy resin. The concentration of aluminum determines the acoustic impedance of the matching layer. The exact composition of matching layers is unknown, because manufacturers hesitate to reveal their secret recipes.

The acoustic impedance of the matching layer is selected to reduce the amount of reflection at the crystal–matching layer and matching layer–tissue interfaces. This is accomplished by taking the geometric mean of the acoustic impedances for the crystal and tissue (the square root of the product of the acoustic impedances):

$$Z_{ml} = \sqrt{Z_c Z_t} \qquad \text{4-12}$$

The acoustic impedance of the matching layer is calculated using Equation 4-12.

$$Z_{ml} = \sqrt{(30 \text{ Mrayls})(1.6 \text{ Mrayls})}$$
$$Z_{ml} = 6.9 \text{ Mrayls}$$

To calculate the improvement in energy transfer from the crystal through the single matching layer to the tissue involves a two-step process.

First, from the crystal ($Z_c = 30$ Mrayls) to the matching layer ($Z_{ml} = 6.9$ Mrayls) the percentage of transmission is found:

$$\%T = 100 - \left\{ \left[\frac{(30 \text{ Mrayls} - 6.9 \text{ Mrayls})}{(30 \text{ Mrayls} + 6.9 \text{ Mrayls})} \right]^2 \times 100 \right\}$$
$$\%T = 100 - 39 = 61\%$$

Next, the percentage of transmission through the matching layer to the tissue ($Z_t = 1.6$ Mrayls) must be calculated:

$$\%T = 100 - \left\{ \left[\frac{(6.9 \text{ Mrayls} - 1.6 \text{ Mrayls})}{(6.9 \text{ Mrayls} + 1.6 \text{ Mrayls})} \right]^2 \times 100 \right\}$$
$$\%T = 100 - 39 = 61\%$$

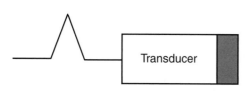

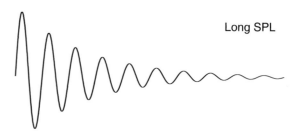

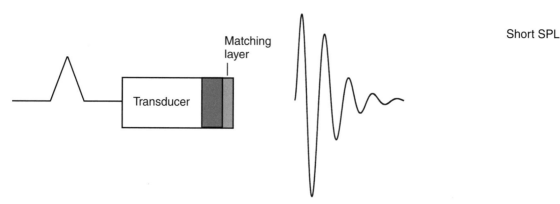

Fig. 4-15 Matching layer (facing material) between crystal and tissue allows greater instantaneous intensity to enter the patient and reduces the pulse length.

Thus, of the total sound energy generated, 61% passes from the crystal to the matching layer, and 37% (the product of transmission coefficients) is transferred into the tissue. The improvement above 19% transmission without the matching layer is evident.

Optimizing Matching Layer Performance

The acoustic impedance of the matching layer should be optimized to give the best axial resolution (shortest pulse possible) with maximum transmitted beam intensity. Optimizing the facing material by considering the transmission properties of the crystal may result in a matching layer acoustic impedance that is not the geometric mean of the crystal and tissue acoustic impedances:

$$Z_{ml} = Z_c^{1/3} Z_t^{2/3}$$

4-13

A specific thickness of the facing material is also necessary. A thickness equal to integer multiples of the quarter wavelength provides maximum reinforcement of the ultrasound wave reflected from the crystal–facing material interface. This enhances the intensity of the ultrasound wave transmitted into the body. Normally, the one-quarter layer (which causes less attenuation than a three-quarter layer or any other quarter multiple) is adjusted for the center frequency of the transducer. A transducer with a quarter-wavelength matching layer is referred to as a quarter-wavelength transducer.

Multiple Matching Layers

Because pulsed systems produce ultrasound waves of many frequencies (frequency distribution described by the bandwidth), and each frequency has its own associated wavelength, the optimal single matching layer for transmission or reception is difficult to design. The quarter-frequency matching layer allows maximum transmission for a single frequency of the ultrasound wave. Additional improvement in performance can be achieved by using multiple matching layers on the face of a transducer (Fig. 4-16). These matching layers taper the acoustic impedance from that of the crystal to that of tissue. Indeed, the efficiency of transmission is so improved that in many cases the backing layer is no longer needed. Ringing does not occur, because the energy is transferred to tissue and does not remain in the crystal for multiple reflections at the crystal interfaces.

The multiple matching layers alter the frequency distribution toward a broader bandwidth. The increased bandwidth enhances the sensitivity of the transducer, which results in improved image quality. The axial resolution is enhanced, because the larger bandwidth normally means a shorter spatial pulse length. Short spatial pulse length allows the echoes from close objects to be processed separately. To form a short spatial pulse, multiple frequency components are necessary. A wide frequency distribution provides a better opportunity to match the crystal to the rest of the ultrasonic system. The low-frequency components of the

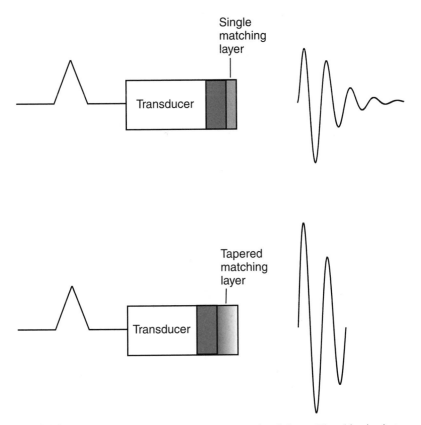

Fig. 4-16 Multiple matching layers between crystal and tissue. The objective is to transfer nearly all of the generated acoustic energy into the tissue for a short duration pulse.

spectrum can be controlled to decrease the far field divergence. The angular divergence of the far field is inversely proportional to the frequency (discussed at greater length later in the next chapter).

Focusing

Divergence of the ultrasonic beam causes a decrease in the intensity (energy per unit area per time) with increasing distance from the transducer. This is easily understood by considering a constant amount of energy spread over a larger and larger area. The amount of energy incident on a unit area reflector will decrease as the distance between the reflector and the transducer increases. The reflected beam will also diverge, returning to the transducer and creating a partial "miss" of the ultrasound wave at the transducer (Fig. 4-17). Thus divergence is responsible for intensity loss for both the transmitted and the reflected beam.

The ultrasound beam can be focused, which concentrates the acoustic energy over a small area at a specific distance from the transducer. Compared with a nonfocused beam, the focused beam produces a stronger echo reflected to the transducer for detection. This is true only for structures within the focal zone of the transducer, however, where less divergence occurs. Focusing techniques and the resulting ultrasonic fields are discussed in Chapter 5.

Tissue Variations

Several nontransducer-related variables influence the overall sensitivity of the system. The intensity of the sound beam is not spatially uniform as the beam leaves the face of the transducer. The intensity of the beam incident on an interface depends on the location of the interface. Because a fraction of the incident energy is reflected, the position of the reflecting interface affects the intensity of the returning echo. In addition, the beam is attenuated with depth; that is, the medium transmitting the sound removes acoustic energy from the beam. Recall from Chapter 1 that the attenuation for tissue is approximately 0.7 dB/cm/MHz. The composition, shape, and size of structures in the medium also contribute to the reflectivity and thus to the sensitivity. When scanning human subjects, the operator cannot control characteristics of the medium. A transducer can be selected, however, that will have properties conducive to the diagnostic information desired from the portion of the body to be scanned.

Q-VALUE

The **Q-value,** or mechanical coefficient, assesses an essential characteristic of the pulsed ultrasound beam–pulse duration and bandwidth. The Q-value can thus be thought of as having two separate definitions relating to the two affected beam characteristics. These definitions are

$$Q = \frac{\text{Energy stored per cycle}}{\text{Energy lost per cycle}}$$ 4-14

and

$$Q = \frac{\text{Center frequency}}{\text{Bandwidth}}$$ 4-15

where *bandwidth* is a parameter that describes the frequency distribution that composes the sound wave.

A high-Q transducer retains energy in the crystal and therefore loses very little each cycle. After being stimulated by the voltage pulse, it vibrates (rings) for an extended duration, producing a long duration pulse. A low-Q transducer, on the other hand, generates a short pulse after excitation, because most of its energy is lost from the crystal and converted to sound during the first few vibrations. Diagnostic pulsed wave ultrasound uses low-Q transducers, the Q-value being approximately 2. High-Q transducers (700 or greater) are good for continuous wave ultrasound. Quartz, with a Q-value of 25,000, is advantageous for therapeutic applications.

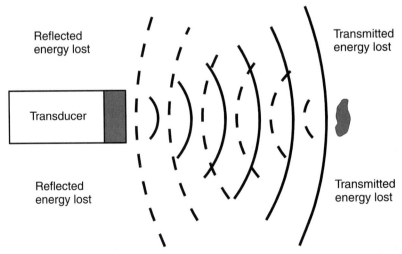

Fig. 4-17 Energy loss due to divergence. Energy is lost in both transmitted *(solid lines)* and received *(dashed lines)* directions.

BANDWIDTH

From Equation 4-15, it can be seen that the Q-value is indirectly proportional to the **bandwidth** or frequency spread of a transducer. Recall that a narrow bandwidth decreases the sensitivity of the transducer. For a transducer operating with a continuous output, only a single frequency is generated. *For a pulsed system, however, because of imperfections in the crystal and the complex nature of the damped pulse, a range of frequencies is generated.* Many waves of differing frequency combine to form the pulse. Fourier analysis enables a complex waveform (e.g., pulsed

ultrasound wave) to be broken into its various frequency components. An algebraic summation of sine waves of varying frequency (Fig. 4-18) yields the original waveform; in other words, any complex waveform can be considered a series of sine waves with different frequencies and amplitudes. (A more complete discussion of Fourier analysis is presented in Appendix B.)

The frequency spectrum can be analyzed by measuring the signal strength as a function of time for an electrical signal induced by an echo returning from a flat steel target located a fixed distance from the transducer in a non-attenuating medium. With Fourier analysis, the signal waveform is converted to energy output and from the time domain to the frequency domain. Frequency domain is a mathematical term meaning that the various frequency components of the signal are identified. Output plotted against frequency shows a spectrum of values, with the center frequency (f_c) having the greatest amplitude (Fig. 4-19). Output in this instance indicates the relative importance of each frequency in the transmitted ultrasound pulse. The relative value of the output represents the fraction of the pulse composed of waves of a particular frequency.

Pulse Duration and Bandwidth

A low-Q transducer has a short pulse length (rapidly damped) and a broad bandwidth (Fig. 4-20).

A high-Q transducer has a long pulse length (from crystal ringing) and a narrow bandwidth. In diagnostic ultrasound imaging, trade-offs exist between good reception and good transmission, but generally low-Q transducers with broad bandwidths are desirable.

Calculation of Bandwidth

The center frequency is the primary operating frequency or the natural resonance frequency of the transducer, which

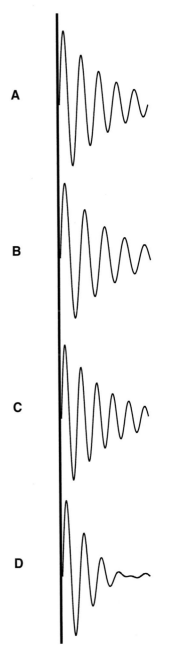

Fig. 4-18 **A** to **C**, Three component frequencies derived from Fourier analysis of a pulsed ultrasound wave, **D.** The amplitude of each sine wave is assumed to decrease at the same rate because of damping. Note that the summation wave has a shorter pulse duration than the component parts.

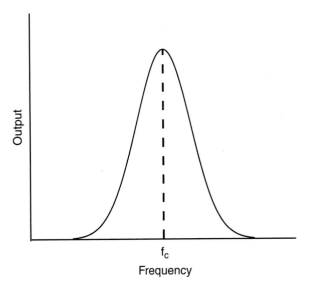

Fig. 4-19 Frequency distribution of the transmitted pulse. The center frequency (f_c) is the dominant component in the transmitted output.

A **B**

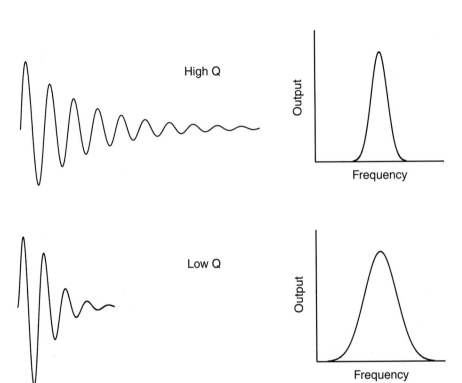

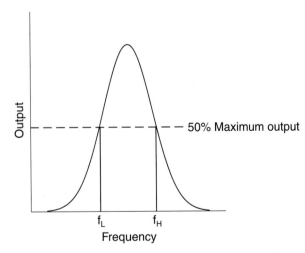

Fig. 4-20 Relationship between Q-value, pulse length, and the frequency spectrum. **A,** Output versus time illustrating pulse length for rapid damping *(low-Q)* versus slow damping *(high-Q).* **B,** Relative importance of various frequencies present in each pulse in **A.** This illustrates the principle that as the pulse duration is shortened, additional frequency components contribute to the transmitted pulse.

depends on the crystal thickness. Rewriting Equation 4-15 with symbols:

$$Q = \frac{f_c}{\Delta f} \qquad \textbf{4-16}$$

where Δf is the bandwidth between the half maximum points on each side of the center frequency (f_c).

A 3 dB loss occurs if the output is reduced to half its original value. From the frequency spectrum, the frequency corresponding to 50% of the maximum output is marked on each side of the center frequency. The bandwidth is calculated by subtracting the low frequency at 50% maximum output from the high frequency at 50% maximum output (Fig. 4-21). This process of determining the width of the frequency distribution at 50% maximum output is called full width at half maximum (FWHM).

A transducer operating at a center frequency of 7.5 MHz with a bandwidth of 3.75 MHz yields a Q-value of 2. When the second definition of Q-value for a transducer is used, it becomes evident (as stated by Equation 4-16) that a high-Q transducer has a very narrow bandwidth, whereas a low-Q transducer has a broad bandwidth.

Fig. 4-21 Determination of bandwidth by subtracting f_L from f_H. The frequency limits f_L and f_H correspond to one half the output at the center frequency.

Fractional Bandwidth

Pulse duration and bandwidth are inversely related. That is, pulse duration is proportional to the reciprocal of the bandwidth.

4-17

$$\Delta f \approx \frac{1}{PD\ (\mu s)}$$

A pulsed wave for imaging with a pulse duration of 1 μs has a bandwidth of approximately 1 MHz. If the pulse duration is reduced by a factor of 2 to 0.5 μs, then the bandwidth increases to 2 MHz. Again, shorter pulsed waves produce higher bandwidths.

Bandwidth is often expressed as a fraction of the center frequency,

4-18

$$\text{Fractional bandwidth} = \frac{\Delta f}{f_c}$$

A transducer operating at a center frequency of 7.5 MHz with a Q-value of 2 yields a fraction bandwidth of 0.5 or 50%.

Fractional bandwidth can be estimated from the number of cycles in the pulse by the following manipulation of Equation 4-17 to achieve an expression for fractional bandwidth:

$$\Delta f \approx \frac{1}{PD\ (\mu s)}$$

Substitute for pulse duration using the number of cycles and the period of the center frequency

$$\Delta f \approx \frac{1}{n\tau}$$

The center frequency is the reciprocal of the period, thus

$$\Delta f \approx \frac{f_c}{n}$$

Divide each side of the equation by the center frequency

4-19

$$\frac{\Delta f}{f_c} \approx \frac{f_c}{nf_c} \approx \frac{1}{n}$$

The fractional bandwidth would be 0.25 and 0.33, respectively, for a four-cycle pulse and a three-cycle pulse.

Matching Layer Effect on Bandwidth

The matching layer enhances the transmission of energy into the patient and shortens the pulse duration. Reduction of the pulse duration introduces additional frequency components into the transmitted pulsed wave. The frequency distribution is broadened by the presence of the matching layer (Fig. 4-22).

Frequency Shift in Tissue

As the beam is transmitted through matter, ultrasound waves of higher frequency are absorbed more rapidly than those of lower frequency, causing a shift in the frequency spectrum toward a lower range (Fig. 4-23). This is similar to the shift toward higher energies as an x-ray beam penetrates the body, because low energies are absorbed more readily. The preferential absorption of the high-frequency components influences the sensitivity of the system. A broadband transducer (as opposed to one with a narrow bandwidth) has greater sensitivity as the sound beam penetrates tissue. A transducer with a broad frequency spectrum is also easier to match electronically with the rest of the ultrasound system, which allows the receiver to be tuned to variable frequencies and maximize the sensitivity at various depths.

IMAGING APPLICATIONS

The desirable characteristics for a transducer used for imaging are summarized in Table 4-3.

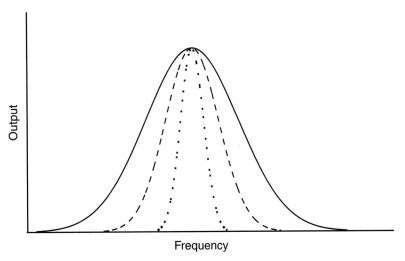

Fig. 4-22 Frequency spectrum produced by transducer: no matching layer (*dotted line*); single matching layer (*dashed line*); multiple matching layers (*solid line*).

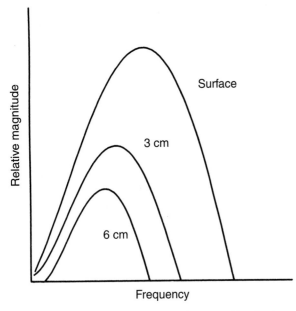

Fig. 4-23 Effect of attenuation on the frequency distribution, illustrating the need for a low-Q (broad bandwidth) transducer.

SUMMARY

The purpose of the transducer is to produce an ultrasound wave of the proper frequency that can be directed into the patient. The transducer also functions as a receiver for the returning echoes. Design criteria for diagnostic imaging include short duration pulsed waves and efficient energy transmission. Matching layers and backing material are incorporated into the transducer to meet these requirements. Pulse duration and spatial pulse length describe the temporal and spatial extent of the ultrasound pulse. The rate of pulse generation is the pulse repetition frequency. The frequency distribution in the transmitted pulse is characterized by the bandwidth and Q-value. Wide bandwidth associated with a short duration pulse is desirable for imaging applications. Sensitivity is enhanced by high conversion efficiencies (electrical energy to acoustic energy and vice versa).

REVIEW QUESTIONS

1. Assume the best resolution of an ultrasound imaging system to be one wavelength. What frequency is required to detect a 0.5 mm object in tissue?
2. What thickness of piezoelectric crystal (c = 5000 m/s) is required to produce a resonant frequency of 5 MHz?
3. What is the wavelength in tissue for the crystal in Question 2?

Table 4-3　Characteristics of Imaging Transducers

Parameter	Characteristic
Waveform	Pulsed
Q-value	Low ($\approx$2)
Frequency	2-15 MHz
Pulse duration	Short (1-5 cycles) ($\approx$1μs)
Frequency distribution	Wide bandwidth (>50%)

4. The maximum pulse repetition frequency (PRF_{max}) is directly proportional to the velocity of ultrasound in a medium and inversely proportional to the _____.
5. Assume the depth of interest to be 15 cm. What is the maximum PRF?
6. What is the pulse repetition period corresponding to the maximum PRF calculated in Question 5?
7. What is the spatial pulse length for a 2.5 cycle pulse if the frequency is 5 MHz?
8. Determine the pulse duration for the transducer in Question 7.
9. Calculate the duty factor for a 5 MHz transducer that produces 2.5 cycles per pulse. The PRF is 2000 per second.
10. Calculate the acoustic impedance of a matching layer assuming Z_c is 40 Mrayls and Z_t is 1.6 Mrayls.
11. Calculate the increase in percentage of transmission for the crystal–matching layer and matching layer–tissue interfaces compared to the crystal-tissue interface alone in Question 10.
12. What is the fractional bandwidth for a two-cycle 5 MHz pulsed wave?
13. What is the approximate pulse duration for a pulsed wave with a bandwidth of 2 MHz?

BIBLIOGRAPHY

Kremkau FW: *Diagnostic ultrasound: principles and instruments,* ed 6, Philadelphia, 2002, WB Saunders.

McDicken WN: *Diagnostic ultrasonics: principles and use of instruments,* ed 3, Edinburgh, 1991, Churchill Livingstone.

O'Brien, Jr, WD: Single-element transducers, *Radiographics* 13:947-957, 1993.

Rose JL, Goldberg BB: *Basic physics in diagnostic ultrasound,* New York, 1979, John Wiley & Sons.

Wells PNT: *Physical principles of ultrasonic diagnosis,* New York, 1969, Academic Press.

Wells PNT: *Biomedical ultrasonics,* New York, 1977, Academic Press.

Whittingham TA: Broadband transducers, *Eur Radiol* 9:S298-S303, 1999.

CHAPTER 5

Single-Element Transducers: Transmission and Echo Reception

The information obtained from ultrasound scanning depends in large part on the beam characteristics, which in turn are governed by transducer design. Numerous parameters are used to describe transducer performance. Physical descriptors and the corresponding symbols introduced in this chapter are listed in Table 5-1.

AXIAL RESOLUTION

The Q-value of a transducer—in conjunction with the matching layer used for transmission of sound into tissue and the frequency of the transducer—determines the spatial pulse length (SPL), which in turn limits the axial resolution achievable by the transducer. The **axial resolution** (also called range resolution and depth resolution) specifies how close together two objects can be along the axis of the beam and yet still be detected as two distinct entities. Axial resolution also specifies the smallest object detectable along the axis of the beam. For a constant wavelength, as the pulse is shortened, the axial resolution improves (Fig. 5-1).

For diagnostic ultrasound imaging at 4 MHz, the resolution (minimum object size detectable) should be on the order of 0.5 mm. Commonly, the SPL is used as a specifier for the axial resolution. The best possible axial resolution is the SPL divided by 2. Fig. 5-2 illustrates this concept. The beam leaves the transducer with a spatial pulse length of 1 SPL and is directed toward two interfaces spaced SPL/2 apart. The beam strikes the first interface, which causes a fraction of the ultrasonic energy to be reflected

Table 5-1 Physical Descriptors and Symbols

Parameter	Symbol
Beam width	w
Degree of focusing	κ
Diameter	D
Far field divergence	φ
Focal length	F
Near field depth	NFD
Radius (transducer)	A
Signal-to-noise ratio	SNR

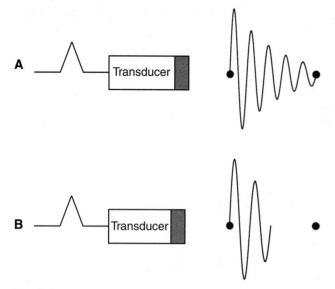

Fig. 5-1 Pulse length versus axial resolution. **A,** A five-cycle pulse includes both objects *(dots)* within the spatial pulse length (SPL). **B,** A two-cycle pulse, which has a shorter SPL, can resolve objects located more closely together.

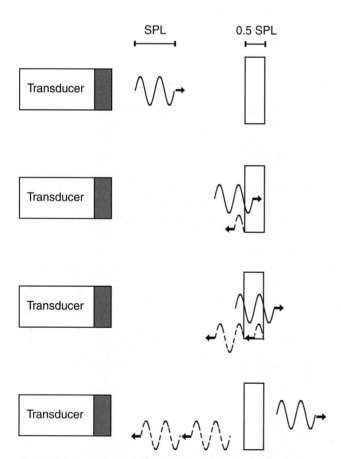

Fig. 5-2 Spatial pulse length (SPL) with minimum resolution. Two objects *(vertical sides of the rectangular box)* are separated by 0.5 SPL. The echo from each interface is shown by dashed lines. The objects are just resolvable.

toward the transducer. The remaining energy of the pulse is transmitted through the interface and progresses to the second interface, at which point some of the energy is again reflected. The echo with the pulse length of 1 SPL leaving the first interface has traveled a distance of SPL/2 when the transmitted pulse strikes the second interface. As the reflected sound wave from the second interface moves toward the first interface, the echo from the first interface is moving toward the transducer. When the echo from the second interface arrives at the first interface, the first echo has moved a distance of 1 SPL, and therefore the echoes from the two interfaces are separated in both distance and time when detected by the transducer.

Several factors, including transducer Q-value (backing material, matching layer, and ringing) as well as frequency, influence axial resolution (SPL). The matching layer enables acoustic energy to quickly and as completely as possible be transferred to the patient. The backing material prevents reflection from the back surface of the crystal by allowing the ultrasound wave to enter the backing material and then rapidly absorbs the ultrasound energy. Oscillations of ultrasound beam in the crystal are inhibited, and thereby the transmitted output is rapidly damped. (SPL consists of a few cycles.) The more efficient the transfer of energy into the patient and into the backing material (Z of the backing approaching Z of the crystal), the shorter the pulse will be. However, as the pulse composition becomes more complex (i.e., frequency components increase), the rate of damping is increased.

The SPL depends on the frequency of the transducer. For a constant number of cycles, as the frequency is increased, the shortened wavelength decreases the SPL and improves the axial resolution (Fig. 5-3). Note that a tradeoff occurs.

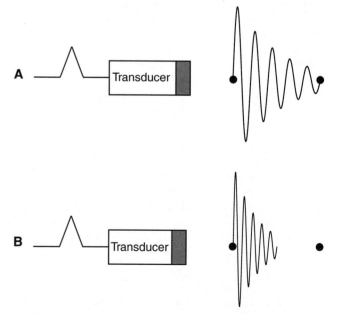

Fig. 5-3 Spatial pulse length (SPL) shortened by increasing the frequency. **A,** The five-cycle pulse from a low-frequency transducer includes both objects *(dots)* within the SPL. **B,** The five-cycle pulse from a high-frequency transducer has a shorter SPL and can resolve objects located more closely together.

■ **Table 5-2**   Parameters Affecting Spatial Pulse Length

Parameter	Change	SPL
Frequency	Increase	Decrease
Q-value	Decrease	Decrease
Damping	Increase	Decrease
Pulse duration	Decrease	Decrease

Although the resolution is enhanced at higher frequencies, the depth of penetration is decreased because of the frequency dependence of the attenuation coefficient.

SPL is established at transmission and is not altered by attenuation along the beam path. *Axial spatial resolution is essentially constant throughout the scan range (independent of depth)*. Factors affecting SPL and hence axial resolution are summarized in Table 5-2.

Focusing of the transducer (discussed later in this chapter) creates a region of higher intensity and thus greater sensitivity within the focal zone. The process of focusing the beam may actually lengthen the measured echo pulse duration, thereby deteriorating the axial resolution. This effect is normally minimal.

BEAM WIDTH AND LATERAL RESOLUTION

One of the original objectives in designing a device for ultrasound production was to generate a beam that would be directional (similar to a flashlight beam) rather than non-directional (e.g., light from a light bulb). If a point source of sound is used, waves are emitted in all directions. The beam from a large-diameter transducer is unidirectional, with planar wavefronts and the lateral extent of the beam nearly the same as the diameter of the crystal (Fig. 5-4).

Lateral resolution describes the ability to distinguish, as separate entities, two objects adjacent to each other oriented perpendicular to the beam axis (Fig. 5-5). It also refers to the ability of the ultrasound beam to detect single small objects perpendicular to the direction of propagation. Decreasing the beam width improves the lateral resolution by allowing objects close together to be resolved and by providing a more accurate presentation of small objects. A single object smaller than the sound beam width produces a signal the entire time it is within the beam; thus the object appears to be the same size as the width of the beam (Fig. 5-6). Small beam width enables small objects to become distinguishable. Lateral resolution is a major factor in the quality of diagnostic ultrasound images.

THE ULTRASONIC FIELD: NEAR FIELD AND FAR FIELD

Another objective in designing a device for ultrasound production was to generate a beam of uniform intensity. A circular sound source with a diameter equal to one wavelength produces spherical wavefronts originating from the

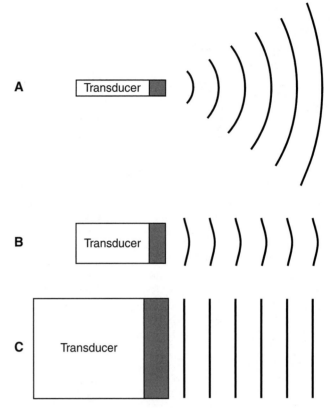

Fig. 5-4   Effect of transducer size on wavefronts. **A,** Spherical wavefronts produced by a small-radius source of sound. **B,** As the size of the source is increased, the wavefronts become less divergent. **C,** Large-radius transducer producing planar (directional) wavefronts.

face of the crystal. The beam diverges rapidly from the crystal face, and the lateral resolution deteriorates. In addition, regions of rarefaction and compression create a nonuniform beam (Fig. 5-7). If the diameter of the sound source is increased to a value of several wavelengths, each small area (one wavelength in size) is considered to be an individual vibrating sound source and thus to produce its own spherical wavefronts. These wavefronts undergo constructive and destructive interference, resulting in a very complex wave pattern (Fig. 5-8), in accordance with Huygens' principle. A nonuniform beam intensity exists in the **near field** (area of nondivergence), and a uniform beam is present in the far field (area of divergence, in which lateral resolution is poor). The far field is called the Fraunhofer zone, and the near field the Fresnel zone (Fig. 5-9).

If the acoustic pressure along the axis of the beam is measured (axial pressure profile) for a high-Q transducer (continuous wave, single frequency), the pressure alternates between a maximum value and zero in the near field and then slowly decreases after the last maximum, which is the beginning of the far field (Fig. 5-10). Cross-sectional intensity measurements (transverse pressure profiles) also reveal a non-uniform beam in the near field (Fig. 5-11). Low-intensity side lobes (adjacent to, but angled away from, the main beam axis) may be produced from these interference phenomena. The side lobes create artifacts in an image by the incorrect

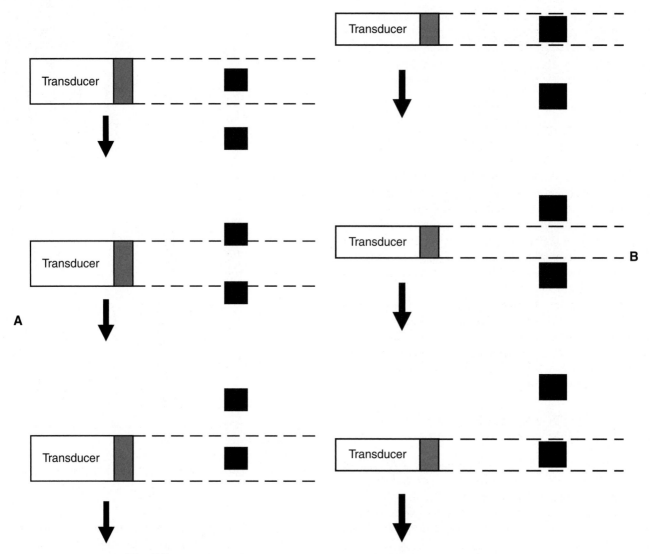

Fig. 5-5 Dependence of lateral resolution on beam width. **A,** Two objects are not resolved with a wide beam. **B,** Two objects can be resolved with a narrow beam when the beam is scanned across the objects.

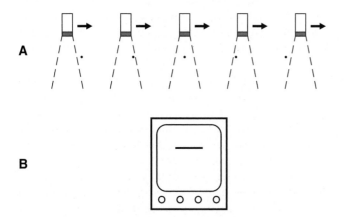

Fig. 5-6 Displayed object size versus beam width. **A,** Sound source scanning small spherical reflector. **B,** The size of an object represented on the display is equivalent to the beam width at the depth of the object. When an object is included within the beam, an echo is produced. A two-dimensional image shows the spherical reflector as a line rather than a dot. The size of the object is misrepresented, because the beam width is larger than the object size.

placement of an interface. This is particularly true for real-time ultrasound, which is discussed in Chapter 8.

A low-Q transducer (broad bandwidth, short pulse length) produces many frequencies rather than just a single frequency. The presence of multiple frequencies tends to make the near field more uniform. Every frequency has a different interference pattern, and when these patterns are superimposed on each other, the result is a smoothing of the overall intensity pattern (Fig. 5-12).

Near-Field Depth

For a nonfocused transducer the near-field depth (NFD), or the distance that the near field extends into the patient, is dependent on the diameter and frequency (or wavelength via $c = f\lambda$) of the transducer according to the following formula:

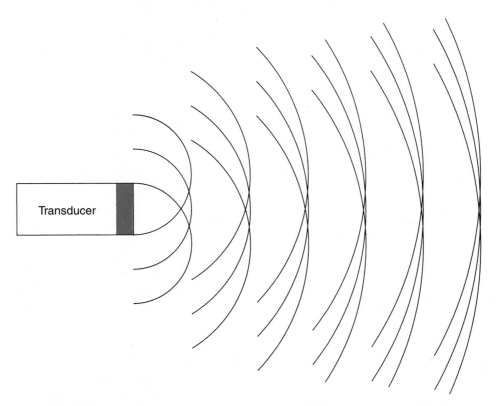

Fig. 5-7 Wavefronts produced from a sound source whose diameter is equal to one wavelength.

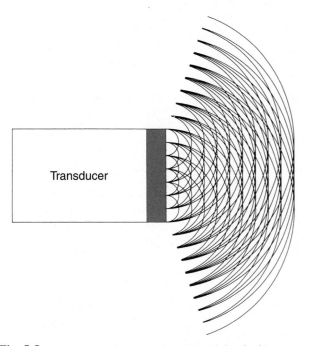

Fig. 5-8 A large sound source acting as multiple, single wavelength sound sources produces a complex pattern of wavefronts.

5-1

$$\text{NFD} = \frac{D^2 f}{4\,c} = \frac{D^2}{4\,\lambda} = \frac{a^2}{\lambda}$$

where f is the frequency of the transducer, D the diameter of the transducer, c the velocity of ultrasound in the medium, λ the wavelength of the ultrasound, and a the radius of the transducer.

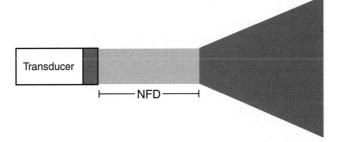

Fig. 5-9 Beam pattern showing the near field *(light gray)* and far field *(dark gray)*. Distance NFD indicates the depth of the near field.

As the frequency increases (with the wavelength decreasing), the NFD increases. In theory, by increasing the frequency, the region of best lateral resolution would be extended. Example 5-1 below illustrates this. In practice, higher frequencies are absorbed more rapidly as the beam propagates through tissue, and, consequently, deep structures may not be visualized, because the reflected ultrasound waves are too weak. At high frequencies lateral resolution associated with narrow beam width in the near field is maintained at increased depth.

Equation 5-1 also indicates that the NFD (area of no divergence) increases rapidly as the diameter of the transducer increases. Example 5-2 demonstrates this effect. The lateral resolution at shallow depths, however, is sacrificed as the crystal diameter is made larger.

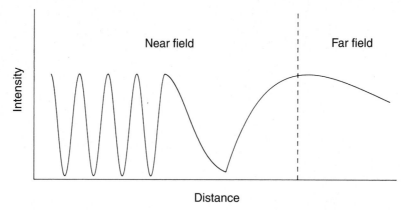

Fig. 5-10 Axial intensity (or pressure) profile from a high-Q transducer. Note the large variation of intensity in the near field.

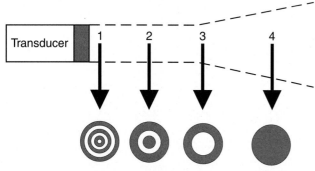

Fig. 5-11 Transverse (cross-sectional) intensity (or pressure) profiles. The profiles are shown at various locations along the axis of the beam. **1,** Depth in the near field in which the axial pressure profile is minimal. **2,** Depth in the near field in which the axial pressure profile is maximal. **3,** Depth of the last minimum in the near field. **4,** Depth in the far field.

■ **Example 5-1**

Calculate the NFD for transducers with frequencies of 1, 2, and 5 MHz. Assume a constant diameter of 20 mm (0.02 m). Using Equation 5-1,

For a frequency of 1 MHz

$$NFD = \frac{D^2 f}{4\,c}$$

$$NFD = \frac{(0.02 \text{ m})^2 (1 \times 10^6 \text{ 1/s})}{4(1540 \text{ m/s})}$$

$$NFD = 0.065 \text{ m} = 6.5 \text{ cm}$$

For a frequency of 2 MHz

$$NFD = \frac{(0.02 \text{ m})^2 (2 \times 10^6 \text{ 1/s})}{4(1540 \text{ m/s})}$$

$$NFD = 0.13 \text{ m} = 13 \text{ cm}$$

For a frequency of 5 MHz

$$NFD = \frac{(0.02 \text{ m})^2 (5 \times 10^6 \text{ 1/s})}{4(1540 \text{ m/s})}$$

$$NFD = 0.325 \text{ m} = 32.5 \text{ cm}$$

This example illustrates that, for a constant-diameter transducer, if the frequency increases (causing the wavelength to decrease), the NFD increases. This extends the useful area of best lateral resolution to greater depths.

■ **Example 5-2**

Calculate the NFD for transducers with diameters of 10, 20, and 30 mm. Assume a constant frequency of 2 MHz. Solve using the same formula as in Example 5-1.

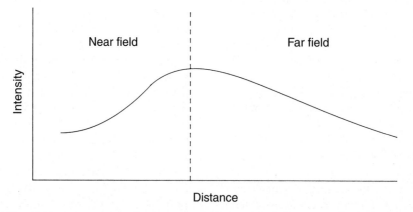

Fig. 5-12 Axial intensity (or pressure) profile from a low-Q transducer. The broad frequency components cause the near field to have less intensity fluctuation.

For a diameter of 10 mm

$$NFD = \frac{D^2 f}{4\,c}$$

$$NFD = \frac{(0.01\ m)^2 (2 \times 10^6\ 1/s)}{4(1540\ m/s)}$$

$$NFD = 0.032\ m = 3.2\ cm$$

For a diameter of 20 mm

$$NFD = \frac{(0.02\ m)^2 (2 \times 10^6\ 1/s)}{4(1540\ m/s)}$$

$$NFD = 0.13\ m = 13\ cm$$

For a diameter of 30 mm

$$NFD = \frac{(0.03\ m)^2 (2 \times 10^6\ 1/s)}{4(1540\ m/s)}$$

$$NFD = 0.292\ m = 29.2\ cm$$

This example illustrates that, for a constant frequency, as the diameter increases, the NFD increases. The increasing beam diameter (i.e., beam aperture, as discussed for real-time scanners in Chapter 8) increases the NFD.

Far-Field Divergence

Beyond the near field is the region called the **far field** (Fraunhofer zone), where the ultrasound beam begins to diverge. The angle φ, a measure of the beam's divergence for a nonfocused transducer, is given as

$$\sin \varphi = \frac{0.61\ \lambda}{a} = \frac{1.22\ \lambda}{D} = \frac{1.22\ c}{Df} \qquad \text{5-2}$$

Therefore

$$\varphi = \arcsin\left(\frac{0.61\ \lambda}{a}\right) = \arcsin\left(\frac{1.22\ \lambda}{D}\right) = \arcsin\left(\frac{1.22\ c}{Df}\right) \qquad \text{5-3}$$

These formulas predict that as the frequency is increased (or wavelength is decreased), the angle of divergence becomes smaller. This is demonstrated by Example 5-3. Also, as the diameter is increased, the beam diverges less rapidly. Example 5-4 illustrates this point.

■ Example 5-3

Calculate the angle of divergence (φ) for transducers with frequencies of 2 and 4 MHz. Assume a constant diameter of 20 mm. Using Equation 5-3, solve for φ.

For a frequency of 2 MHz

$$\varphi = \arcsin\left(\frac{1.22\ c}{Df}\right)$$

$$\varphi = \arcsin\left[\frac{(1.22)\ (1540\ m/s)}{(0.02)(2 \times 10^6\ 1/s)}\right]$$

$$\varphi = 2.7\ degrees$$

For a frequency of 4 MHz

$$\varphi = \arcsin\left[\frac{(1.22)\ (1540\ m/s)}{(0.02)(4 \times 10^6\ 1/s)}\right]$$

$$\varphi = 1.3\ degrees$$

This example illustrates that the angle of divergence for nonfocused transducers with a constant diameter decreases as the frequency increases. The result is reduced beam width in the far field.

■ Example 5-4

Calculate the angle of divergence (φ) for transducers with diameters of 10 and 20 mm. Assume a constant frequency of 2 MHz. Using Equation 5-3, solve for φ.

For a diameter of 10 mm

$$\varphi = \arcsin\left[\frac{(1.22)\ (1540\ m/s)}{(0.01)(2 \times 10^6\ 1/s)}\right]$$

$$\varphi = 5.4\ degrees$$

For a diameter of 20 mm

$$\varphi = \arcsin\left[\frac{(1.22)\ (1540\ m/s)}{(0.02)(2 \times 10^6\ 1/s)}\right]$$

$$\varphi = 2.7\ degrees$$

This example illustrates that if the diameter of nonfocused transducers can be increased (for a constant frequency), the angle of divergence decreases. This results in reduced beam width in the far field.

The influence of crystal size and operating frequency on NFD and far-field divergence is further demonstrated by the calculated results from Equations 5-1 and 5-3, which are listed in Table 5-3.

The lateral resolution deteriorates in the far-field region because of divergence of the beam. Therefore scanning areas of interest should be confined to the near field if possible. An exception to this practice may occur when scanning large patients.

Transducer Selection

The depth of the structures of interest is a primary consideration when selecting the optimum transducer. The objective is to enhance lateral resolution by scanning the area of interest with a narrow beam. Evaluation of the NFD and far-field divergence indicates that transducers with high frequencies and large diameters maintain beam shape to greater depths. Although large-diameter transducers have a large near-field beam width and thus provide poor lateral resolution at shallow depths, the near field extends to greater depths in the body compared with a smaller diameter transducer. The divergence of the beam in the far field is less, which makes the larger transducer preferable for deep-lying structures (Fig. 5-13).

A similar effect is observed with frequency; that is, with other factors constant, an increased frequency results in a deeper near field and a less diverging far field. This may compensate for the loss in penetration (Fig. 5-14).

The following guidelines are for single-element transducers, which for the most part have been replaced by new transducer designs with multiple elements. If shallow structures and irregular surfaces are of interest, a small-diameter high-frequency transducer should be used. Abdominal

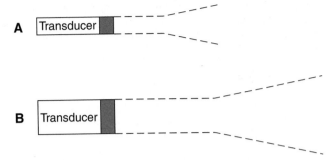

Fig. 5-13 Effect of transducer diameter on lateral resolution. **A,** A small-diameter transducer can maintain a narrow beam width only at shallow depths. **B,** At greater depths the large-diameter transducer has a smaller beam width and better lateral resolution.

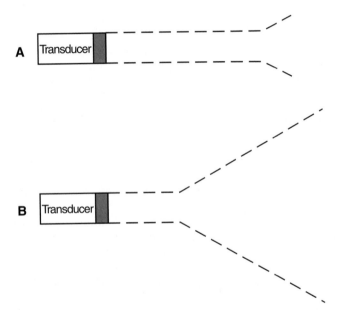

Fig. 5-14 Effect of frequency on lateral resolution. **A,** The high-frequency transducer extents the near field compared with the low-frequency transducer, **B.** The regions at increased depth may not be probed by high-frequency sound waves because of rapid attenuation of the beam, in which case a low-frequency transducer must be used.

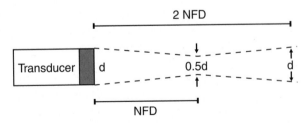

Fig. 5-15 Self-focusing effect. Beam width for a nonfocused transducer in the presence of a nonattenuating medium. A beam width of half the crystal diameter (w = 0.5d) occurs at the limit of the near-field depth *(NFD)* and increases to equal the crystal diameter at twice the NFD *(2 NFD).*

■ **Table 5-3** Near-Field Depth and Far-Field Divergence as a Function of Crystal Diameter and Center Frequency

Frequency (MHz)	Transducer Diameter (mm)	Near-Field Depth (cm)	Far-Field Divergence (degrees)
1	8	1	13.6
1	10	1.6	10.8
1	15	3.6	7.2
1	20	6.5	5.4
2	8	2.1	6.7
2	10	3.2	5.4
2	15	7.3	3.6
2	20	13	2.7
3.5	8	3.6	3.8
3.5	10	5.7	3.1
3.5	15	12.8	2
3.5	20	22.7	1.5
5	8	5.2	2.7
5	10	8.1	2.2
5	15	18.3	1.4
5	20	32.5	1.1
7.5	8	7.8	1.8
7.5	10	12.2	1.4
7.5	15	27.4	1
7.5	20	48.7	0.7
10	8	10.4	1.4
10	10	16.2	1.1
10	15	36.5	0.7
10	20	64.9	0.5

studies usually entail medium-frequency medium-diameter transducers, whereas larger patients or harder to penetrate areas may require low-frequency large-diameter transducers. Various methods to enhance sensitivity permit the use of a higher frequency transducer.

Self-Focusing Effect

Before we leave this topic, the assumption that, in the near field, the beam width is equal to the transducer crystal diameter should be clarified. The nonfocused single-crystal transducer has a self-focusing effect so the beam width actually decreases to a minimum value at the transition point between the near field and far field and then begins to diverge. In fact, the beam width at the transition point is equal to half the diameter of the crystal (Fig. 5-15). The maximum acoustic pressure actually occurs at the transition point, because the same power is distributed over a smaller area. At a distance equal to twice the NFD, the beam diameter diverges to a size equal to the crystal diameter. The following formulas describe the near-field beam width (w_N) and the far-field beam width (w_F).

5-4

$$w_N = D - \frac{2\lambda z}{D}$$

5-5

$$w_F = \frac{2\lambda z}{D}$$

where D is the crystal diameter, λ is the wavelength of the ultrasound, and z is the depth of interest.

Two special cases are considered in the following examples.

■ Example 5-5

Calculate the beam width at the transition point, where $z = \text{NFD}$, the depth of the near field:

$$w_N = D - \frac{2\,\lambda z}{D}$$

and

$$z = \frac{D^2}{4\,\lambda}$$

Therefore

$$w_N = D - \frac{2\,\lambda D^2}{4\,\lambda D}$$

$$w_N = \frac{D}{2}$$

This example illustrates that the beam width at the transition zone is half the crystal diameter, rather than equal to the crystal diameter, as is normally assumed.

■ Example 5-6

Calculate the beam width at a distance in the far field that is equal to twice the near-field depth, where $z = 2\ \text{NFD}$.

$$w_F = \frac{2\,\lambda z}{D}$$

and

$$z = \frac{2\,D^2}{4\,\lambda}$$

Therefore

$$w_F = \frac{2\,\lambda\,(2\,D^2)}{4\,\lambda D}$$

$$w_F = D$$

This example demonstrates that the beam width in the far field is less than or equal to the crystal diameter up to a distance of twice the NFD.

Thus the lateral resolution, based on beam width, is better than normally expected for nonfocused transducers. Typically, however, the beam shape changes in the presence of an attenuating medium, and therefore the beam width is assumed equal to the crystal diameter in the near field.

SIDE LOBES

Side lobes are secondary projections of ultrasonic energy that radiate away from the main ultrasound beam (Fig. 5-16). Immediate echoes (reverberations at the transducer-tissue interface), pulse shape, transducer design, and radial mode vibration all contribute to the formation of side lobes. Radial mode vibration (nonthickness mode) refers to the expansion and contraction of the circular disk along the radial direction (Fig. 5-17). The position (angle) and intensity of side lobes can be predicted from directivity functions obtained by solving the wave equation.

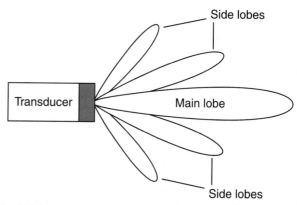

Fig. 5-16 Side lobes. Sound energy radiates in multiple directions. The intensity of the side lobes is less than that of the main lobe.

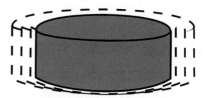

Fig. 5-17 Radial mode vibrations of a circular transducer contribute to side lobe formation.

The intensity of side lobes is normally 60 to 100 dB below that of the main ultrasound beam, which usually does not pose significant problems. If present at high intensity levels, however, side lobes create artifacts (presentation of off-axis structures) and noise in the image. Clutter, a type of acoustic noise, consists of low-amplitude signals from weak echoes that originate from secondary lobes striking off-axis structures.

Broad bandwidth (low-Q) transducers create fewer and less intense side lobes than do high-Q transducers, although the main lobe intensity pattern is widened.

FOCUSING

Lateral resolution (a major consideration for diagnostic ultrasound imaging) can be improved by focusing the transducer crystal (Fig. 5-18). Focusing limits the useful NFD, because the beam diverges rapidly beyond the focal zone. The **focal zone** is defined as the region where intensity has a value within 3 dB of the maximum along the transducer axis. Manufacturers may also quote a larger focal zone based on intensity measurements within 6 dB of the maximum. The focal zone or focused area is closer to the face of the transducer than the nonfocused NFD, provided the transducers are of equal diameter and frequency. The focal zone may not be symmetrical around the focal point, which is the point of maximum intensity. At the focal point the beam is most narrow. The intensity of an ultrasound beam at the focal point is expected to be greater than that for the same diameter of nonfocused transducer, because the cross-sectional area of the beam is less for the focused than for the nonfocused beam.

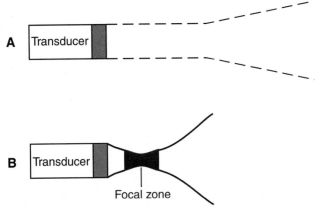

A Transducer

B Transducer

Focal zone

Fig. 5-18 Ultrasonic field for focused versus nonfocused transducers. **A,** Nonfocused transducer; **B,** focused transducer. Note that the focal zone is within the near field on the nonfocused transducer.

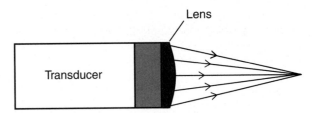

Lens

Transducer

Fig. 5-19 Focused transducer with an acoustic lens.

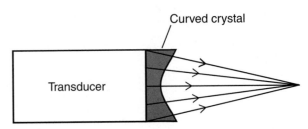

Curved crystal

Transducer

Fig. 5-20 Focused transducer with a curved piezoelectric crystal.

The magnitude of an intensity increase produced by focusing may be as high as a factor of 100. Attenuation will shift the maximum intensity from the transition point to a location closer to the face of the nonfocused transducer. Attenuation may also dramatically affect the intensity of focused beams. When a patient is being scanned, the lack of tissue uniformity may have a dramatic effect on the position of the focal zone compared with that observed in a uniform phantom. The axial resolution may be somewhat worse for the focused beam in the focal zone, because the stronger echoes are detected over a lengthened time interval (the received signal is elongated).

Focusing Methods

To improve the lateral resolution, a single-element transducer can be focused in two ways. Sound follows many of the same principles as light. It can be focused by an acoustic lens that works in a manner similar to a light lens. Acoustic lenses are formed from polystyrene, nylon, or aluminum and placed in front of the piezoelectric crystal (Fig. 5-19). The velocity of sound in the lens is greater than that in tissue; thus sound waves are bent toward a point in tissue (principle of refraction). This is an example of external focusing.

The most common form of focusing for transducers with frequencies of less than 5 MHz uses a curved crystal (Fig. 5-20), which is an internal focusing method. For frequencies above 5 MHz, external focusing methods are normally used, because the crystals become extremely thin and are difficult to form into curved shapes of proper uniformity without breaking. With a velocity of 4000 m/s for PZT, a 5 MHz crystal has a wavelength of 0.8 mm and a 10 MHz crystal has a wavelength of 0.4 mm. The crystal thickness is equal to half the wavelength. Therefore the thickness of the crystal is 0.4 mm for the 5 MHz transducer and 0.2 mm for the 10 MHz transducer. Real-time ultrasound scanning systems employ electronic focusing methods in addition to the mechanical methods just outlined. (See Chapter 8 for details.)

Degree of Focusing

The distance from the front face of the transducer to the focal point is called the **focal length** (F). The degree of focusing can be changed to vary the focal length by increasing the radius of curvature of the crystal or by increasing the curvature of the acoustic lens. This allows transducers operating at the same frequency to be made with focal zones at different depths, depending on the degree of focusing (Fig. 5-21). As the degree of focusing becomes stronger, the beam width is made more narrow, but the focal zone is drawn closer to the face of the transducer.

The **degree of focusing** (κ) is expressed quantitatively as the ratio of NFD to focal length.

5-6

$$\kappa = \frac{\text{NFD}}{\text{F}} = \frac{a^2}{\lambda F}$$

In this scheme, weak focusing has a value of less than 6, medium focusing a value of 6 to 20, and strong focusing a value greater than 20.

■ Example 5-7

Calculate the degree of focusing (κ) for a 3-cm diameter crystal operating at a frequency of 3 MHz if the focal length is 7 cm.

$$\kappa = \frac{a^2}{\lambda F}$$

$$\kappa = \frac{(15 \text{ mm})^2}{(0.51 \text{ mm})(70 \text{ mm})}$$

$$\kappa = 6$$

Weak-focused transducers (also called long-focused) composed of a single element have a focal length of 7 to 19 cm, medium-focused transducers a focal length of 4 to 10 cm, and strong-focused (short-focused) transducers a focal length of 1 to 4 cm. Focusing, particularly for real-time scanners, has been one of the major reasons why ultrasound

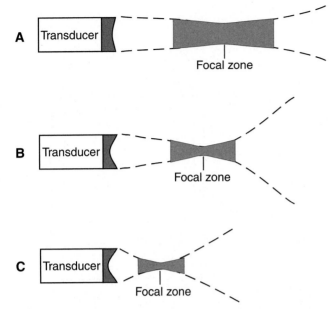

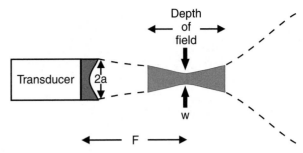

Fig. 5-22 Parameters describing the ultrasonic field for a focused transducer, 2a aperture, depth of field, focal length, and beam width.

■ **Table 5-4** Beam Width versus Frequency for Constant Aperture (2a = 20 mm) and Constant Focal Length (F = 4 cm)

Frequency (MHz)	Wavelength (mm)	Focal Length (cm)	Beam Width (mm)
2	0.77	4	2.2
4	0.38	4	1.1
6	0.26	4	0.72
8	0.19	4	0.54
10	0.15	4	0.43

■ **Table 5-5** Beam Width versus Focal Length for Constant Frequency (4 MHz) and Constant Aperture (2a = 20 mm)

Frequency (MHz)	Wavelength (mm)	Focal Length (cm)	Beam Width (mm)
4	0.38	2	0.5
4	0.38	4	1.1
4	0.38	6	1.6
4	0.38	8	2.2
4	0.38	10	2.6

Fig. 5-21 As the focusing is made stronger, the beam width decreases, the focal zone moves closer to the face of the transducer, and the intensity increases in the focal zone. **A,** Weak or long focusing; **B,** medium focusing; **C,** strong or short focusing.

is so widely accepted today as a clinical imaging modality. (Methods of checking the transducer focus are discussed in Chapter 24.)

Beam Width

One of the major advantages of focusing is to reduce the beam width in the focal zone (Fig. 5-22).

The **beam width** in the focal zone is determined by aperture (2a), focal length (F), and wavelength (λ):

$$w = \frac{1.4\,\lambda F}{2a} = \frac{1.4\,Fc}{2\,af} \tag{5-7}$$

As frequency and aperture size (diameter of the crystal) are increased, beam width at a designated focal length is reduced, which is illustrated in Examples 5-8, 5-9, and 5-10.

■ Example 5-8

Calculate the beam width in the focal zone for a 1-cm diameter transducer operating at 3 MHz. The focal length is 6 cm.

$$w = \frac{1.4\,\lambda F}{2a}$$

$$w = \frac{1.4\,(0.51\text{ mm})(60\text{ mm})}{10\text{ mm}}$$

$$w = 4.3\text{ mm}$$

■ Example 5-9

Calculate the beam width in the focal zone for a 1-cm diameter transducer operating at 5 MHz. The focal length is 6 cm.

$$w = \frac{1.4\,(0.31\text{ mm})(60\text{ mm})}{10\text{ mm}}$$

$$w = 2.6\text{ mm}$$

■ Example 5-10

Calculate the beam width in the focal zone for a 2 cm diameter transducer operating at 3 MHz. The focal length is 6 cm.

$$w = \frac{1.4\,(0.51\text{ mm})(60\text{ mm})}{20\text{ mm}}$$

$$w = 2.1\text{ mm}$$

Tables 5-4, 5-5, and 5-6 summarize calculations of beam width versus frequency, focal length, and aperture, respectively. To illustrate the effect of one parameter (frequency, focal length, or aperture) on beam width, the remaining parameters are held constant.

F-Number

Another parameter used to characterize focusing is the **f-number** or the ratio of focal length to the aperture

$$\text{f-number} = \frac{F}{2a} \tag{5-8}$$

■ **Table 5-6** Beam Width versus Diameter for Constant Frequency (4 MHz) and Constant Focal Length (F = 4 cm)

Frequency (MHz)	Wavelength (mm)	Aperture (cm)	Beam Width (mm)
4	0.38	4	0.5
4	0.38	3	0.7
4	0.38	2	1.1
4	0.38	1	2.1

Stronger focusing is indicated by decreased f-number. (The focal zone is moved closer to the transducer without changing aperture size.)

Depth of Field

The focal zone is the region within the ultrasonic field that provides the best lateral resolution. The length of the focal zone (or **depth of field**) is given by

5-9

$$\text{Depth of field} = 7.1\,\lambda\ (\text{f-number}) = \frac{7.1\,\lambda F^2}{4a^2}$$

■ **Example 5-11**

What is the depth of field for the transducers in Examples 5-8, 5-9, and 5-10?

For a 1-cm diameter transducer operating at 3 MHz with a focal length of 6 cm

$$\text{Depth of field} = \frac{7.1\,\lambda F^2}{4a^2}$$

$$\text{Depth of field} = \frac{7.1(0.51\ \text{mm})\,(60\ \text{mm})^2}{(10\ \text{mm})^2}$$

$$\text{Depth of field} = 13\ \text{cm}$$

For a 1-cm diameter transducer operating at 5 MHz with a focal length of 6 cm

$$\text{Depth of field} = \frac{7.1(0.31\ \text{mm})\,(60\ \text{mm})^2}{(10\ \text{mm})^2}$$

$$\text{Depth of field} = 7.9\ \text{cm}$$

For a 2-cm diameter transducer operating at 3 MHz with a focal length of 6 cm

$$\text{Depth of field} = \frac{7.1(0.51\ \text{mm})\,(60\ \text{mm})^2}{(20\ \text{mm})^2}$$

$$\text{Depth of field} = 3.2\ \text{cm}$$

Depth Dependence of Lateral Resolution

Lateral resolution is not constant throughout the scan range. Since the beam width changes with depth, the ability to represent small objects as small objects changes with depth (Fig. 5-23). The ability to resolve adjacent structures will also depend on their location in the ultrasonic field.

Factors affecting beam width and hence lateral resolution are summarized in Table 5-7.

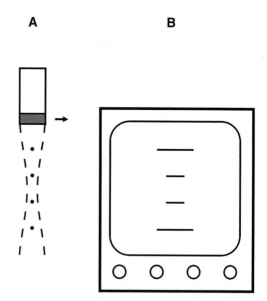

Fig. 5-23 Depth dependence of beam width. **A,** Beam width changes with depth for a focused transducer. The small reflectors at different depths are not displayed with equal lateral extent, **B.**

■ **Table 5-7** Effects on Beam Width

Parameter	Change	Effect on Beam Width
Frequency	Increase	Decrease
Aperture	Increase with F constant	Decrease
Aperture	Increase with f-number constant	No change
Focusing	Increase degree of focusing	Decrease
Focal length	Decrease	Decrease

RECEPTION

Any discussion of ultrasonic instrumentation must include the basic A-mode scanner, from which all other scanning systems are derived by incorporating various modifications. A-mode scanning is an echo-ranging technique in which an ultrasound beam is directed along a single path into the body. Detected echoes from interfaces along this path are displayed as a series of spikes. The position of the spikes along the horizontal display axis denotes the depth of the interface; the height of the spikes denotes the strength of the echo. The A-mode scanner is used here as a model to demonstrate the fundamentals of echo reception and signal processing.

A system has been devised in which a transducer is used to generate an ultrasound beam via the converse piezoelectric effect and then to direct that beam into the body. As the ultrasound wave strikes various interfaces in the body, some of the energy is transmitted, and some is reflected, in accordance with the reflection formula (Equation 1-8). The reflected echo returns to the transducer, and the pressure wave incident on the crystal is converted into an electrical signal and processed for display.

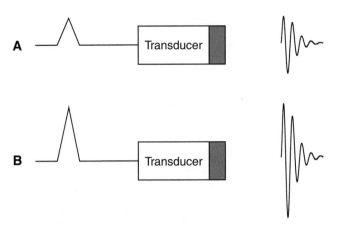

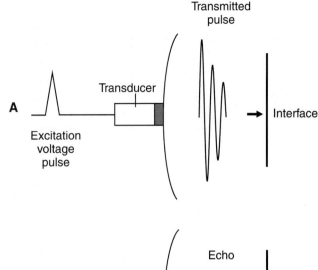

Fig. 5-24 Excitation voltage regulates the transmitted beam intensity. **A,** Low voltage. **B,** High voltage.

Transmit Power or Gain

Most ultrasound units include an output, power, or transmit gain control that adjusts the voltage spike to the crystal to produce an acoustic pulse of higher intensity. This results in a stronger echo (Fig. 5-24). The typical excitation voltage pulse is about 150 volts. Frequently, the control is adjustable in 1 to 3 dB increments.

Increased sound wave intensity enhances the detectability of weak reflectors. However, higher intensity levels increase patient exposure, and unlimited power gain does not continue to improve sensitivity. In addition, high intensity distorts the sinusoidal pressure wave (nonlinear propagation), altering both the acoustic velocity and the reception of sound waves. Nonlinear propagation has developed into an imaging modality (tissue harmonic imaging), which will be discussed in Chapter 9.

Amplification

The echo, in the form of mechanical pressure waves, strikes the crystal and induces a radiofrequency (RF) signal via the piezoelectric effect (Fig. 5-25). The waveform of the RF signal mimics the ultrasound waveform, since the voltage variations are in response to pressure-induced thickness changes in the crystal. A preamplifier located very near the piezoelectric crystal provides initial signal amplification to enable signal transfer to the amplifier without significant degradation from spurious electronic signals. The preamplifier also isolates other components from the transmitter during excitation to prevent damage to these components. In the amplifier the microvolt or millivolt RF signal is increased to 1 to 10 volts for processing and display purposes. The amount of amplification is designated by the term *gain,* which equals the ratio of the output signal to the input signal. Combinations of linear, exponential, logarithmic, and variable amplifications can be used.

The most common type of receiver gain is logarithmic. The amount of amplification or gain is adjustable by the operator. Weak signals undergo greater amplification than do strong signals. The disparity between weak and strong reflectors is diminished. **Dynamic range** (usually expressed

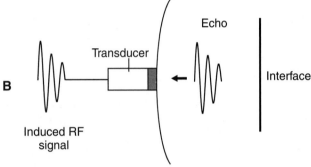

Fig. 5-25 Transmission of pulsed wave and reception of echo. **A,** Acoustic wave initiated by the excitation pulse applied to the transducer striking an interface. **B,** The echo on return to the transducer induces the radiofrequency signal.

in decibels) is the ratio of the largest to the smallest signal that can be accommodated by a system component. Logarithmic amplification reduces the dynamic range of the induced RF signals. Decreasing the dynamic range is called compression.

Most gain controls adjust only the amplification of the received signals and have no effect on the intensity of the generated ultrasound beam. The improved sensitivity in these cases is the result of extra amplification only and possible tuning of the receiver to allow detection of weaker signals.

Time Gain Compensation

One problem that must be considered is the attenuation of an ultrasonic beam with depth. Equally reflective interfaces produce different signal levels, depending on their relative distances from the transducer. It is often advantageous to display reflectors of similar size, shape, and reflection coefficients with equal signal strengths or brightness levels.

Time-dependent exponential amplification (called time gain compensation [TGC], depth gain compensation [DGC], swept gain control, depth-varied gain, distance-attenuation compensation, and sensitivity-time control) is used to correct the signals for attenuation. This can be easily demonstrated: Assume that a phantom is composed of alternating layers of water and gelatin (Fig. 5-26, *A*) that are very similar in acoustic impedance. Each layer is 1 cm thick.

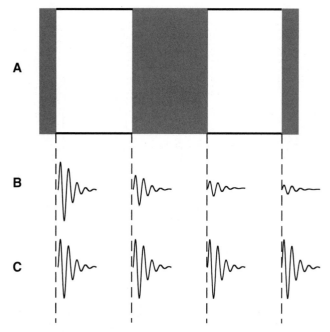

Fig. 5-26 Effect of time gain compensation (TGC). **A,** Phantom composed of alternating layers of water *(white)* and gelatin *(gray)*. All interfaces have the same composition. **B,** Signal amplitude versus depth without TGC. **C,** Signal amplitude versus depth with TGC.

A small fraction of the incident beam is reflected at each interface, and the percentage reflected is constant for every interface in the phantom. Recall that the reflection formula (Equation 1-8) does not distinguish which medium contains the incident beam.

Because of attenuation, however, the display shows exponentially decreasing signal strengths (Fig. 5-26, *B*) rather than signals of equal amplitude. To compensate for this attenuation, a TGC control is used to increase the amplitude of processed signals with time or depth (Fig. 5-26, *C*). The amplification could be a reverse exponential function, because the signals decrease exponentially (Fig. 5-27). TGC also contributes to signal compression. When the liver is scanned with TGC, all echoes should be of nearly the same amplitude, unless an abnormality is present or vessels are observed.

Automatic TGC (also called adaptive gain control, auto-gain control, and auto-sensitivity control) adjusts the time-varying gain without operator intervention. The amount of amplification is determined by the general decrease in echo-induced signal amplitude. This assumes that the detected structures have similar reflectivity.

Time Gain Compensation Controls

Different tissues have varying rates of attenuation. The frequency response of the attenuation rate depends on the tissue type. This, along with the capability to enhance a particular area of interest, makes a variable gain control desirable. Some diagnostic ultrasound units have a combination of three TGC controls (Fig. 5-28). The near gain or

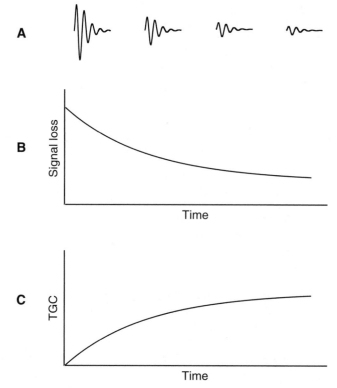

Fig. 5-27 Time gain compensation (TGC). **A,** Signal amplitude versus depth without TGC. **B,** Exponential loss in signal caused by attenuation. **C,** Reverse exponential TGC used to modify the signal levels in **A.**

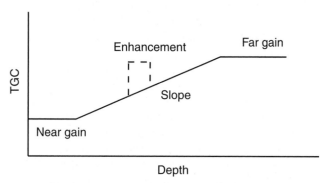

Fig. 5-28 Control adjustments for time gain compensation.

mean gain adjusts the level at which the initial signals are amplified. The delay regulates the depth at which the TGC begins. Often it is convenient not to amplify signals originating close to the transducer, because they have high amplitude levels. The slope of the TGC indicates the amount of compensation that is applied with depth. The far gain represents the maximum amount that signals can be amplified. In this zone the signals are amplified by a constant amount, but they exhibit an exponential decrease because of attenuation. A completely variable gain control may also be included to permit a particular area of interest to be enhanced beyond the amplification provided by TGC.

Variable TGC controls are commonly configured in a slider knob arrangement in which each knob corresponds to a particular depth, and movement of the knob left to right increases the applied gain at that depth. The association of each knob with depth depends on the scan range. Often, the variation of gain with depth is displayed on the monitor to provide feedback to the operator. This allows adjustment for smooth transition from one knob-controlled region to the next.

The variable TGC controls permit adjustable compensation for different frequency transducers, allowing greater amplification when high frequencies are used. Remember: Attenuation in soft tissue is frequency dependent. As the frequency is increased, more amplification is required to counteract the accelerated loss of beam intensity.

Flexibility in the TGC controls enables higher quality images to be obtained. Nevertheless, the sonographer must be more aware of the functions of the different controls; furthermore, he or she must also interact more with the system during scanning. A scanner with selectable TGC controls can produce poor quality images when operated by an inexperienced individual. Automation of the TGC controls provides more consistent images, but they are often poorer in overall quality.

SIGNAL PROCESSING

The RF signal induced in the transducer by the returning echoes could be amplified and then displayed, but it would then appear similar to the acoustic pulse sent out. If numerous interfaces are present, the interpretation of the received signals becomes confusing. For viewing ease, the goal is to process the signal before displaying it. The processing lowers the information content (smaller dynamic range) while, at the same time, facilitates the association of final output with physical structures.

The normal processing procedure involves rectification (converting the negative portion of the RF signal to positive) after the signal has been amplified and has undergone TGC amplification (Fig. 5-29). Alternatively, the negative component of the RF wave can be eliminated rather than flipped to positive. The peaks of the RF waves are "electronically" surrounded or enveloped, resulting in a processed signal that could be further amplified for display purposes (Fig. 5-30). Enveloping is often referred to as demodulation and is generally accomplished by passing the signal through a circuit with a slow time response. The overall outline of the pulse is retained, but the internal fast oscillations are lost. This is not the true meaning of demodulation, but it shows how the term is used in this context. Demodulation normally involves removing a signal that has undergone interference with a carrier wave, which is important in Doppler ultrasound (as discussed in Chapter 14).

Usually the area under the enveloped signal is electronically measured. Determination of the area is called integration. This area is then represented as a spike for A-mode scanning or as a dot for other scanning techniques. An increase in the amplitude of the induced RF signal results in a larger area under the curve and therefore an increase in displayed echo signal (Fig. 5-31).

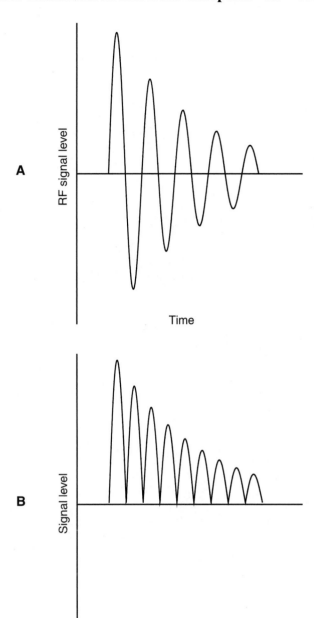

Fig. 5-29 Rectification. **A,** The crystal response to an incident sound wave induces a radiofrequency signal in the receiver circuit. **B,** In the rectified signal negative components are flipped to become positive.

A reject control (also called threshold or suppression control) may be added to eliminate low-level signals and noise below a certain level, as selected by the operator (Fig. 5-32). The reject control is similar to the lower level discriminator used in radiation counting systems. Rejection of signals decreases the dynamic range.

DISPLAY

For the simplest scanning system (A-mode), echoes received from different depths are displayed on a cathode ray tube (CRT). A voltage to the horizontal plates moves the time base sweep across the display at a constant rate that correlates

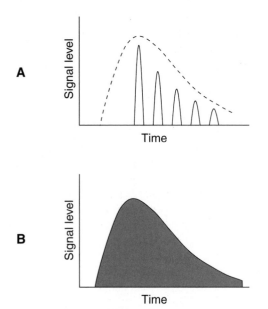

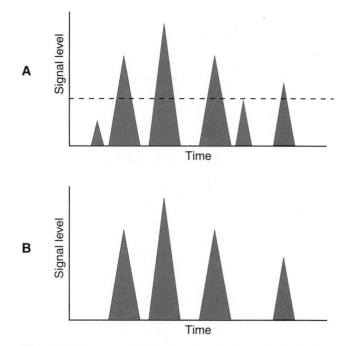

Fig. 5-30 Enveloping. **A,** The induced radiofrequency signal that has been enveloped (i.e., an electronic surrounding of the peaks). **B,** Resultant enveloped signal.

Fig. 5-32 Reject control. The four signals above the threshold (*dotted line,* **A**) are processed and ultimately displayed (**B**); the others, below the threshold, are not.

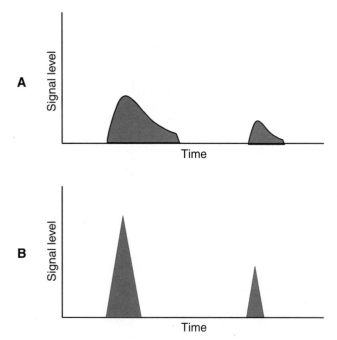

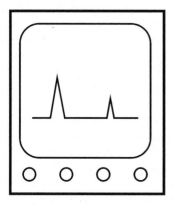

Fig. 5-31 Integration. **A** is two enveloped signals; **B** is the area under each enveloped signal (represented as a spike).

Fig. 5-33 Cathode ray tube trace showing two interfaces.

with the speed of ultrasound in tissue. The sweep, which must advance the equivalent of 1 cm on the distance scale for every 13 μs, is initiated by a pulse from the master synchronizer, and as it progresses across the display, the signal detected for each interface is amplified and sent to the vertical deflection plates to control the electron beam's vertical position.

For example, assume that an interface generates a 5-volt pulse to the vertical deflection plates. This would deflect the electron beam upward. Because the duration of the induced pulse is short, the voltage on the vertical deflection plates

would return to zero, and the electron beam would move back to the baseline in but a fraction of a second. The electron beam would again be deflected vertically when the next interface was encountered, and the signal would be sent to the display (Fig. 5-33). This whole process occurs repeatedly many times per second for the single line of sight, which thus defines the direction of sampling.

As long as the transducer is directed along the same line of sight (scan line), the displayed signals remain unchanged, because the scan is repeated many times each second. The sampling rate is equal to the pulse repetition frequency (PRF) of the unit (200 to 2000 times per second). If the transducer is positioned toward a new line of sight, the displayed signals change in accordance with the interfaces encountered along this line. Once again, the scan is displayed at the rate of the PRF. Fig. 5-34 is a typical A-mode display showing a plot of echo amplitude versus time or depth.

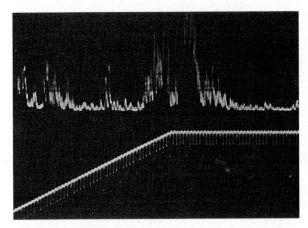

Fig. 5-34 A-mode display of the liver *(top curve)* with the accompanying time gain compensation *(lower curve).*

DYNAMIC RANGE

The **dynamic range,** which is a measure of the signal magnitudes (expressed in dB) that can be identified and manipulated by various components of the ultrasound system, needs to be considered in more detail. Strong signals greater than a certain level produce the same response (saturation). Weak signals below a certain amount (threshold) are not detected. Echo amplitudes may be as much as 100 to 150 dB (or a factor of 10^{10} to 10^{15}) below the original intensity sent into the body depending on the depth of sampling and frequency of the transducer. This wide range of echo strengths is also present in the induced signals from the receiver section.

TGC and logarithmic amplification reduce the dynamic range to about 80 dB. Depending on the processing method, the dynamic range may be further reduced. The output device (CRT or TV) decreases the dynamic range to 20 to 40 dB. The signals normally undergo greatest compression in the display system. The recording device reduces the useful range even further, to 10 to 20 dB. Fig. 5-35 summarizes the compression of information.

Compression by TGC and thresholding is desirable, because these signal-processing steps attempt to correlate displayed signal level with reflectivity. Compression is necessary, however, between detection and display, because system components have limited capacity to preserve the range of signal magnitudes. The best example of this limitation is the brightness levels available on a CRT. Suppose eight brightness levels are available. The entire dynamic range of signals must then be depicted as one of eight values when the echo data are displayed. Ultimately, signals must be combined in groups so they can be managed by the CRT.

If the original data could be maintained without loss, then noninvasive tissue characterization might be possible. Much research has been devoted to reducing data compression and increasing the dynamic range of ultrasound systems. Fourier analysis, as well as special feature analysis using multiple frequency images, may play a major role in tissue characterization. The ultimate aim is to identify malignant, benign, and normal tissues without surgical intervention.

NOISE

If a reflector is probed repeatedly with a series of pulsed ultrasound waves, each wave creates an echo characteristic of the object. The returning echoes are detected by the transducer. Under these conditions induced signals of equal strength are expected. In practice, however, the signal amplitude is not constant but fluctuates from one measurement to the next. This variation is known as **noise** (or random noise).

Noise is inherent in the measurement process and cannot be totally eliminated. System electronics also contributes to it. External sources of noise include environmental RF interference and power line voltage fluctuations. Signals must be processed and displayed in the presence of noise (Fig. 5-36). As weaker and weaker signals approach the noise level, they become more difficult to identify. The relative amplitude of the signal compared to the noise variation is delineated by the signal-to-noise ratio (SNR).

High SNRs indicate strong signals, which are easily detected. A minimum SNR of 3 to 5 is necessary to distinguish weak echoes from the noise. The sensitivity of an ultrasound instrument is often quantified by measuring the SNR from a well-defined reflector.

Improvements in equipment design have reduced the noise level and improved the sensitivity of modern scanners.

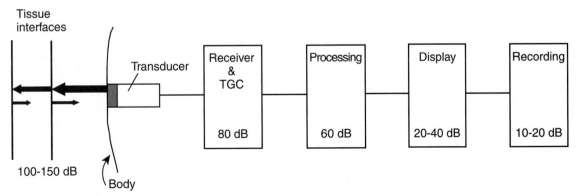

Fig. 5-35 Dynamic range associated with the various components of an ultrasound system.

A

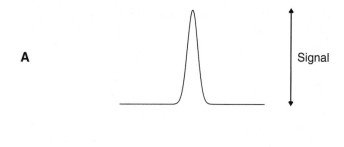

Signal

B

Noise

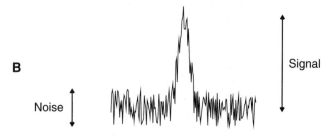

Signal

Fig. 5-36 Effect of noise on the processed signal. **A,** Ideal signal (no noise). **B,** Noise masking the true signal.

Since noise is random, signal processing cannot isolate the signal from the noise; that is, mathematical corrections applied to the detected signal to eliminate the noise are not possible. When averaged together, however, the induced signals from multiple samplings of an interface increase the SNR. This is called frame averaging or persistence and is discussed in Chapter 10.

SUMMARY

A piezoelectric material is electronically stimulated to produce an ultrasonic pressure wave via the converse piezoelectric effect. The ultrasound wave enters the patient's body, and a small portion is reflected at the various interfaces in accordance with the percentage reflection relation presented in Chapter 1. Returning echoes strike the transducer and, because of the piezoelectric effect, induce a voltage (RF signal). The RF signals undergo both amplification and TGC. The latter compensates for attenuation of the sound wave with depth. The electronically amplified and processed signal is represented as a voltage spike on the CRT. The height of the spike is proportional to the amplitude of the originally detected signal. The master synchronizer initiates the excitation voltage pulse to the transducer as well as the start signals to activate the timer mechanisms for TGC and special electronic processing. It also provides electronic signals for the time base sweep of the CRT.

The display format for the CRT consists of amplitude in the vertical direction versus distance or time in the horizontal direction. A linearly increasing voltage is applied to the horizontal deflection plates from the master synchronizer so the electron beam moves at a rate of 1 cm every 13 μs. All electronic trigger signals must be synchronized for the correct depth (time) measurement of each interface to be displayed on the screen. Sweeps across the CRT are repeated 200 to 2000 times per second, and thus the pattern of deflections appears stationary to the human eye.

REVIEW QUESTIONS

1. What transducer factors affect the axial resolution?
2. What transducer factors affect beam width?
3. Near-field depth is directly proportional to the frequency and the square of the _____.
4. Far-field divergence for a nonfocused transducer is decreased as the _____ is increased.
5. Calculate the depth of the near field for a 20-mm-diameter, nonfocused, 3 MHz transducer.
6. Calculate the far-field divergence for a 20-mm-diameter, nonfocused, 3 MHz transducer.
7. Why is the ultrasound beam focused?
8. Name two focusing methods.
9. Time gain compensation (TGC) is a variable amplification technique that corrects for _____ along the beam path.
10. List in order from echo reception the processing techniques of TGC, rectification, reject, enveloping, and integration that are applied.
11. Why is broad dynamic range important in ultrasound detection?
12. Noise affects system sensitivity and inhibits the detection of _____ echoes.
13. What are side lobes? The intensity of side lobes can be reduced by _____ the Q-value.
14. What effect do logarithmic amplification and TGC have on dynamic range of echo signals?

BIBLIOGRAPHY

Bushberg JT et al: *The essential physics of medical imaging,* ed 2, Baltimore, 2002, Lippincott Williams & Wilkins.

McDicken WN: *Diagnostic ultrasonics: principles and use of instruments,* ed 3, Edinburgh, 1991, Churchill Livingstone.

Thomenius KE: Instrumentation of B-mode imaging. In Goldman LW, Fowlkes JB, eds. *Medical CT and ultrasound: current technology and applications,* Madison, Wisc, 1995, Advanced Medical Publishing.

Turnbull DH: Fundamentals of acoustic transduction. In Goldman LW, Fowlkes JB, eds. *Medical CT and ultrasound: current technology and applications,* Madison, Wisc, 1995, Advanced Medical Publishing.

Zagzebski JA: *Essential of ultrasound physics,* St Louis, 1996, Mosby-Year Book.

CHAPTER 6

Static Imaging Principles and Instrumentation

A-mode
B-mode
C-mode
Line of sight

Position generator
Registration arm
Scan converter

Ultrasound as a clinical modality began in the mid-1950s with the use of A-mode scanning for examination of the eye and for echoencephalography. In the early to mid-1970s ultrasound instrumentation changed significantly with the advent of analog and digital **scan converters,** which made two-dimensional static B-mode gray-scale imaging possible. The evolution of ultrasound instrumentation continued with the introduction of real-time scanners in the late 1970s, followed by spectral Doppler and Doppler imaging in the 1980s, and three-dimensional scanning today.

Sonar (sound navigation and ranging) played a major role in the development of medical diagnostic ultrasound instrumentation, particularly in A-mode scanning. The previous two chapters described transducer design, pulse generation, and echo reception. This chapter discusses the modifications and refinements required to convert the basic unit into systems that are used for static imaging techniques. A-mode instrumentation is considered only briefly, because the basic unit described in Chapter 5 is the typical A-mode scanner. Static B-mode gray-scale imaging and specific gated scanning techniques are the main subjects of this chapter, along with transmission-mode scanning, the only technique that does not rely on the echo-ranging principle. Most static imaging systems have now been replaced by real-time, Doppler, and M-mode scanning techniques, which are the subjects of subsequent chapters.

Static imaging has a very limited role in current clinical practice. Nevertheless, the principles of static imaging are essential for understanding techniques and instrumentation having applications in diagnostic ultrasonography. The discussion of static imaging in this chapter includes multiple examples to illustrate these concepts.

A-MODE SCANNING

A-mode (amplitude-mode) scanning is based on the echo-ranging principle, similar to sonar. A pulsed ultrasound wave is directed into the patient's body, and the echoes generated at various interfaces along the beam path are detected. Only structures that lie along the direction of propagation within the ultrasound beam are interrogated. This sampling according to the beam path is called the line of sight or scan line.

Although the basic scanner is electronically complex, a block diagram (Fig. 6-1) describes the main system components and operation of the unit. All these subsystems must be synchronized in time. The clock measures the elapsed

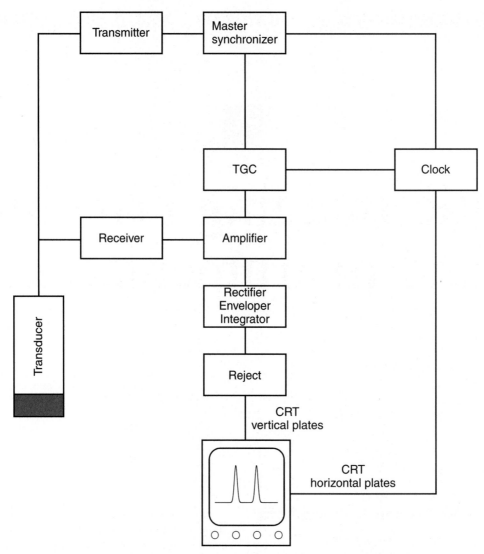

Fig. 6-1 Block diagram of the A-mode scanner. The signal processing steps of time gain compensation (TCG), amplification, integration, and reject occur before display. The cathode ray tube trace is controlled by elapsed time in the horizontal direction and signal level in the vertical direction.

time from generation of the ultrasound pulse to reception of the echoes. The block diagram shows an electroacoustic conversion device (transducer) connected to the transmitter-receiver section of the scanner. The transducer is responsible for the generation of an ultrasound beam and the detection of returning echoes. A pulsed ultrasound beam is generated and sent into the body. It undergoes various interactions (discussed in Chapter 1), and when an interface is encountered, a fraction of the beam's energy is reflected back toward the transducer. The transducer, acting as a receiver rather than a transmitter, converts the ultrasound wave (returning echo) to an electronic signal that is processed and displayed. The displayed signal must be related to interaction that has taken place in the body.

System Components

The master synchronizer initiates the scanning process by commanding the transmitter to send a voltage pulse to the

transducer. The excitation of the crystal generates a pulsed ultrasound wave (via the converse piezoelectric effect) that is directed into the body. Coincidentally, the master synchronizer sends a command to activate the clock that measures the elapsed time from transmission of the ultrasound pulse to reception of the echo. This time determines the depth of the interface based on the constant velocity of ultrasound in tissue (1540 m/s). When the transducer is excited, the master synchronizer sends a command to the display to begin moving the electron beam (time base sweep) across the screen of the cathode ray tube (CRT). The sweep rate corresponds to 1 cm every 13 μs.

As the ultrasound pulse propagates away from the transducer, part of the energy is reflected at each interface encountered along the beam path. This sampling is restricted laterally by the width of the beam. The reflected energy returns toward the transducer in the form of an echo. As the echo strikes the transducer, an electrical signal is induced in the crystal (piezoelectric effect), and this is processed for display. To correlate the amplitude of the induced signal with the depth of the interface, the time interval between the time that an ultrasound pulse leaves the transducer and the time the echo returns must be known. Any special amplification based on elapsed time, such as time gain compensation (TGC) and gating applied to the detected signals, also requires knowledge of the exact time of travel for the pulse. The processed signal is applied to the vertical deflection plates in the CRT to shift the electron beam upward during the time base sweep. The height of the deflection indicates the strength of the received echo; the position along the horizontal denotes the depth of the interfaces.

Signal Level

The term *amplitude* refers to the signal strength of a detected echo. A-mode displays the amplitude of the signal as a spike in the vertical dimension versus depth or time of reception in the horizontal dimension. Depth and time are interchangeable, because they are directly proportional. An increase in the strength of the signal gives rise to an increase in the height of the spike. This variation in signal level is due to the reflectivities of different interfaces and the attenuation of the beam as the ultrasound wave travels to and from the various interfaces. TGC attempts to correct for attenuation loss. Without TCG, strong reflectors far from the transducer may produce lower amplitude signals than weak reflectors nearer the transducer. The A-mode scan also contains spatial information; that is, it registers the distance between interfaces.

Multiple interfaces encountered along the sampling direction are detected by a series of echoes. Fig. 6-2 shows three interfaces as three separate spikes. Interface I generates a larger signal than interface II or interface III. A-mode scanning preserves the spatial relationship of the observed structures. Interface II is located closer to interface III than to interface I.

A-Mode Display

The A-mode "image" is a one-dimensional portrayal of the amplitude of the signal versus depth. A narrow beam samples the structures along the line of sight. *Only one line can be observed at any given instant on the display.* As long as the transducer and detected interfaces are stationary, the trace appears unchanged, because the CRT screen is refreshed at the rate of the pulse repetition frequency (PRF). For a different line of sight to be observed, the transducer must be moved to a different position.

A-Mode Applications

A-mode scanning is used in echoencephalography for detection of midline shift (Fig. 6-3) and for the localization of foreign bodies in the eye. A-mode information may be valuable for tissue characterization, because the detected echoes can be displayed in unaltered form. (Signal processing can be bypassed.) A greater dynamic range of signals is preserved compared with other imaging techniques.

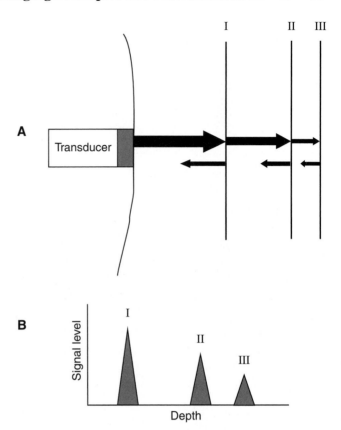

Fig. 6-2 A-mode scan and display. **A,** Three interfaces (*I, II,* and *III*). **B,** Corresponding display of the interfaces.

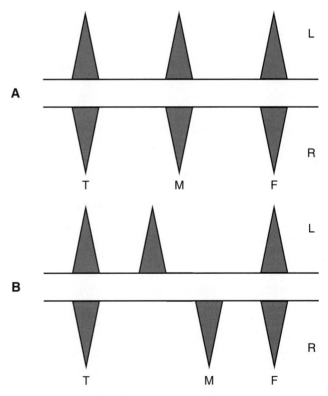

Fig. 6-3 Clinical application of the A-mode scanner. **A,** Normal echoencephalogram showing a similar pattern from the left (*L*) and right (*R*) sides. *T,* Transducer; *M,* midline; *F,* far side. **B,** Abnormal echoencephalogram with the midline spikes not aligned.

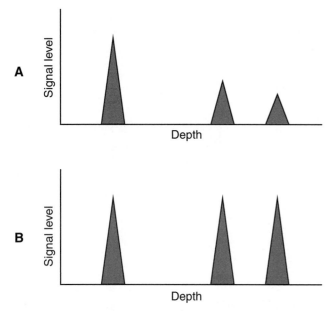

Fig. 6-4 Signals from identical reflectors located at different depths. **A,** No time gain compensation (TGC). **B,** TGC applied during signal processing.

Identification of cysts in the breast is occasionally facilitated by A-mode scanning. Nonmedical applications include nondestructive testing in industry.

ILLUSTRATIVE A-MODE SCANS

The A-mode scan can be used to illustrate the concepts of TGC, receiver gain, axial resolution, focusing, lateral resolution, and sensitivity.

Without TGC, identical reflectors at different depths have exponentially decreasing signal levels as the beam path is increased. TGC provides variable amplification based on elapsed time to correct for the effect of attenuation loss on the echo signal; thus the displayed signal level for each reflector is equal regardless of the depth of the reflector (Fig. 6-4).

Receiver gain is applied equally to all echo-induced signals so that each signal is increased in magnitude by the same factor (Fig. 6-5). This generally enhances the presentation of weak signals. The reject control eliminates weak signals with amplitudes less than the threshold value. Amplification may now display additional weak signals. Also, log compression tends to emphasize differences in weak signals, which are now available for display.

When the interfaces are located close together along the direction of propagation, the spikes in the display overlap (Fig. 6-6). The two echoes appear as one spike, which is consequently interpreted as a single interface. Echoes are more likely to be resolved if the spatial pulse length is kept short (high frequency and few cycles).

Focusing alters the intensity in the ultrasound field. The highest intensity is in the focal zone. Transducer design and instrument settings determine the beam width. Reflectors with identical acoustic properties produce different signal levels depending on their locations in the field (Fig. 6-7).

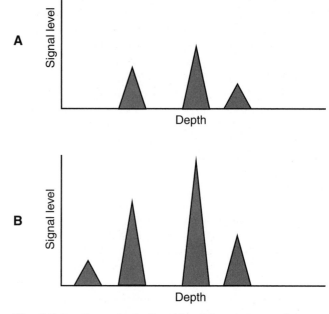

Fig. 6-5 Receiver gain. **A,** Signal levels from reflectors located at different depths. **B,** Application of a factor of 2 in receiver gain. Additional weak signal is displayed.

An echo is generated for each object within the ultrasonic field. If multiple objects are present at a certain depth, then multiple echoes are formed. However, echo ranging places the echo-induced signals at the same point on the time axis, and only one signal spike is observed (Fig. 6-8). By narrowing the beam, only one small object in the focal zone is interrogated.

The ability to detect weak echoes is improved by increasing the power setting (Fig. 6-9), although this effect is relatively small since doubling the intensity results in a sensitivity change of only 5%.

STATIC B-MODE SCANNING

Image Formation

In **B-mode** imaging the amplitude of the signal (detected echo strength) is represented by the brightness of a dot. The A-mode spike on the CRT display is converted into a dot, which can be demonstrated by rotating the spike 90 degrees out of the plane of the paper (i.e., the axis of rotation is the horizontal axis). The amplitude or strength of the signal is designated by the brightness of the dot. The position of the dot represents the depth (time) of the interface from the transducer (Fig. 6-10). The information contained in the two-dimensional A-mode display has been condensed to one dimension in the B-mode display, but the relative signal level and spatial relationship of the interfaces have been maintained.

Normally we are interested in constructing a two-dimensional image of the area of interest rather than acquiring data from a single scan line or line of sight. This is accomplished by compound B-scanning, whereby multiple

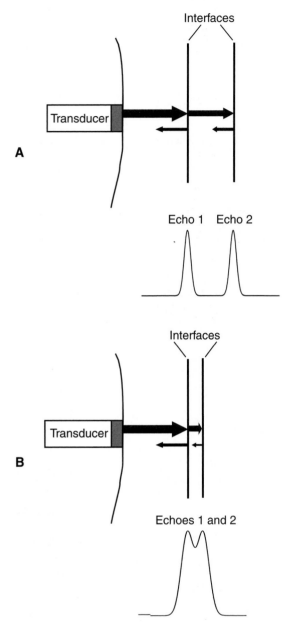

Fig. 6-6 Axial resolution in A-mode scanning. **A,** Interfaces separated by a distance greater than half the spatial pulse length are depicted as two distinct spikes. **B,** When interfaces are located close together, the returning echos strike the transducer at nearly the same time. The signals overlap and are combined into one spike.

sets of dots are combined to delineate the echo pattern from internal structures within the body. The transducer is moved across the patient so that the patient is scanned from many different directions. A single line of sight through the patient is acquired at each position of the transducer when the pulser is activated (Fig. 6-11). The scan line is composed of a series of bright dots representing the interfaces encountered along that line of sight. The superimposition of multiple scan lines creates a composite two-dimensional image, which has the advantage of portraying the general contour of the patient and the internal organs (Fig. 6-12). Compound B-mode scanning produces a static image that can be envisioned as a stop-action photograph of the reflecting surfaces.

Scanning Requirements

Two technical requirements with B-mode scanning not present with A-mode are registration (i.e., the two-dimensional placement of an echo's origin) and storage of the scan-line information. Knowledge of transducer position is essential to the proper placing of dots from different scan lines at the correct locations within the image. To build up the image, information from previous scan lines must be retained in some manner.

Registration. For the accurate localization of an interface (i.e., the origin of its echo), the horizontal and vertical position of the transducer, as well as its angulation, must be known. Thus the transducer is mounted on a special scanning or registration arm (Fig. 6-13) that indicates its precise location so the time-of-flight (depth) measurements along the beam axis can be accurately displayed. Because the transducer changes its orientation frequently during scanning, this arm must be flexible; however, at the same time, it must be stable to accurately correlate collected information within the image.

The interface location (dot) on the display is moved to the appropriate location by biasing the CRT deflection plates with voltages from the position generator. Sensors mounted in the registration arm define the position of the transducer with respect to a reference point established at the time of scanning. This information is communicated to the position generator, which calculates the appropriate deflection plate voltages as a function of elapsed time. Registration arms can be mechanical in nature, using voltage signals obtained through potentiometers to indicate the position of the transducer. A change in position of one segment of the registration arm is sensed by a change in resistance within the potentiometer, which alters the voltage sent to the position generator. Registration arms can be made using electromagnetic or optical arrangements that do not require moving electrical contacts. Some systems are computer controlled for more precise determination of transducer position.

Multiple images of the entire pelvis and abdomen in any plane (transverse, longitudinal, or sagittal) can be acquired in this manner. The registration arm is responsible for ensuring that the echo information from a particular interface is displayed at the same location, regardless of transducer orientation; that is, the interface should be in exactly the same location on the display when the subject is viewed from many different directions, as shown in Fig. 6-14. This arm should be checked periodically to ensure that echo data are displayed properly with respect to position. Otherwise, false placement of interface position can cause the image to become blurred and distorted.

Signal storage. The second requirement with B-mode scanning involves storing the signal levels at the appropriate locations for display. By moving the transducer in A-mode scanning, the trace on the CRT display can be changed. The information obtained from the previous transducer position

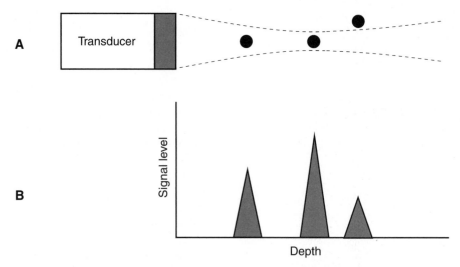

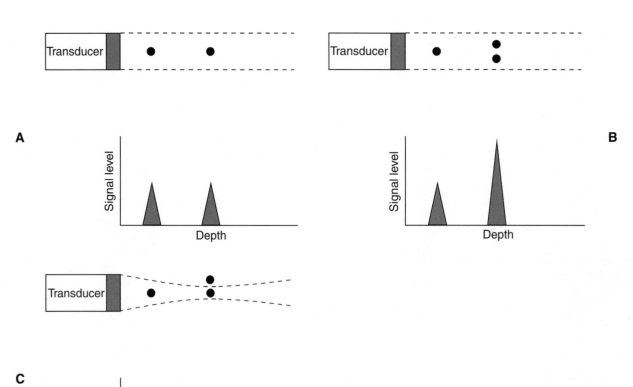

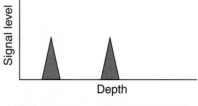

Fig. 6-7 Nonuniform beam intensity causes variation in signal level. **A,** Three identical reflectors located in the ultrasonic field of a focused transducer. **B,** A-mode scan of the reflectors. Note that the highest signal corresponds to the focal zone and that intensity does not immediately decrease to zero at the boundary of the ultrasonic field. The lowest signal is generated by a reflector located outside the indicated beam width (designating regions where the intensity is within 6 dB).

Fig. 6-8 Effect of beam width. **A,** Signal level from reflectors located at different depths. **B,** The addition of another reflector at one depth does not yield a separate signal for that reflector but rather an increase in signal level corresponding to that depth. **C,** Focusing the beam allows the reflector within the focal zone to be the primary contributor to the observed signal.

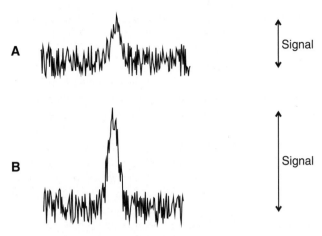

Fig. 6-9 Effect of transmitted power on the signal-to-noise ratio. **A,** Signal from a weak reflector at a low power setting. **B,** Signal from the same reflector at a high power setting. The signal-to-noise ratio is increased, and sensitivity improved. The change in signal has been exaggerated to illustrate this effect.

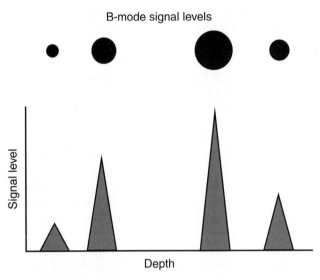

Fig. 6-10 Comparison of B-mode and A-mode displays. A-mode display of four interfaces encountered along the line of sight, which are converted to dots of varying brightness in the B-mode display. Because multiple gray levels cannot be reproduced effectively in diagrams, signal level is represented by varying the size of the dot. Brighter dots are not physically larger in the B-mode display.

is not retained on the screen. To maintain the trace, the transducer must be kept in the same position—pointed along a single line of sight. The display is continually updated with the same information (i.e., the scan is repeated over and over at the rate of the PRF). If a scan were acquired all the way around a patient, as is the case for static B-mode scanning, the initial traces would disappear from the screen before the total scan was completed. (Five to 10 seconds are required to perform a B-mode scan.) Indeed, as soon as the ultrasound beam is directed along a new line of sight, the prior trace is lost. In addition to the scanning arm modifications already discussed, a modification in the display system is necessary.

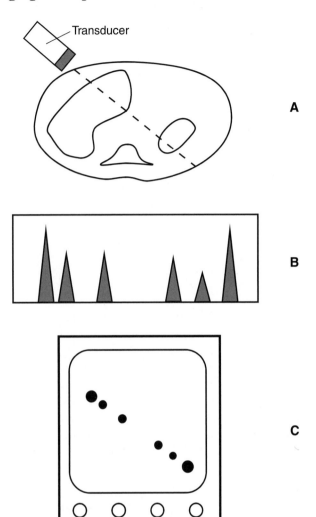

Fig. 6-11 Single scan line in B-mode. **A,** The transducer position defines the line of sight sampled. **B,** In A-mode the interfaces are represented as spikes of varying height. **C,** In B-mode the interfaces are represented as dots of varying brightness along the line of sight.

Analog Scan Converter

A-mode scan information is limited to depth and signal level only. Static B-mode, however, has three variables—two-dimensional spatial location within the scan plane and the signal level.

Initially, storage CRTs were used to display static B-mode images. These CRTs exhibit only an "on" or "off" mode. If the detected signal is strong enough, it is displayed as a light-emitting area on the phosphorescent screen. Otherwise, weak signals are read as no signals, and no light is emitted from the corresponding areas on the screen. This produces the so-called bistable image (Fig. 6-15). Most of the internal detail of organs is absent, however. Because the nonspecular reflections lost in a bistable image (i.e., when the amplitude is too low to be recorded) are desirable for analyzing normal and abnormal tissues, new storage/display technology was developed in the 1970s to show the finer detail of internal structures. Called analog scan converters, these devices enabled different echo amplitudes (i.e.,

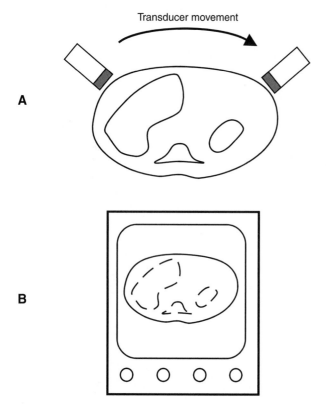

Fig. 6-12 Compound B-mode scanning. **A,** The transducer is moved to probe the patient along several lines of sight. **B,** In the display the interfaces are formed as a composite of dots along the lines of sight.

detected signal strengths) to be displayed in varying shades of gray so the fine internal structure of various organs could be visualized (Fig. 6-16). They represented a major innovation in the evolution of ultrasound.

Rapid alternating between the read (display) mode and the write (collect) mode enables the image to be viewed as it is being formed; that is, the scan converter switches back and forth from line-by-line acquisition during collection to raster-by-raster scanning during display. This characteristic is responsible for the name of the device—the scan converter. Once the data are collected, the image can be viewed by operating the device in a continuous read mode.

Digital Scan Converter

During the 1970s digital scan converters were developed. These devices are essentially solid-state computer memories that are inexpensive, reliable, and versatile. Because they do not use evacuated tubes, instability and drift associated with the analog systems is eliminated. Prolonged viewing of acquired image data is now possible, and day-to-day variations are reduced. Digital scan converter resolution is superior to the fuzzy images obtained from analog systems. Spatial resolution, however, is determined primarily by the spatial pulse length and ultrasound beam width. Raster scanning may contribute to blurring if a low number of raster lines is used.

The area scanned is divided into small rectangular or square picture elements called pixels, which make up a two-

dimensional matrix. Each pixel contains a digital number to represent the amplitude of the received echo. The placement of echo amplitudes within the matrix is designated by the position generator (Fig. 6-17). The out-of-plane width of the sound beam means that each pixel actually signifies a three-dimensional volume of tissue, called a voxel. The matrix size denotes the number of rows and columns in the pictorial representation. For example, a 512×512 matrix has 512 rows and 512 columns. The image is composed of 262,144 individual pixels. The physical extent of each pixel is typically less than 0.5 mm. The output of the computer memory (digital scan converter) is read in a raster fashion and converted back into an analog signal, which provides the input to the television cathode for display.

Signal Processing

Another feature of the scan converter system is the overwrite-protect circuit. Each interface is scanned from many orientations or directions during a B-mode acquisition. A variety of signal levels is detected for each pixel depending on the transducer orientation. When a signal is received, the appropriate location in the scan converter is identified via sensors in the registration arm and the position generator. The scan converter would replace the value that already exists in memory with the new signal amplitude if the overwrite-protect system is not present. Overwrite-protect processing permits the maximum-strength signal to be displayed for a particular location while not recording other low-amplitude signals that may be received for that same location.

The overwrite-protect circuit works in the following manner: When the interface is scanned for the first time, the associated signal level is stored in the scan converter. As the scan continues, the ultrasound wave's approach to the interface may be closer to normal incidence, resulting in a stronger detected signal. This signal level replaces the first in the scan converter for that pixel. At another scan line the interface may yield a lower signal level, which is discarded, because a higher value has previously been recorded for that location. Thus an image is generated in which the maximum signal level is recorded for each pixel. A buildup of signal levels, which would result in an all-black or all-white image, is prevented; if not, contrast would be decreased, because most pixels would contain the same numerical value for the echo amplitude.

Many other algorithms are possible for manipulating the incoming signal levels to determine the numerical value placed at a particular pixel location. These preprocessing techniques are applied before data storage. The presentation of the image on the display also can be manipulated via various postprocessing techniques (see the discussion in Chapter 10).

Spatial Resolution

For a well-designed ultrasound scanner, spatial resolution is determined by spatial pulse length and beam width only.

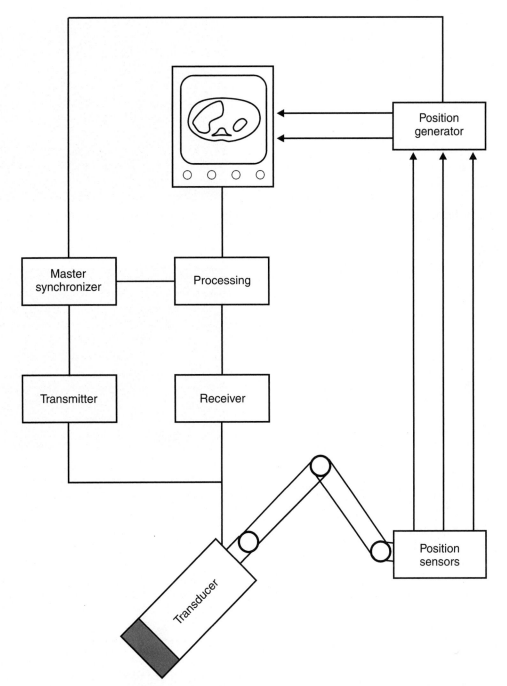

Fig. 6-13 B-mode scanner. The basic A-mode scanner modified to include a scanning arm, position generator, and storage display.

However, the digital scan converter and television system may degrade the spatial resolution beyond the limits imposed by pulse length (axial resolution) and beam width (lateral resolution). For example, assume that a patient measures 20 cm in the anterior-posterior dimension and 30 cm in the lateral dimension. This area (20 × 30 cm) is represented by a 20 × 20 digital matrix (400 pixels). The physical dimensions depicted by each pixel are 10 × 15 mm. If the pixel size is compared with the axial resolution and beam width (0.7 mm and 5 mm) obtained with a nonfocused transducer (3 MHz, 10 mm diameter, three cycles per pulse), the computer matrix size becomes the limiting factor in the image resolution.

■ **Example 6-1**

Calculate the total number of pixels (n) in a matrix that is 512 × 512.

n = Number of pixels in row × Number of pixels in column

$$n = 512 \times 512$$
$$n = 262,144$$

■ **Example 6-2**

Calculate the pixel size (x and y) if the 20 × 30 cm field of view is digitized using a 512 × 512 matrix:

$$x = \frac{\text{length in one dimension}}{\text{number of pixels in that direction}}$$

$$x = \frac{20 \text{ cm } (10 \text{ mm/cm})}{512}$$

$$x = 0.4 \text{ mm}$$

$$y = \frac{30 \text{ cm } (10 \text{ mm/cm})}{512}$$

$$y = 0.6 \text{ mm width}$$

A matrix size of 512×512 decreases the pixel size to 0.4×0.6 mm. The ultrasound beam is now the major determinant of image resolution. Some manufacturers improve the resolution of their digital scan converters by using an asymmetric matrix; that is, the number of pixels in each direction is not equal (i.e., 350×750).

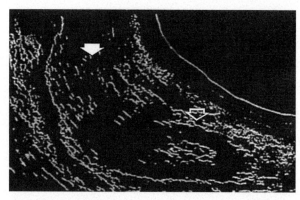

Fig. 6-15 Bistable image of a kidney *(open arrow)* and the liver *(solid arrow)*.

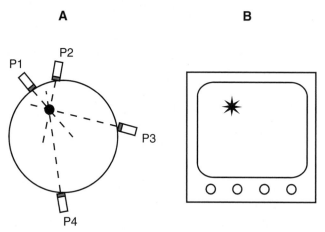

Fig. 6-14 Registration of an interface with compound B-mode. **A,** Scan of the interface from four positions *(P1, P2, P3,* and *P4)*. **B,** Display of the interface.

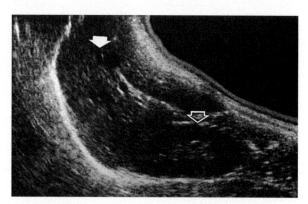

Fig. 6-16 Gray-scale image of a kidney *(open arrow)* and the liver *(solid arrow)*. Note the increased detail of these structures in this image compared with those in the bistable image shown in Fig. 6-15.

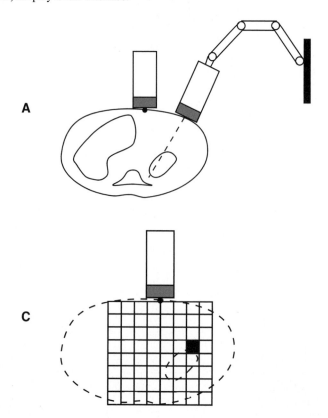

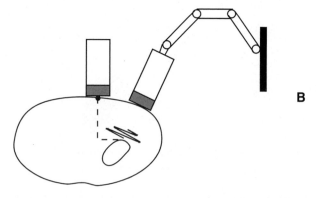

Fig. 6-17 Placement of a detected interface in the digital scan converter. **A,** Sensors in the registration arm determine the transducer location with respect to a reference point. **B,** The position generator, using the time of flight, identifies the location of the generated echo with respect to the reference point. **C,** Pixel location for the digital scan converter. Row and column are specified relative to the reference point.

A single television frame consists of 525 lines. The limit imposed on the resolution of the imaging system is similar to that contributed by the digital scan converter. This means that the vertical direction cannot depict spatial detail finer than the physical dimensions of each line.

Character Generator

The display monitor also contains a character generator, which is a device that translates coded electrical signals into light patterns that form characters on the screen. The placement of text with image data on the screen is a valuable aid in the identification of patient and the scan parameters.

Temporal Resolution

One major problem with B-mode (and other static imaging techniques) is the poor temporal resolution. Moving interfaces create blurred B-mode images. The inability of static B-mode scanning to rapidly update the displayed image with new scan data has caused the almost total replacement of this modality by real-time imaging.

Clinical Significance of Static B-Mode

The most important clinical features of static B-mode imaging are summarized in Box 6-1.

GATED-MODE SCANNING

Gated scanning is a type of B-mode imaging that requires the usual B-mode registration arm, transducer, and digital scan converter. The only difference is the additional electronics needed for gating purposes. *Gating uses a temporal marker or physiologic signal to trigger data collection.* In static B-mode scanning, short (microsecond) pulses of ultrasound are directed into the body, and all the returning echoes along that line of sight are collected before the next pulse is sent out. Occasionally, however, echoes outside the plane of interest will interfere with the desired information, or interface motion will cause significant deterioration of the image.

C-Mode Scanning

Interference from overlying and underlying structures in static B-mode scanning is partially eliminated by using constant-depth scanning (**C-mode** scanning), in which

---

Box 6-1 Important Clinical Features of Static B-mode Imaging

Large field of view
Multi-angle sampling (high signal-to-noise ratio)
Long acquisition time
Subject-to-motion artifacts
Restricted transducer movement
Single-depth focusing

---

additional gating electronics is incorporated into the standard B-mode unit.

An interface reflects part of the ultrasound beam energy (percentage reflection formula, Chapter 1). All interfaces along a scan line contribute to the normal B-mode image. The gating electronics of C-mode scanning reject all returning echoes except those received during a specified time interval. Thus only scan data obtained from a specific depth are displayed. Induced signals outside the allowed period are not amplified and thus are not processed and displayed. Detected signals within the specified period are processed and displayed, thereby creating a plane of interest or a slice (tomogram). Ultrasound tomograms are obtained in any orientation.

For example, if we were interested in a plane of depth between 5 and 6 cm, this would correspond to a time of flight (transmit and return time) of 65 μs to 78 μs (5 × 13 cm μs/cm to 6 cm × 13 μs/cm). Echoes arriving at the transducer between 65 μs and 78 μs after the transmitted ultrasound pulse would be amplified and displayed. All other echoes would not be amplified and thus would be lost (Fig. 6-18). Scanning over the region of interest produces a tomogram of the plane of interest. The gate can be adjusted to select both slice location and slice thickness.

■ **Example 6-3**

Determine the thickness of the tomographic slice if the range gates are set for 26 μs and 52 μs.

The time of travel for 1 cm is 13 μs. The start recording for displaying corresponds to a depth of 26 μs divided by 13 μs/cm, or 2 cm. The end recording for display corresponds to a depth of 52 μs divided by 13 μs/cm, or 4 cm. The slice thickness is equal to the difference between these depths, or 2 cm.

This type of gated scanning is not presently practiced for static imaging, but similar principles apply for pulsed Doppler scanning (as discussed in Chapter 14).

Electrocardiograph Gating

Electrocardiograph-gated scanning is designed to reduce motion artifacts obtained from static B-mode scanning of the heart. The motion of the heart creates a blurred image, because the positions of the structures are not constant during the time needed to collect the B-mode image. To eliminate the problem, the electrocardiogram (ECG) wave (P-QRS-T complex) acts as a gate to trigger the acquisition of scan data. By selecting the Q part of the wave as the gating point, an image of the heart at the beginning of the ventricular contraction is formed. The assumption is made that the heart walls are in the same spatial configuration during every Q portion of the wave; therefore if the information is collected, amplified, processed, and displayed only during the time of the Q gate, the heart walls will appear stationary. Repeated short samplings during a well-defined phase of the cardiac cycle prevent blurring of the heart walls in the image. During the remainder of the cardiac cycle the received echoes are not amplified and processed for display.

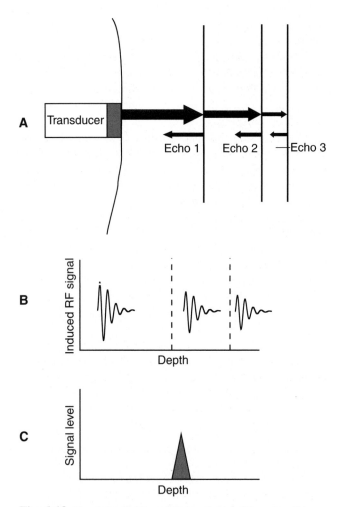

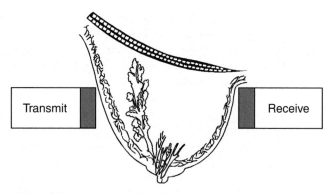

Fig. 6-19 Transmission mode scanning system. The receiver transducer is directly opposite the transmitting transducer and moves in concert.

Fig. 6-18 Gated-depth (C-mode) scanning. **A,** Three interfaces encountered along the line of sight. **B,** Time display of received echoes. Time interval for gating is shown as the region between the dotted lines. **C,** The echo received within the gated time interval is received, processed, and displayed, whereas signals generated outside that region are received but not processed or displayed. A change in the gating time allows sampling at different depths. Slice thickness can also be adjusted.

The gate can be changed to acquire data for different phases of the cardiac cycle. Images from systole and diastole are used for measuring the ejection fraction and wall thickness.

With ECG gating a patient is exposed to the ultrasound beam when no information is being processed for display. A longer scanning time is required to collect the image. Neither C-mode nor ECG-mode scanning has received widespread use.

TRANSMISSION MODE SCANNING

All ultrasound systems discussed thus far have relied on the detection of reflected echoes (echo-ranging principle) to characterize structures along the beam path. *Transmission-mode scanning is the only ultrasound scanning method that detects the transmitted beam through the patient.* The transmitting and receiving transducers are separated by an angle of 180 degrees and move in concert (Fig. 6-19). This is comparable with x-ray computed tomography (CT) scanning, in which the x-ray source (transmitter) and x-ray detector

(receiver) rotate around the patient at an angle of 180 degrees opposite each other. In transmission-mode scanning, projection data are collected, and the image is formed by applying computerized reconstruction techniques (e.g., back projection and Fourier transform) analogous to those used in x-ray CT.

In most circumstances the transmitted ultrasound wave is of such low intensity that detection is impossible. The intensity of the transmitted ultrasound wave is reduced by reflections at bowel gas–soft tissue interfaces (99.9%) and soft tissue–bone interfaces (43%), absorption through bone, refraction, and scattering. In spite of these difficulties, transmission-mode scanning may prove beneficial in examining more uniform structures (e.g., the breast). Attenuation measurements are used to differentiate dense fibrotic masses or less dense cystic masses from normal tissue. In addition, velocity measurements have potential applications, because, generally, the velocity of ultrasound is higher in dense than in less dense objects. Combinations of attenuation and velocity measurements may be of benefit in characterizing benign and cancerous lesions from normal tissues. Transmission-mode scanning may be extended to include refracted and scattered ultrasound waves. Because scattering is frequency dependent (f^4 to f^6), scattering may aid in tissue characterization. Dual-frequency examinations with special subtraction techniques are also possible.

The male genitals and the infant head are other possible anatomical sites upon which transmission-mode scanning may have a significant impact.

Reflux Transmission Imaging

An imaging technique called reflux transmission imaging (RTI) has been developed for use in conjunction with ultrasound lithotripsy systems. Reflected ultrasound from a specified depth beyond the focal zone is indicative of the ultrasound transmission through overlying tissues. This technique offers a significant advantage for the identification of gallstones before, during, and after lithotripsy.

SUMMARY

Static imaging techniques, particularly B-mode gray-scale scanners, were the mainstay of ultrasound departments through the mid-1970s. The development of scan converters greatly hastened the acceptance of diagnostic ultrasound in the medical community. B-mode scanners have provided the foundation for extensive applications of ultrasound as a noninvasive diagnostic tool.

Although real-time and Doppler devices with superior temporal resolution have a limited field of view and lower signal-to-noise ratio, they have now replaced most static imaging systems. Many of the same principles of operation, however, still apply.

REVIEW QUESTIONS

1. A cathode ray tube (CRT) display of an A-mode scan shows a plot of the time in one dimension versus _____ in the other dimension.
2. The CRT time base sweep rate corresponds to _____ μs/cm.
3. In A-mode scanning the CRT trace is updated at a rate _____ to the pulse repetition frequency (PRF).
4. In static B-mode scanning the signal level controls the _____ of the pixel displayed on the monitor.
5. The _____ in a static B-mode scanner provides information regarding transducer position and orientation.
6. The _____ is so named because this device, which holds two-dimensional echo data, switches back and forth from the line-by-line acquisition during collection to the raster readout during display.
7. What are the physical dimensions of a pixel in which a 400 × 400 matrix represents a 10 × 20 cm field of view?
8. A _____ allows selection of received echoes for processing based on the elapsed time between transmission of the pulsed wave and reception of the echo.

BIBLIOGRAPHY

McDicken WN: *Diagnostic ultrasonics: principles and use of instruments,* ed 3, Edinburgh, 1991, Churchill Livingstone.

Rose JL, Goldberg BB: *Basic physics in diagnostic ultrasound,* New York, 1979, John Wiley & Sons.

Wells PNT: *Physical principles of ultrasonic diagnosis,* New York, 1969, Academic Press.

Wells PNT: *Biomedical ultrasonics,* New York, 1977, Academic Press.

Image Formation in Real-Time Imaging

Field of view
Frame rate
Line of sight
Pulse repetition frequency (PRF)

Scan converter
Scan line
Scan range

In real-time scanning the displayed image is continuously and rapidly updated with new scan data as the beam is swept repeatedly throughout the **field of view.** The rate at which new information is displayed can be 30 or more times each second. The widespread acceptance of real-time imaging is the result of improvements in transducer technology, digital electronics, and ultrasound beam focusing. But probably just as important as these technical advances is the advantage of increased user-friendliness—the transducer can be moved to any orientation without the restriction in movement imposed by the reference arm. Consequently, real-time ultrasound imaging, with superior spatial resolution and temporal resolution but limited field of view and lower SNR, has almost totally replaced static B-mode imaging and now is often referred to as B-mode imaging.

The rapid **frame rates** in real-time imaging eliminate difficulty with motion artifacts, which greatly compromise static imaging. Indeed, the ability to depict motion now makes dynamic studies possible. The total examination time is reduced, because the sonographer receives instant feedback with respect to anatomical structures included within the field of view. The scan plane can be changed rapidly to a new orientation.

The major disadvantage is that the limited field of view makes anatomical identification more difficult. Real-time images also appear more nonuniform, because the signal-to-noise ratio (SNR) is reduced compared with static imaging. Recall that in static B-mode a structure is often interrogated from several different directions, and this multiple sampling lowers the noise level (i.e., images appear less grainy).

PRINCIPLES OF REAL-TIME IMAGING

To understand the basic requirements of a real-time ultrasound imaging system, we must first appreciate the limitations of A-mode and static B-mode scanners.

In A-mode scanning a transducer is placed over the area of interest. An ultrasound beam is sent out by exciting the crystal. The pulse lasts approximately 1 μs, and then the transducer is "silent" for 999 μs, waiting for the return echoes before it generates the next pulse. The returning echoes are amplified and displayed as a cathode ray tube

(CRT) trace of amplitude versus depth along this single **line of sight.** To see a different line of sight, we must move the transducer to a different position. Only one line of sight can be observed at any given instant on the display. As long as the transducer and interfaces are stationary, the trace appears unchanged, because the CRT screen is refreshed at the rate of the pulse repetition frequency (PRF).

In static B-mode gray-scale imaging the transducer is placed at the starting position, and information is recorded along a single line of sight. All echoes from a single pulse are assumed to originate from reflections along this line of sight. The amplitude of each signal is represented by the brightness of the dot.

To build up a two-dimensional image (similar to a single stop-action photograph or conventional x-ray film), the sonographer moves the transducer manually to a different position or orientation to acquire information along a new line of sight. The previous line of sight data are retained in the digital **scan converter.** The image thus is created by obtaining a large number of lines of sight over a 5- to 10-second period. The lateral resolution of the image is improved as the number of lines of sight is increased. Static scanning depends on the object not moving, because lines of sight are acquired at different times and then combined to form a single image.

Real-time gray scale imaging depicts the reflectivity of structures within the field of view and continually updates this information for display by repeating the data acquisition process. A succession of two-dimensional images is formed rapidly to give the perception of motion, if structures are moving within the sampled region. It can be compared with other dynamic modalities (x-ray fluoroscopy or motion-picture films) in which a series of stop-action shots is taken and then viewed rapidly one after another to depict motion.

Data collection for each frame is a combination of echo-ranging and directional beam scanning. The time delay between the transmitted pulse and the received echo determines the distance of the interface from the transducer. This distance is measured along the beam axis (direction of propagation). A series of echoes following the transmitted pulse allows placement of multiple interfaces encountered by the beam along a single line of sight. Only structures that lie along the direction of propagation within the beam are interrogated. This linear sampling according to the beam path is called line of sight or **scan line.** An image is composed of multiple scan lines by acquiring echo-ranging data along different paths by scanning the beam (Fig. 7-1). Displayed brightness for a reflector is controlled by the intensity of the received echo.

A pulsed-wave, narrow beam is first directed along a straight-line path, and after the echoes are received, the ultrasound beam is then moved to a new sampling direction. Beam orientation is controlled by mechanical or electronic means in a repetitive, automated fashion without intervention by the sonographer. A single image is formed by sweeping pulsed sound beams along different sampling directions throughout the field of view. This process is repeated to produce successive images of the region.

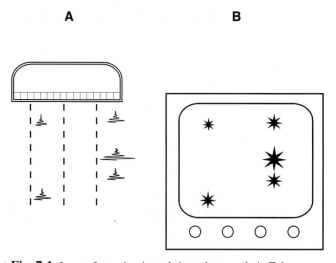

Fig. 7-1 Image formation in real-time ultrasound. **A,** Echo-ranging data measured with three scan lines allows spatial mapping of detected echoes. The origin and amplitude of each echo along the respective beam paths *(dashed lines)* are shown. **B,** Image display on monitor. The brightness of the dot represents the strength of the detected echo.

Lines of Sight

Real-time gray-scale imaging requires the acquisition of data in a very rapid fashion to give the perception of motion. The ultrasound beam is "swept" or steered through the area of interest (by mechanical or electronic means) in a repetitive, automated fashion. Instead of a single sonogram with multiple lines of sight, as in static B-mode scanning, multiple images are formed one after another, each composed of multiple lines of sight. Every scan line requires one pulse of ultrasound waves to probe interfaces along its path.

The ultrasound beam is first directed along one line of sight, and after the echoes are received, it is automatically moved to a new line. A single image is formed by sweeping through the entire region. This process is repeated to produce successive images of the region. As motion becomes more rapid within the field of view, a faster frame rate is necessary to display the structures without jerkiness (abrupt transitions from one location to another, or blurring). The time for the pulse to travel to the depth of interest and back to the transducer—along with the need for good spatial resolution provided by a large number of lines of sight in each image—imposes a restriction on the frame rate. Frame rates of 5 to 40 images per second are available. The number of scan lines in a frame is usually between 50 and 200 depending on scan conditions. Commonly 120 to 150 scan lines are used.

SCAN CONVERTER

Multiple lines of sight are the building blocks for each image. As discussed shortly, each line of sight represents a particular position of the crystal or activation of a group of crystals in the transducer array, which is established by the scanning mechanism. The ultrasound beam is directed into the patient in a well-defined pattern. Hence, no articulated arm is necessary to determine the position of the line of sight, as in static B-mode imaging. Because the data are collected and displayed in real time, permanent archiving is possible by recording the real-time images on videotape. A storage device is not needed; however, most real-time units incorporate a scan converter to obtain better gray-scale images and provide "freeze frame" capability. The use of digital scan converters also allows for manipulation of the image data to aid interpretation.

TIME CONSTRAINTS

For each line of sight one pulse of ultrasound waves is used to detect interfaces located along the beam path. A finite amount of time is necessary for the ultrasound wave to move away from the transducer, probe the region of interest, and return as an echo to the transducer (13 microseconds for every centimeter of tissue). Every transmitted pulse produces a similar sequence of events. Extending the scanning depth requires increased measurement time to acquire the echo-ranging data for each scan line (Fig. 7-2).

The following analogy illustrates the concept of image formation in real-time ultrasound. A company wants to determine the effectiveness of advertising in attracting customers to its stores. Imagine that three stores are each located one block away from a central starting point in the directions of north, east, and west. A sonography student, who is also an employee of the company, is assigned to monitor the number of customers in each store and then report this finding. The student walks east to the first store, counts the customers, and returns to the starting point where the information is recorded. Other stores are evaluated sequentially in the same manner. However, customer number is only accurate for the time at which the observation occurred. Customers will enter and leave a store. To obtain the current status the student must return to each store repeatedly.

In this analogy the number of customers indicates the reflectivity of the interface, and the directions east, north, and west represent different beam paths (a total of three scan lines). Obviously, the data are not obtained instantaneously; travel time to and from each store limits the rate at which the information is attained.

By constraining the sonography student to walk at a constant velocity, the time required to collect customer data from all stores is well defined. Similarly, the acoustic velocity of ultrasound in soft tissue is constant and imposes a restriction on the frequency of sampling. The **scan range** is set at one block. However, if the stores were located farther away, then the sonography student must travel a longer distance, and the information updates would be less frequent. As scan range is increased, more time must be allotted to accumulate data for a scan line. Compare the total time to collect an image consisting of eight scan lines for the different scan ranges shown in Fig. 7-2. The total time for a scan range of 5 cm and 15 cm is 520 μs and 1,560 μs, respectively.

Frame Rate Limitations

Since a finite amount of time is necessary to form one image, the number of images that can be acquired and displayed each second (frame rate) is limited. The maximum frame rate (FR_{max}) is given by the following equation:

7-1

$$FR_{max} = \frac{c}{2\,Rn} = \frac{PRF}{n}$$

where c is the velocity of ultrasound in the medium, R the scan range, n the number of lines of sight per frame (lpf), and PRF the pulse repetition frequency. Equation 7-1 indicates that, if the scanning depth and/or number of lines of sight are increased, the maximum frame rate must decrease. The number of frames per second is ultimately limited by the velocity of ultrasound in tissue (1540 m/s).

For instance, assume that the field of view extends to a depth of 10 cm. The data collection time for each line of sight is 130 μs (13 μs/cm × 10 cm). If only one line of sight is desired (as in A-mode), the maximum frame rate would be:

$$FR_{max} = \frac{1540\ m/s}{2\,(0.1\ m)\,(1\ lpf)}$$
$$FR_{max} = 7700\ fps$$

By increasing the number of lines of sight to 100 lines per image, the maximum frame rate becomes

$$FR_{max} = \frac{1540\ m/s}{2\,(0.1\ m)\,(100\ lpf)}$$
$$FR_{max} = 77\ fps$$

Extending the depth of interest results in a reduced maximum frame rate. If 100 lines of sight are to be maintained for a change in scan range from 10 cm to 20 cm, the maximum frame rate is decreased:

$$FR_{max} = \frac{1540\ m/s}{2\,(0.2\ m)\,(100\ lpf)}$$
$$FR_{max} = 38\ fps$$

■ Example 7-1

What is the maximum frame rate (FR_{max}) if the depth of scanning is 15 cm and 150 lines compose each frame?

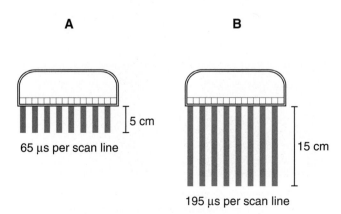

A　　　　　　**B**

5 cm

65 μs per scan line

15 cm

195 μs per scan line

Fig. 7-2 Time to acquire a scan line depends on scan range. **A,** 5-cm scan range. **B,** 15-cm scan range.

Using Equation 7-1

$$FR_{max} = \frac{c}{2\,Rn}$$

$$FR_{max} = \frac{1540\ m/s}{2\,(0.15\ m)\,(150\ lpf)}$$

$$FR_{max} = 34\ fps$$

■ **Example 7-2**

How many scan lines (n) can be acquired for each frame if the scan range is 10 cm and the frame rate is 24 per second?

Rearranging Equation 7-1

$$n = \frac{c}{2\,R\,(FR_{max})}$$

$$n = \frac{1540\ m/s}{2\,(0.1\ m)\,(24\ fps)}$$

$$n = 320\ lpf$$

■ **Example 7-3**

If 200 scan lines compose each frame acquired at a rate of 18 frames per second, what is the range of scanning (R)?

Rearranging Equation 7-1

$$R = \frac{c}{2\,n\,(FR_{max})}$$

$$R = \frac{1540\ m/s}{2\,(200\ lpf)\,(18\ fps)}$$

$$R = 0.21\ m\ or\ 21\ cm$$

To achieve a faster frame rate, the scanning depth and/or number of lines of sight must be reduced. The decreased penetration enables a higher frequency transducer to be used for better axial resolution. Real-time scanners usually operate at a PRF of between 2000 and 5000 pulses per second but can be as high as 12,000 pulses per second to preserve lateral resolution while maintaining a high frame rate. Some sacrifice in scanning depth may be required at higher PRFs. Table 7-1 demonstrates the relation between number of lines of sight, depth of scanning, and maximum frame rate.

The manufacturer of real-time equipment sets the frame rate based on the field of view, depth of interest, and number of lines of sight required for the desired image quality. Several approaches are possible to compensate for an increase in scanning depth. The real-time unit may automatically decrease the frame rate but maintain the same number of lines. On the other hand, both frame rate and number of lines may be adjusted downward. The number of lines may be reduced without a loss in resolution by narrowing the field of view. Often, several transducers of different frequencies are available for use with a single ultrasound unit. Each frequency is optimized with respect to the number of lines of sight and frame rate as a function of sampling depth. It is imperative that the sonographer understand these principles when selecting and operating the equipment.

BEAM WIDTH

The objectives in designing a transducer for imaging are to transmit a beam that would be directional with a narrow beam width. These characteristics are desirable, because small objects can be located and distinguished as separate entities.

A single object smaller than the beam width produces an echo when it is intercepted by the transmitted pulsed wave. An echo is created regardless of the lateral position of the object in the ultrasonic field (Fig. 7-3). The lateral dimension of the object in the image is defined as the same size as the beam width. Multiple small objects equidistant from the transducer are not resolved when encompassed by the beam (Fig. 7-4). Remember, axial displacement of objects can be detected by altered echo times. Multiple samplings with successive narrow beams enable the objects to be observed as separate structures (Fig. 7-5).

Focusing reduces the beam width at a specific depth to enhance the spatial mapping of received echoes. Sampling is restricted laterally by the width of the beam. Objects located outside the beam do not contribute signals for that scan line. Scanning the narrow beam throughout the field of view enables all structures to be examined.

■ **Table 7-1** Maximum Frame Rate versus Depth and the Number of Lines of Sight

Depth (cm)	Maximum Frame Rate			
	25 LS	**50 LS**	**100 LS**	**200 LS**
5	616	308	154	77
10	308	154	77	38
15	205	103	51	26
20	154	77	38	19
25	123	61	30	15
30	103	51	25	12

LS, Lines of sight.

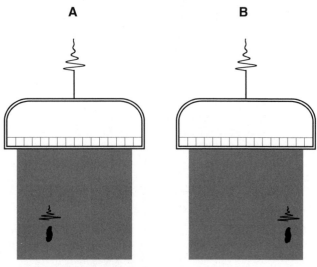

Fig. 7-3 Generation of an echo by small object within the ultrasonic field using a broad beam *(gray region)*. **A** and **B,** At constant depth the induced signal is the same regardless of lateral location.

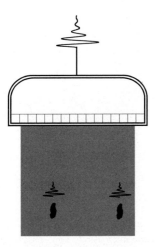

Fig. 7-4 Generation of echoes by two small objects within the ultrasonic field using a broad beam *(gray region)*. Since the depth is the same and the echoes arrive at the transducer simultaneously, the induced signal does not indicate the presence of two structures. The signal strength is twice that in Fig. 7-3.

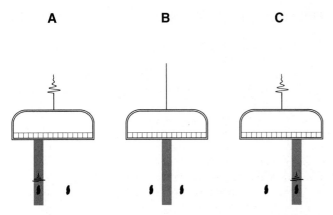

Fig. 7-5 By narrowing the beam and collecting echo-range data along multiple scan lines *(three separate gray regions)* separated in time, signals that indicate the lateral positions of the objects are generated. **A, B,** and **C,** Time sequence for signals received along different beam paths. Time interval for each scan line equals scan range multiplied by 13 μs/cm.

LATERAL RESOLUTION

Lateral resolution describes the ability to resolve two objects adjacent to each other that are perpendicular to the beam axis. Decreasing the beam width improves the lateral resolution by allowing objects close together to be resolved and by providing a more accurate presentation of small objects. *Line density also affects lateral resolution.*

Returning to the analogy involving the student sonographer, suppose, instead of three stores in the survey, numerous stores are distributed throughout the city. If travel is restricted to the directions of north, east, and west, respectively, then only stores located along these three paths are encountered—other stores are missed. To include all stores in the survey, the student sonographer must walk in many different directions. For real-time image formation, increasing the number of scan lines improves the spatial

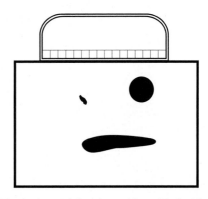

Fig. 7-6 Phantom containing three objects. Each object has a unique size and shape.

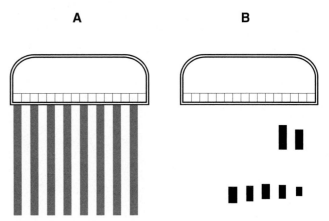

Fig. 7-7 Effect of line density on lateral resolution. **A,** Scan lines *(total of eight denoted by gray regions)*. **B,** Image formed by probing the phantom along the scan lines in **A.** Note that the smallest object is not observed, because low scan line density creates sampling voids within the field of view.

sampling in the direction perpendicular to beam propagation. The effect of line density on image quality is illustrated in Figs. 7-6, 7-7, and 7-8.

In practice, lateral resolution is affected when the separation between two scan lines is greater than the beam width. Reducing the number of scan lines to achieve a high frame rate sometimes creates this situation (Fig. 7-9). Furthermore, if the scan range and frame rate are unchanged, expanding the width of the field of view decreases the scan line density (Fig. 7-10). Extending the scan range has a similar effect (Fig. 7-11).

TEMPORAL RESOLUTION

As motion becomes more rapid within the field of view, a faster frame rate is necessary to display the structures without jerkiness (abrupt transitions from one location to another). The finite transit time for the ultrasound pulse to travel to the depth of interest and back to the transducer, as well as the need for good spatial resolution provided by a large number of lines of sight in each image, impose a restriction on the frame rate. Frame rates of 15 or more images per second are typically available.

A   **B**

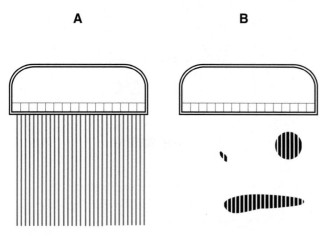

Fig. 7-8 Lateral resolution is improved by increasing line density. **A,** Scan lines *(total of 31 denoted by gray regions).* **B,** Image formed by probing the phantom in Fig. 7-6 along the scan lines in **A.**

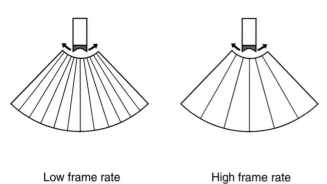

Low frame rate   High frame rate

Fig. 7-9 A reduction in the number of scan lines allows frame rate (low versus high) to increase. The scan range and field of view are unchanged.

SUMMARY

Real-time gray-scale imaging has become the dominant scanning mode used in medical diagnostic ultrasound. Image formation is based on echo ranging and beam scanning. A major advantage of real-time ultrasound is excellent temporal resolution for the study of fast-moving structures. Frame rate depends on scan range and number of

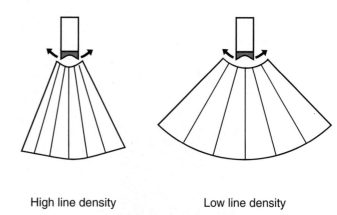

High line density   Low line density

Fig. 7-10 If the scan range, frame rate, and number of scan lines remain unchanged, an increase in field of view (small versus large) results in a lower line density.

scan lines. To optimize image quality for different clinical applications, the scan parameters of frame rate, scan range, width of the field of view, and line density are adjusted.

REVIEW QUESTIONS

1. Calculate the maximum frame rate if the scan range is 15 cm and 120 lines compose each frame.
2. Consider an image with 100 scan lines. How much time is required to form this image if the depth of interest is 10 cm?
3. If scan line density is increased by a factor of 2 and the scan range is unchanged, what is the effect on the maximum frame rate?
4. Line density and beam width affect _____ resolution.
5. How many scan lines compose a real-time image?
6. What is the pulse repetition frequency for real-time scanners?
7. What is a common frame rate for real-time scanners?

BIBLIOGRAPHY

Hedrick WR, Hykes DL: Image formation in real-time ultrasound, *J Diagn Med Sonography* 11:246-251, 1995.
Hykes DL, Hedrick WR: Real-time ultrasound instrumentation, *J Diagn Med Sonography* 6:257-268, 1990.
McDicken WN: *Diagnostic ultrasonics: principles and use of instruments,* ed 3, Edinburgh, 1991, Churchill Livingstone.

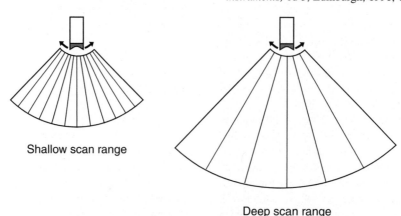

Shallow scan range

Deep scan range

Fig. 7-11 If the field of view and frame rate remain unchanged, an increase in the scan range (shallow versus deep) lowers the total number of scan lines.

Real-Time Ultrasound Transducers

Real-time ultrasound imaging techniques have almost totally replaced static B-mode gray-scale imaging. The increased use of real-time imaging is the result of progress in transducer technology, miniaturization of electronics through the development of digital circuitry, advances in computer software, and improved ultrasonic focusing. The final result has been better image quality and higher information content for real-time ultrasound.

The most common classification of real-time transducers is based on the method by which the ultrasound beam is focused and swept through the field of view. Mechanical **sector scanners**, the first major class, are normally the simplest and least expensive. Mechanical motion of single or multiple crystals sweeps the beam back and forth over the region of interest to collect different lines of sight for images in rapid succession. Focusing is achieved by fixed mechanical means. The second major class, multiple-element transducers, steers and focuses the beam electronically. The annular array is a mixture of the two classifications in which an electronically focused beam is steered mechanically through the field of view.

MECHANICAL SCANNERS

The mechanical sector scanner uses one or more piezoelectric crystals attached to a stepping motor that moves the crystals to various locations. The changing positions of a crystal allow scan data to be collected from multiple lines of sight. In addition to the previously mentioned pulse repetition frequency (PRF) limitations on frame rate, the mechanical motion of a crystal restricts the acquisition rate to about 30 frames per second. Mechanical real-time units typically employ one or more of the static B-mode focused crystals and are classified as either contact or liquid path scanners.

Contact Scanners

Contact scanners are those in which the transducer makes physical contact with the patient. Often the crystal is mounted within a liquid medium to eliminate any air interfaces between the moving crystal and the protective front surface of the transducer. The ultrasound path across the liquid medium is narrow (<3 mm). Gel is also placed between the transducer face and the patient to remove air-tissue interfaces.

One of the first real-time mechanical systems employed a disk-shaped crystal (usually focused) attached to a motor (Fig. 8-1). It oscillated or wobbled back and forth during data collection and with a frame rate of 15 frames per second subtended an arc of 15 to 60 degrees. Some of the early systems vibrated so much, in fact, that they were uncomfortable for both the patient and the sonographer.

When the crystal is at the extreme left position, data collection begins. The crystal is excited, and the ultrasound beam moves outward along that line of sight, a fraction of its energy being reflected at various interfaces along its path. After an interval equal to the time needed for the wave to travel to the maximum depth of interest and return to the transducer (13 μs per centimeter), the crystal is moved to the next line of sight by the stepping motor and re-pulsed. This sequence repeats itself until the last line of sight is collected for one image (i.e., the crystal is at the extreme right position). The time required to collect one image depicting information from a depth of 15 cm with 200 lines of sight is 39 milliseconds (ms), and the process is repeated for the next image, which in the present example achieves a frame rate of 26 images per second. The time to collect scan data for each frame establishes the upper limit of the frame rate.

$$FR_{max} = \frac{1000 \text{ ms/s}}{39 \text{ ms/frame}} = 26 \text{ fps}$$

Equation 7-1 confirms this analysis:

$$FR_{max} = \frac{1540 \text{ ms/s}}{2 \, (0.15 \text{ m}) \, (200 \text{ lpf})} = 26 \text{ fps}$$

Focusing to a specific depth along each line of sight is done mechanically. The focal zone for a particular transducer is fixed and cannot be changed. Because beam width is not constant along the scan line, lateral resolution is not uniform throughout the field of view. The focal length of the transducer must be matched to the depth of the structures of interest. In the clinical setting this requires multiple, interchangeable transducers, each with a different focal length. Lateral resolution is also affected by scan line density. Line density is varied by adjusting the speed of rotation of the crystal. Mechanical sector transducers offer the advantage of high line density.

In another version of the mechanical scanner, multiple crystals are mounted on a rotating wheel (Fig. 8-2). The technique for acquiring echo data is very similar to that used with the oscillating sector scanner. A crystal is positioned at the extreme left and is excited, and the ultrasound beam probes interfaces along that line of sight. The wheel then moves, and the crystal is excited for the next line of sight. When the crystal moves to the extreme right, the last line of sight is collected for one frame. The neighboring crystal on the rotating wheel is then in position at the extreme left to begin the acquisition for the next frame. This technique may allow for faster frame rates, especially if **parallel processing** of information is used. In parallel processing two separate crystals collect data in slightly different areas (nonadjacent lines of sight) simultaneously. The increased rate of sampling allows for more rapid updating of image data. Multiple crystals, each with a different frequency, may also be used to obtain images of the same area with varying spatial detail and contrast.

Characteristics of Contact Scanners

Oscillating or rotating wheel contact scanners produce an image with a sector or pie-shaped format. The field of view is narrow near the transducer and expands with depth. Because these sector scanners are physically small, scanning in tight areas between ribs, behind ribs, and elsewhere is possible. The limited number of crystals and mechanical steering enable manufacture of these transducers at relatively low cost.

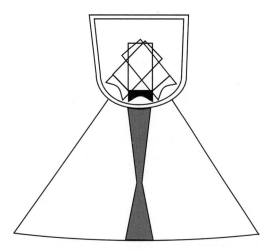

Fig. 8-1 Mechanical sector transducer. A single crystal with a fixed focal length is swept back and forth across the field of view by a motorized arm.

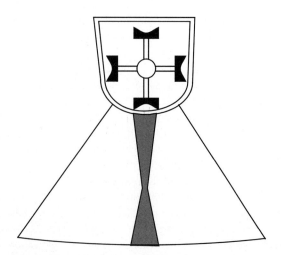

Fig. 8-2 Rotating wheel contact transducer.

Problems with sector transducers do exist, however: Their small size limits the field of view and may make anatomical identification difficult. Their fixed focal length restricts the best lateral resolution to a limited range of depths. The scan line density is reduced with distance from the transducer face. There are more lines of sight crossing a given area near the top of the sector than in an equal area near the bottom.

The nonuniform scan-line density is illustrated in Fig. 8-3. Streams of water radiating from a showerhead demonstrate a similar effect. Near the source they are close together, and they become less concentrated as distance from the showerhead increases. Line density can be varied by changing the speed of rotation of the crystal. One advantage of mechanical sector transducers is that high line density can be achieved.

In practice, lateral resolution is affected when the distance between two lines is greater than the beam width. Reducing the number of lines to achieve high frame rate sometimes creates this situation. Furthermore, increasing the sector angle to encompass a larger field of view decreases scan-line density (provided that the scanning range and frame rate are unchanged) and degrades lateral resolution.

Liquid Path Scanners

Another type of mechanical scanner is the liquid-path scanner, in which the crystals are placed in a liquid bath (usually a water and alcohol mixture). These scanners are further classified as nonreflecting liquid-path or reflecting liquid-path. Single or multiple transducer crystals are incremented in a linear or a sector fashion for data collection.

The nonreflecting liquid-path and mechanical contact scanners are said to be in-line transducers. The ultrasound beam travels directly from the crystal through the liquid into the patient and back through the liquid to the crystal without

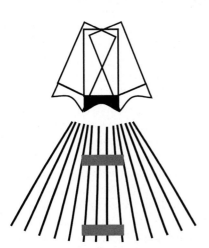

Fig. 8-3 In sector scanning the lateral resolution becomes poorer at increasing depths. High line density is obtained in the region near the transducer. The line density decreases at greater depths, since the number of lines of sight per unit area decreases. Compare the number of lines of sight through the rectangular blocks, which are equal in size.

striking a mirror. The reflecting liquid-path scanner uses an acoustic mirror to alter the ultrasonic path for purposes of sweeping the beam. Directing the beam is accomplished by moving the crystal while reflecting the beam from a stationary mirror or by reflecting the beam from a moving mirror while the crystal remains stationary. The reflecting liquid-path systems are said to be offset, because the ultrasound beam must be reflected from the mirror during both transmission and reception.

The liquid path reduces reverberations from shallow structures and allows for strongly focused large-diameter transducers to be used to improve the lateral resolution at the desired depth. The large trapezoidal field of view enhances anatomical identification compared to that obtainable with sector scanners (although static B-mode is superior in this respect).

Advantages and Disadvantages

Liquid-path transducers are larger and bulkier than contact scanners and are more difficult to apply to small or irregularly shaped areas. The maximum frame rate is also reduced, because the liquid path must be traversed twice by the ultrasound beam. (The penetration distance is increased by twice the length of the liquid path.)

Generally, mechanical systems are less expensive and easier to operate (except for the inconvenience of changing transducers) than electronic systems. Good-quality images are produced, but mechanical wear may limit the overall lifetime of the transducers. Turning the transducer off when not in use can reduce mechanical wear. The mechanical motion also limits the frame rate.

LINEAR ARRAYS

An important advance in medical diagnostic ultrasound instrumentation occurred in the late 1970s with the development of electronic, multiple-element transducers. These systems produce high-quality images with high frame rates and the possibility of high line density without the limited lifetime caused by mechanical wear. More importantly, the transducer is manipulated electronically to focus, as well as to sweep the ultrasound beam throughout the field of view. Multiple element transducers were initially introduced as **linear arrays** or **linear phased arrays.** Both types are expensive compared with mechanical sectors, although there can be some overlap in pricing.

Sequential Linear Arrays

The first type of electronic transducer was the sequential or nonsegmented linear array. As the name implies, multiple rectangular crystals are arranged in a straight row. Each crystal produces an ultrasound beam and then receives the returning echoes for data collection along one line of sight. The crystals are activated in a sequential fashion to form the individual lines of sight (Fig. 8-4). The number of crystals in the array determines the number of lines of sight for each

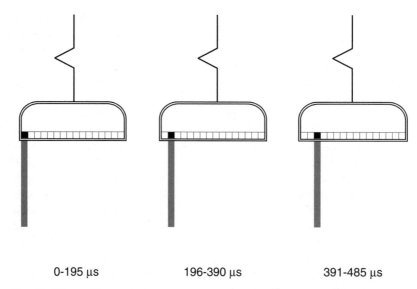

| 0-195 µs | 196-390 µs | 391-485 µs |

Fig. 8-4 Beam scanning with a sequential linear array. The beam direction is determined by element selection during transmission. The first three scan lines are shown. For a scan range of 15 cm, each crystal is fired 195 µs after the preceding crystal.

image. If the array contains 130 individual crystals that are fired (excited) one at a time in sequence, 130 lines of sight are acquired.

The first crystal in the array is excited, and then a time delay for collection of the returning echoes is imposed before the next crystal is fired. The duration of the delay is set by the maximum scanning depth (13 µs is required for every centimeter of depth). For example, assume that a maximum viewing depth of 15 cm is desired. The first crystal is electronically stimulated to produce an ultrasound beam, and 195 µs later (13 µs/cm × 15 cm) the second crystal is excited. After another 195 µs, the third crystal is fired. This sequence continues until all 130 crystals are fired to form one image. The process is repeated for the next image. The rate at which this sequence of firing all 130 crystals is repeated determines the frame rate. Fig. 8-4 illustrates the timing pattern for a sequential linear array. The 15 cm depth limits the PRF to 5000 pulses per second (pps). With 130 lines per frame (lpf) a maximum frame rate of 38 images per second is obtained:

$$FR_{max} = \frac{5000 \text{ pps}}{130 \text{ lpf}} = 38 \text{ fps}$$

Recall that the physical dimensions of the crystal dictate the width of the ultrasound beam. Linear arrays consist of many small crystals along a row. The major problem with a sequential linear array is that the small crystal size produces a short, narrow near field and a rapidly diverging far field. As discussed in Chapter 5, larger crystals produce a deeper near field and a less diverging far field (Fig. 8-5).

Segmental Linear Arrays

When a group (segment) of crystals in the linear array is stimulated, it acts in concert to produce a deeper near field

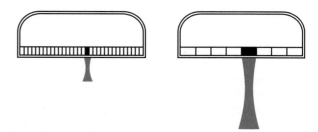

Fig. 8-5 Crystal size in the transducer array affects the beam pattern. Small crystals create a short near field and a rapidly diverging far field. Large crystals produce a wider but deeper near field and a less diverging far field.

and a less divergent far field compared with a small, single crystal acting alone. This segmental linear array, however, creates fewer lines of sight for the same scan plane width, which causes the spatial mapping to deteriorate, although the resultant ultrasonic field provides a more favorable beam pattern. For example, assume that 16 individual crystals are fired in groups of four. The first four crystals are excited simultaneously and then 195 µs (corresponding to the time required to sample 15 cm in depth) elapse before the next four crystals in a group (numbers 5 through 8) are fired. By using adjacent blocks of four crystals, four lines of sight that are spaced widely apart can be created (Fig. 8-6). This is less than ideal, although the overall beam pattern for sampling each line of sight at increased depth is improved.

To achieve good lateral resolution throughout the field of view, a combination of narrow beam width associated with the near field and high line density is required. This is accomplished by using a step-down segmental array. Fig. 8-7 shows the excitation sequence for the first three lines of sight for a 16-crystal linear array. The number of lines of sight is increased by firing crystals 1 through 4, waiting 195 µs, and then firing crystals 2 through 5. After

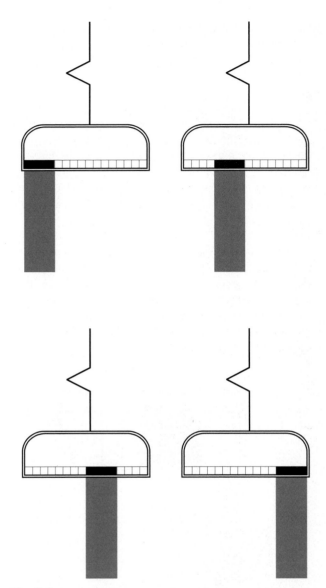

Fig. 8-6 Segmental linear array. For a 15-cm scan depth, each group of four crystals is fired 195 μs after the preceding group. For a 16-element array, four lines of sight are produced.

another 195 μs, crystals 3 through 6 are excited. In other words, a set of four crystals is fired as a group or segment to produce the desired beam pattern, and, by overlapping groups, the number of lines of sight can be increased. The step-down segmental array produces 13 lines of sight for the 16 crystals shown, rather than 4 lines of sight obtained by the sequential segmental array.

If in an array of 64 crystal elements four crystals are fired at a time and each group is offset by one crystal, a total of 61 lines of sight will be acquired for each image. Assuming that 15 cm is the desired depth (195 μs between firing each segment), we can see that a maximum of 84 images could be generated each second:

$$FR_{max} = \frac{1540 \text{ m/s}}{2 \ (0.15 \text{ m})(61 \text{ lpf})} = 84 \text{ fps}$$

The step-down segmental array with 64 to 200 piezo-electric elements produces good temporal resolution (high frame rate) and good spatial resolution (beam width and number of lines of sight). The field of view is presented in a rectangular format, with the in-plane width equal to the physical length of the array. The linear array has a flat face, which causes difficulty in maintaining transducer-patient contact when a wide field of view is desired. Nevertheless, this step-down technique improved the image quality of real-time scanners dramatically, although additional adjustments in focusing are necessary to narrow the beam width further so the spatial resolution will be optimal.

ELECTRONIC FOCUSING TECHNIQUES

As shown in Chapter 5, a circular transducer crystal produces a symmetrical ultrasound beam pattern with a relatively narrow near field and a diverging far field. Fortunately, a rectangular shape creates a similar beam pattern, regardless of whether a single crystal is excited or a group of crystals is fired together (Fig. 8-8). The beam pattern for a linear array is not symmetrical, and therefore

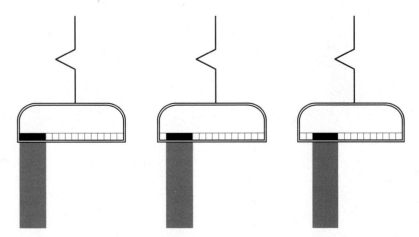

Fig. 8-7 Lines of sight for a segmental linear array. Four elements compose a group, and the group is shifted by one element for each successive transmission. The total number of lines of sight for the 16-element array is increased to 13 by overlapping segments.

the dimension along the row of crystals (in-plane) and perpendicular to the row of crystals (elevation) must be specified separately. As previously stated (in Chapter 5), ultrasound beams are focused to improve the lateral resolution and sensitivity. Because a linear array has a rectangular format, focusing must be applied in two directions as shown in Fig. 8-9. The in-plane direction is also referred to as the azimuth direction, which is perpendicular to the direction propagation. Focusing along the elevation direction (out of plane) determines the thickness of tissue represented by the cross-sectional image (Fig. 8-10).

Mechanical focusing narrows the ultrasound beam in the elevation direction. Mechanical focusing is achieved either by curving the crystal or, more commonly, by placing an acoustic lens in front of the crystal. The beam is most narrow at a specified depth, which is fixed by the lens or curvature of the crystal. Focusing in the elevation direction is applied uniformly to each crystal in the array. The **slice thickness** in the focal zone is typically 3 to 10 millimeters.

Electronic focusing creates an in-plane beam width of one millimeter or less, and the depth of focus can be varied (Fig. 8-11).

Focusing Dynamics

The sequence of firing one group of crystals (stepping down) and then firing the next group prohibits mechanical focusing of the ultrasound beam in the in-plane direction. The relative position of a crystal in the group dictates the focusing requirements for that crystal. *Because most crystals in the array belong to multiple firing groups, the focusing requirements change and cannot be achieved by static mechanical means.* For example, in a step-down segmented array, crystal 3 is the center of a five-crystal firing sequence involving crystals 1 through 5; when crystals 2 through 6 are fired, crystal 3 occupies the second position; and when 3 through 7 are fired, crystal 3 moves to the first position. This changing position dictates different focusing requirements for that crystal and thus prevents mechanical focusing in the in-plane direction.

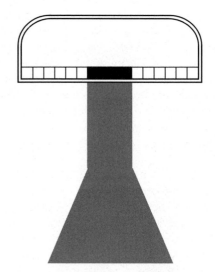

Fig. 8-8 The beam shape from a segment of crystals in an array is similar to that from a single crystal circular transducer.

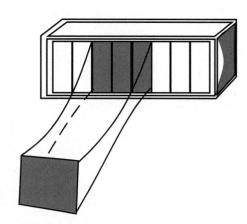

Fig. 8-10 Mechanical focusing of an array in the elevation direction using an acoustic lens or curved crystal elements.

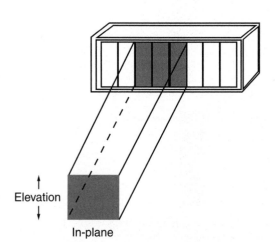

Elevation

In-plane

Fig. 8-9 Rectangular beam pattern along the in-plane and elevation directions produced by a segment of crystals.

A　　　**B**

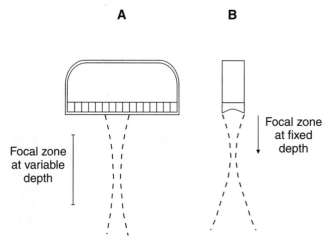

Focal zone at variable depth

Focal zone at fixed depth

Fig. 8-11 Dual focusing. **A,** In-plane focusing creates a narrow beam width perpendicular to the direction of propagation, and the focal length is variable. **B,** Mechanical focusing in the elevation direction determines the slice thickness.

Fortunately, linear arrays are electronically focused in the in-plane direction, which (when combined with mechanical focusing in the elevation direction) creates a narrow beam (Fig. 8-12). Focusing in the in-plane direction is variable, which allows narrow beam width in this direction at any specified depth along the line of sight, whereas the beam width in the elevation direction is not changeable (Fig. 8-13).

Note that focusing of an ultrasound beam depends on the uniformity of the tissues interrogated. Most scanning of human subjects involves a diverse array of tissue types interrogated by the ultrasound beam at any given time. This places severe restrictions on the quality of the electronically synthesized beam in comparison with the theoretical images seen when uniform phantoms are used.

Principle of Focusing

Electronic focusing involves the superimposition (algebraic summation) of ultrasound waves. Each crystal produces a

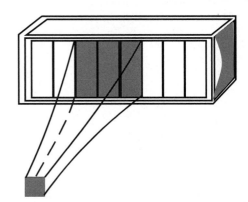

Fig. 8-12 Resultant beam pattern from both mechanical focusing and electronic focusing. Cross-sectional beam *(gray)* is shown at a depth within the focal zone of the mechanically focused crystals.

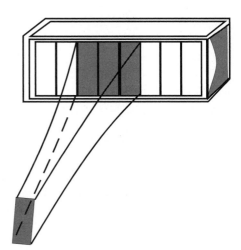

Fig. 8-13 Resultant beam pattern from both mechanical focusing and variable electronic focusing. Cross-sectional beam *(gray)* is shown at a depth outside the focal zone of the mechanically focused crystals. Note the difference in beam dimension in the elevation direction compared with Fig. 8-12.

particular wave pattern, and the overall pattern derived from a group of crystals is the summation of all the wave patterns from the individual crystals (Huygens' principle). Electronic focusing is accomplished by offsetting the firing of various crystals in a group by a small time delay (10^{-9} second). This delay is small compared with the time required for the sound beam to travel to the depth of interest. For a group of crystals the beam direction is normally centered at the middle crystal. The nanosecond timing is accomplished by delay lines, which are special electronic devices that hold the signal from the pulser for a specified period. The exact nanosecond timing sequence depends on the crystal position and the focal zone depth desired. The wavefront generated by each crystal in the group is made to arrive at a specific point in the phase, and the result is a focused beam at that point.

Fig. 8-14 demonstrates electronic focusing with five crystals of an array. The positions of the crystals are arranged so the distance from either crystal 1 (d_1) or crystal 5 (d_5) to the object or point of interest is the same but greater than the distance from either crystal 2 (d_2) or crystal 4 (d_4). Distances d_2 and d_4 are equal but greater than d_3 (the distance from crystal 3 to the object). For the waves from each crystal to be in phase at the point of interest, constructive interference must occur. Each wavefront must arrive at the point at exactly the same time. This is accomplished by firing crystals 1 and 5 first, delaying a short time (50 to 100 ns) before firing crystals 2 and 4, and finally waiting another short time before firing crystal 3. The ultrasound beam thus is reinforced or focused in the in-plane direction, producing a narrow width over a limited depth near the point of interest. The next segment of crystals (2 through 6) is fired in the same manner (2 and 6, 3 and 5, then 4) to produce another focused beam, but directed along a different line of sight. The remaining segments are also focused by this delayed firing technique. A narrow beam is swept throughout the transducer array to collect an image using a set focal length. The firing sequence is repeated for the next image in the real-time acquisition. Improved spatial detail (lateral resolution) is thus obtained within the focal zone.

Transmit Focusing

Unlike mechanical sector scanners (in which depth of the focal zone is fixed), many linear array units allow the operator to select one of several possible focal lengths (transmit focal zones) within the scan plane. *The depth of the focal zone is altered by varying the delay times between crystal excitations.* The scanning of the region of interest is conducted with a depth of focus selected by the operator. After review of the real-time image, a new focal zone may be selected (by modifying the delay line timing) to rescan the same area with different focusing in the scan plane. The beam is focused to a new depth simply by changing the delay times. This technique is called transmit focusing, and the transducers that have this capability are described as **phased linear arrays.** Electronic phasing of the elements allows variable focusing along the scan line, which, in turn, controls beam width in the in-plane direction (Fig. 8-15).

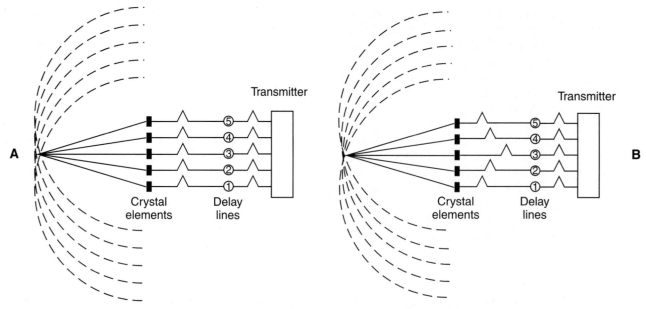

Fig. 8-14 Electronic focusing. **A,** If five crystals are stimulated simultaneously, the wavefronts do not arrive simultaneously at the target, because the distances d_1, d_2, d_3, d_4, and d_5 are not equal. **B,** Transmit delay lines are used to excite the crystals at slightly different times (nanosecond delays between firings). The wavefronts arrive exactly simultaneously at the target point, and the result is a focused beam. Crystals 1 and 5 are stimulated first, then 2 and 4, and then 3. Changing the time delays allows other points to become the center of focus.

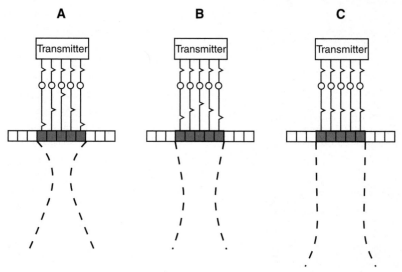

Fig. 8-15 Variable delay lines allow focusing at different depths. The delay lines stagger the timed-excitation pulses to the crystals, depending on the degree of focusing desired. **A,** Short focus. **B,** Medium focus. **C,** Long focus.

High-resolution images with multiple focal zones throughout the image are also possible using these adjustable delay lines (Fig. 8-16). Multizone transmit focusing slows the frame rate, because data must be collected for all the lines of sight across the array with a set focal zone depth before the lines of sight are repeated with a different focal zone depth. For example, assume that the unit can be focused to three different depths for the same "image." In reality, three separate images, each focused to a particular depth, must be collected before they are combined into one

"final image" for viewing. This reduces the frame rate by a factor of three. For six separate focal zones the frame rate is reduced by a factor of six. Equation 7-1 for maximum frame rate (FR_{max}) is modified to read:

8-1

$$FR_{max} = \frac{c}{2\ Rnn_z}$$

where n_z is the number of focal zones used to produce one image, c the velocity of ultrasound, R the depth of interest, and n the number of lines of sight per frame.

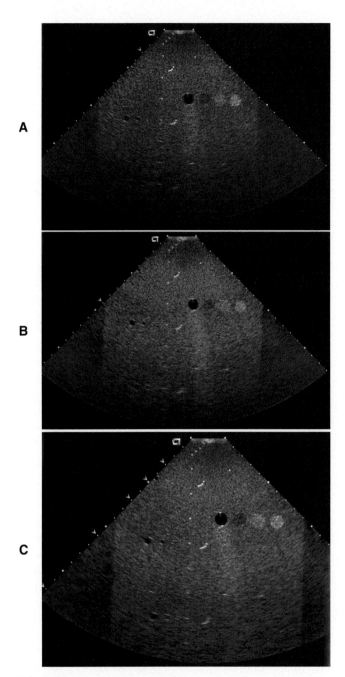

Fig. 8-16 Image quality improvement with transmit focusing. **A,** Single focal zone that does not correspond with the depth of interest (9 cm) in the phantom. **B,** Single focal zone that corresponds with the depth of interest (9 cm) in the phantom. **C,** Multiple transmit focal zones throughout the scan range.

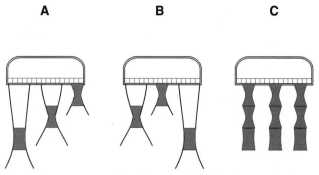

Fig. 8-17 Parallel processing. **A** and **B,** Information for three focal zones is collected and processed simultaneously for three nonadjacent lines of sight. **C,** Once all the segments of a scan line are collected, the data are displayed as one composite scan line. The frame rate is higher than that for multifocal zones acquired individually.

Equation 8-1 is a conservative estimate for maximum frame rate when multiple transmit focal zones are acquired. This equation assumes that all lines of sight are sampled throughout the entire scan range. In order to reduce the acquisition time, data collection is limited to the depth of focus for short and medium focal lengths. This technique improves frame rate performance without sacrificing image content (the information beyond the focal zone is excluded from the final image).

Combining multiple zones to form one image may cause a discontinuity at the boundary between the focal zone areas, called the stitch-line artifact. Parallel processing of the echoes can restore the frame rate to near the original value. The rate of data collection is increased by simultaneously acquiring multiple lines of sight. Selected portions of each line of sight corresponding to the focal depth are retained for the final image. While the line of sight corresponding to the short focused depth is being collected at one location along the array, other lines of sight with different focal depths are being generated at other locations along the array. Because the data for all three zones have been obtained concurrently, the frame rate is not decreased (Fig. 8-17).

Aperture Focusing

Electronic focusing during transmission is also accomplished by varying the number of crystals fired in the segment (Fig. 8-18). For example, two crystals are fired as a group to produce a very short, narrow near field and a rapidly diverging far field (designed to enhance the focal zone near the transducer). If more crystals are added in the group, then the depth of the near field is extended, and the beam width near the transducer is broadened. This method is a focusing technique based on beam aperture. *Large aperture extends the depth of focus.*

Aperture focusing is characterized by the f-number, which is defined as the ratio of the focal length (F) to the size of the aperture along the row of crystal elements (d):

$$f\text{-number} = \frac{F}{d}$$

8-2

Optimal focusing occurs with an f-number of 2. In reality many manufacturers employ combinations of time-delayed firing and changing beam aperture to optimize focusing at different depths. The normal trade-off is a decrease in frame rate (loss of temporal resolution) when multiple focal zones compose the image unless parallel processing is used.

Focusing must occur within the near field of the excited crystal group. The depth of the near field (NFD) is a

A   **B**   **C**

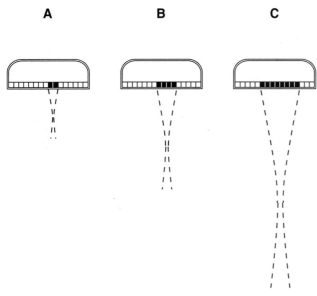

Fig. 8-18 Aperture focusing. Two crystals are fired for short focus **(A),** four crystals for medium focus **(B),** and eight crystals for long focus **(C).**

function of the dimensions of the active elements and the wavelength (λ):

$$NFD = \frac{d^2}{4\,\lambda}$$ **8-3**

where *d* is the aperture, the distance along the length of the array that encompasses elements activated for beam transmission. The aperture is increased to maintain minimum beam width for longer focal lengths.

Focusing narrows the beam width in the region around the focal point (Fig. 8-19). The extent of the focal zone (depth of field) for a multi-element array is determined by aperture size (d), focal length (F), and wavelength (λ).

$$\text{Depth of field} = \frac{7.1\,\lambda F^2}{d^2}$$ **8-4**

To maintain the depth of field as focal length is increased, the aperture must also increase. This is accomplished by using a small group of crystals at short focal lengths and more elements at longer focal lengths. Since the depth of field is inversely proportional to the square of the aperture, at a specific focal length increasing aperture size creates a strongly focused beam and improves lateral resolution. However, some scatterers of interest may be located outside the transmit focal zone, which requires that the transmit focal zone be altered to a new focal length.

Dynamic Receive Focusing

Another means to reduce the effective sampling volume is dynamic focusing in the receive mode. The principle of receive focus is difficult to conceptualize. The following analogy may help: Three runners of equal ability begin a race at the same starting point but follow different routes to the finish line. At the finish line an observer is assigned to each runner and must shout the point of origin when the

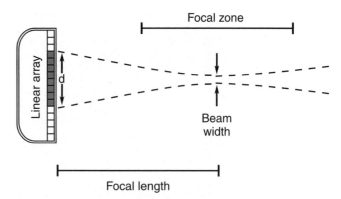

Fig. 8-19 Depth of field. Beam width is most narrow with the focal zone, which is affected by aperture size *(d),* focal length, and wavelength.

runner crosses the finish line. Because the distance traveled by each runner is not identical, three separate shouts are heard as the race is completed. If an obstacle, such as a wall, is placed in the path of each runner, the sequence of finish can be regulated. The height of the wall is adjusted depending on the distance between the starting point and finish line. To increase the delay before crossing the finish line, the obstacle is made greater. In this case, the shortest route would incorporate the tallest wall. For a certain combination of obstacles, the runners finish the race simultaneously, and one loud shout is heard from all the observers identifying the point of origin. The race can be made more complex by varying the starting point. The heights of the obstacles can be adjusted according to the change in distance. Now the observers are given a chart that denotes the starting point based on the elapsed time of the race. This is possible because the participants run at the same speed. The shouts of the observers at the finish line are still synchronized; only the words to identify the starting points vary. **Dynamic receive focusing** works in a similar manner.

By means of delay circuitry in the receiver, the returning sound beam–induced signals are refocused when multiple crystals receive the echo. Dynamic focusing is not limited to one fixed depth per transmitted pulse, as transmit focusing is, but operates at all depths. In Fig. 8-20 five crystals are activated to receive the ultrasound beam reflected toward the transducer from the object. The ultrasound beam diverges during its return to the transducer. The wavefront intercepts crystal 3 first, then crystals 2 and 4, and finally crystals 1 and 5. Through the use of receive-time delays, the echo-induced signal at crystal 3 is delayed, before being sent for processing to the receiver electronics, until the wavefront reaches crystals 1 and 5. Similarly, the echo-induced signals from crystals 2 and 4 are delayed until the wavefront reaches crystals 1 and 5, although the delay time is shorter than for crystal 3. The actual time delay is determined for each crystal by simple geometry and an assumed constant velocity of ultrasound in soft tissue. The wavefront from the object appears to be in phase for all five crystals, resulting in a "focused" beam from that depth of interest. This delay and sum strategy is called **beam formation.**

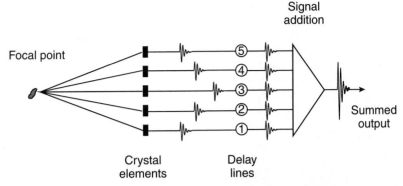

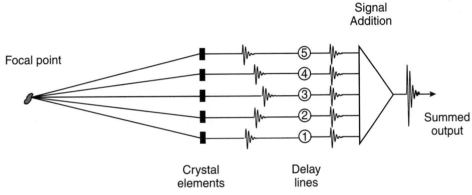

Fig. 8-20 Dynamic receive focusing. The echo wavefront from the object arrives at crystal 3 first, then at 2 and 4, and finally at 1 and 5. By delaying the individual echo signal at each crystal until the wavefront has arrived at all five crystals, focusing is applied to the received signals to produce a summed output.

Fig. 8-21 Dynamic receive focusing. The delay times change with respect to depth. Compare the signal spacing in time with Fig. 8-20.

The same principle applies to an object located farther from the transducer in Fig. 8-21, but because of the greater depth, the wavefront strikes the crystals with less variability. A shorter receive delay focuses the detected signals from the object. The master synchronizer sends timing messages to the receiver-delay lines to indicate the elapsed time from transmission to reception. The elapsed time determines the delay times (in nanoseconds, just as in transmit focusing) for each crystal. The depth for receive focus is always known, and thus receive-delay times are constantly changed to yield a continually focused beam at all depths. That is, during acquisition of image data the receive time delays are varied dynamically to sweep the focal zone to each point along the scan line. Hence, the name of this technique is dynamic receive focusing.

The received beam width is uniformly narrow along the line of sight. In essence, therefore, lateral resolution is improved by restricting the tissue volume that contributes to each building block in the image. A dynamic aperture adjusts the number of receiving crystals along the array as a function of depth. This acquisition technique optimizes focusing at a particular depth. Additional elements are included in the aperture as the depth of the focal zone is increased (Fig. 8-22). *Dynamic receive focusing is achieved without a loss in frame rate or line density.*

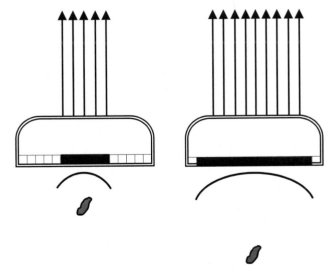

Fig. 8-22 Receive aperture. The number of elements used in beam formation increases with depth.

Each independent element with the associated electronics for transmission and reception constitutes a **channel.** Focusing is improved as the number of channels is increased. Compare the spatial resolution at a depth of 8 cm for the sonograms obtained with 64 versus 128 receive channels (Fig. 8-23).

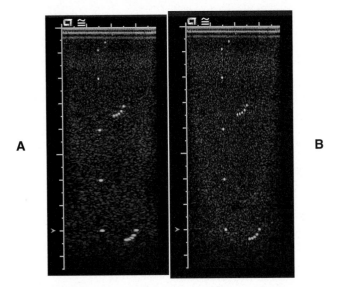

Fig. 8-23 Effect of channel number. Sonograms of a resolution phantom with 64 receive channels (**A**) and 128 receive channels (**B**). (Courtesy Rob Steins.)

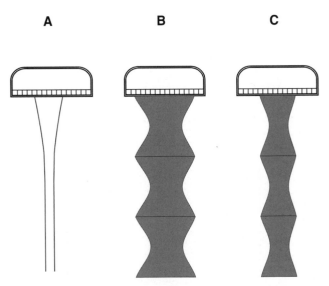

Fig. 8-24 Effective beam width, **C,** is a product of the transmit focal zone, **B,** and the received beam width, **A.**

Effective Beam Width

Linear arrays use both transmit focusing and dynamic receive focusing. The effective beam width is the product of the transmit focal zone beam width and the received beam width (Fig. 8-24). As the number of fixed transmit focal zones increases, the composite effective beam width becomes more narrow (Fig. 8-25). Each segment along the line of sight is optimized for a certain focal length. Since the ultrasound beam diverges rapidly beyond the focal zone, multiple transmit focal zones are necessary to maintain a narrow beam width. The improvement in spatial detail for linear array has contributed to the rapid acceptance of real-time ultrasound in the clinical environment.

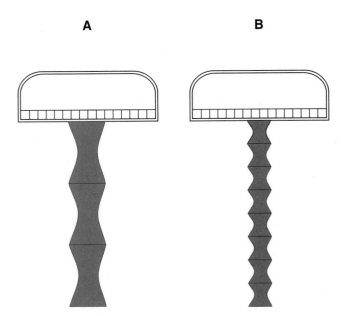

Fig. 8-25 The effective beam width is made narrower by increasing the number of transmit focal zones. **A,** Three zones; **B,** eight zones.

Multiplexers

Communication between the transducer and the transmitter/receiver is through a cable connected to the scanner. In theory each crystal element would have an electrical connection from it to the transmitter/receiver. The number of wires in the cable would, at a minimum, equal the number of crystal elements. In order to reduce the bulk of the cable as well as cost, the number of wires is reduced to carry only the necessary signals for transitory beam formation. For example, suppose a linear array contains 200 crystals, but a maximum of 10 are excited at any one time for beam formation. A cable consisting of 10 wires (instead of 200) could carry signals from the transmitter to the transducer, and at the transducer these signals are directed by a multiplexer to the appropriate crystals for the transmitted pulse.

A multiplexer (demultiplexer) is a switching device with multiple input (output) lines, one of which is connected to the output (input) identified by binary signals applied to the select lines (Fig. 8-26). Three select lines allow the input to be directed to one of eight output lines. Each select line has either a 0 or 1 signal, resulting in eight possible combinations. Additional select lines increase the number of possible output lines. The cable to the transducer must also include the select lines for proper direction of the signals.

CURVILINEAR ARRAYS

In the past few years **curvilinear** (also called convex, curved linear, or radial) **arrays** that produce large sector formats have been developed. Crystal elements are arranged along an arc in a linear fashion. The radius of curvature is usually 25 to 100 mm. A large radius of curvature extends the width of the field of view. As with other types of arrays,

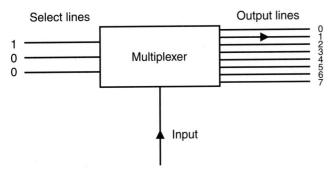

Fig. 8-26 Multiplexer. Input signal is directed along one of eight possible pathways depending on the value specified by the select lines. Binary code 001 selects output line 1.

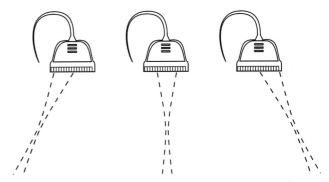

Fig. 8-28 Beam steering with linear phased arrays. The direction of propagation can be varied from one transmitted pulse to the next. Three scan lines are shown.

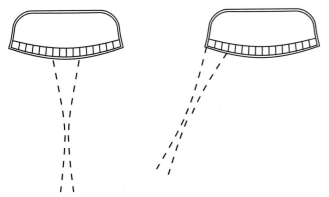

Fig. 8-27 Curvilinear array. Ultrasonic beams are directed perpendicular to the array surface.

the physical dimensions of the crystal elements influence the beam pattern.

As regular linear arrays do, curvilinear arrays sweep the beam by firing multiple crystals in a group, stepping down after the appropriate delay, and then firing the next group. The curved crystal arrangement provides lines of sight that are perpendicular to the array surface (Fig. 8-27). No loss of focus occurs at the edges of the field of view; however, beam divergence may limit the useful depth. Analogous to sector scanning, with curvilinear arrays line density is decreased at depth, and a loss of lateral resolution can occur. As discussed shortly, curved arrays also reduce grating lobes.

LINEAR PHASED ARRAYS

The second type of electronic real-time system, the linear phased array, was developed to overcome certain limitations inherent in the segmental linear array. Image formation with a linear array produces a rectangular format in which the width of the field of view is determined by the physical length of the row of elements in the array, and the maximum number of scan lines corresponds to the number of elements in the array. The relatively low scan lines per frame allow high frame rates, but lateral resolution is sacrificed. The large physical size (several centimeters in length) prevents access to structures where a narrow acoustic window is available (e.g., between the ribs for cardiac imaging).

The linear phased array can be a small transducer with few crystals (16). To generate and direct the ultrasonic beam, all (or most) of the crystals in the array are excited nearly simultaneously (Fig. 8-28). This contrasts with segmental linear arrays, in which the crystals are fired in groups. The design produces a sector format with a sector angle as large as 90 degrees. In the sector format, scan lines diverge with depth, and therefore line density is not constant throughout the field of view. A small sector angle (e.g., 30 degrees) allows a higher frame rate or increased line density. For example, an image composed of 150 scan lines can be updated 30 times per second if the range is 15 cm. A large number of very small crystals (up to 256) may be used to improve spatial resolution. Linear phased arrays are commonly employed in echocardiology, because their small size (10 to 30 mm in length) allows better access to the heart.

Steering the beam throughout the field of view allows for data collection along different lines of sight. Small time delays, on the order of nanoseconds, are used for transmit focusing purposes as the beam is steered. The linear phased array can also be dynamically focused in the receive mode. Outside the central field of view, spatial resolution deteriorates, because electronic focusing becomes more difficult when large-angle beam steering is performed. As with linear arrays, linear phased arrays are mechanically focused in the elevation (slice thickness) direction.

Transmit Steering

The entire linear phased array produces only one line of sight each time the crystal elements are excited. Electronic steering relies on the interference of waves for reinforcement to produce planar wavefronts, thus the name phased steering or phased array. By altering the timing sequence of the excitation pulses, the direction of propagation of the transmitted beam can be varied to any desired scan angle (Fig. 8-29). The scan angle is denoted as the angle between the direction of propagation and the normal to the central element in the array.

Fig. 8-30 illustrates the principle of transmit steering using a five-element linear array. Elements 1 through 5 are

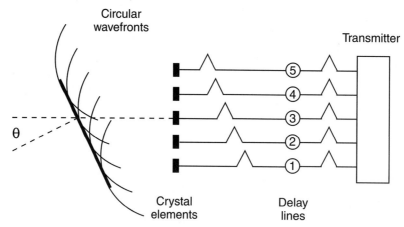

Fig. 8-29 Principle of beam steering. Each crystal after stimulation produces a circular wavefront. The wavefronts from all crystals combine to create a planar wavefront that propagates through tissue at a scan angle θ.

stimulated in sequence with the same time delay between excitations. Each crystal produces a circular wavefront, which moves into tissue. Since the origins of the individual wavefronts are shifted with respect to location and time, they will add together to create a resultant planar wavefront. The planar wavefront propagates through tissue at a constant scan angle.

The acoustic beam is reoriented to any scan angle θ by changing the time delay. For a linear phased array with element separation equal to one half of the wavelength, the time delay is given by:

8-5

$$\text{Time delay} = \frac{\sin \theta}{2\,f}$$

where *f* is the frequency of the transducer. Steering at a scan angle of 30 degrees with an operating frequency of 2.5 MHz requires a 0.1 microsecond delay between excitation of successive elements. For large steering angles the time delay is increased (see Table 8-1).

Transmit Focusing

The concept of beam formation can be extended to include focusing of the transmitted beam at a specific depth along the direction of propagation. In Fig. 8-31 the distance (r_i) between each array element (i) and the point of interest (focal point) is different. The time for sound to travel from element 5 to the focal point is shorter than that for element 4, and the time for sound to travel from element 4 to the focal point is shorter than that for element 3 and so forth. If the delay time between elements is set equal to the time difference for travel, then the wavefronts arrive simultaneously at the focal point.

Mathematically, this relationship is expressed as:

8-6

$$\text{Time delay} = \frac{r_1 - r_i}{c}$$

where *c* is the velocity of sound in tissue and *subscript i* represents crystal elements 2 to 5. The time delay can be

■ **Table 8-1** Time Delay for Steering at Various Scan Angles for 2.5 MHz Transducer

Scan Angle (degrees)	Time Delay (µs)
0	0
5	0.017
10	0.035
15	0.052
20	0.068
25	0.084
30	0.10
35	0.11
40	0.13
45	0.14

calculated from the Law of Cosines using the scan angle, focal length, velocity of sound, and interelement center-to-center spacing. A timing sequence for a 16-element array operating at 2.5 MHz is shown in Table 8-2. Note that the respective time delays between elements are not linear, but rather spherical. The magnitude of the time delay is decreased for longer focal lengths (Fig. 8-32).

As with linear arrays, transmit focusing is limited to one focal point for each transmitted beam. Once data have been collected along this scan line, the focal point can be changed (by modifying the delay line timing) to rescan this line of sight with a new focal point. In this manner the focal point can be positioned at different depths. This improves the lateral resolution. However, multizone transmit focusing slows the frame rate, because multiple transmit pulses are necessary to compose each scan line.

Dynamic Focusing

Dynamic focusing during reception is also possible. Analogous to transmit focusing with respect to the timing sequence, the time-of-flight of the echo created in the focal zone to an array element depends on the focal length, scan angle, and position of the element in the array. By delaying the output from each element by a time specified

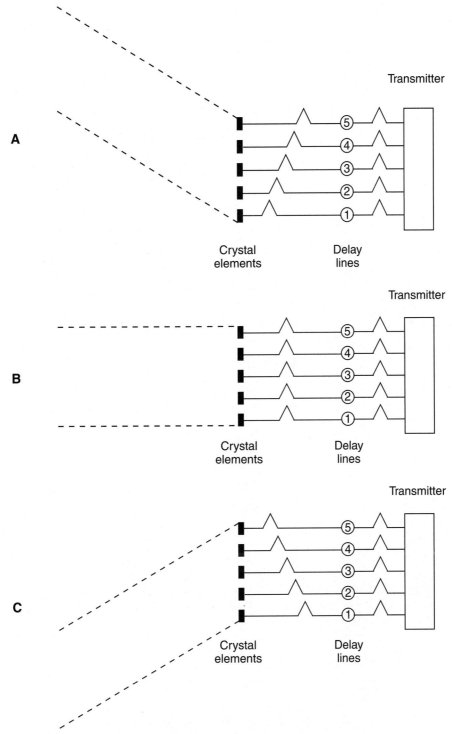

Fig. 8-30 Beam steering with a five-element linear phased array. Each crystal is connected to an adjustable delay line. **A** through **C,** The excitation sequence is changed to steer the beam in different directions.

by Equation 8-6, the signals induced by echoes originating from within the focal zone are synchronized in time. The outputs from all received elements are then summed to produce a large amplitude signal (beam formation).

Fig. 8-33 illustrates that the array is initially focused to a single spatial location during reception. After all echoes

associated with this focal region have been received, the time delay for each channel is changed to create a new focal zone distal to the previous focal zone (Fig. 8-34).

Dynamic focusing improves lateral resolution by restricting the tissue volume that contributes to each summed output. Echoes originating from points outside the focal zone

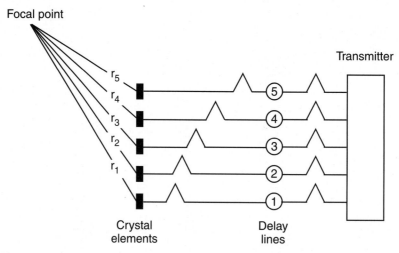

Fig. 8-31 Transmit beam focusing. The distance between the focal point and the element (r_i) determines the delay time before excitation for that element ($i = 1, 2, 3, 4,$ or 5).

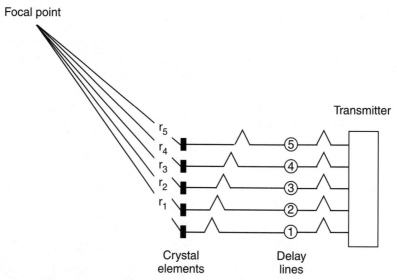

Fig. 8-32 Transmit beam focusing. If the focal point is established farther from the transducer, then the transmitted delay times are changed. Compare the time spacings with those in Fig. 8-31.

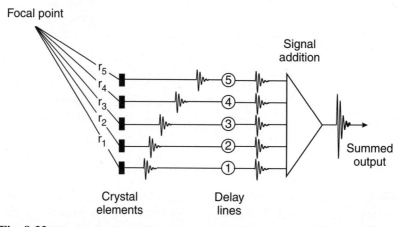

Fig. 8-33 Receive focusing. Echoes generated at the focal point reach elements in the array at slightly difference times. Each induced signal is delayed by an amount corresponding to the difference in travel distance. The signal from element 5 is detected first and must undergo the longest delay before signal addition.

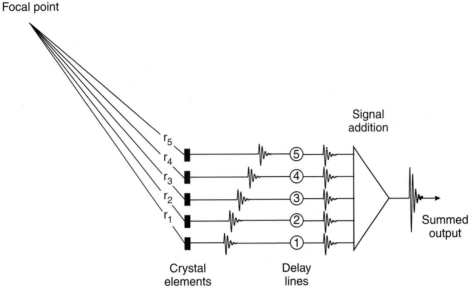

Fig. 8-34 Receive focusing at a focal point distal to that shown in Fig. 8-33. The time sequence of the induced signals in the crystals is less varied.

■ **Table 8-2** Time Delay for Different Focal Lengths (2.5 MHz, Element-to-Element Spacing Equals $1/2\lambda$, and Scan Angle of 0 Degrees)

Element Number	Time Delay (ns)	
	Focal length = 5 cm	Focal length = 10 cm
1	0	0
2	0.618	0.313
3	2.46	1.24
4	5.55	2.77
5	9.86	4.92
6	15.4	7.7
7	22.2	11.1
8	30.2	15.1
9	22.2	11.1
10	15.4	7.7
11	9.86	4.92
12	5.55	2.77
13	2.46	1.24
14	0.618	0.313
15	0	0

will induce signals, but after the time delays these signals are not coherent, and thus the summed amplitude is low.

Channels

Grating lobes are avoided if the interelement spacing is one half of the wavelength. Consequently, phased arrays are constructed with a high number of very small crystal elements. Since each element requires a communication pathway from the transducer to the scanner, the cable becomes larger and more bulky as the number of channels is increased. The associated electronics required for each channel cause phased array to be more expensive than other types of transducers.

COMPOUND LINEAR ARRAYS

Compound linear arrays (also called vector arrays) have been developed to incorporate characteristics from both the linear array and the linear phased array. Multiple crystals are fired at one time to steer the beam in various directions. Scan lines for the central field of view are obtained by directing the beam perpendicular to the array. At the extremes of the field of view the ultrasound beam is steered at wide angles by the phased method. The timed excitation of a large number of crystals is controlled by delay lines. An enlarged effective field of view that extends beyond the physical length of the array is created. Areas of overlapping data are manipulated by the scan converter to form a composite image. The **footprint** is smaller than that for the curvilinear array, and the field of view is trapezoidal in shape.

ANNULAR PHASED ARRAYS

Annular phased array transducers, when viewed end on (Fig. 8-35), have a central crystal surrounded by concentric rings of additional crystals. For each transmitted pulse, each crystal is excited in such a fashion as to permit electronic focusing to a very small region (1 to 3 mm) at a specified depth along the beam axis. Changing the timing sequence sweeps the focal zone through multiple depths along the beam axis. Dynamic receive focusing is also possible, although an annular phased array must be mechanically steered to collect different scan lines.

Steering is accomplished by reflecting the beam from a moving mirror or by rotating the transducer mechanically without a mirror. The mirror systems are usually liquid path. The ultrasound beam converges symmetrically to the focal point (Fig. 8-36). The beam width is the same in both the slice-thickness direction and the in-plane direction (similar to a circular transducer). This symmetrical beam should

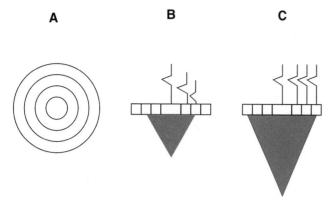

Fig. 8-35 Annular array. **A,** Top view of an annular array showing four crystal elements. Note that all except the innermost crystal are doughnut shaped. **B,** Side view to show focusing at shallow depth. **C,** Side view to show focusing at increased depth.

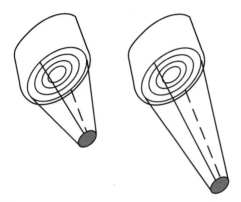

Fig. 8-36 Electronic focusing with annular arrays. The dimensions of the beam at the focal point are symmetrical and unchanged at different depths.

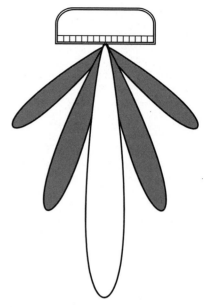

Fig. 8-37 Side lobes (*shaded regions*) at various angles with respect to the main beam.

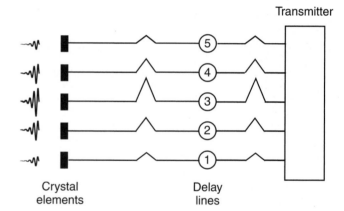

Fig. 8-38 Apodization demonstrated by varying the strength of the voltage pulse to each crystal (represented by different peak heights in a five-crystal segment). The highest voltage is applied to the center crystal.

be contrasted with ultrasound beams generated by linear arrays, which have varying dimensions depending on the focusing technique, pulsing sequence, and crystal size.

PROBLEMS WITH ELECTRONIC ARRAYS

A major problem with electronic arrays is the formation of secondary lobes of ultrasound energy. Secondary lobes originate at the transducer and radiate outward at various angles to the main beam. Artifacts in the image are created by the misregistration of interface position, since all returning echoes are assumed to originate along the main beam axis. Secondary lobes are also responsible for clutter (induced signals from echoes formed along the path of the secondary lobes), which inhibits the detection of weak echoes. There are two types of secondary lobes: **side lobes** and **grating lobes.**

Side Lobes

Side lobes (Fig. 8-37), which are present with all transducers (single or multiple crystals), result from width and length mode vibrations (radial mode vibrations for circular and annular transducers), immediate reverberations at

crystal-tissue interfaces, and interference phenomena. They are typically of low intensity compared with the main beam. A technique called **apodization** lowers their intensity for electronic arrays. Apodization employs a variable-strength voltage pulse to the crystals across the aperture during delay line focusing. The excitation voltage to the individual crystals of each segment is maximized at the center and reduced toward the periphery (Fig. 8-38). During reception the contribution to the overall signal from crystals located toward the outer edges of the aperture is also reduced.

Increasing the number of similar elements in the active area of an array (effectively creating a larger generating aperture) reduces the intensity of side lobes. When the side lobes are approximately 60 dB below the main beam intensity, no serious misregistration artifacts in the image are created. Clutter is still present, however, which influences

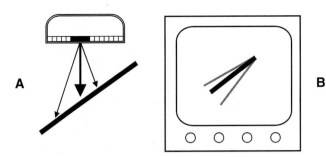

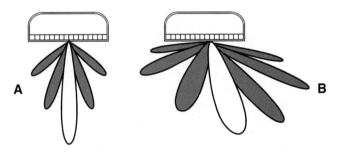

Fig. 8-39 Grating lobe artifacts. **A,** Since the interface is at an angle to the main beam, two additional reflected echoes are produced. They correspond to the grating lobes striking the interface before and after the main beam. **B,** The object is registered at three locations in the displayed image. True location is shown in black, and the false locations are shown in gray.

sensitivity. High-frequency transducers reduce the number and intensity of the side lobes.

Grating Lobes

Another significant secondary lobe problem unique to linear arrays is grating lobes, which are caused by the regular periodic spacing of elements within the array. Grating lobes create artifacts in the image by measuring the time of flight (distance) to an object located outside the main beam and placing the detected echo as if the interface were located along the ultrasound path of the main beam. All ultrasound scanners assume that the registered echoes travel in a straight line along the axial line of sight. If grating lobes are present, artifacts appear closer to and/or farther behind the true position of the object depending on whether the grating lobe strikes the object before or after the main beam (Fig. 8-39). This occurs because the grating lobes are traveling at an angle to the main beam. These artifacts are very prominent at highly reflective interfaces (e.g., the diaphragm behind the liver). Grating lobes also contribute to clutter and reduce image contrast.

The specific angular location of the grating lobes is given by the following formula:

8-7

$$\sin \theta = \frac{m\lambda}{x}$$

where θ is the grating lobe angle from the central axis, m an integer denoting order of the grating lobes (1, 2, 3, etc.), λ the wavelength, and x the center-to-center distance between adjacent array elements.

Equation 8-7 demonstrates that the only way to modify the grating lobes for a given frequency is to change the spacing distance (x). When this element-to-element distance is decreased to less than one wavelength, the angle of the grating lobes becomes greater than 90 degrees with respect to the main beam, and thus the grating lobes are eliminated.

Unfortunately, the elements of the array are often spaced greater than one wavelength from center to center; however, design engineers have found that the grating lobes can be reduced or eliminated by a technique called **subdicing.** In

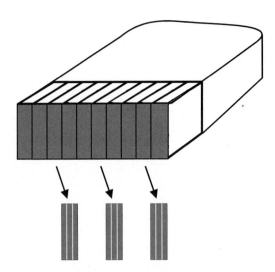

Fig. 8-40 Electronic linear array showing the subdiced crystal elements.

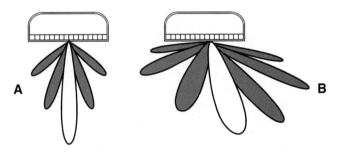

Fig. 8-41 Comparison of grating lobes for a stepdown segmental linear array, **A,** and a linear phased array, **B.** The number and intensity of grating lobes are increased for the steered linear phased array.

this technique, the normal element of an array is divided into many smaller subelements with the subelements electronically wired together to form the original-size element (Fig. 8-40). The subdiced elements act in concert as a single crystal. This effectively reduces the center-to-center distance between elements and makes the grating lobes occur at an angle of greater than 90 degrees.

Linear phased arrays have a more severe problem with grating lobes, because the steering of an ultrasound beam at large angles increases the number and intensity of grating lobes as compared with the nonsteered beam from a stepdown segmental linear array (Fig. 8-41). The grating lobes are a result of the summation of side lobes from the individual crystals. When multiple crystals are pulsed for steering, low-intensity side lobes are added together and create significant secondary lobes of energy. Curvilinear arrays partially eliminate grating lobes since the beam is not steered.

Crystal Element Isolation

One additional problem with linear array systems is inter-element isolation, which is a measure of how one element of an array affects adjacent elements. When a voltage pulse excites one element, the other elements should not respond.

The same holds true when a crystal receives an echo. No communication (cross-talk) should take place between a supposedly isolated crystal element and neighboring crystals. Electrical and mechanical coupling exists between the array elements and cannot be completely eliminated. The quality of real-time images deteriorates when the crystal elements are not electrically and mechanically isolated from each other. Fortunately, ways to reduce the effects of coupling have been developed.

The array elements are isolated electrically by separate ground wires and separate signal electrodes for each element (including subdiced elements). Nevertheless, the elements are not completely isolated electronically, because they act as tiny capacitors (devices that store electrical charge). If the voltage changes in one crystal (due to an excitation or induced radiofrequency [RF] signal from an echo), the neighboring crystals are affected because of the capacitance of the elements, although this effect can be made quite small.

Mechanical isolation is a much more difficult problem to overcome, because the elements are mechanically coupled by the matching layers, focusing lenses, and backing material. Even the housing itself, which is used for electrical and acoustic insulation, serves to couple the elements together. Return echoes pass through the matching layers and focusing lens before striking the crystal element to induce an RF signal. The return echoes are dispersed (similar to light from a cassette screen in radiology) and also strike the adjacent crystals; thus low-amplitude signals are induced in these elements.

Furthermore, crystals must be mechanically isolated to prevent cross-talk (ultrasound transfer between crystals). Air, as a spacing material, partially eliminates this coupling. Any sound produced by a crystal from length mode vibrations is reflected back into the crystal rather than transmitted to the adjacent crystals. An alternative method of isolating crystals is to design the width and length dimensions to be dramatically different from the thickness. If any width or length mode vibration does occur, the vibration is at a different frequency from the center frequency of the transducer (which is caused by thickness mode vibration). The bandwidth of the receiver, normally sensitive to thickness mode frequencies, is tuned to be insensitive to the width and length mode frequencies. An aspect ratio (thickness/length or thickness/width) of 2:1 provides significant cross-talk reduction. As mentioned, total mechanical isolation cannot be achieved, because the continuity of matching layers, lenses, and backing material extends over the array.

Other factors that influence the transducer design—the electromechanical coupling coefficient, the Q-value, and the acoustic impedance discussed in Chapter 4—also affect the performance of electronic real-time transducers.

DIGITAL BEAM FORMER

The function of focusing during transmission and reception is executed by a digital beam former. The complex combination of time delays, aperture, and apodization are applied with digital electronics during both transmission and reception. Compared with analog devices, digital beam formers allow greater flexibility in beam manipulation with regard to ultrasonic field shape, beam width, direction, and intensity.

SMALL-FOOTPRINT TRANSDUCERS

Linear phased arrays with small physical dimensions (miniature probes) are desirable for neonatal applications and small parts scanning. However, these transducers have, by necessity, a limited area for assembling the piezoelectric elements. The size of their active radiating surface is their footprint.

Electronic focusing becomes suboptimal as scanning range is extended beyond a depth equal to twice the active length of the array. For an aperture of 14 mm × 8 mm, this corresponds to a depth of 28 mm. Miniature probes, because of their limited range, operate at high frequency (5 to 15 MHz) and have excellent axial resolution (Fig. 8-42). Additional advantages of small-footprint transducers are their reduced weight and relatively wide field of view (90-degree sector format).

COMPOSITE MATERIAL TRANSDUCERS

A composite material transducer is formed by dicing the piezoelectric material into an array of rectangular pillars and filling the interspace with epoxy resin. Each pillar is small, measuring one third of a wavelength in cross-section. The pillar-to-pillar separation is twice the dimension of the pillar. The electromechanical coupling coefficient is increased to 0.6 to 0.7, because each pillar in the composite operates in a rodlike rather than a thickness vibration mode. Epoxy is less dense and more flexible than the replaced piezoelectric material, which causes a reduction in the acoustic impedance to 10 to 20 megarayls (Mrayls). Since acoustic impedance more closely approaches tissue, good transmission is obtained with a single matching layer. It is also easy to shape the composite material for the desired geometric focusing.

The epoxy fill improves element isolation—lateral resonance and coupling between elements is reduced,

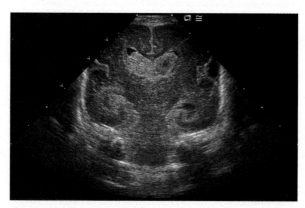

Fig. 8-42 Sonogram of a neonate head acquired with a small footprint transducer (1.5-cm aperture).

resulting in a more uniform frequency response. The combination of high electromechanical coupling coefficient and relatively low acoustic impedance improves sensitivity.

BROADBAND TRANSDUCERS

Composite piezoelectric materials have been formulated for lowering the acoustic impedance of the crystal. This design change, in combination with improved matching layer performance, has enabled ultrasound pulses with higher-frequency components to be generated. The additional frequency components broaden the bandwidth (hence the name **broadband transducers**). The fractional bandwidth is increased significantly to 60% to 80% and may be as high as 160%. As a numerical example, the frequencies included within 3 dB of the maximum on the frequency response curve range from 3 MHz to 7 MHz for a center frequency of 5 MHz and 80% fractional bandwidth.

These transducer modifications result in a shortened pulse length for better axial resolution and higher conversion efficiencies for increased sensitivity. Lateral resolution depends primarily on beam width. Increased sensitivity allows broadband transducers to operate at higher frequency for a particular application, resulting in smaller beam width and thus improved lateral resolution.

The frequency distribution of the transmitted pulse also affects the beam intensity pattern. High-frequency components tend to increase the intensity maximum in the focal zone and cause a rapid decrease of intensity with depth. The presence of low-frequency components extends the depth of penetration. Thus a trade-off exists between axial resolution and depth of penetration.

An innovation made possible by broadband transducers is the manipulation of transmit frequency bandwidth and received frequency bandwidth to optimize image data acquisition. The specific adjustments depend on the desired information. Excellent spatial detail using the high frequency portion of the bandwidth can be obtained.

ENDOSONOGRAPHY

The miniaturization of electronics and the refinement of real-time transducers have led to the development of specialized probes. **Endosonography** transducers, such as endovaginal (transvaginal), endorectal, and transesophageal, are specially designed real-time mechanical, linear array, or phased array transducers mounted on probes that can be inserted into various body cavities (even the sinuses).

Beam Steering and Focusing

Several endovaginal probes are available in which a single, focused crystal is mounted at the end of the probe. This crystal is mechanically swept up and down to produce a 45- to 110-degree sagittal sector. By rotating and tilting the probe different planes are imaged, although transverse views are not possible. Other endovaginal probes, by mounting the crystal on the top (top mounted) or side of the probe (side mounted), are able to acquire transverse planes (Fig. 8-43). The plane of imaging is changed by moving the probe to a different depth. At least one mechanical system allows for collection of sagittal and transverse planes and all planes in between by attaching the crystal to a base that rotates over a 180-degree arc. The sonographer manually turns the base controls while the probe is in place to select the desired plane. The crystal is mechanically swept in an arc through the selected plane. Fetal anatomy is often more clearly presented when endovaginal scanning is used to supplement the more traditional transabdominal scanning (Fig. 8-44).

Linear array and linear phased array endosonography transducers work in the same manner as the corresponding contact real-time transducers; they are just much smaller. Multiple lines of sight for each image are collected, either by mechanically sweeping the beam back and forth or by electronically sweeping or steering the beam over the region of interest. Because the crystals are close to the tissues of interest, and there is thus minimal sampling depth, many lines of sight can be collected to improve the spatial mapping. The obvious necessity of keeping the transducer crystal(s) small creates problems in maintaining a narrow beam, but restricted sampling depth overcomes this difficulty.

Both electronic focusing and dynamic receive focusing are possible. High-frequency transducers are used to optimize axial and lateral resolution. By pulsing at very high PRFs, rapid framing rates can be obtained, which is particularly valuable for transesophageal imaging of the heart. Scan data from multiple planes are acquired throughout the area of interest by rotating or moving the probe within the body cavity.

Multiple arrays can be incorporated into the same probe so orthogonal planes are visualized without reorienting the probe. The dual-headed probes emit two frequencies for

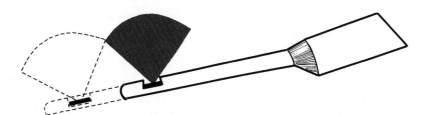

Fig. 8-43 Endosonography transducer probe showing a side-mounted mechanically sectored crystal. Scan data are collected in the transverse plane *(shaded region).* By moving the probe, different transverse views are obtained *(dotted region).*

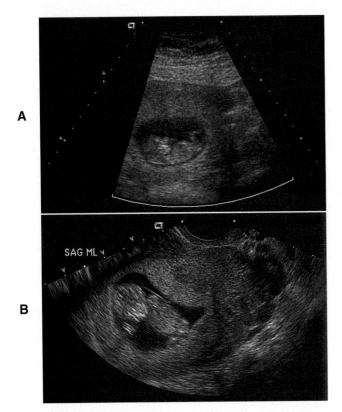

Fig. 8-44 Sonogram of a fetus. **A,** Transabdominal scan. **B,** Endovaginal scan. Note the improved tissue contrast compared with sonogram in **A.**

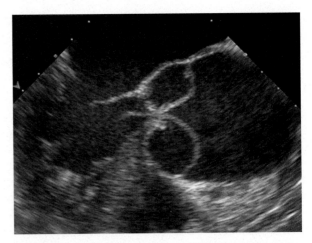

Fig. 8-45 Sonogram of an aortic valve obtained with a transesophageal probe. (Courtesy Bridget Marsolo.)

collecting two frequency-dependent images of a single plane. Multiple-frequency acquisitions may be of value for tissue characterization.

Scanning Techniques

During endorectal and endovaginal imaging the probe is normally covered with a plastic sheath or condom filled with water to enhance acoustic coupling. These probes have special attachments that are desirable for ultrasound-guided biopsy or amniocentesis. Intraoperative imaging, particularly for brain, liver, pancreas, and gallbladder procedures, is also possible. A special sterilization cover is placed over the probe for intraoperative scanning. Extremely high-detailed images are obtained intraoperatively, and puncture biopsies can be performed with precision using the endoprobes. Operator-controlled angle offsets of the mechanically moved crystal or electronic array are available to define the spatial relations between the anatomic structures of interest more accurately.

Transesophageal Probes

Special endosonographic transducers for examination of the heart have been developed. These typically small electronic linear or phased arrays are inserted down the esophagus to acquire two-dimensional images of the heart (Fig. 8-45). Mechanical sector probes are somewhat more difficult to construct with the small dimensions necessary for transesophageal applications. Because the transducer is close to the heart, high frequency, high line density, and high frame rates are achievable. Acoustic coupling devices (e.g., water-filled condoms) are not necessary, because the esophagus tends to collapse around the probe.

TRANSLUMINAL TRANSDUCERS

The miniaturization of electronics and transducer arrays has led to the development of transvascular (transluminal) ultrasound transducers. Extremely small crystal arrays are mounted on the end of a catheter to inspect the interior of vessels visually for vascular plaques (Fig. 8-46). These transducers, which operate at 10 to 20 MHz, produce very-high-detail images that aid in the placement of balloons for plaque reduction or laser obliteration. Such probes have proven to be valuable in echocardiology for assessing valves and cardiac vessels, particularly in postinfarction procedures. Placement of catheters through the umbilical cord to the fetal heart may have applications in fetal cardiology. Transluminal probes are also inserted into the fallopian tubes to evaluate the status of a fertilized oocyte.

1.5D ARRAY TRANSDUCERS

The major weakness of multiple-element linear arrays is the inability to employ dynamic focusing techniques to reduce the slice thickness of the transmitted beam. Focusing in the elevation plane is commonly accomplished by acoustic lenses with fixed focal length. Within the focal zone the slice thickness is 3 to 5 mm, but outside the focal zone slice thickness can increase to 10 mm. Compare this to a beam width of about 1 mm, which is achievable by electronic focusing in the scan plane. This relatively large beam width creates partial volume artifacts when imaging small lesions. Contours may be blurred, and the detected signal level is a combination of the lesion and the surrounding tissue. The 1.5D array transducer was developed to allow electronic focusing in the elevation plane.

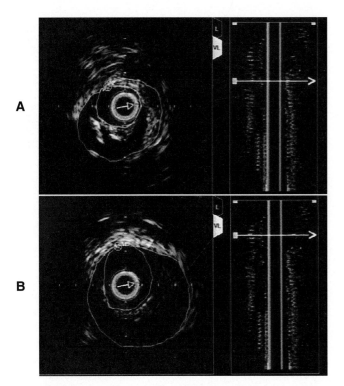

Fig. 8-46 Transvascular probe placed in a vessel with transverse and longitudinal views. **A,** Plaque present in vessel. **B,** Following treatment in which the plaque was ruptured.

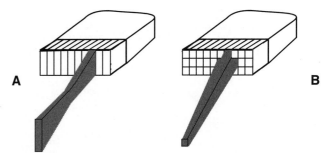

Fig. 8-47 1.5D transducer. **A,** For a linear array, focusing in the elevation direction is fixed to a particular depth. **B,** By subdividing the crystals along the width direction of the 1.5D array, focusing in the elevation direction at different depths is possible.

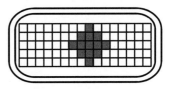

Fig. 8-48 Cross-sectional view of a 1.5D transducer showing the active elements for one scan line.

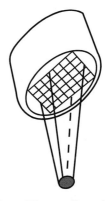

Fig. 8-49 2D transducer. The two-dimensional array of crystal elements enables focusing and steering of the beam throughout the sampled volume.

The single row of elements in the conventional linear array is replaced by three to seven rows of smaller elements in the 1.5D array (Fig. 8-47). The interelement spacing is one half of the wavelength and the interrow spacing is 10 times the wavelength. Beam direction is determined by element selection—no beam steering via time delay occurs. The small number of additional elements and even fewer delay channels enable electronic focusing in the elevation plane. A cross-sectional view of the active elements for one scan line is shown in Fig. 8-48. Portrayal of small lesions is improved and more uniform at all depths.

HANAFY LENS

An alternative method to control beam width in the elevation plane is to use a variable-thickness crystal called a Hanafy lens. The central portion of the crystal in the elevation direction is thin, resonates at high frequency, and forms a superficially focused beam. The crystal becomes thicker, resonates at lower frequency, and contributes to focusing at progressively deeper depths as the outer boundary of the crystal is approached. This technique produces an extremely broad bandwidth pulse with narrow slice thickness along the scan line.

2D ARRAY TRANSDUCERS

Electronic steering in three dimensions producing a volumetric image without moving the transducer is the motivation for current research to develop 2D array transducers. The 2D array is formed by a matrix of crystal elements with

a similar number of rows and columns. One design consists of a 64 × 64 matrix containing 4096 total elements of 300 μm each. Each element must have an electrical connection to participate in beam formation. The beam can be focused in both the elevation and azimuth planes as the beam is steered (Fig. 8-49). Several factors, including cost, complexity of beam formation, and high information content, have delayed the commercial availability of 2D arrays.

TRANSDUCER CARE

Many external transducers are not watertight, and thus immersion in liquids can damage the transducer. The preferred cleaning method is a damp cloth moistened with soap and water, isopropyl alcohol, or diluted bleach. If decontamination of bodily fluids is required, then disinfecting and

■ **Table 8-3** Transducer Characteristics

Type	Scanning Mechanism	In-plane Focusing	Slice Thickness	Image Format	Footprint
Mechanical sector	Mechanical	Mechanical	Mechanical	Sector	Pointed
Linear array	Electronic sequencing	Electronic	Mechanical	Rectangular	Flat
Phased linear array	Electronic sequencing	Electronic	Mechanical	Rectangular	Flat
Curvilinear array	Electronic sequencing	Electronic	Mechanical	Sector	Curved
Linear phased array	Electronic steering	Electronic	Mechanical	Sector	Pointed
Compound array	Electronic steering	Electronic	Mechanical	Trapezoidal	Flat
Annular phased array	Mechanical	Electronic	Electronic	Sector	Pointed

sterilizing solutions usually containing glutaraldehyde are used. Intracavitary probes are soaked in the disinfecting liquid. Check the manufacturer's recommendations for cleaning.

Gas sterilization, ultraviolet sterilization, dry heat sterilization, autoclaving, and soaking in chlorine bleach can damage the transducer and must be avoided. If sterility is required, then the transducer is placed in a sterile sleeve filled with sterile coupling gel.

Chemical agents containing acetone, mineral oil, iodine, and oil-based perfume can also damage the transducer. Coupling gels with these chemical agents should not be used. Also, certain coupling gels may be toxic to human reproductive cells. The manufacturer usually provides a listing of approved products.

SUMMARY

Many different types of transducers have been developed for real-time imaging, including mechanical sector, linear array, linear phased array, phased linear array, curvilinear, annular phased array, and compound array. All these transducers with the exception of the mechanical sector contain multiple crystal elements, which are individually controlled for beam formation during transmission of the ultrasound beam and reception of tissue generated echoes. Characteristics of each transducer type are summarized in Table 8-3.

Electronic sequencing/steering and focusing for a multi-element array are applied only within the scan plane. Geometric focusing with a lens or curved crystal elements determines slice thickness. The curvature of the elements determines the depth of focus in this dimension, which is unchangeable.

Transmit focusing is limited to one focal zone for each transmitted pulse directed along a specific scan line. Dynamic receive focusing is applied to echo-induced signals from multiple elements to focus the resultant signal to a particular point along the scan line. Beam formation during reception is a dynamic process in which focusing is swept along all depths of the scan line as a function of elapsed time. After data collection for one scan line is completed, then the transmitted pulse is directed along a new scan line, and the beam formation processing is repeated.

Multizone transmit focusing improves the lateral resolution of B-mode image by minimizing the beam width throughout the scan line. This is accomplished by using multiple focal zones, each with a different depth of focus along a single scan line.

Gray-scale presentation of the acoustic properties of individual tissues has been improved by more precise in-plane and out-of-plane focusing of the ultrasound beam, reduced contributions from side lobes and grating lobes, diminished cross-talk between crystals, more uniform matched performance of crystals in arrays, and greater sensitivity.

REVIEW QUESTIONS

1. What is the method of focusing for electronic linear array in the elevation direction (out-of-plane or slice thickness)?
2. Name three methods of focusing during transmission for linear arrays.
3. For a linear array, what method is used to direct the beam across the region of interest?
4. For a linear phased array, what method is used to steer the beam across the region of interest?
5. For an annular phased array, what method is used to scan the beam across the region of interest?
6. Name two components of dynamic receive focusing.
7. Consider a linear array with 150 scan lines. How much time is required to form one image if the depth of interest is 8 cm?
8. Calculate the f-number for a focal length of 5 cm using an aperture 3 cm in length.

BIBLIOGRAPHY

Hangiandreous NJ: B-mode US: basic concepts and new technology, *Radiographics* 23:1019-1033, 2003.

Hykes DL, Hedrick WR: Real-time ultrasound instrumentation, *J Diagn Med Sonography* 6:257, 1990.

Kremkau FW: Multiple-element transducers, *Radiographics* 13:1163-1176, 1993.

McDicken WN: *Diagnostic ultrasonics: principles and use of instruments,* ed 3, Edinburgh, 1991, Churchill Livingstone.

Rizzatto G: Evolution of ultrasound transducers: 1.5 and 2D arrays, *Eur Radiol* 9:S304-306, 1999.

Thomenius KE: Instrumentation for B-mode imaging. In Goldman LW, Fowlkes JB, eds: *Categorical course in diagnostic radiology physics: CT and US cross-sectional imaging,* Oak Brook, Ill, 2000, Radiological Society of North America.

Von Ramm OT, Smith SW: Beam steering with linear arrays, *IEEE Trans Biomed Eng* 30:438-452, 1983.

Wells PNT: *Physical principles of ultrasonic diagnosis,* New York, 1969, Academic Press.

Wells PNT: *Biomedical ultrasonic,* New York, 1977, Academic Press.

Whittingham TA: Broadband transducers, *Eur Radiol* 9:S298-303, 1999.

Real-Time Ultrasound Instrumentation

3D ultrasound
4D ultrasound
Cine loop
Coded waveforms
Elasticity imaging
Extended field of view
Frequency averaged image

Harmonic frequencies
Nonlinear propagation
Phase aberration
Spatial compounding
Tissue harmonic imaging
Voxel

The transducer forms and directs the ultrasound beam into the patient and then detects the returning echoes. But the transducer must be incorporated into an electronic environment that controls transducer functions, manipulates the radiofrequency (RF) signals, and composes the image. All signal and image processing must be completed in real-time. The conversion to digital electronics has increased processing speed and capabilities. The result has been improved image quality and expanded types of real-time instrumentation.

IMAGE ACQUISITION

Fig. 9-1 is a block diagram of the image acquisition components of a B-mode scanner. A mechanical sector has a single crystal with one pulser and one transmit/receive switch. The complexity increases dramatically for multiple-element arrays. A system with 128 channels requires 128 pulsers, 128 transmit/receive switches, and 128 crystals in the array. The transmit/receive switch is designed to isolate the sensitive amplification stage from the high voltages associated with crystal excitation.

On command, the pulsers generate a square wave burst of one to three cycles, which is directed by transmit/receive switches and multiplexers to the appropriate crystals within the transducer for beam formation. Beam formation in the transmit mode consists of both beam steering/sequencing and focusing including aperture selection, generation of time delays, and apodization. The stimulated crystals generate an ultrasound pulse of short duration and send it into the body. During reception the transducer converts the returning echoes from interfaces along the scan line to electronic signals that can be subsequently processed and displayed. The processing sequence for the received signal is time gain compensation (TGC), gain, beam formation (receive mode), signal processing, scan conversion, image processing, image storage, and display.

TGC is variable gain applied as a function of elapsed time to compensate for attenuation caused by sound propagation through tissue. The amplifier increases the relatively weak received signals (microvolts to a few millivolts) to the range of 1 volt for analog-to-digital conversion (ADC). ADC usually takes place in the beam former, which is described as a digital beam former. The function of the beam

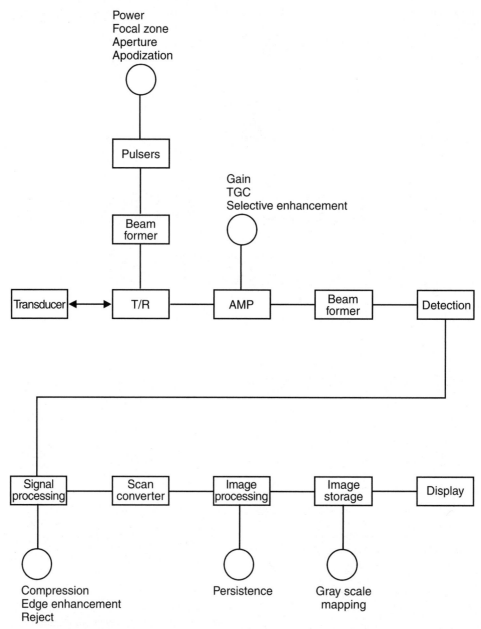

Fig. 9-1 Image-acquisition components of a real-time scanner. Circles indicate operator controls.

former is to perform dynamic receive focusing of the detected echo across several crystal elements. The beam-sum signal is then modified by applying logarithmic compression and edge enhancement before envelope detection.

Scan data are acquired line by line in a sector or rectangular grid format that must be converted into the raster format for display. This takes places in the scan converter, which is essentially an image matrix in computer memory. Once the image is formed, additional processing such as gray scale mapping and persistence are executed. Finally, the digital signals in computer memory are converted to analog video signal for display.

Signal and image processing are discussed in more detail in the next chapter. Digital beam former, scan converter, operator controls, and system design are examined in the following sections.

BEAM FORMER

In the digital beam former, time-gain–compensated RF signals from the crystals undergo analog to digital conversion before interpolation, time delay, apodization, and summing (Fig. 9-2). Analog to digital conversion occurs at a sampling rate of 20 to 40 million times each second with 8 to 12 bits. The dynamic range after TGC and gain amplification is 50 to 80 dB. Digitalization in 12 bits reduces the dynamic range to 36 dB. Interpolation increases the effective sampling rate by a factor of 4 to allow nanosecond time delays for dynamic receive focusing. Channel-specific time delays are applied as a function of elapsed time so that echoes from the receding transmitted pulse stay continuously in focus. Weighting of the channel signals (dynamic apodization) minimizes side-lobe levels and enhances focusing.

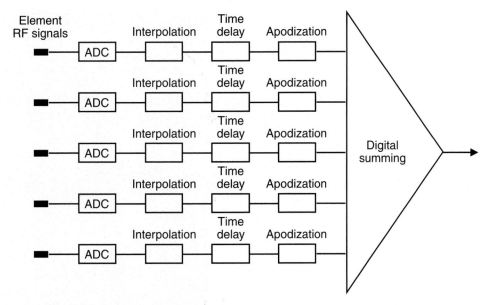

Fig. 9-2 Digital beam former.

In a hybrid design, analog processing of multiple channels with appropriate analog time delays occurs before digital conversion and beam summing. The number of ADCs is reduced to lower cost. In general, analog delay lines degrade beam former performance, resulting in limited accuracy and variations with time and temperature. Digital beam formers are more stable and offer greater flexibility.

IMAGE MATRIX

For the digitized representation of the echo signal to be placed at the correct location in the image matrix, the spatial coordinates (row and column) must be specified. This is accomplished by a position generator, which uses the time of travel for the ultrasound pulse and position sensors (single-element transducers) or element selection/phasing (multielement arrays) for beam direction. The beam sweeps through the region of interest either electronically or mechanically in a repetitive fashion. The signal amplitude and position coordinates for multiple lines of sight are placed temporarily in the buffer before transfer to the scan converter. The format is changed from signal levels along successive lines of sight to the matrix notation, which represents a composite of all scan data. The buffer also serves to hold the scan data acquired at a very rapid rate until the computer can store the information in memory.

Fig. 9-3 shows two successive line-of-sight samplings of an object. Three reflecting structures of varying amplitude are detected. The contents of the buffer corresponding to the two lines of sight are listed in Table 9-1, where the signal level is recorded as a function of the Cartesian spatial coordinates. Alternatively, the beam angle and elapsed time could be placed in the buffer to indicate position (with the spatial coordinates calculated from these two parameters).

The signal amplitudes are assigned to the appropriate pixels in an 8 × 8 matrix (Fig. 9-4). The spatial coordinates

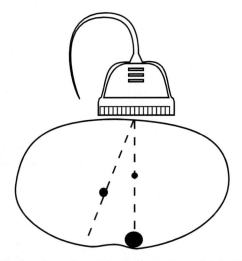

Fig. 9-3 Sampling of a patient along two lines of sight. Note that the two interfaces are detected along the central line of sight. The size of the black dot is directly proportional to the intensity of the reflected echo.

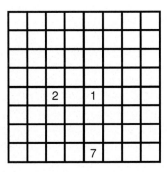

Fig. 9-4 An 8 × 8 matrix depicting the three structures observed in Fig. 9-3. Note that the pixels corresponding to the various interfaces are assigned different values based on the intensity of the reflected echoes.

■ **Table 9-1** Contents of the Buffer for Successive Scan Lines

Signal Amplitude	X Position	Y Position
000	5	1
000	5	2
000	5	3
000	5	4
001	5	5
000	5	6
000	5	7
111	5	8
000	5	1
000	5	2
000	4	2
000	4	3
000	3	4
010	3	5
000	2	6
000	2	7
000	1	8

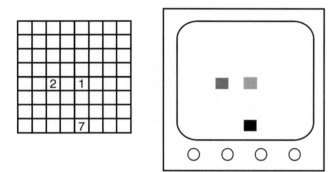

Fig. 9-5 Image matrix in digital format is converted to gray levels pixel by pixel for display.

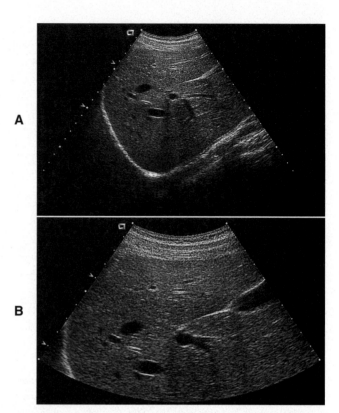

Fig. 9-6 Depth control allows adjustment of the scanning range in the acquisition of a sonogram of the liver. **A,** Depth of 18 cm. **B,** Depth of 10 cm.

dictate the location within the matrix (also the address in memory), and the signal level dictates the numerical value of the pixel. In this example the pixel locations corresponding to the various interfaces are assigned different values based on the intensity of the reflected echoes, which are depicted as different shades of gray in the displayed image on the monitor (Fig. 9-5).

OPERATOR CONTROLS

Several operator-adjustable controls are available to optimize the two-dimensional (2D) image. The most important instrument settings are scan range, transmit power, transmit focal zone, gain, TGC, log compression, edge enhancement, reject control, persistence, and gray scale. Additional preprocessing and postprocessing manipulation of the scan data may also be selected (as discussed in Chapter 10).

Transmission

The depth control sets the maximum range of the field of view (FOV) (Fig. 9-6). It also influences the frame rate and

line density. These parameters, not typically under direct operator control, are the result of an array of instrument settings.

The power control adjusts the intensity of the ultrasound beam transmitted into the patient. Power levels are commonly expressed in decibels (e.g., 0 dB corresponds to the maximum level, and –30 dB to the minimum). Increased intensity improves the signal-to-noise ratio (SNR) and enhances sensitivity (weak reflectors can be observed as shown in Fig. 9-7). On many scanners a change in the power setting is accompanied by an automatic commensurate adjustment of the gain so the overall image brightness remains constant.

The transmit zone selection control adjusts the depth of focusing. Variable transmit zones allow the operator to designate a region within the FOV where enhanced axial resolution is desired. Multiple-transmit focal regions may improve the axial resolution throughout the FOV; however, the frame rate will be reduced unless parallel processing is used (Fig. 9-8).

Gain Control

Receiver gain modifies the amplification of signals during signal processing and often is expressed in decibels. TGC is also a type of receiver gain that is varied according to time delay (or depth). TGC must be readjusted when the depth of scanning is changed. The SNR is unchanged by gain. Consequently, gain is used to establish the proper brightness

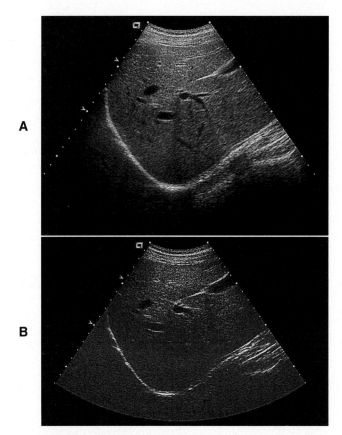

Fig. 9-7 Effect of power setting in the acquisition of a sonogram of the liver. **A,** High power. **B,** Low power. Note the loss of weak tissue scatterers at a depth of 10 cm.

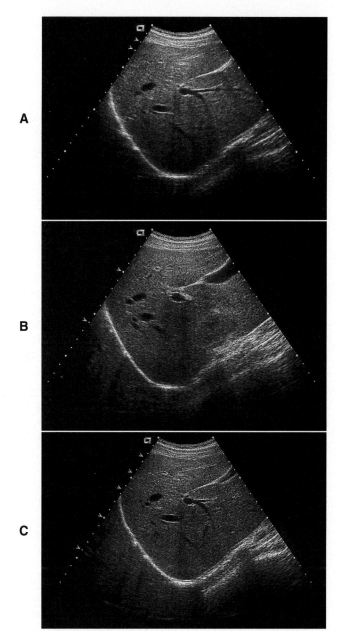

Fig. 9-8 Illustration of selectable fixed transmit focal zone. The arrows along the left depth markers indicate the transmit focal zones. **A,** Short focus. **B,** Medium focus. **C,** Multizone focus.

level for echoes of varying strength, but it cannot improve detection of subtle differences between scatterers.

Signal Processing

Because the scan converter and display device are unable to process an extremely wide range of signal levels, compression is necessary. In general, the digitized signal levels are placed in the scan converter as 8 bits. With 8 bits a total of 256 values is available to quantify the signal amplitude. If a linear representation is used, the maximum signal can be only 256 times the weakest signal. The range of values of the received signals after beam formation, however, may extend over four or more orders of magnitude. A logarithmic transformation of the signal levels is employed to compress the signal levels to a narrower range (0 to 255). Weaker signals are enhanced by log compression. That is, subtle differences between weak scatterers are emphasized, because low signal levels occupy a proportionally greater portion of the 0 to 255 compressed values. Increasing the depth beyond 8 bits would allow a greater range of values to be processed and stored, but the signal levels are ultimately compressed to the dynamic range of the display device.

Ultrasound imaging is ideally suited to the detection of interfaces or boundaries between structures. Edge enhancement is a filtering technique that can be applied to the line-

of-sight data to further emphasize a change in signal level generated at an interface.

The reject control, by accepting signals greater than a prescribed amplitude, reduces low-amplitude noise. Weak signals from scatterers along the scan line are also eliminated. In some circumstances (e.g., a high-reflectivity object located off axis) acoustic noise exceeds the threshold value and contributes to the image.

Image Processing

The individualized pixel values in the image matrix can be altered by various image processing techniques, including digital filtering, temporal averaging, and contrast enhancement. A more complete discussion of image processing is presented in Chapter 10.

Persistence

Persistence (a type of image processing) is a noise-reduction technique that applies temporal averaging to individual pixels. The operator selects the number of frames during which an average is obtained. Variations in noise at each pixel location tend to offset each other with time, whereas echo-induced signals tend to be reinforced. Fast-moving objects become blurred in the image when persistence is increased.

Freeze Frame

Real-time imaging depicts motion of moving interfaces, which is lost during freeze-frame display of one real-time image. The freeze-frame option allows the operator to select an image of interest for prolonged viewing. A single frame is held in the output buffer, and scan data acquisition is discontinued while the freeze-frame option is activated. The video buffer is repeatedly read in raster fashion, which allows the monitor to be constantly refreshed with the same information. The framing rate for the TV display is 30 frames per second, but because the same image data are shown over and over, the image appears unchanging to the observer.

Cine Loop

The **cine loop** function of acquired images allows the operator to review the dynamic relationships. Many frames (150 or more, corresponding to an acquisition time of several seconds) can be stored in computer memory for immediate playback using the cine loop function. The rate of playback can be adjusted to either coincide with or deviate from the real-time acquisition rate. The slow-motion review capability allows the sonographer to select an appropriate image for study as well as hard copy recording, if desired.

SYNTHETIC APERTURE

Lateral resolution is improved as the number of processing channels is increased. A linear array can easily contain 256 elements. However, to maintain 256 processing channels in the beam former is expensive. The number of channels in the beam former can be reduced to half the number of elements if a two-pulse sequence is used for transmission-reception (synthetic aperture). Half the elements, in this example 128, participate in beam formation in the first pulse sequence and form a series of echo-induced signals along the scan line. These scan data are stored and delayed until the echo-induced signals from the second pulse sequence are similarly acquired and processed by the beam former. The two sets of echo data are then added (Fig. 9-9). The high crystal number is maintained with the synthetic aperture for

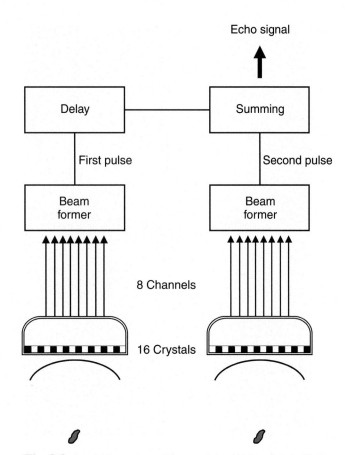

Fig. 9-9 Synthetic aperture. The number of channels is half of the number of crystals. Radiofrequency signals from two transmitted pulses are summed to compose the received focused echo signal along one line of sight.

excellent lateral resolution, but the image composition time is increased.

MULTIPLE BEAM FORMERS

All the previous discussions regarding beam formation and transmit focusing have emphasized that the maximum sampling rate is one scan line per transmitted pulse. Multiple beam formers now provide the ability to acquire multiple scan lines per transmitted pulse (up to four). The beam width of the transmission beam is expanded to include an area that would be sampled by multiple scan lines. Dynamic receive focusing of the returning echoes by each of the different beam formers permits the transmitted beam width to be subdivided into smaller effective beam widths. Each beam former then contributes one scan line to the image. An example of parallel beam formation is illustrated in Fig. 9-10.

Multiple scan line generation per transmitted pulse reduces the acquisition time per frame and can increase frame rate. Alternatively, lateral resolution can be improved by increasing scan line density. Parallel processing with multiple beam formers in transmit mode using multiple focal zones also can improve lateral resolution without a loss in frame rate.

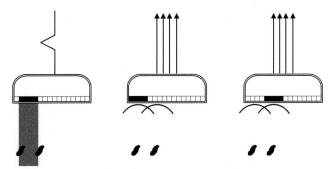

Fig. 9-10 Multiple beam formers permit multiple receive scan lines for each transmitted pulse. The transmitted beam extends over several crystals. Echoes from reflectors at the same depth strike the array at different center points. Two receive apertures of four crystals each acquire data along different lines of sight. Independent time delays for each aperture focus the signal along the respective scan line.

COHERENT IMAGE FORMATION

Parallel receive beam formation with multiple scan lines from a single excitation creates a subtle geometric distortion. The narrow receive focusing and the more broad transmission beam do not share a common axis but rather are offset from one another. The net effect is that sampling along the scan line is curved (Fig. 9-11). Mapping of the echoes in the image matrix assumes parallel scan lines. Image composition with curved scan lines degrades spatial detail (Fig. 9-12).

Coherent image formation corrects scan line curvature by manipulating the sampling data from multiple receive beams to form synthetic straight scan lines. The time-varying summed signal from each beam former is retained and assembled in two dimensions (Fig. 9-13). Coherent image processing includes both axial data along individual scan lines and lateral data from adjacent scan lines. Since time-varying information is used, this technique is often described with the term *phase*.

The echo amplitudes for a pair of oppositely curved interrogation lines are averaged, depth-by-depth, to produce the fabricated RF signal along the synthetic line (Fig. 9-14). This processing occurs before rectification and enveloping and is a good approximation for the signal that would have been obtained for a straight scan line located midway between the acquired curved scan lines.

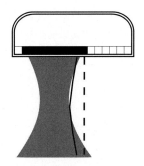

Fig. 9-11 The receive scan line *(dotted line)* with multiple beam formers is offset from the transmitted beam. The effective sampling path *(solid line)* is a curved combination of the transmitted beam width and receive aperture.

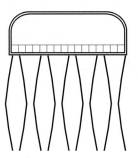

Fig. 9-12 Scan line geometry for multiple beam formers. Nonparallel scan lines compose the image.

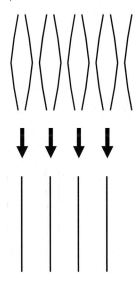

Fig. 9-14 Curved scan lines are acquired across the field of view. Lines with opposite curvature are paired and combined together to form a synthetic scan line. The synthetic scan lines are used to compose the image.

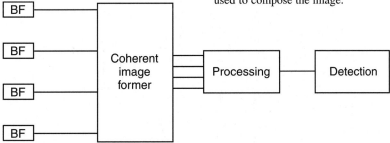

Fig. 9-13 Coherent image formation. Adjacent scan lines from multiple beam formers are processed simultaneously.

Any phase change between the pair of interrogation lines caused by beam steering or aperture must be corrected before averaging. The same method of delay and summing of RF signals used in beam formation also applies. Since processing includes spatial phase information, accurate echo signal data in the lateral dimension are possible.

PHASE ABERRATION

Beam forming applies time delays based on geometric considerations (path length differences from point of focus to the respective elements) and an assumed constant acoustic velocity. However, acoustic velocity in tissue can differ from 1450 m/s in fat to 1665 m/s in collagen. If the tissue velocity is not uniform along the path, such as when fat is present near the skin layer, then the ultrasound pulse arrives at a later time than expected (Fig. 9-15). This delay causes a loss of signal coherence during beam formation, which is called **phase aberration** (Fig. 9-16). Phase aberration reduces the SNR and degrades the sensitivity.

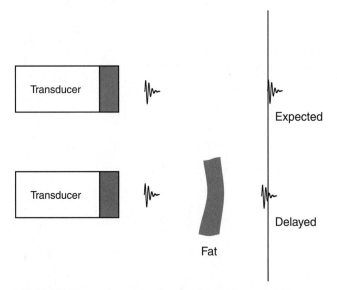

Fig. 9-15 Phase aberration. Fat has an acoustic velocity 8% slower than that of soft tissue. Fat along the beam path causes a delay compared with the anticipated arrival time based on a uniform path of soft tissue only.

Correction for phase aberration is performed by adjusting the time delay applied independently to each element in the active aperture of a multirow crystal array transducer. This more sophisticated control of time delay focusing is described as a 1.75D transducer.

The most common method to determine the time delay for phase aberration correction is the neighbor element technique using the near-field, thin-phase screen model. In this model aberrations are caused by a thin disruptive layer located on the transducer surface. The cross-correlation of signals from adjacent elements is calculated. In essence, the signal from one crystal element is shifted in time until a maximum sum signal from the two elements is obtained. The time shift is equal to the time delay necessary to produce time-coincident signals. This process is repeated for all elements in the active array. The respective time shift for each element can be applied during both transmit and receive beam forming to refocus the transducer. Remember, the aberration layer disrupts the transmit and receive focusing, since both the transmitted pulse and returning echo must travel through this layer.

Alternative methods have been proposed to improve phase aberration correction. Generally, these methods vary in how the reference signal is formed for the cross-correlation calculation. The signal from each element can be aligned with the signal from the central array element or the sum signal from a group of previously corrected elements. In theory these methods provide a more accurate correction for phase aberrations.

Phase aberration time-delay corrections are applied in real time. Contrast is improved (e.g., veins are darker and spectral reflectors are brighter). These corrections are computationally intense and require immense computing power.

BROADBAND TECHNIQUES

Real-time units with limited bandwidth have relatively poor axial resolution and cannot perform signal and image processing based on frequency information. Broadband transducers provide flexibility in operation such that image acquisition parameters can be changed during scanning. As the frequency bandwidth becomes wider, the possibility of

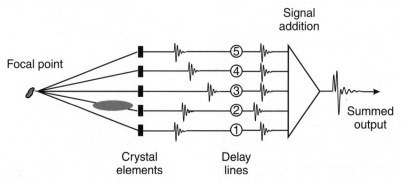

Fig. 9-16 Loss of signal coherence in beam formation when phase aberration is present.

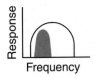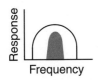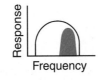

Fig. 9-17 Bandwidth of a transducer is divided into three transmit frequency bands, which are selectable by the operator.

matching optimal image acquisition parameters with the desired clinical information is improved. Broadband techniques include multifrequency imaging, confocal imaging, dynamic frequency filtering, frequency compounding, and tissue harmonic imaging.

MULTIFREQUENCY IMAGING

In multifrequency imaging the available broad bandwidth is subdivided into two or more frequency ranges for transmission and reception of sound waves (Fig. 9-17). The operator selects the center frequency appropriate for the present examination. The high-frequency portion provides good spatial detail. The low-frequency portion affords maximum tissue penetration. An intermediate-frequency bandwidth between these two extremes is also possible.

The outcome of multifrequency imaging is the same as if three independent transducers, each with a different center frequency, were supplied within the same case. The distinct advantage is one of convenience in that one variable-frequency transducer views the patient's anatomy while the center frequency is adjusted. The optimal frequency range can be selected without losing the clinical point of interest in the scan plane.

CONFOCAL IMAGING

Confocal imaging is an extension of transmit-zone focusing, except that the focal zone at each depth is formed with a different center frequency. In this imaging scheme the available broad transmit bandwidth is split into multiple frequency ranges. Multiple small transmit bandwidths with different center frequencies are used to collect echo data along each line of sight. This technique provides a very narrow beam width with good spatial detail at all depths.

Since multiple transmit pulses are necessary for each line of sight, frame rate decreases unless additional measures are taken (high pulse repetition frequency, parallel processing). Rapid firing of the crystals causes echoes from different transmit pulses to be incident on the transducer simultaneously. This causes range ambiguity artifacts, because each detected echo is assumed to come from the most recent transmit pulse. Parallel processing of the echo data can reduce range ambiguity artifacts and still allow high frame rates.

DYNAMIC FREQUENCY FILTERING

Dynamic frequency filtering uses the total transducer bandwidth for the transmitted pulse and then adjusts the receiver center frequency and bandwidth to lower frequencies as deeper depths are sampled. Since tissue attenuation is frequency dependent (higher frequencies are absorbed more rapidly), a frequency shift occurs as the ultrasound wave propagates through tissue. The center frequency and bandwidth of the echo decrease as the depth increases. By continuously and automatically matching the receiver electronics with the frequency characteristics of the detected echo based on elapsed time, this technique provides additional focusing at various depths and improved noise reduction. Noise is proportional to receiver bandwidth. Therefore by progressively narrowing the bandwidth with increased depth, a lower noise level is achieved.

High definition imaging can alter the transmitted bandwidth depending on the scanning range in conjunction with dynamic frequency filtering. High-frequency components may be eliminated in the transmitted pulse to extend the depth of penetration. Lateral resolution at shallow depths is improved by removal of the low-frequency components.

FREQUENCY COMPOUNDING

If the bandwidth of the receiver is matched with that of the transmitter, then the short echo pressure pulses can be faithfully converted into RF signals with broad bandwidth. The echo frequency spectrum is subdivided into frequency bands by filters, then processed separately before being recombined to form a **frequency averaged image** (Fig. 9-18). Speckle at different frequencies is independent. The summing of multiple frequency images reduces speckle and electronic noise to improve contrast resolution.

CODED EXCITATION

Long **coded waveforms** during transmission are used to improve the SNR and/or penetration depth. Two methods are used—frequency modulation (chirp) and binary encoding. Since the total transmission time is 20 μs or longer, axial resolution would be poor unless the received signal is manipulated mathematically to compress the pulse. These decoding techniques are described as matched filtration or deconvolution.

Binary Encoding

The applied voltage for a single transmitted pulse is represented by a square wave in the voltage waveform. A combination of two excitation pulses in a specific time sequence creates two possible patterns, which are labeled either as 0 or 1. These binary coded pulses now comprise the burst during transmission (Fig. 9-19). Coded pulse length for the burst transmission is 8 to 22 binary pulses.

The transmission burst has a known binary-coded sequence. Each reflector along the scan line will produce a similarly coded sequence in the echo train. Long duration echoes from nearby reflectors will overlap one another. The time-varying, echo-induced signal is analyzed (called deconvolution) for the coded pattern to yield a short, well-defined echo of a few cycles for each reflector. This

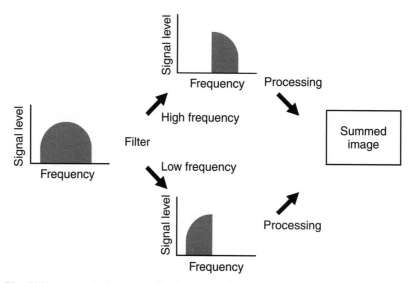

Fig. 9-18 Dynamic frequency filtering. The summed image is formed after independent processing of signal levels from separate frequency bands.

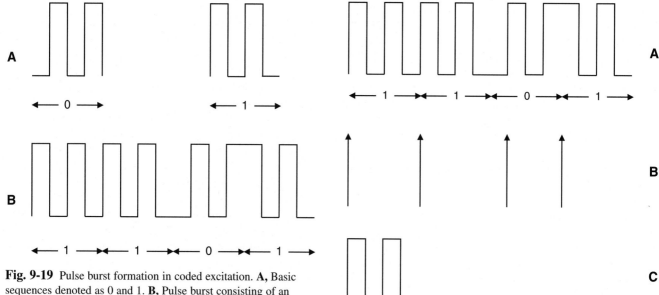

Fig. 9-19 Pulse burst formation in coded excitation. **A,** Basic sequences denoted as 0 and 1. **B,** Pulse burst consisting of an 1101 coded sequence.

Fig. 9-20 Pulse compression in coded excitation. **A,** Pulse burst consisting of an 1101 coded sequence. **B,** Decoding sequence. Lines are located at the first maximum of each 0 or 1 segment. **C,** Decoded short duration pulse. The compressed pulse in **C** convolved with the decoding sequence in **B** yields the original pulse burst in **A.**

corresponds to the echo-induced signal if a short duration transmission pulse (1 μs) were used.

Sometimes the reverse process is easier to understand. Suppose there are two reflectors separated by a few centimeters along the beam path. During echo ranging with a short duration pulse, each reflector generates a short duration echo, which is separated in time in the echo wavetrain. If a binary encoded burst were to replace the short duration transmitted pulse, each echo would be similarly elongated by the same coded sequence, and the echoes could easily overlap. Mathematically, if each reflector location were replaced by the coded sequence, then the echo wavetrain during reception would be obtained (Fig. 9-20). Fortunately, mathematical techniques and knowledge of the coded sequence allow the processing of the echo wavetrain to identify the individual reflector components without prior knowledge of the reflectors along the beam path.

An increase in SNR of 14 dB has been reported for a 2.6 μs binary code duration at a center frequency of 10 MHz and a fractional bandwidth of 0.38. Side lobe intensity was 40 dB less than the main beam. Axial resolution was slightly degraded.

Frequency Modulation

Frequency modulation of the transmitted pulse is achieved by varying the emitted frequency with time (Fig. 9-21). Imagine that the initial transmitted frequency is at the lower

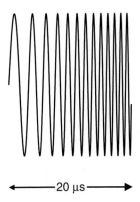

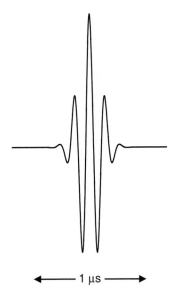

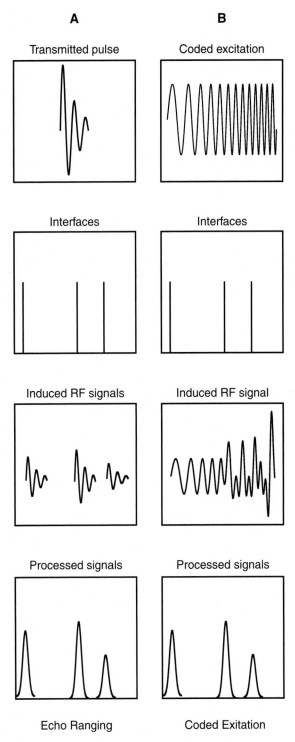

Fig. 9-21 Frequency-modulated transmitted pulse in coded excitation. The frequency increases during transmission time. Pulse duration is 20 μs.

Fig. 9-22 Decoding the frequency-modulated transmitted pulse yields the compressed pulse. Mathematically, all frequency components are shifted in time to the same initial transmission point.

Fig. 9-23 Comparison of echo ranging and coded excitation.

limit of the bandwidth and is subsequently increased linearly with time. This creates a long duration pulse (20 μs), but all frequency components within the bandwidth are contained in the pulse. If transmission of each frequency is matched in time (e.g., time offset is equal to zero), then the traditional short duration pulse is obtained (Fig. 9-22). In this method frequency is used to encode the pulse. Upon reception the frequency encoding is removed to form the compressed pulse. This is accomplished by the convolution of the received signal with the time-reversed transmitted pulse (Fig. 9-23).

Axial resolution does not depend on the chirp pulse duration, but rather the fractional bandwidth. Since the transmitted pulse is composed of all frequencies throughout the bandwidth, axial resolution is maintained. An increase in SNR of 10 to 20 dB and a corresponding penetration depth of 20 cm is possible at a center frequency of 5 MHz. Side lobe intensity was 65 dB less than the main beam.

Compared with traditional echo ranging, more energy per unit time without higher peak intensity is present in the coded waveform. This is the source of the SNR improvement. Since the spatial pulse length is 3 cm for a 20 μs pulse, image formation at shallow depths less than 1.5 cm is compromised. Traditional echo ranging is more appropriate for superficial structures. Artifacts in the form of repeating echoes from strong reflectors are sometimes encountered. Side lobes are a major consideration and can be reduced by proper weighting of each frequency and the window function (range of frequencies) in pulse formation.

TISSUE HARMONIC IMAGING

Tissue harmonic imaging (THI) is a relatively new imaging technique that relies on the detection of the **harmonic frequencies** created by beam propagation through tissue. Even though the detected signal is weaker than traditional echo ranging, contrast is often improved by the suppression of interfering signals from clutter and multiangle scattering.

Nonlinear Propagation

Under conditions of relatively high pressure amplitude, the speed of the sound wave (c) is not constant but varies over the propagation path (z):

9-1

$$c(z) = c_o + \left(1 + \frac{B}{2A}\right) u(z)$$

where c_o is the average acoustic velocity in the medium, $c(z)$ is the acoustic velocity at a point along the propagation path, $u(z)$ is the particle velocity at that point, and $(1 + B/2A)$ is the coefficient of nonlinearity. Equation 9-1 shows that the acoustic velocity at each point over the waveform is modulated by the particle velocity. Further, this contribution to wave velocity also depends on the medium via the ratio B/A.

During the compressional phase particle velocity is positive, and the speed of sound increases during this portion of the wave cycle. However, particle velocity is negative during the rarefaction phase, and the speed of sound decreases (Fig. 9-24). Consequently, because the speed of sound is not constant during the wave cycle, the sinusoidal shape

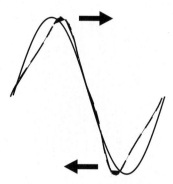

Fig. 9-24 Particle velocity varies during compression (speeds up) and rarefaction (slows down).

becomes distorted as the wave propagates through the medium (Fig. 9-25).

The distortion in the sound waveform at high intensity can be illustrated by a ball attached to a spring. If the ball is moved a small distance from the equilibrium position, the spring compresses. When released, the ball oscillates back and forth with relatively smooth sinusoidal motion (Fig. 9-26). If, on the other hand, the spring is compressed as much as possible before releasing the ball, the ball initially moves at very high velocity through the equilibrium position and then slows markedly as the spring is stretched. The sinusoidal motion becomes distorted (Fig. 9-27).

The change in shape from sinusoidal corresponds to a change in frequency components of the sound wave. As shown in Fig. 9-28, energy is transferred from the fundamental frequency (f_o) to harmonic frequencies (integral multiples of the fundamental frequency, such as $2f_o$, $3f_o$). If the fundamental frequency (also called first harmonic) is 2 MHz, then the next multiple or second harmonic is 4 MHz. *As the sound wave propagates through the medium,*

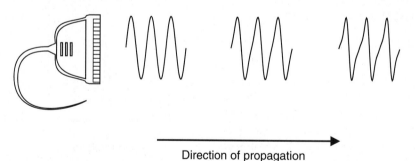

Direction of propagation

Fig. 9-25 Nonlinear propagation distorts the sinusoidal waveform. The effect becomes more pronounced with depth.

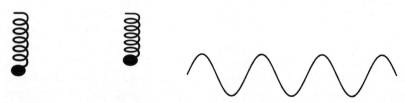

Fig. 9-26 Ball connected to a spring exhibits smooth sinusoidal motion if the ball is displaced a small amount and released. The waveform shows the displacement of the ball versus time.

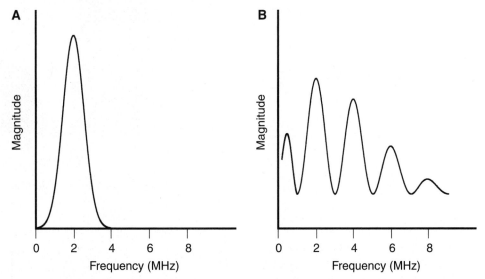

Fig. 9-27 Example of nonlinear propagation. When the spring is compressed completely before the ball is released, the initial fast movement is slowed considerably as the spring is stretched. The waveform shows the displacement of the ball versus time.

Fig. 9-28 Frequency spectrum of the transmitted pulse at the transducer (**A**) and after a path length of a few cm (**B**).

harmonic components intensify, and the waveform becomes more distorted. Attenuation causes the fundamental frequency sound wave to lose pressure amplitude and revert to linear propagation. Energy is no longer transferred to the harmonic frequencies. Meanwhile, the high-frequency harmonics are very rapidly attenuated in the medium (Figs. 9-29 and 9-30). **Nonlinear propagation** due to the high-frequency components exhibits more rapid pressure amplitude loss than predicted by the attenuation equation.

Presently, the relatively weak amplitudes of the third and higher harmonics limits tissue harmonic imaging to the detection of the second harmonic. The amplitude of the second harmonic (p_2) depends on the acoustic pressure (p), frequency (f), nonlinearity coefficient, density of the medium (ρ), acoustic velocity (c), and the distance of propagation (z):

9-2

$$p_2 = \left(1 + \frac{B}{2\,A}\right)\left(\frac{\pi\,f}{\rho\,c^3}\right) z\,p^2$$

The sound wave must propagate a few centimeters in the medium before a transfer in energy to the second harmonic can occur. Little pulse distortion is present near the transducer, and this region is free of harmonics. A further increase in depth enhances harmonic production. High-intensity sound beams via the squared relation between acoustic pressure and second harmonic formation produce large harmonic components.

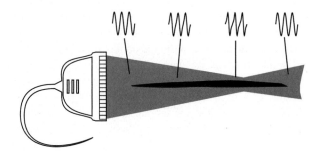

Fig. 9-29 Harmonics are present in the central portion of the transmitted beam but offset from the transducer face.

Two methods, harmonic band filtering and pulse phase inversion, are used in tissue harmonic imaging to isolate the second harmonic component and form the image. The intensity of the second harmonic is 10 to 20 dB lower than the fundamental. A low-noise, wide dynamic range receiver is necessary to preserve the relatively weak signal.

Harmonic Band Filtering

An object within the ultrasonic field where the second harmonic is present will be interrogated by both the fundamental frequency and the harmonic frequency. Harmonics are created as a result of propagation through tissue and are not produced upon reflection. An exception to this statement

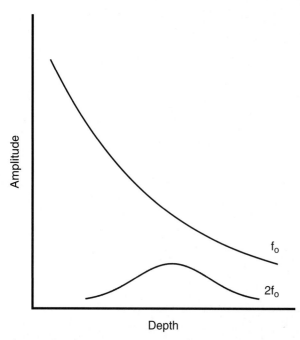

Fig. 9-30 Relative intensity of the fundamental frequency and second harmonic frequency as a function of distance from the transducer.

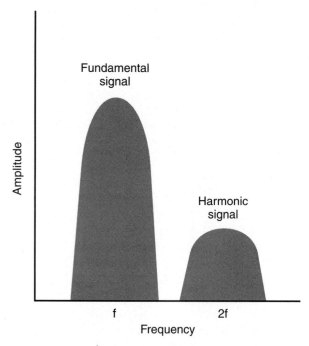

Fig. 9-31 Frequency components of the received echo.

is microbubble contrast agents, which are discussed in Chapter 18. The returning echo and thus the detected signals have a fundamental frequency component and a harmonic frequency component (Fig. 9-31). The propagation of echoes at relatively low intensity does not generate additional harmonic components. *A filter is applied to remove the fundamental echo signal, and only the tissue harmonic component is processed for image formation.*

The fundamental and harmonic bands should not overlap. The transmitted pulse must be carefully shaped and controlled to prevent high frequency components within the harmonic region. If these high frequencies are present, they will give rise to echoes of the same frequency (including noise and clutter), and the purity of the harmonic component generated from native tissue will be corrupted. To separate the fundamental and harmonic bands, a narrow transmission bandwidth is formed by elongating the transmission pulse (Fig. 9-32). This may degrade the axial resolution, but the increased detection frequency of the second harmonic compensates to some extent for the longer transmitted spatial pulse length.

Pulse Phase Inversion

A two-pulse sequence is transmitted along the same path in which the second pulse is shifted 180 degrees in phase. The echo-induced signal from the first pulse is stored until the signal from the second pulse is received. The received signals from each transmitted pulse are then summed. For linear propagation the two received signals have the same amplitude but an 180-degree phase difference and cancel completely when summed. If nonlinear propagation occurs, harmonics are added in the same proportion to each

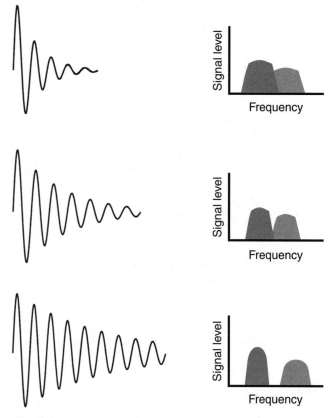

Fig. 9-32 Effect of spatial pulse length on harmonic separation from the fundamental frequency band.

waveform following transmission. The received signals are not identical in amplitude and produce the harmonic component when summed (Fig. 9-33). Note that the summed result has a frequency that is two times the fundamental frequency. SNR is increased, since the measurements of the

0-Degree pulse   180-Degree pulse   Summation

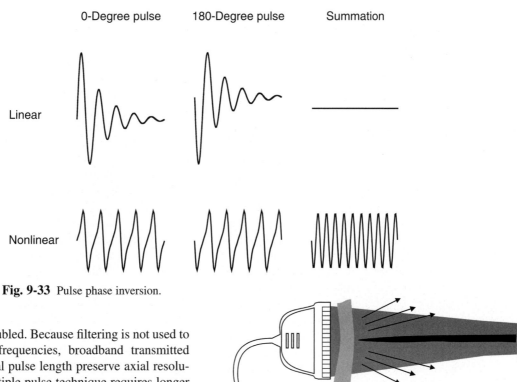

Linear

Nonlinear

Fig. 9-33 Pulse phase inversion.

harmonic signal are doubled. Because filtering is not used to isolate the harmonic frequencies, broadband transmitted pulses with short spatial pulse length preserve axial resolution. However, the multiple pulse technique requires longer sampling/processing time and is subject to motion artifacts.

Advantages of Tissue Harmonic Imaging

Clutter, grating lobes, and side lobes are generated at the fundamental frequency. Echoes from these sources are also at the fundamental frequency and are suppressed in the tissue harmonic image. Multiple scattering produces low amplitude sound waves, which do not form harmonics.

Reverberation artifacts are reduced. Echoes in general do not generate harmonics because of their low amplitude. The harmonic content of reverberation echoes is established by the transmission path to the target and is consequently much lower than that present in tissue echoes of equal transit time.

Subcutaneous fat, particularly in large patients, defocuses the beam and masks the signals from deep-lying structures (Fig. 9-34). Once more, distortion and scattering are at the fundamental frequency and are suppressed in the tissue harmonic image.

The reduction of acoustic noise from the previously mentioned sources enhances contrast resolution and border delineation (Fig. 9-35). The detection and characterization of low-contrast solid lesions are improved. Acoustic enhancement and shadowing are more easily demonstrated. Liquid cavities are depicted with less fill-in.

High acoustic pressure occurs near the main beam axis and within the focal zone. This is the source of harmonic production. The width of the harmonic beam is effectively narrower than the main beam at the fundamental frequency. Reduced beam width improves lateral resolution.

The overall penetration in THI is less than that obtainable in the conventional mode at the fundamental frequency because of higher attenuation rates for harmonics. The penalty is not as severe as anticipated, since harmonics

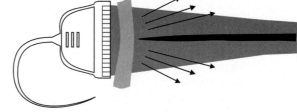

Fig. 9-34 Subcutaneous fat creates distortions and clutter at the fundamental frequency.

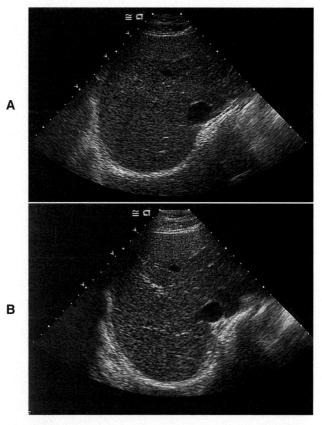

A

B

Fig. 9-35 Comparison of tissue harmonic imaging (THI) with fundamental imaging. Sonograms of the liver obtained at 4 MHz. **A,** Fundamental. **B,** Harmonic. Note the improved image contrast with THI.

travel only a portion of the total path length. Often, the fundamental frequency in THI is lowered to image deeply-lying structures. If visualized, these structures are depicted with greater contrast and spatial detail.

SPATIAL COMPOUNDING

The amplitude of the echo-induced signal depends on the angle of incidence and the geometry of the boundary. Normal incidence maximizes the signal. During the examination the sonographer reorients the transducer, changing the relative beam direction with respect to an interface to maximize the reflectivity from a particular interface. In so doing, however, the less favorable beam orientation for other interfaces throughout the FOV causes their respective signals to be decreased. **Spatial compounding,** by acquiring multiple beam angles and averaging the data, improves the presentation of boundaries throughout the FOV.

A linear array with a high number of elements (>192) and at least 64 channels is required. A group of elements is stimulated as a phased array to direct the beam at a specific angle. The active aperture is moved along the length of the array until all scan lines with that beam angle are obtained. The procedure is repeated for different beam angles. One frame of the FOV is acquired at each beam angle. The

steering angles may range ± 20 degrees. Fig. 9-36 illustrates the sampling for three beam angles.

Averaging of the frames for display is accomplished in real time. Fig. 9-37 shows a sequence of sampled frames using three beam angles. The displayed image is an average of the three most recently acquired frames. In this manner the displayed image is always composed of pixels insonated from multiple directions. Since the displayed image is refreshed when a new frame is obtained, no reduction in frame rate occurs.

Spatial compounding improves depiction of tissue boundaries and reduces noise variations (Fig. 9-38). Shadowing from strong reflectors and enhancement from weak reflectors are less pronounced. Increasing the number of angles of insonification amplifies the compounding effect. However, since the sampling occurs over more frames, the potential for motion blurring also increases.

A wideband transducer is necessary to lower the center frequency for large angle steering in order to reduce grating lobes. The fully compounded region does not occupy the entire FOV; the scan lines for all beam angles do not overlap at the periphery, which becomes more pronounced with depth. In this case the displayed image is formed on scan data from a reduced number of beam angles. The extent of the fully compounded region depends on system design

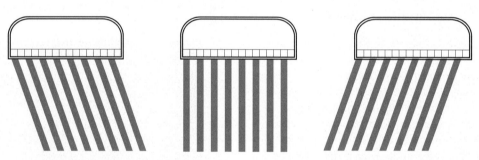

Fig. 9-36 Spatial compounding with the transmitted beams oriented at three different angles.

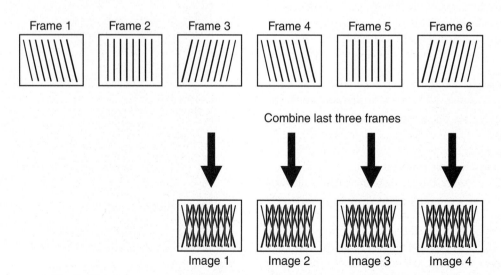

Fig. 9-37 Frame composition and averaging during spatial compounding. In this example the previous two frames are combined with the current frame to compose the displayed image.

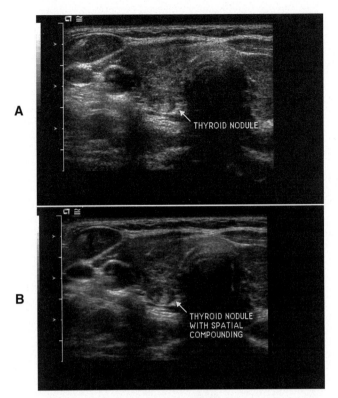

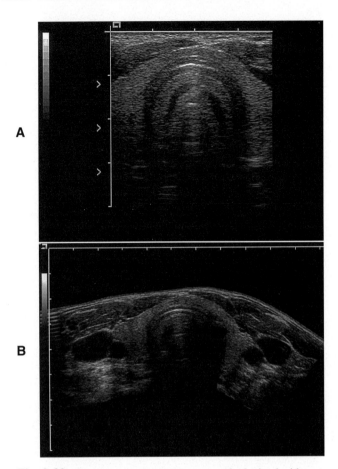

Fig. 9-38 Example of spatial compounding. **A,** Sonogram of the thyroid without spatial compounding. **B,** Sonogram of the thyroid with spatial compounding. Note the improved definition of the nodule.

Fig. 9-39 Sonogram of a normal human neck obtained with a 10 MHz linear array transducer. **A,** Standard field of view with a width of 4 cm. **B,** Extended field of view with a width of 11 cm.

considerations including the number of elements, transmitted frequency, distance between elements, width of the spacing between elements, and element angular response.

A weighted average of the scan lines is necessary to compensate for differences in amplitude caused by sensitivity variation in the angular response of the elements, differences in aperture, and changes in center frequency. Maximum amplitude detection from all scan lines at each pixel may be used as an alternative to averaging, but noise reduction is diminished.

EXTENDED FIELD OF VIEW

The advantages of real-time ultrasound include excellent temporal resolution (high frame rate), focusing using multiple element arrays, and elimination of the articulated scanning arm. However, static B-mode enabled a large anatomical region to be displayed in a single image. Real-time FOV is limited by transducer width (linear array) or sector scanning angle (mechanical sector, annular phased array, linear phased array, curvilinear array). To establish spatial relationships throughout a large region, the sonographer must often acquire several small FOV frames and then compose a mental picture of the anatomy.

Extended FOV real-time ultrasound attempts to overcome this limitation by combining successive frames to form a panoramic image as the transducer is moved across the patient. The FOV of the panoramic image is larger than the FOV of a single real-time frame and can be generated in

real time. An alternative method acquires real-time images in a cine clip and then processes the successive frames to form the panoramic image. Standard and extended FOVs of a normal human neck acquired with a linear transducer are shown in Fig. 9-39.

In static B-mode lines of sight are mapped in the image based upon the location and orientation of the transducer. The positional information is obtained by sensors in the articulating arm after a reference point has been defined. The presence of position-sensing devices inhibits flexibility. Extended FOV real-time imaging employs computer analysis of image features to determine transducer location without sensors or an articulating arm.

Image Registration

As the transducer is moved slowly across the patient, individual frames are obtained at a rapid rate (15 to 20 frames per second). Sequential frames have many common image features, because much of the anatomy examined by each frame is the same. The overlapping region for two frames acquired sequentially as the linear array is translated to the right is shown in Fig. 9-40. Each frame is depicted individually in Fig. 9-41 and then superimposed on one another in Fig. 9-42. Examination of the superimposed image identifies the club and triangle as common image features,

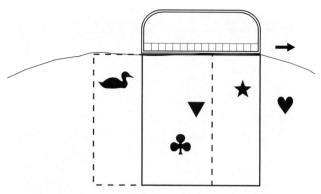

Fig. 9-40 Multiple frames are obtained as a linear array moves across the patient. First frame is denoted with the dashed line border. Second frame is denoted with the solid line border.

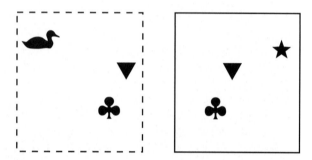

Fig. 9-41 Image features present in each frame acquired in Fig. 9-40.

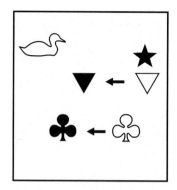

Fig. 9-42 Individual frames in Fig. 9-41 superimposed on one another. Structures in the first frame are denoted by the solid line outline of the geometric shape. Arrows indicate the change in position of common image features.

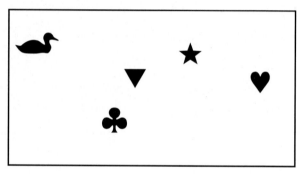

Fig. 9-43 Extended field of view of scan data acquired in Fig. 9-40.

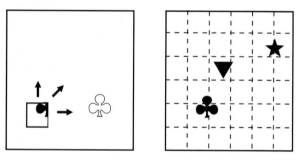

Fig. 9-44 Image feature matching. The second frame is divided into blocks. A search of the reference frame starting at the block location is conducted to find a region with similar properties. Arrows indicate search directions. The process is repeated for each block in the second frame.

which have moved linearly right to left from the first to second frame (direction opposite to the motion of the transducer). The speed of the transducer movement determines the magnitude of the displacement of common image features.

By measuring the geometric shift and rotation of common image features, the motion of the probe can be established. Once the probe motion is known, each successive frame can then be registered with respect to all previous frames that form the panoramic image. Fig. 9-43 depicts the extended FOV as the probe is moved across the region shown in Fig. 9-40.

Computer matching of image features in successive frames is accomplished by dividing the most recently acquired frame into blocks and then searching the prior frame for a region with similar properties that correspond to an individual block (Fig. 9-44). The search initiates at the location of the block and proceeds radially outward. The change in position of the common image features is small if the sampling rate is rapid and tissue motion is minimal. The matching region is expected to be near the block location and thus is the logical point to begin the search. Parallel processing allows multiple blocks to be analyzed simultaneously, which reduces the time to register the frame.

Each block is assigned a motion vector based on matching with the reference image. A map of local motion (velocity) vectors is created. If the probe moves linearly as illustrated in Fig. 9-40, then image feature displacements are in the same direction and the same distance throughout the superimposed frames (see Fig. 9-42). However, a curved

body surface would cause the probe to rotate as it is moved across the patient (Fig. 9-45). If the probe translates and rotates, then the image feature displacements change with depth (Fig. 9-46). The effect of translation and rotation is shown in Fig. 9-47. Image feature displacements are not the same for all blocks throughout the velocity map. The difference in local motion vectors near the top versus near the bottom of the velocity map allows determination of the overall probe motion. The current frame is translated and rotated to properly position the image data within the panoramic image.

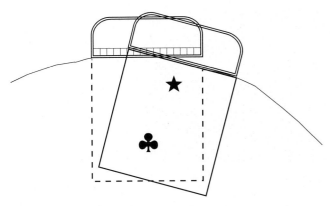

Fig. 9-45 Multiple frames are obtained as a linear array is translated and rotated. First frame is denoted with the dashed line border. Second frame is denoted with the solid line border.

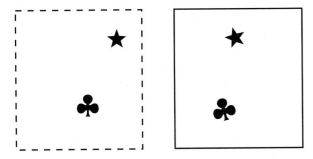

Fig. 9-46 Image features present in each frame acquired in Fig. 9-45.

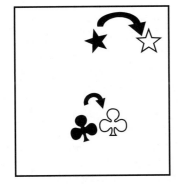

Fig. 9-47 Individual frames in Fig. 9-46 superimposed on one another. Structures in the first frame are denoted by the solid line outline of the geometric shape. Arrows indicate the change in position of common image features.

The extended FOV, if composed in real time, has both real-time and static components. The real-time component advances with the probe motion and shows the anatomy currently being imaged. The static component displays the anatomy that has been scanned. Using Fig. 9-40 as an example, the extended FOV image combines frames left to right as the probe advances, but the right side portion displays the current real-time image. All frames used to compose the extended FOV image are placed in cine memory so that the individual frames may be viewed.

Extended FOV imaging provides a method to expand the viewing area as real-time transducers are moved across the

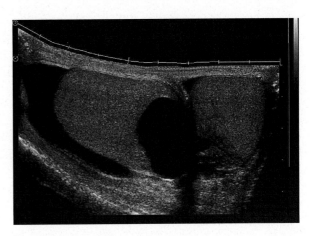

Fig. 9-48 Extended-field-of-view sonogram of the testicle. (Courtesy Ken Barrett, RDMS, RVT.)

body surface. The basis for this technique is image feature matching applied to sequential frames, which assumes that many of the same anatomical structures are present in both frames. Accurate registration of the current frame is practicable following translation and in-plane rotation of the probe. In-plane rotation is rotation around an axis perpendicular to the image plane.

The fidelity of registration process is corrupted by actions that reduce image feature similarity. The primary factors that can cause artifacts are large-scale tissue motion and off-plane rotation. Tissue motion contributes to the displacement of common image features and results in improper registration of the current frame. Off-plane rotation shifts the imaging plane at an angle into or out of the plane of the reference image. The sampled anatomical region is changed, which eliminates common image features. Small-scale off-plane rotation inherent in freehand scanning is usually tolerated in extended FOV imaging.

Clinical applications of the extended FOV technique include breast, abdominal, pelvic, extremity, and vascular imaging (Figs. 9-48 and 9-49). The relationship of a large mass or abnormality with surrounding structures can be depicted in a single image. A large FOV enhances the potential of subsequent examinations to reproduce prior findings.

HIGH-FREQUENCY IMAGING

Transducers operating at a center frequency above 10 MHz are very desirable to improve spatial resolution. A 20-MHz transducer has achieved an axial resolution of 100 µm and a lateral resolution of 300 µm. The major concern is the ability to obtain good penetration, since beam intensity is rapidly reduced by attenuation. High sensitivity by suppressing noise and expanding the dynamic range is required. The maximum imaging frequency is limited by the digitization rate according to the Nyquist sampling theorem. The Nyquist limit for frequency is equal to half of the sampling rate. For a 20-MHz transducer the analog-to-digital converter must operate at 40 MHz.

High-frequency imaging at frequencies above 10 MHz is now routinely performed for superficial organs including

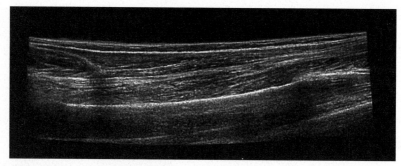

Fig. 9-49 Extended-field-of-view sonogram of the forearm.

muscles, tendons, breasts, thyroids, and testicles. A scan range of several centimeters is possible. Applications in dermatology and ophthalmology, where the scan range is a few millimeters, can be expanded to higher frequencies.

THREE-DIMENSIONAL IMAGING

In three-dimensional (3D) imaging the spatial relationships of structures within a scanned volume are represented by an image or a set of images. Following data collection echo information is processed for display as a static image. Real-time scanning of the tissue volume is called four-dimensional (4D) imaging and is discussed in the following section.

Limitations of 2D Real-Time Scanning

In 2D imaging the sonographer must mentally form a 3D impression of the anatomy from a series of acquired 2D images. This process is time consuming, subjective, and inconsistent. Depending on operator proficiency, spatial relationships are often distorted or misrepresented.

Patient management decisions often rely on measurements of organ or tumor volume. Real-time 2D imaging provides an accurate measurement of area within the scan plane, but in order to project the structure into three dimensions for the calculation of volume, some idealized shape must be assumed. This technique is potentially inaccurate if the organ/tumor shape deviates from the projected outline. Also, monitoring of therapeutic regimens often requires repeated measurements, separated by long-time intervals, of the same 2D image plane placed in the same location.

Acquisition Methods

Most **3D ultrasound** systems acquire a series of 2D images throughout the volume of interest. The 2D images may be arranged in a set of parallel slices, in a wedge, in a cone, or in an arbitrary orientation (Fig. 9-50). The position and orientation of the transducer for each 2D image must be accurately known to avoid geometric distortions in the 3D image. Mechanical and freehand scanning methods have been developed to sample the volume of interest. An alternative approach is to use a 2D array transducer, which acquires the 3D data set without moving the transducer.

Linear motion. The transducer is mounted in a mechanical assembly that translates the transducer linearly over the patient's surface. The 2D images are acquired parallel to one another and at well-defined intervals. Since the scanning geometry is known, short reconstruction time is possible. The scanning direction is along the elevation direction of the transducer.

Tilt motion. The transducer is tilted about an axis by the mechanical assembly. Images are acquired at constant angular intervals and are arranged in a fanlike wedge. The line of convergence for the image planes is either at the transducer face or at a line parallel to the transducer face but above the skin surface. The distance between sampled planes increases with depth. Tilting is also along the elevation direction of the transducer. These factors combine to reduce the resolution in the scan direction. Tilt scanning is often used with transesophageal and transrectal transducers. For example, a side-firing linear array is rotated around the long axis of the probe through an angle of 100 degrees to image the prostate.

Rotational motion. A motor rotates an end-mounted crystal array around the tip of the probe. The resulting 2D images sweep out a conical volume in a propeller-like fashion. Since the images intersect along a line extended from the probe, spatial sampling is not uniform but is highest near the center of the conical volume. Resolution is a complex function of distance from the transducer, distance from the center of the sampled volume, and elevational beam width.

Freehand scanning without position sensing. The transducer is moved manually across the patient without any sensing device. The transducer movement must be uniform and conform to the predefined scanning geometry. Deviations from the assumed scanning motion introduce geometric distortion in the reconstructed volume. This technique is limited to qualitative assessment, since measurements of distance, area, and volume are generally not accurate.

Freehand scanning with position sensing. Four position-sensing techniques have been used: articulated arm, magnetic field sensor, acoustic ranging, and image-based correlation.

Articulated arm: The transducer is mounted on an articulated arm as described in static B-mode imaging. Potentiometers located in the arm provide information to determine the position and orientation of the transducer.

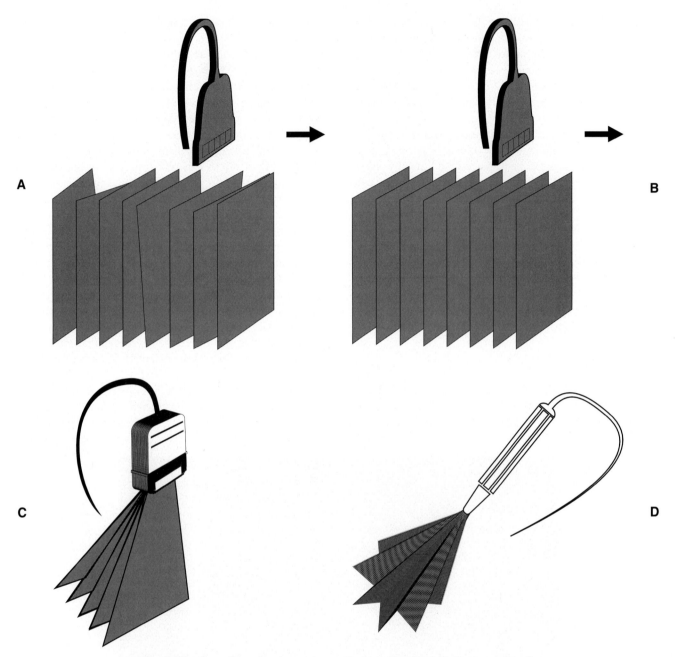

Fig. 9-50 Three-dimensional scanning methods. **A,** Freehand. **B,** Linear motion. **C,** Tilt motion. **D,** Rotational motion.

Magnetic field sensor: A transmitter near the transducer generates a spatially varying magnetic field. A set of orthogonal coils in the transducer measures the local magnetic field strength in three directions, which allows assessment of transducer position and angulation. Electromagnetic interference from cathode ray tubes, power cabling, and other electronic devices can alter the magnetic field measurements. Also, the presence of metal can distort the magnetic field and affect positional accuracy.

Acoustic ranging: Sound emitting devices (spark gaps) on the transducer are activated during scanning. An array of fixed microphones above the patient detect the sound from the spark gaps. The position of the sound source is determined by the time of flight to the respective microphones using an assumed value for the velocity of sound in air.

Image-based correlation: Successive images are analyzed with respect to the spatial energy pattern. The change in image characteristics is indicative of the shift in relative position of the adjacent images.

Rectangular arrays. An alternative approach is to use a rectangular-array transducer. Ultrasound beam sampling direction is electronically controlled with the appropriate crystal-firing sequence. Parallel processing reduces sampling time. Matrix arrays offer the potential for data collection in orthogonal planes.

Image Reconstruction

The most common method to form the 3D volume data set is voxel-based reconstruction. A **voxel** is a three-dimensional picture element with length, width, and thickness. The dimensions in each direction are not necessarily the same. Each pixel in the set of 2D images is placed at the proper location within the 3D volume. If a voxel was not sampled by a 2D image, then the value for that voxel is calculated by interpolation using the values from neighboring voxels.

The original data set of 2D images is preserved. That is, if the appropriate plane in the 3D volume is selected, then the acquired 2D image can be displayed. Additionally, other views not present in the set of acquired 2D images can be displayed. Since these additional views depend on interpolation of the sampling data set, a distance greater than one half of the elevational thickness between 2D images degrades spatial resolution and misrepresents anatomy.

To adequately sample the tissue volume, large data files are generated. A single 3D scan of the liver may require 16 MB but may increase to as much as 512 MB for imaging the heart through the cardiac cycle. Other scanning modes such as power Doppler further enlarge the storage requirements.

Image Display

After reconstruction the 3D volume is viewed interactively using computer graphics. The 3D volume contains massive quantities of data, which cannot be viewed all at once.

Information must be extracted from the volume data set and then displayed. The process of selecting and manipulating data for visualization is called rendering. Three types of rendering form 3D images for display: multiplanar formatting, surface rendering, and volume rendering.

Multiplanar reformatting. The 3D data set is composed of voxels that are stacked together as a pile of bricks. Similar to isolating the bricks that comprise one layer, the operator can view a single plane in the 3D volume. Imagine that the pile of bricks can be cut in any orientation and a single layer of bricks extracted. Following their removal, another single layer of bricks with the same orientation but one layer offset from the first is extracted. The 3D volume can be rotated so that the operator can view its contents along any line of sight. Once the line of sight is established, the visualized 2D images are formed using one layer of voxels in the plane perpendicular to this line of sight. In this manner successive parallel plane images are generated at equal intervals along the operator's line of sight, and the operator can scroll through the set of 2D images. Typically, three orthogonal planes are displayed simultaneously with indicators regarding their orientation and intersection (Fig. 9-51).

In an alternate approach a polyhedron representing the boundaries of the reconstructed volume is displayed (Fig. 9-52). Each face of the polyhedron depicts the 2D

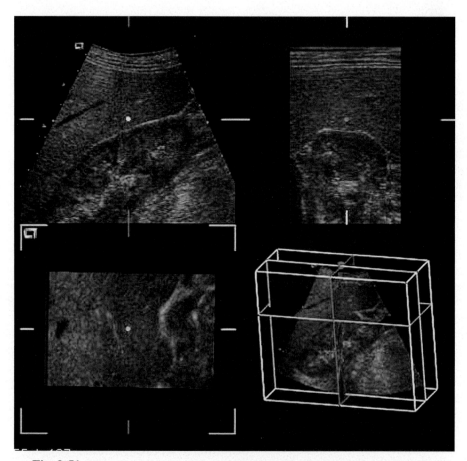

Fig. 9-51 Three-dimensional multiformat. Three orthogonal planes through the kidney are displayed. The reference image denotes the orientation. (Courtesy Siemens Medical Solutions USA, Inc., Ultrasound Division, Malvern, Penn.) (See Color Plate 1.)

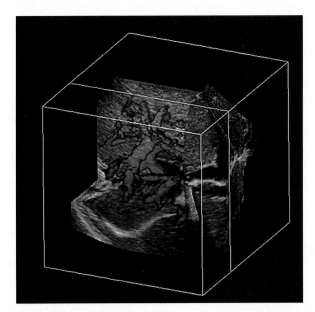

Fig. 9-52 Three-dimensional polyhedron image display showing liver vasculature in a child. (Courtesy Siemens Medical Solutions USA, Inc., Ultrasound Division, Malvern, Penn.) (See Color Plate 2.)

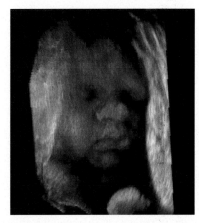

Fig. 9-53 Three-dimensional surface rendering of a fetal head. (Courtesy Siemens Medical Solutions USA, Inc., Ultrasound Division, Malvern, Penn.)

image for that plane. The polyhedron can be rotated to any desired orientation, and the plane of reference moved in or out. The 3D image set is then mapped to that face. The relative position of the reference plane with respect to other anatomy must be indicated.

Surface rendering. Surface rendering depicts the surface of organs or other structures for display. The boundaries of the structure are identified by the operator or by computer contouring. The points within the boundary are interconnected by a wire mesh formed in triangular or polygonal segments. Once the surface is established, the texture and lighting are changed depending on the operator's viewing perspective (Fig. 9-53). Interactive display of the surface-rendered data is possible.

The surface-rendered image can contain artifacts and must be viewed in conjunction with the planar images. Spatial detail is lost unless a high-resolution mesh is used.

Volume rendering. Multiformat planar and surface rendering form a 2D planar image that does not depend on information in the 3D data set outside of the 2D image. Volume rendering, on the other hand, forms a 2D projection image based on data throughout the 3D volume set. Volume rendering is computationally intensive and may require dedicated hardware for interactive rendering.

The viewing direction must first be established. Then, a set of parallel rays is cast through the 3D volume. Each ray corresponds to one pixel in the volume-rendered image. The voxels encountered along each ray are identified, the values are multiplied by factors, and their products are summed to obtain the final value for that ray (pixel). The array of pixels is configured in a 2D projection image.

One common approach is to generate a maximum intensity projection image. This type of volume rendering retains only the maximum voxel value along each ray. All other voxel values are excluded.

The translucent/opacity rendering technique weights the voxel values along each ray by opacity and color factors. The opacities, shades, and colors encountered along the ray are blended to produce the final pixel color and luminance in the 2D projection image. The opacity and color factors are adjustable to depict the desired anatomical structures. Volume rendering has been very successful in the display of fetal and vascular anatomy.

4D IMAGING

Display of a surface-rendered plane or multiple planes of the sampled volume in real time is called **4D ultrasound.** The fourth dimension of time is combined with volumetric sampling to depict the dynamic spatial relationships of structures in three dimensions. Mechanically steered multielement array and 2D array transducers have been developed to rapidly acquire volumetric data.

Multielement Arrays

The first approach mechanically sweeps a 1.5D crystal array back and forth across the beam port of the transducer. The direction of movement is perpendicular to the crystal rows. This is very similar to a mechanical sector scanner, except that the single crystal has now been replaced with a multirow crystal array. The crystal array allows electronic steering of the beam within any plane defined by the mechanical position of the crystal array. Instead of a single scan line directed from the crystal at each sampling position along the arc in a mechanical sector scanner, the array can direct the beam in and out of the page to acquire a plane at each sampling position along the arc. This interrogates a 3D volume. The crystal array is encased in fluid within the transducer housing to provide good energy transmission into tissue. Different transducer types including curvilinear, linear, and endocavity (end-fire and side-fire) are available.

A frame rate of five volumes per second is possible. Time constraints prohibit scan lines from being acquired plane by plane as the crystal array is swept across the volume. Rather, the beam is directed along selected lines of sight within a plane before the array is moved to the next position. Since fewer scan lines are acquired compared with 3D ultrasound, some loss in spatial resolution occurs in 4D ultrasound. Also, resolution deteriorates with distance from the transducer (lower scan line density).

2D Arrays

The alternative method to acquire volumetric data uses a 2D array transducer to electronically steer the beam throughout the volume without moving the transducer. Approximately 4000 crystal elements comprise the 2D array. The FOV is smaller, but the frame rate is higher than that obtainable with the combination mechanical/electronic steering. The maximum frame rate is 20 volumes per second. To achieve this frame rate, the number of scan lines that compose the image are limited, and the sampling volume is restricted in size. Similar to other real-time systems, a tradeoff exists among frame rate, scan lines, and sampling volume.

The future of 4D ultrasound will depend on the technological advances in the design of 2D array transducers. Specifically, more crystal elements at lower cost are needed to make 4D ultrasound with 2D arrays clinically viable.

Limitations

One major drawback of this 4D imaging method, however, is the lack of orthogonal scan planes. Reconstruction of scan data sets into the 3D display is more abstruse than the methods used for computed tomography (CT) or magnetic resonance imaging. High-speed computer systems are required.

4D imaging must overcome slow frame rates/limited scan lines and relatively long computation times because of large data sets. The latter problem will be solved as the current capabilities of computers are expanded. A more subtle difficulty is that the relationship between the echo-induced signal amplitude and the physical situation is not well defined by a single parameter. Unlike CT, in which one physical characteristic (electron density) determines the measured value, in ultrasound many factors contribute to the reflectivity of an interface. The lack of a common unifying factor, speckle, and small differences in signal levels makes some data manipulation techniques difficult to apply.

ELASTICITY IMAGING

Elasticity imaging is a relatively new technique that creates a visual display of information that would be obtained by manual palpation. A quantitative map of tissue stiffness throughout the region of interest is presented. Tissue changes shape or volume when a force is applied over a surface area. Stiffness is a measure of how likely the tissue will maintain its shape when the force is applied.

This deforming force per area is called the stress. The relative displacement of tissue when subjected to stress is the strain. If the strain is proportional to the stress, then the

material exhibits elastic behavior. The amount of stress required to cause a given displacement depends on the tissue type. The proportionality constant is called the elastic modulus of the material. Removal of the low-level stress restores the material to the original shape and dimensions.

Breast tissue is considered elastic for the compression force applied during freehand scanning. However, at increased stress, breast tissues exhibit a nonlinear stress-strain relationship and change stiffness as they are deformed. Elastic moduli of breast tissue types are not uniform in magnitude (fat < glandular tissue < invasive ductual carcinoma < fibrous tissue). That is, breast tissue types have different stiffness.

Strain imaging depicts the relative tissue displacement between precompression and compression measured by ultrasound. The RF signal for each line of sight is acquired before and after deformation. The A-line echo signal in each data set is divided into short segments (fraction of a millimeter), and each segment is sampled over time. The compression RF signal is then shifted in time to match the predeformation RF signal (Fig. 9-54). The amount of time shift yields the displacement for that segment of tissue. Comparison with adjacent segments provides the rate of change of the displacement (also called the gradient), which is depicted in the strain image. In essence, the shift in position caused by overlying tissues is eliminated, and the

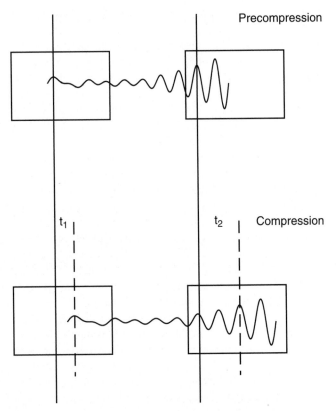

Fig. 9-54 Elasticity imaging. Radiofrequency (RF) signals from tissue (precompression and compression) are divided into small segments indicated by the rectangles. The time shifts (t_1 and t_2) for the displacement of the RF signal during tissue compression are shown (*distance between solid and dotted lines*).

displacement for the stress acting on this small tissue element is revealed.

Image contrast is based on the mechanical properties of the different tissue types and has the potential to produce high contrast when measuring strain. Contrast is likely to change when elevated stress is applied, since the media are no longer elastic. Multiple A-lines and short RF segments allow 2D tracking in the lateral and axial directions. This increases the contrast-to-noise ratio. Lesions less than 3 mm in diameter with a stiffness three times that of glandular breast tissue have been resolved.

Elasticity images and B-mode images are shown side by side in a split screen format in real time (seven frames per second). The operator denotes the region of interest for the strain images.

The relative lesion size in B-mode versus elasticity images may allow tissue differentiation. Fibroadenomas and cysts are nearly equal in size in both image types (Fig. 9-55), whereas invasive ductal carcinomas are two to three times larger in the strain image compared with the B-mode image (Fig. 9-56). Elasticity imaging may improve ultrasound's ability to identify lesions for biopsy.

Elasticity imaging provides quantitative measurement of tissue stiffness, which is more sensitive and less subjective than palpation. Since the image data are in digital format, other advantages include ease of comparison with other imaging modalities, electronic storage, and electronic transfer.

PORTABLE DEVICES

Hand-held, portable, real-time scanners weighing less than 6 pounds are now commercially available. These small and less expensive scanners provide image quality and features

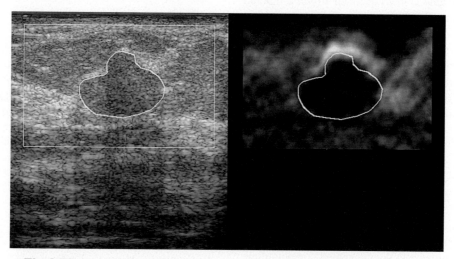

Fig. 9-55 B-mode image *(left)* and elasticity image *(right)* of a fibroadenoma. The lesion is traced on the B-mode image, and that tracing is superimposed on the elasticity image. The size and shape of the lesion in the two images is very similar. (Courtesy Timothy Hall, PhD, University of Wisconsin.)

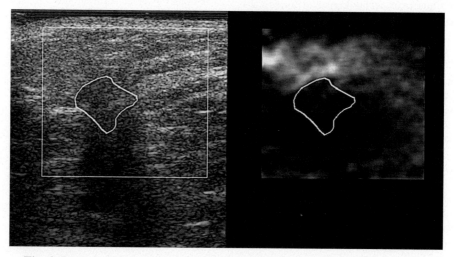

Fig. 9-56 B-mode image *(left)* and elasticity image *(right)* of a scirrhous invasive ductal carcinoma. The lesion is traced on the B-mode image, and that tracing is superimposed on the elasticity image. The size of the lesion is larger on the strain image. (Courtesy Timothy Hall, PhD, University of Wisconsin.)

that, in many ways, are comparable with full-size scanners. The modes of operation include tissue harmonic imaging and Doppler (pulsed wave, continuous wave, color Doppler, and power Doppler). Stated applications from the manufacturers include general imaging, obstetrics/gynecology, small parts, endocavitary, vascular, and cardiac.

In one manufacturer's product the transducer is attached to an electronics module, which is interfaced to a laptop computer. The computer becomes the operator control panel, display monitor for real-time images, archive for image storage, and means to postprocess images. Multi-element broadband transducers are available including 5-10 MHz linear array with 128 elements, 4-2 MHz curvilinear array with 128 elements, 4-2 MHz linear phased array with 64 elements and 8-4 MHz endocavity with 128 elements.

In another product the entire real-time scanner except for the transducer and cable is self-contained within a module measuring approximately 13 inches × 7.5 inches × 2.5 inches. Multiple curvilinear arrays of varying frequency, a 10-5 MHz linear array, and 8-4 MHz endocavity transducers are available. Specifications include high frame rate (up to 100 fps), 256 gray levels for display, and a maximum displayed scan range of 24 cm. Postprocessing and freeze image capabilities are not offered.

SUMMARY

Advances in real-time instrumentation (broadband frequency response, minification of electronics, high-speed digital components, and increased SNR) have improved real-time image quality and led to the development of new scanning techniques, such as tissue harmonic imaging, coded excitation, extended FOV, and spatial compounding. Three-dimensional imaging and 4D ultrasound provides tomographic presentation of the scanned volume. Ultrasound is one of the fastest growing and most exciting areas of diagnostic imaging, and its clinical utility is expanding rapidly. Broadband transducer technology and associated instrumentation is still evolving.

REVIEW QUESTIONS

1. What is a channel in the beam former?
2. What is the advantage of spatial compounding?
3. Beam formation is based on channel-specific time delays, which are applied to the received radiofrequency signals. How are these timed offsets derived?
4. What is phase aberration?
5. Nonlinear versus linear propagation is related to ultrasound _____.
6. Where is harmonic production most likely to occur within the transmitted beam?
7. Name two methods to isolate the second harmonic signal in tissue harmonic imaging.
8. Multiple beam formers allow the acquisition of _____ during each transmit/received cycle.
9. Which imaging technique depicts the displacement of tissue when a force is applied?
10. What is the advantage of coded excitation?

BIBLIOGRAPHY

Behar V: Techniques for phase correction in coherent ultrasound imaging systems, *Ultrasonics* 39;603-610, 2002.

Claudon M et al: Advances in ultrasound, *Eur Radiol* 12:7-18, 2002.

Duck FA: Nonlinear acoustics in diagnostic ultrasound, *Ultrasound Med Biol* 28:1-18, 2002.

Fenster A, Downey DB, Cardinal HN: Three-dimensional ultrasound imaging, *Phys Med Biol* 46;R67-R99, 2001.

Hall TJ: Beyond the basics: elasticity imaging, *Radiographics* 23:1657-1671, 2003.

Hedrick WR: Extended field of view real-time ultrasound: a review, *J Diagn Med Sonography* 16:103-107, 2000.

Jedrzejewicz T: Digital technology for solving acoustic problems, *Eur Radiol* 9:S315-S317, 1999.

Jedrzejewicz T: System architecture for various image reconstruction and processing techniques, *Eur Radiol* 9:S334-S337, 1999.

Jespersen SK, Wilhjelm JE, Sillesen H: Multi-angle compound imaging, *Ultrason Imaging* 20:81-102, 1998.

Kremkau FW: Clinical benefit of higher acoustic output levels, *Ultrasound Med Biol* 15(suppl 1):69-70, 1989.

Lencioni R, Cioni D, Bartolozzi C: Tissue harmonic and contrast-specific imaging: back to gray scale in ultrasound, *Eur Radiol* 12:151-165, 2002.

Misaridis TX et al: Potential of coded excitation in medical ultrasound imaging, *Ultrasonics* 38:183-189, 2000.

Nelson TR: Three-dimensional US imaging. In Goldman LW, Fowlkes JB, eds: *Categorical course in diagnostic radiology physics: CT and US cross-sectional imaging,* Oak Brook, Ill, 2000, Radiological Society of North America.

Pedersen MH, Misaridis TX, Jensen JA: Clinical evaluation of chirp-coded excitation in medical ultrasound, *Ultrasound Med Biol* 29:895-905, 2003.

Pesque P, Sonquet J: Digital ultrasound: from beamforming to PACs, *Eur Radiol* 9:S312-S314, 1999.

Tranquart F et al: Clinical use of ultrasound tissue harmonic imaging, *Ultrasound Med Biol* 25:889-894, 1999.

Wells PNT: *Physical principles of ultrasonic diagnosis,* New York, 1969, Academic Press.

Wells PNT: *Biomedical ultrasonic,* New York, 1977, Academic Press.

Weng L et al: US extended field of view imaging technology, *Radiology* 203:877-880, 1997.

Whittingham TA: Transducer and signal processing developments, *Radiography* 1:61-73, 1995.

Whittingham TA: New and future developments in ultrasonic imaging, *Br J Radiol* 70:S119-S132, 1997.

Whittingham TA: Broadband transducers, *Eur Radiol* 9:S298-S303, 1999.

Whittingham TA: Tissue harmonic imaging, *Eur Radiol* 9:S323-S326, 1999.

Digital Signal and Image Processing

The adaptation of the digital format for signal and image processing has resulted in substantial performance advantages compared with specifically designed electronic components used for analog processing. The same digital hardware can perform different tasks depending on the software instructions. Essentially, if a processing technique can be described mathematically, then it is now possible to implement that algorithm. This expands the processing options available. Upgrades for new and revised processing using the same hardware are instituted by changing software. Scan data can be stored and processed repeatedly by several pathways in parallel. Digital components are more reliable than analog devices and are not subject to electronic drift with temperature change. Additionally, digital hardware often incorporates diagnostic testing of instrument condition to identify failed components and minimize downtime.

Quantitative manipulation and analysis of the received echoes are possible in an expeditious fashion using current computer technology. Time gain compensation (TGC), edge enhancement, logarithmic compression, frame averaging, and gray-scale mapping are all examples of techniques used in the clinical environment for processing the scan data.

DATA MANIPULATION

Signal processing is the manipulation of echo-induced radiofrequency signals before their input to the scan converter (Fig. 10-1). The scan data are typically in analog format until after TGC and amplifier gain reduce the dynamic range of the signals. Digitalization and dynamic focusing occur in the beam former before detection (enveloping). Following detection, additional signal processing subject to operator control (edge enhancement, logarithmic compression, and weak-signal reject) are applied.

The incorporation of a digital scan converter in real-time instruments has dictated that images be manipulated in the matrix format. A large amount of information can be presented in a compact and more easily recognized form. Received echoes configured in a pictorial format, as light and dark regions on a display monitor, are more readily comprehended than a series of voltage spikes on an A-mode cathode ray tube display. Changing the shade of gray associated with a particular received echo in accordance with

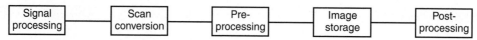

Fig. 10-1 Signal and image processing.

well-defined processing techniques may enhance the observer's ability to interpret the scan data.

Image processing techniques are applied after scan conversion and are classified according to when they occur with respect to the computer storage of scan data in a matrix format. Preprocessing refers to the manipulations that take place during data collection before the scan data are stored in computer memory. Postprocessing denotes the operations applied after storage. Changing the manner in which the stored information is displayed constitutes a postprocessing technique.

SIGNAL PROCESSING

The most common types of signal processing include TGC, selective enhancement, gain, reject, logarithmic compression, and edge enhancement.

Time Gain Compensation

The attenuation of an ultrasound beam with depth causes equally reflective interfaces to produce different signal levels depending on their relative distances from the transducer. It is often advantageous to display reflectors of similar size, shape, and reflection coefficients with equal amplitude (see the discussion in Chapter 5). Exponential amplification as a function of elapsed time from the transmitted pulse is used to correct the received signals for attenuation; that is, the reduction in signal level caused by the increased depth at which echoes are generated is compensated by applying time-dependent amplification to the received signal. This processing technique is called TGC.

Adaptive Time Gain Compensation

Two weaknesses of TGC are: (1) the same variable depth gain is applied to each scan line without consideration of the nonuniformity of tissue along the path, and (2) the operator must continually make manual adjustments as the scan plane is changed. Adaptive TGC addresses these problems by calculating a unique gain function for each scan line and then automatically adjusting the TCG in real time. At all sampling points along a particular scan line, the locally applied gain at a specific depth is compared with the average gain from all scan lines at the same depth. For example, if the local gain function is greater than the global gain function, then the local gain function is set equal to the global gain function. And if the local gain function is less than the global gain function, then the local gain function is set to a weighted average of the two gain functions. A unique TGC is thus applied to each part of the image.

Selective Enhancement

Amplification of the received signal (in addition to TGC) may be applied in a nonuniform manner to highlight echoes generated within a particular region of interest. In this technique, referred to as selective enhancement, the amplification is applied as a function of depth. The operator uses a series of slide control keys to set the depth, each key corresponding to a certain depth; the displacement of a key denotes the amount of amplification.

Gain

Receiver gain increases the amplitude of signals during signal processing and provides the necessary signal strength for analog-to-digital conversion. The application of gain is uniform. *That is, all signals and noise are increased by the same factor.* Gain, in conjunction with the power setting, is used to establish proper brightness levels for echoes of varying strength.

Reject Control

Reject, by passing signals greater than a prescribed amplitude, removes weak signals and noise. Noise reduction is desirable for improving image quality. However, weak signals corresponding to interfaces at deep depths or subtle differences in the composition of interfaces may be lost. In some circumstances (e.g., high reflectivity object located off axis), the signal level exceeds the threshold value and will contribute to the final image.

Logarithmic Compression

In general the digitized signal amplitudes are stored in computer memory as 8 bits. With 8 bits, a total of 256 values is available to quantify the signal amplitude. If a linear representation is used, the maximum signal can be only 256 times the weakest signal. The range of values of the received signals after TGC and amplification, however, may extend over four or more orders of magnitude. *This high information content of signal magnitudes cannot be preserved by other system components.* High and low signals would be lost. Consequently, the dynamic range must be reduced by a technique called logarithmic **compression,** or signals must be combined in groups before display and image recording.

A logarithmic transformation of the signal levels (e.g., 1 to 10^4) is employed to compress the signal levels to a narrower range (0 to 255). The equation defining the transformation from signal level (B) to compressed signal level (B_c) is

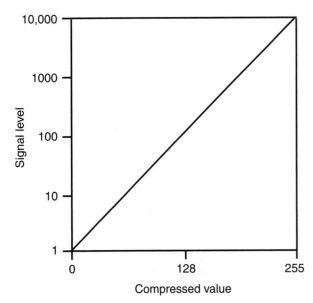

Fig. 10-2 Log compression. Signal levels over four orders of magnitude are assigned values between 0 and 255 for an 8-bit scanner. The vertical scale is logarithmic.

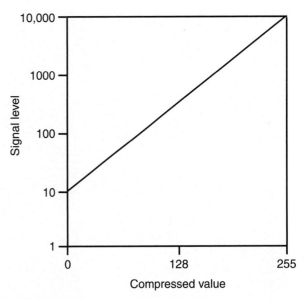

Fig. 10-3 Log compression. Signal levels over three orders of magnitude are assigned values between 0 and 255 for an 8-bit scanner. Weak echoes are discarded.

$$B_c = 255 \left(\frac{\log B}{\log B_{max}} \right)$$ **10-1**

where B_{max} is the maximum signal level that can be compressed (equal to 10^4 in this example). Fig. 10-2 illustrates the relationship between signal level and the stored pixel value.

Log compression enhances the differences between weaker signals within the dynamic range. Half the pixel values ranging from 0 to 128 represent signal levels 1 to 100, where the remaining 50% of pixel values represent signal levels 100 to 10,000. A proportionally larger fraction of compressed signal range is devoted to low signal strengths.

The amount of compression is expressed by a logarithmic scale denoted in dB. The dynamic range for Fig. 10-2 is 40 dB. If the maximum signal level were increased to 10^5, then the dynamic range would be 50 dB. Compression over the entire dynamic range allows very low strength echoes to be depicted in the image.

The operator can adjust log compression. Changing the compression control to a lower decibel setting reduces dynamic range and removes weak echoes and noise. Suppose the dynamic range for compression in Fig. 10-2 is reduced to 30 dB. The logarithmic transformation of the signal levels (10 to 10^4) is now applied to compress the signal levels to the 0 to 255 range (Fig. 10-3). Mathematically, this is accomplished by modifying Equation 10-1 to specify the lowest signal level accepted for inclusion in the image matrix (B_{min}):

$$B_c = 255 \left(\frac{\log \dfrac{B}{B_{min}}}{\log \dfrac{B_{max}}{B_{min}}} \right)$$ **10-2**

The advantage of this technique is that differences in the high signal levels are enhanced (compare the pixel values corresponding to the range 10^3 to 10^4 in Figs. 10-2 and 10-3). However, most often differences in low signal levels are of interest clinically, and improper setting of compression can prevent the visualization of small, low-contrast structures. Sonograms with different settings for log compression are presented in Fig. 10-4.

Because the display monitor and other devices are unable to process an extremely wide range of signal levels, compression is necessary. Increasing the depth beyond 8 bits allows a greater range of values to be stored, but the increased signal levels are ultimately compressed by the display or recording device. Scan data must be selectively excluded from the final displayed image.

Edge Enhancement

Ultrasound imaging is ideally suited to the detection of interfaces or boundaries between structures. **Edge enhancement** is a filtering technique that can be applied to the line-of-sight data (or in some applications to the matrix image data) to emphasize further a change in signal levels across an interface. Suppose that eight pixels along one line of sight have the initial values shown in Table 10-1. The filtering process uses a kernel (i.e., a collection of weighting factors or convolution coefficients) applied to the original values. In this example the kernel is applied to three sequential pixels with weighting factors of −1, 3, and −1. To calculate the edge-enhanced value for pixel number 4, the kernel is centered on pixel number 4. The sum of each weighting factor times the respective original value of each pixel in the three-pixel sequence (pixel number 4 and the adjacent pixels) is calculated. This yields a new value of 300 for pixel 4. The numeric operations are

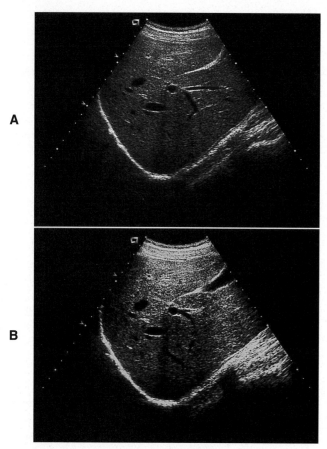

Fig. 10-4 Sonograms of the liver with different levels of compression. **A,** 75 dB. **B,** 40 dB. Note the loss of weak scatterers when the dynamic range is reduced.

■ **Table 10-1** Numerical Example of Edge Enhancement

Pixel No.	1	2	3	4	5	6	7	8
Original value	200	200	200	200	100	100	100	100
Kernel			-1	3	-1			
Edge-enhanced value	200	200	200	300	0	100	100	100

$$(-1 \times 200) + (3 \times 200) + (-1 \times 100) = 300$$

The edge-enhanced values for the remaining pixels in the original data set are determined in a similar manner, by moving the center of the kernel to each pixel along the line of sight. Centering the kernel at pixel 5, for example, yields an edge-enhanced value of 0:

$$(-1 \times 200) + (3 \times 100) + (-1 \times 100) = 0$$

Note that the original value and not the new filtered value for pixel 4 was used in this calculation. The kernel always operates on the original data; the edge-enhanced results must be maintained separately from the initial values. Fig. 10-5 is a graphic representation of edge enhancement. Changing the magnitude or number of weighting factors used in the filtering process can modify the amount of edge enhancement.

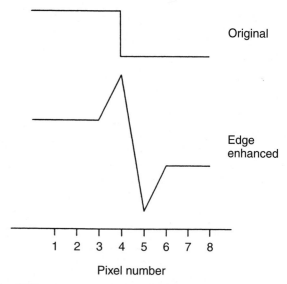

Fig. 10-5 Edge enhancement. The original change in signal level detected along a particular line of sight is manipulated mathematically to produce a more dramatic difference at the boundary.

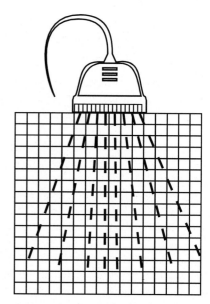

Fig. 10-6 Lines of sight *(dotted)* superimposed on the matrix to demonstrate that not all pixels are sampled by the sound beam. The value assigned to the unsampled pixels is calculated by averaging signal amplitudes in the neighboring pixels.

SCAN CONVERSION

The scanned area is probed by a series of ultrasound pulses directed along various lines of sight. The angle and depth information (polar coordinates) must be converted to the matrix format (rectangular coordinates) for display. By superimposing all the lines of sight on the image matrix, it can be demonstrated that several pixels are not sampled by the ultrasound beam (Fig. 10-6). If these blank pixels were each displayed with a zero signal level, a disconcerting checkerboard image would result. Manufacturers avoid this by averaging the signals from nearby pixels that are sampled to generate a fill-in value for the blank pixel. A value for the blank pixel can thus be inferred by examining the surrounding region.

Fill-In Interpolation

The most widely used scan conversion method is **bilinear interpolation.** Two algorithms, which can be executed in real time, have been developed to interpolate the scan data along the axial and angular directions. In the first technique a synthesized scan line through the pixel of interest is generated by interpolating angularly between sampling points on adjacent scan lines (Fig. 10-7). Axial interpolation between two points on the synthesized scan line, which encompass the pixel, establishes the pixel value. In the alternative technique additional axial values are calculated by interpolation along each scan line (Fig. 10-8). Angular interpolation between these new axial points establishes the pixel value.

PREPROCESSING

Manipulation of scan data in the matrix format includes image updating, write zoom, and panning. These preprocessing techniques complete data acquisition and create the image data placed in memory for postprocessing and display.

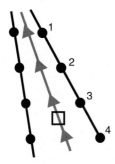

Fig. 10-7 Fill-in interpolation. A synthetic scan line *(gray)* through the pixel of interest is calculated by interpolating angularly between sampling points *(1, 2, 3,* and *4)* on adjacent scan lines. Axial interpolation along the synthetic scan line establishes the pixel value.

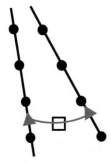

Fig. 10-8 Fill-in interpolation. Additional axial values are calculated by interpolation along each scan line *(gray triangles).* The pixel value is calculated by angular interpolation between these new axial points.

Image Updating

Because the ultrasound beam sweeps repeatedly through the patient, new information is constantly becoming available. The most recent scan data are held in the buffer for updating the image data in memory. Several techniques by various manufacturers are employed for this purpose. Most simply, the old value at a particular location stored in memory is replaced by the current value for that pixel location. This is referred to as last-value mode. The image data are updated continuously and rapidly with the newest echo data (Fig. 10-9). The average of the old value and current value may also be used to replace the stored scan data.

Write Zoom

Write zoom (also called regional expansion, reduced field of view [FOV], and zooming) is a magnification technique applied during data collection. The operator designates a

A

0	0	5	0	0
0	0	4	0	0
0	0	3	0	0
0	0	2	0	0
0	0	1	0	0

B

0	0	5	0	0
0	0	4	0	0
0	0	7	0	0
0	0	2	0	0
0	0	1	0	0

C

0	0	5	0	0
0	0	4	0	0
0	0	5	0	0
0	0	2	0	0
0	0	1	0	0

Fig. 10-9 Image updating. **A,** Old matrix data. **B,** Last-value mode or most recent matrix data. **C,** Pixel-by-pixel average of these two matrices.

region within the FOV to be magnified. The signals received from this designated region are placed in pixels to generate the image matrix. *Because the physical dimensions of the zoomed region are much smaller than the original FOV, and an equal number of pixels compose the image matrix, improved spatial resolution is now possible.*

For example, in Fig. 10-10, a 5 × 5 matrix is used to store an image of an object that has physical dimensions of 1 cm × 1 cm. By designating the central region for expansion, the same 5 × 5 matrix can be made to represent a 0.5 cm × 0.5 cm portion of the object. The same number of pixels is available in each case, but in the magnified mode the pixels are distributed over a smaller FOV. In the magnified mode the physical size of the object represented by a single pixel decreases from 0.2 cm × 0.2 cm to 0.1 cm × 0.1 cm. Spatial

detail is thus enhanced with the application of regional expansion.

The disadvantage of write zoom is that the FOV is limited. The portraits of Abraham Lincoln displayed with the same number of pixels in normal and magnified modes illustrate the effect of write zoom (Fig. 10-11). The normal and magnified views of a breast containing a cyst (Fig. 10-12) demonstrate write zoom. In practice, the improvement in resolution is usually limited by the beam width and spatial pulse length.

Panning

Panning is an image-acquisition technique that allows the operator to shift the expanded region to a new anatomic

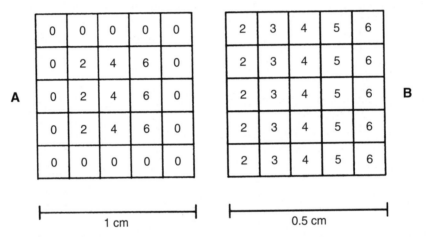

Fig. 10-10 Write zoom. **A,** Original sampled region. **B,** Central portion of the original region scanned in write-zoom mode. Although the number of pixels is constant, a smaller region is sampled in write zoom, and thus each pixel corresponds to a smaller physical size.

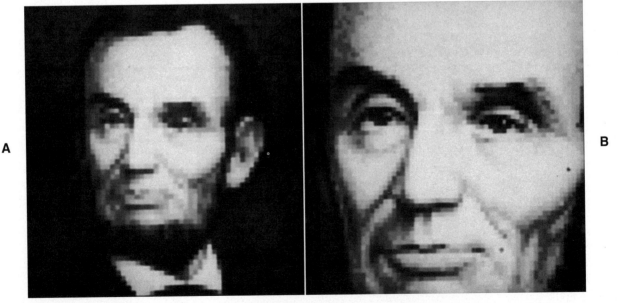

Fig. 10-11 A, Portrait of Abraham Lincoln in normal mode. **B,** Write-zoom mode. The number of pixels in each matrix is identical, but in write-zoom mode spatial detail is improved.

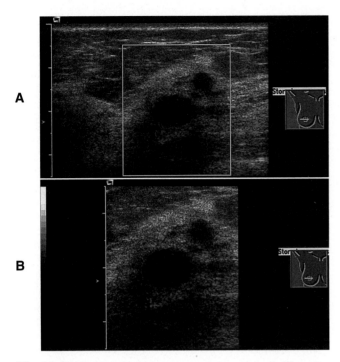

Fig. 10-12 Sonogram of a breast containing a cyst. **A,** Normal mode. **B,** Write-zoom mode.

location during scanning. The maximum FOV for a particular transducer is well defined. During panning, a portion of this FOV is displayed, and the sonographer can move the expanded region to a new position within the FOV of the transducer. In essence, panning provides a write-zoom image that can be translated vertically and horizontally under operator control to sample different regions.

POSTPROCESSING (DISPLAY)

The image data stored in memory after further processing are converted into a video signal (digital to analog conversion) and sent to a video monitor for display (Fig. 10-13). The standard video signal implies a specific format for information transmittal. A frame consists of 525 raster lines subdivided into two fields. Alternate raster lines are assigned to each field; thus half of the total raster lines are placed in a field. At the monitor the fields are interlaced to re-form the original frame. The transmission rate is 30 frames per second.

Computer monitors offer the possibility of increased information transfer rates (more pixels or lines with faster refresh rates), since the television video format does not apply. As the demand for hard copy devices with video input has decreased, ultrasound scanners have incorporated computer monitors.

Gray-Scale Mapping

The image data are transferred to an output buffer or video card, which is read in a raster fashion. The signal amplitudes are converted back into analog signals via a digital-to-analog converter (DAC) and fed into the monitor. Postprocessing options enable the operator to manipulate the image data before viewing. Each pixel is displayed uniformly as a particular shade of gray depending on the pixel value (Fig. 10-14). The translation of signal amplitude into brightness level is according to a gray-scale map. The gray-scale map encodes each pixel value to a brightness level. However, multiple pixel values may be displayed with the same shade of gray. The gray-scale map is selectable by the operator.

The number of values that can be stored at any one location in computer memory is determined by the number of bits. If each memory location could store 1 bit of information, each pixel would be "on" or "off" (0 or 1), and a bistable image would be created. A system that was 2 bits deep could represent four different values (four combinations of 1s and 0s—00, 01, 10, 11—equivalent to the decimal numbers 0, 1, 2, and 3). Most units are 8 bits deep, creating up to 256 numeric representations in memory, and these stored values can be translated into various shades of gray on the display screen. A 2-bit system displays 0 as black, 1 as dark gray, 2 as light gray, and 3 as white. Systems with more bits can exhibit more shades of gray.

At this point, it is important to differentiate between the number of values that can be stored in computer memory and the number of gray levels that can be displayed on the output device. The gray scale on most monitors consists of 32 or 64 levels. If the signal amplitude is expressed as 8 bits (with 256 numeric configurations possible), obviously each value cannot be represented as a separate and distinct shade of gray. A range of numeric values must be associated with

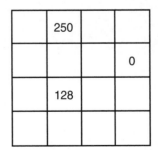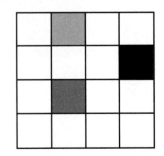

Fig. 10-14 Display of pixels. Each pixel is assigned a value representing a signal level. Each pixel is depicted on the monitor as a uniform shade of gray based on the pixel value. Brightness levels for three pixels are shown.

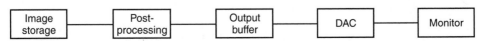

Fig. 10-13 Image output components of a real-time scanner.

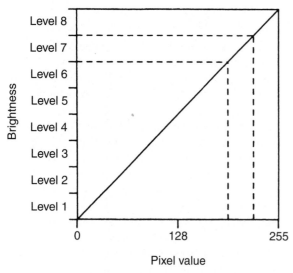

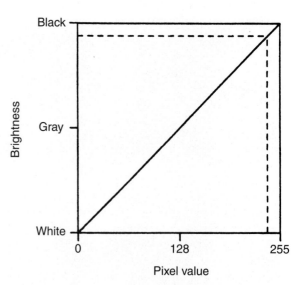

Fig. 10-15 A gray-scale map provides the translation of stored pixel values to different brightness levels. For this system, eight brightness levels are possible. Usually level 1 is black, and level 8 is white. Pixels with values from 191 to 223 are all displayed with brightness level 7.

Fig. 10-16 Black/white inversion. The brightness levels on the gray-scale map are inverted. High pixel values such as 240 are displayed as near black.

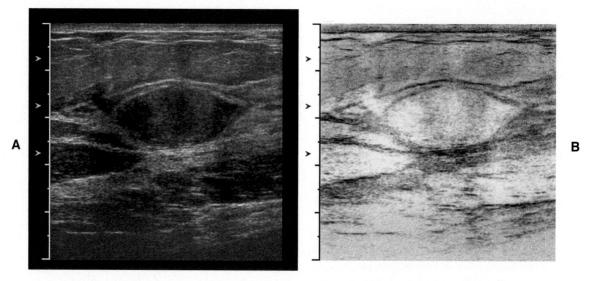

Fig. 10-17 Sonogram of the breast with a mass, **A,** and with black/white inversion, **B.**

each gray level. The translation of the range of pixel values (stored values in image memory) to brightness levels is called gray-scale mapping. Fig. 10-15 is a gray-scale map in which eight brightness levels are available. Pixels with values between 191 and 223 are all displayed as brightness level 7. Several methods, including linear, logarithmic, and enhancement algorithms, can be selected by the operator as postprocessing options for converting the digitized amplitudes into various shades of gray. Pixels with similar values are displayed with either the same or different brightness levels depending on the gray-scale mapping. Altering the gray-scale mapping does not change the stored value in image storage; rather, it modifies how that pixel is displayed

based on its stored value. (This is discussed in more detail on p. 165.)

Black and White Inversion

In black and white inversion the brightness levels on a gray-scale map are inverted to extend from white (at the low signal amplitude) to black (at the high signal amplitude). A pixel value of 240, which is normally displayed as near white, is depicted as near black on the inverted image (Figs. 10-16 and 10-17). Note the reversal of brightness levels on the vertical scale in Fig. 10-16 (black represents high signal levels).

Freeze Frame

The **freeze frame** option allows the operator to select an image of interest for prolonged viewing. The data collection of scan lines is suspended and the last frame acquired is displayed on the monitor. This enables the operator to analyze the image with various processing tools (text labeling, region of interest, distance measurements, area measurements) or to record the image on a hardcopy device.

Frame Averaging or Persistence

Noise is the variation in signal level introduced by the interactions of ultrasound with tissue and by limitations in the detection system. In other words, multiple measurements of the reflected echo from a particular interface yield not the same but slightly different values. Thus a uniform object would be depicted by nonuniform pixel values throughout the image.

Real-time scanners acquire images at a rate of several frames per second (15 to 20 fps). **Frame averaging** (also called **persistence**) allows successive frames (as many as four or more) to be held in a buffer and then added together to increase the signal-to-noise ratio (SNR). Image quality is improved, because the variations in signal level from regions of comparable-strength echoes are reduced. However, because, in effect, the sampling occurs over a longer time interval, temporal resolution is poorer. The rate of movement of the interfaces must be small; otherwise, motion will induce lag or blurring. During imaging of the heart, high persistence levels are not appropriate, because the small, rapid motions of the valves cannot be perceived when several frames are added together. The technique of frame averaging does allow high-quality abdominal scans to be obtained.

A series of temporary storage areas (called buffers) that sequentially accept the most recent frame is created. The displayed image is the average of all accepted frames in the storage areas (Fig. 10-18). Note that the memory requirements for four frames, each with a 512 × 512 matrix, are 4 × 256 kilobytes.

Adaptive Frame Averaging

Frame averaging is designed to reduce noise, but it can create blurring of fast moving structures. Adaptive frame averaging is a modification of this technique in which the image is subdivided into many small regions. The time variance of the pixel values in each of these small regions is assessed. More averaging is applied in regions with little change from frame to frame and less averaging is applied in regions with high variation. The amount of averaging with previous measurements for the respective interfaces is variable throughout the image. In this manner the SNR for slow-moving structures is increased without the penalty of lag for the fast-moving structures.

Read Zoom

Read zoom is a display magnification technique applied to the scan data after image storage. The pixels that compose the image are shown in a larger format on the monitor; that is, the portion of the monitor screen associated with each pixel is enlarged. The number of pixels throughout the scanned area remains constant, and the area of tissue represented by each pixel does not change. Unlike write zoom, this technique cannot improve spatial detail. Figs. 10-19 and 10-20 illustrate the change in display format when read zoom is selected. Read zoom is called display zoom or magnification by some manufacturers.

To increase the number of pixels in the displayed matrix during read zoom, a technique known as image interpolation is applied. The original image data are unaltered. Every pixel in the read zoom matrix is replaced by four smaller pixels. One pixel is set equal to the value of the original large-size pixel. The remaining three pixels are each assigned a value by averaging the values of the nearby pixels (Fig. 10-21). The most frequently used method creates a linear variation between original pixels. Image interpolation provides a more pleasing image since the individual pixels are less discernible. Spatial resolution, however, is not improved by increasing the displayed matrix size. Fig. 10-22 illustrates the effect of image interpolation on the matrix data.

POSTPROCESSING (DATA MANIPULATION)

Additional manipulation and analysis of the echo data are possible, because the image information has been digitized and stored in computer memory. The postprocessing techniques of contrast enhancement and filtering can be performed. Pixels with similar values over a narrow range

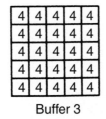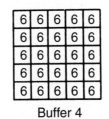

Buffer 1   Buffer 2   Buffer 3   Buffer 4   Displayed image

Fig. 10-18 Frame averaging. Four samplings of a scanned area are temporarily held in a buffer. The displayed image is a pixel-by-pixel average of the samplings (0 + 2 + 4 + 6 = 12, which, divided by the four banks equals 3). In this example, the signal amplitude at each pixel (numbers in the boxes) increases as a function of time.

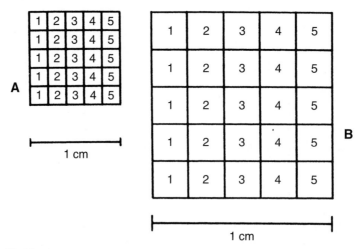

Fig. 10-19 In read-zoom mode the original displayed image, **A,** is presented in a larger format, **B.** The number of pixels and the physical dimensions of the scanned object represented by a pixel remain unchanged.

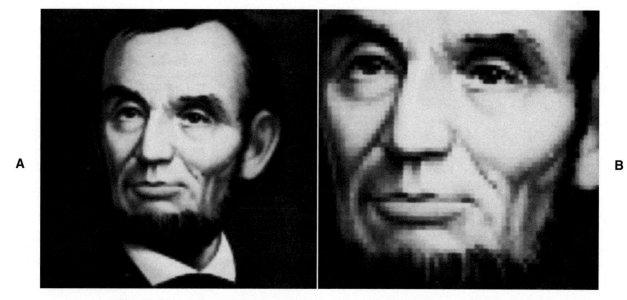

Fig. 10-20 Portrait of Abraham Lincoln in normal-size mode, **A,** and in read-zoom mode, **B.** In read-zoom mode the central portion of the image has been magnified by a factor of 2.

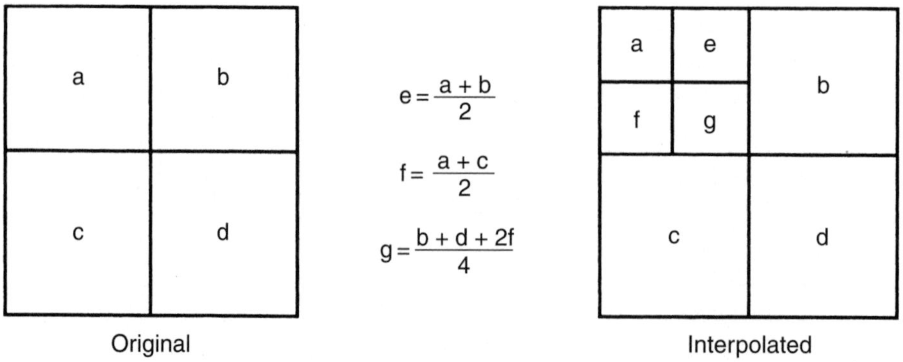

Original

$$e = \frac{a + b}{2}$$

$$f = \frac{a + c}{2}$$

$$g = \frac{b + d + 2f}{4}$$

Interpolated

Fig. 10-21 Matrix interpolation. Each original pixel is replaced by four smaller pixels. The values assigned to the originals are calculated from values in the surrounding pixels.

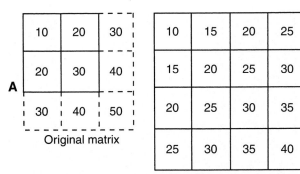

Fig. 10-22 A 2 × 2 portion of the original data matrix, **A,** is expanded to contain more pixels (16) by linear interpolation, **B.** Values for neighboring pixels in the original matrix required for the interpolation calculation are shown by the dotted lines.

■ **Table 10-2** Change in Values Associated with Various Gray-Scale Levels Using Contrast Enhancement

Original Values	Gray Level	New Values
181 to 210	7 white	189 to 210
151 to 180	6	167 to 188
121 to 150	5	145 to 166
91 to 120	4	123 to 144
61 to 90	3	101 to 122
31 to 60	2	79 to 100
1 to 30	1	57 to 78
0	0 black	0 to 56

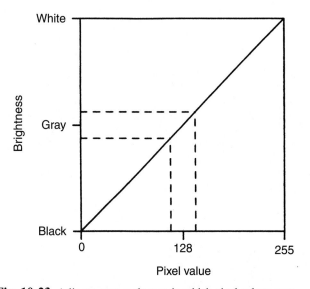

Fig. 10-23 A linear gray-scale map in which pixel values near 128 are displayed as intermediate shades of gray.

can be displayed with differing brightness levels via contrast enhancement. Thus these pixels can be distinguished from each other on the displayed image. Digital filtering is used extensively in other imaging modalities. Filtering refers to the modification of a pixel value based on the values of surrounding pixels. Smoothing and edge enhancement are forms of digital filtering.

Contrast Enhancement

Contrast enhancement is an especially powerful technique. For example, if the echo data in computer memory range from 0 to 210, and the pixel values are to be visualized in eight shades of gray, every pixel with a value of 0 will be depicted as black, and the remaining pixels will be linearly distributed over seven levels of gray. Each gray level is associated with a specific spread of values. Thus pixels with values between 61 and 90 are all displayed in the same shade of gray (level 3). Suppose values less than 56 (weak echo signals) are not of interest and can be eliminated for viewing purposes. By depicting these pixels as black and redistributing the gray scale over a new range of values (57 to 210), image contrast is enhanced. The range of pixel values associated with each gray level is then decreased from 30 to 22 following contrast enhancement, and pixels with similar values are more likely to be separated by being displayed at different gray levels. Whereas pixels with relative signal amplitudes of 65 and 85 were displayed as gray level 3 initially, after contrast enhancement they are presented as gray level 1 and gray level 2 (Table 10-2).

Contrast enhancement can also be illustrated with the aid of gray-scale mapping. Fig. 10-23 is a linear gray-scale map used to translate pixel values from 0 to 255 to the different brightness levels in a linear fashion. Pixels with values near 128 are displayed with intermediate shades of gray. If the gray-scale map is changed so pixel values from 0 to 160 are distributed linearly over the various brightness levels, and if values above 160 are displayed as white, pixels with values near 128 will be displayed with very light shades of gray

(Fig. 10-24). There are more brightness levels available to display a fixed range of values for the contrast-enhanced gray-scale map (e.g., see Fig. 10-24) than for the original gray-scale map (see Fig. 10-23). In other words, the distance along the vertical axis corresponding to a particular range of pixel values is greater for the enhanced gray-scale map than for the initial map.

The gray-scale map is not restricted to a linear relationship. Logarithmic, inverse logarithmic, exponential, squared, and square root gray-scale maps are also available. Fig. 10-25 illustrates three gray-scale maps. The linear map distributes gray levels equally throughout the range of pixel values (echo strengths). The logarithmic map enhances the contrast of weak echoes. The threshold linear map eliminates the weak echoes and emphasizes variations in high-strength echoes. Usually these gray-scale maps, available as postprocessing options in the scanner, are used to enhance contrast so its effect on the image can be visualized before recording.

Fig. 10-26 is a sonogram of the liver displayed with different gray-scale maps. The stored pixel values remain unchanged. The operator-selected gray-scale maps alter the presentation of data.

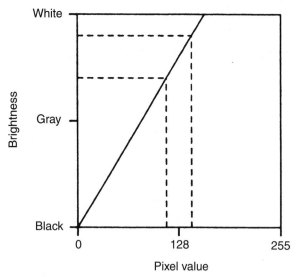

Fig. 10-24 An enhanced gray-scale map in which pixel values near 128 are displayed as near white. The range of brightness levels for pixel values near 128 is wider than in Fig. 10-23. Types of gray-scale mapping are linear, logarithm, and threshold linear. Weak echoes are enhanced with a logarithm gray-scale map. Strong echoes are enhanced by a threshold change in linear gray-scale map.

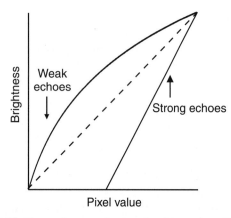

Fig. 10-25 Types of gray-scale mapping. Linear, logarithm, and threshold linear gray-scale maps. Weak echoes are enhanced with a logarithm gray-scale map. Strong echoes are enhanced by a threshold change in linear gray-scale map.

Image Equalization

Image equalization is a method to automatically adjust brightness levels throughout the image to enhance contrast. Multiple techniques have been employed for image equalization. Histogram analysis of the pixel values within a small region of interest provides a feedback mechanism to change contrast and gain for image optimization. Alternatively, regional statistical analysis is used to perform region-by-region adjustments to the acquisition gain parameters.

Smoothing

Smoothing is an image-processing technique for the reduction of noise. Noise is the variation in signal level

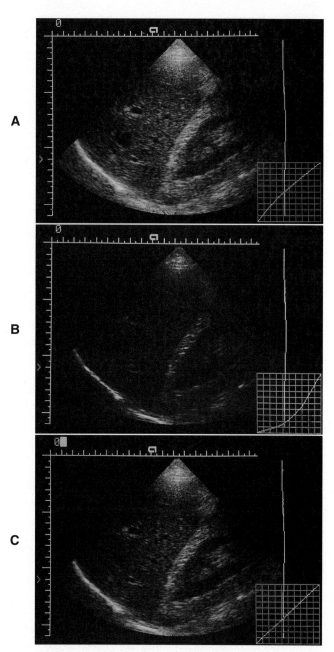

Fig. 10-26 Sonogram of the liver displayed with different gray-scale maps in **A, B,** and **C.** The gray-scale map for each image is presented in the lower right. The data in image memory are unchanged, but the translation of pixel values to brightness levels is altered to produce radically different images.

associated with a particular interface. It has no well-defined spatial pattern, which prohibits using a mathematical correction to eliminate its contribution in the image. Noise can be reduced, however, by averaging the values in nearby pixels if the pixels are representative of the same physical entity. This assumption fails at sharp boundaries, where a rapid change in pixel value occurs.

The digital portion (i.e., conversion to the digital format with subsequent digital processing) of the scanner does not introduce electronic noise to the image.

Smoothing is a two-dimensional spatial averaging technique whereby values in the surrounding pixels are used to calculate a new value for the pixel of interest. The most common smoothing operation employs a nine-point spread function, or kernel. A set of weighting factors is arranged in a 3 × 3 minimatrix as shown:

$$\begin{matrix} 1 & 2 & 1 \\ 2 & 4 & 2 \\ 1 & 2 & 1 \end{matrix}$$

The center of the kernel is superimposed on the pixel of interest in the raw data matrix. The smoothed value for that pixel is calculated as a weighted sum of the value of the pixel of interest and the values of the neighboring eight pixels. Specifically, the sum of the product of each weighting factor and the corresponding pixel value is divided by the sum of the weighting factors to generate a new value for the pixel of interest. The kernel is subsequently placed over every pixel (except those along the edge) to produce the smoothed values. Each application of the kernel on the raw data matrix creates one new pixel value for the new matrix of smoothed values. All calculations are applied to the raw data, which requires that the smoothed matrix be generated separately from the raw data matrix.

Fig. 10-27 illustrates the nine-point smoothing operation applied to a 5 × 5 image matrix. Calculations for pixel CH (column C, row H) and pixel DH (column D, row H) are shown. The new value for pixel CH is found by

$$\begin{aligned} &[(1 \times 50) + (2 \times 40) + (1 \times 30) + \\ &(2 \times 40) + (4 \times 50) + (2 \times 40) + \\ &(1 \times 30) + (2 \times 40) + (1 \times 50)]/16 \end{aligned}$$

The factor *16* is the sum of the weighting factors. To complete the smoothing operation on this 5 × 5 matrix, the kernel must be applied a total of nine times (the pixels along the border are not included). For each calculation the same weighting factors are used to modulate the contribution of the surrounding pixels to the pixel of interest. For a larger-sized matrix the kernel would be applied many more times.

The degree of smoothing is modified by changing the weighting factors or by increasing the size of the kernel (e.g., a 5 × 5 instead of a 3 × 3 minimatrix). Weighting factors of equal magnitude or those averaging a greater number of surrounding pixels produce a stronger smoothing effect.

The disadvantage of smoothing is that some spatial detail is lost, because the smoothed value represents the averaging over the nearby region. Compare the portrait of Abraham Lincoln and the sonogram of the breast after undergoing the smoothing operation with the respective original (Figs. 10-28 and 10-29).

Edge Enhancement

Edge enhancement (also called sharpness) is a filtering technique that can be applied to the matrix image data to increase the visibility of small high-contrast structures. However, the application of the edge filter is accompanied by an increase in image noise.

The filtering process uses a kernel applied to the original values in the same manner as described for smoothing. The set of weighting factors, however, arranged in a 3 × 3 minimatrix assumes different values:

$$\begin{matrix} 0 & -1 & 0 \\ -1 & 5 & -1 \\ 0 & -1 & 0 \end{matrix}$$

Fig. 10-30 shows the effect on a sonogram of the breast processed with edge enhancement. The amount of edge enhancement can be modified by changing the magnitude or number of the weighting factors used in the convolution.

IMAGE ANALYSIS

Since the scan data were digitized to improve and expand processing options, a secondary benefit is the ability to quantify the characteristics of the image and manipulate the image based on these numeric parameters.

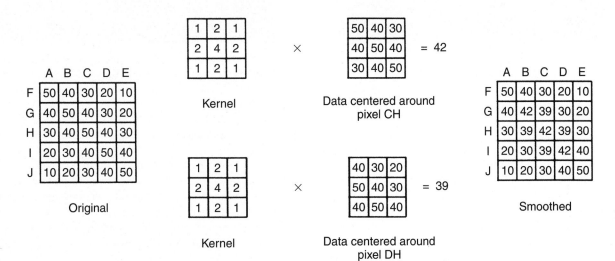

Fig. 10-27 A kernel (collection of weighting factors) is applied to the original matrix data to generate the smoothed matrix data.

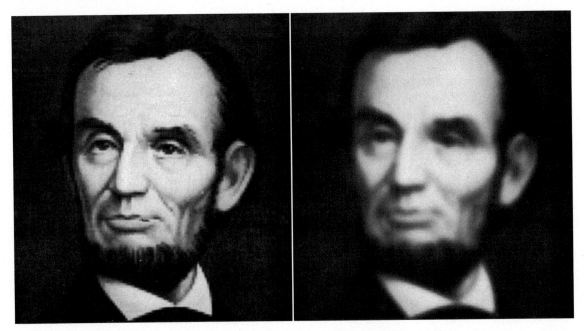

Fig. 10-28 Digital filtering applied to the portrait of Abraham Lincoln. The smoothed image is on the right.

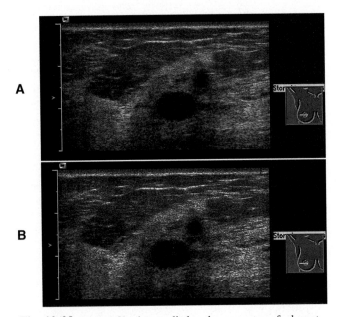

Fig. 10-29 Digital filtering applied to the sonogram of a breast containing a cyst. **A,** None. **B,** Smooth.

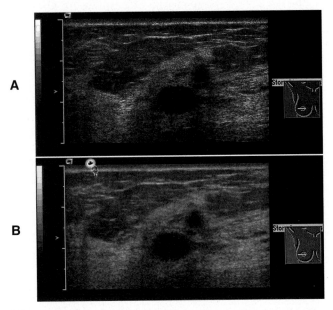

Fig. 10-30 Digital filtering applied to the sonogram of a breast containing a cyst. **A,** None. **B,** Edge enhancement.

Region of Interest

Region-of-interest definition enables the operator to specify a portion of the image for special consideration. The region of interest on the displayed image is denoted by defining the boundary of the desired area. This is accomplished by moving a visible cursor on the screen via a mouse or track ball. Pixels within the boundary are now designated for special consideration (Fig. 10-31). For example, the average pixel value and the statistical variation within a particular area of the liver can be determined.

Distance Calculation

The image matrix is calibrated in terms of physical size. The side of one pixel corresponds to a known length (e.g., 1 pixel equals 0.2 mm), which is dictated by the transducer and the collection parameters (matrix size and FOV). Therefore the distance between any two points of interest on the displayed image is readily calculated by the computer. The operator must identify the two locations, which is usually accomplished by moving a visible cursor on the screen via a track ball. Once the separation in number of pixels is determined,

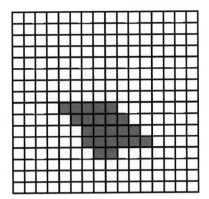

Fig. 10-31 Region of interest. The boundary of the region of interest is marked with the mouse. Pixels within this boundary denoted in *gray* are included in the region of interest.

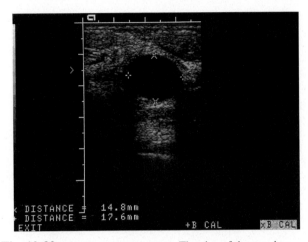

Fig. 10-32 Distance measurements. The size of the cyst in a breast is determined by marking the boundary of the cyst with cursors in two directions.

the actual distance is calculated by the computer using the product of the number of pixels and the calibration factor (0.2 mm per pixel). Distance measurements of femur length, crown–rump length, biparietal diameter, and many other structures are routinely performed in the clinical environment (Fig. 10-32). Accuracy of distance measurements is compromised when a matrix with few pixels is used for imaging.

PERSONAL COMPUTERS

High-level programming languages provide the individual user with the ability to solve problems by directing the computer to execute a series of instructions. The solution to a particular problem requires a precise and unambiguous statement of the exact sequence of tasks to be performed. This description of the necessary steps in the solution process is called an algorithm, and it must be translated into the terminology of a specific programming language.

A personal computer can be very effective in the clinical environment. Various parameters (crown–rump length, femur length, head circumference, abdominal circumference, and biparietal diameter) have been shown to be excellent

predictors of fetal age. The computer can be programmed to calculate fetal age based on the measurements of a particular structure. The equation relating fetal age and the measured parameter is assimilated into an algorithm that is then translated into program code.

A simple BASIC program designed to calculate menstrual age (MA), given measurements for biparietal diameter (BPD), femur length (FL), head circumference (HC), and abdominal circumference (AC), is listed in Box 10-1. For readers who want to learn BASIC, Marateck has written an excellent textbook providing practical instruction on programming techniques (see Bibliography). For readers already familiar with BASIC, the program is divided into four sections: initialization (lines 10 to 60), data input (lines 70 to 460), calculation (lines 470 to 640), and data output (lines 650 to 1310). Data input allows for both patient demographics (lines 70 to 260) and measurements of the various parameters (lines 270 to 460). If a particular parameter is not of interest, a zero entered will cause the program to ignore the MA calculation using that parameter. A sample report generated by this program is shown in Box 10-2.

Although the sample program in Box 10-2 does accomplish the designed purpose of calculating fetal age based on ultrasonically measured parameters, its usefulness in the clinical environment would be enhanced if it were modified. Changes would include the ability to edit the input data, identify the hospital on the printed report, and select calculation alternatives (e.g., fetal weight and multiple variable analyses for fetal age). In addition, storage of the information (examination date, patient demographics, and measured parameters) for subsequent retrieval and analysis is very desirable.

Real-time scanners are microprocessor based, which means that most of their functions are computer controlled. Many units allow for direct calculation of fetal age by incorporating equations relating the age of the fetus with measured parameters into the scanner. Some units even allow the operator to modify these equations. Because several equations are available based on the work of different researchers, the operator should know which ones are used by his or her scanner.

DATABASE MANAGEMENT

The database is a collection of data pertaining to a particular project. The data are stored in files and maintained as a source of reference. They often include identification, statistical and historic information, physical measurements, and images. The files must be updated when new data become available. Data extracted from the files can be used to compare results and produce a report.

Database management will become increasingly important during the next few years in ultrasound imaging. Although the computers used to manage a database will be separate from the imaging devices, quick retrieval of the results from previous examinations saves personnel time and aids the diagnostic process. Personal computers could easily be employed to accomplish this task by using BASIC

Box 10-1 BASIC Program to Calculate Fetal Age

```
10 REM INITIALIZE
20 REM FETAL AGE CALCULATION
30 REM FEBRUARY 1990
40 DIM PTDATA$(10), MA (10)
50 KEY OFF
60 REM *****************************************
70 REM PATIENT DATA INPUT
80 CLS
90 PRINT : PRINT
100 PRINT "ENTER PATIENT'S FIRST NAME";
110 INPUT PTDATA$(1)
120 PRINT "ENTER PATIENT'S LAST NAME";
130 INPUT PTDATA$(2)
140 PRINT "ENTER PATIENT'S ID NUMBER";
150 INPUT DATA$(3)
160 PRINT "ENTER PATIENT'S AGE";
170 INPUT DATA$(4)
180 PRINT "ENTER REFERRING PHYSICIAN";
190 INPUT PTDATA$(5)
200 PRINT "ENTER RADIOLOGIST";
210 INPUT PTDATA$(6)
220 PRINT "ENTER SONOGRAPHER";
230 INPUT PTDATA$(7)
240 PRINT "ENTER HISTORY";
250 INPUT PTDATA$(8)
260 REM *****************************************
270 CLS
280 PRINT : PRINT
290 PRINT "ENTER BIPARIETAL DIAMETER
MEASUREMENT IN CM";
300 INPUT BPD
310 PRINT
320 PRINT "ENTER MEASUREMENTS FOR HEAD
CIRCUMFERENCE";
330 PRINT "ENTER OCCIPITO-FRONTAL DIAMETER IN
CM";
340 INPUT OFD
350 PRINT "ENTER HEAD DIAMETER IN CM";
360 INPUT HD
370 PRINT
380 PRINT "ENTER MEASUREMENTS FOR ABDOMINAL
CIRCUMFERENCE";
390 PRINT "ENTER ABDOMINAL DIAMETER #1 IN CM";
400 INPUT AD1
410 PRINT "ENTER ABDOMINAL DIAMETER #2 IN CM";
420 INPUT AD2
430 PRINT
440 PRINT "ENTER FEMUR LENGTH MEASUREMENT";
450 INPUT FL
460 REM *****************************************
470 REM CALCULATE CIRCUMFERENCE
480 AC = 3.1416*SQR( (AD1^2 + AD2^2) / 2)
490 HC = 3.1416*SQR( (HD^2 + OFD^2) / 2)
500 REM *****************************************
510 REM CALCULATE FETAL AGE
520 REM REFERENCE HADLOCK ET AL., RADIOLOGY
152, 497-501, 1984
530 FOR I = 1 TO 4
540 MA(I) = 0
550 NEXT I
560 IF BPD<9.4 OR BPD>1.7 THEN 580
570 MA(1) = 9.54 + 1.482*BPD + .1676*BPD^2
580 IF HC> 34.6 OR HC<6.8 THEN 600
590 MA(2) = 8.96 + 0.54*HC + 0.0003*HC^3
600 IF AC>35.3 OR AC<4.6 THEN 620
610 MA(3) = 8.140001 + 0.753*AC + 0.0036*AC^2
620 IF FL>7.7 OR FL<7 THEN 640
630 MA(4) = 10.35 + 2.46*FL + 0.17*FL^2
640 REM *****************************************
650 REM OUTPUT BEGINS HERE
660 CLS
670 PRINT : PRINT
680 PRINT "SELECT OUTPUT DEVICE"
690 PRINT "0 TO QUIT"
700 PRINT "1 FOR PRINTER"
710 PRINT "2 FOR SCREEN"
720 INPUT FLAG
730 IF FLAG = 0 THEN 1320
740 IF FLAG = 1 THEN OPEN "LPT1:" FOR OUTPUT AS #2
750 IF FLAG = 2 THEN OPEN "SCRN:" FOR OUTPUT AS #2
760 PRINT #2,CHR$(12) : PRINT #2,"  "
770 PRINT #2," "
780 PRINT #2,TAB(45);DATE$
790 PRINT #2," "
800 PRINT #2, TAB(22);"PATIENT LAST NAME: ";
810 PRINT #2, PTDATA$(2)
820 PRINT #2, TAB(21);"PATIENT FIRST NAME: ";
830 PRINT #2, PTDATA$(1)
840 PRINT #2,TAB(22);"PATIENT ID NUMBER: ";
850 PRINT #2, PTDATA$(3)
860 PRINT #2,TAB(28);"PATIENT AGE: ";
870 PRINT #2, PTDATA$(4)
880 PRINT #2,TAB(20);"REFERRING PHYSICIAN: ";
890 PRINT #2, PTDATA$(5)
900 PRINT #2, TAB(28);"RADIOLOGIST: ";
910 PRINT #2, PTDATA$(6)
920 PRINT #2,TAB(28);"SONOGRAPHER: ";
930 PRINT #2, PTDATA$(7)
940 PRINT #2, TAB(32);"HISTORY: ";
950 PRINT #2, PTDATA$(8)
960 PRINT #2," " :PRINT #2," "
970 REM FETAL AGE OUTPUT
980 IF MA(1) = 0 THEN 1050
990 PRINT #2, TAB(10);"For a BPD of";
1000 PRINT #2, USING "#.#";BPD;
1010 PRINT #2, " cm, the age is ";
1020 PRINT #2, USING "##.#";MA(1);
1030 PRINT #2, " weeks."
1040 PRINT #2," "
1050 IF MA(2) = 0 THEN 1120
1060 PRINT #2, TAB (10);"For a HC of ";
1070 PRINT #2, USING "##.#";HC;
1080 PRINT #2, " cm, the age is ";
1090 PRINT #2, USING "##.#";MA(2);
1100 PRINT #2, "weeks."
1110 PRINT #2," "
1120 IF MA(3) = 0 THEN 1190
1130 PRINT #2, TAB(10);"For a AC of ";
1140 PRINT #2, USING "##.#";AC;
1150 PRINT #2, " cm, the age is ";
```

Box 10-1 BASIC Program to Calculate Fetal Age—cont'd

```
1160 PRINT #2, USING "##.#";MA(3);
1170 PRINT #2, " weeks."
1180 PRINT #2," "
1190 IF MA(4) = 0 THEN 1260
1200 PRINT #2, TAB(10);"For a femur length of ";
1210 PRINT #2, USING "##.#";FL;
1220 PRINT #2, " cm, the age is ";
1230 PRINT #2, USING "##.#";MA(4)
1240 PRINT #2; " weeks."
```

```
1250 PRINT #2," "
1260 CLOSE #2
1270 IF FLAG = 1 THEN GOTO 660
1280 PRINT : PRINT
1290 PRINT "STRIKE ANY KEY TO CONTINUE"
1300 RES$ = INKEY$:IF RES$ = " " THEN 1300
1310 GOTO 660
1320 END
```

Box 10-2 Sample Report Generated by Sample BASIC Program

04-27-2003

PATIENT LAST NAME: JOHNSON
PATIENT FIRST NAME: CATHY
PATIENT ID NUMBER: 888888
PATIENT AGE: 26
REFERRING PHYSICIAN: JONES
RADIOLOGIST: SMITH
SONOGRAPHER: FINLEY
HISTORY: FETAL AGE DETERMINATION

For a BDP of 6 cm, the age is 24.5 weeks
For an HC of 20.1 cm, the age is 22.3 weeks
For an AC of 19.8 cm, the age is 24.5 weeks
For a femoral length of 3.8 cm, the age is 22.5 weeks

■ **Table 10-3** Contents of Data File

Record No.	Patient	ID No.	HC (cm)	AC (cm)	Date
1	C. Smith	123456	10.8	9.2	10/05/02
2	P. Jones	111111	12.8	10.6	01/02/03
3	C. Smith	123456	20	17.3	11/25/02
4	A. Adams	222222	15	13	02/10/03
5	P. Jones	111111	20.9	19.6	02/19/02
6	C. Smith	123456	27.3	25	02/01/03
7	P. Smith	333333	17	14.7	02/15/03

HC, Head circumference; *AC*, abdominal circumference.

■ **Table 10-4** Evaluation of Growth Rate*

Record No.	HC (cm)	AC (cm)	Date	Fetal Age[†] (weeks)
1	10.8	9.2	10/05/02	15.2
3	20	17.3	11/25/02	22.5
6	27.3	25	02/01/03	32.1

*Information from database pertaining to C. Smith.
[†]Fetal age established by examination on 10/05/02.

programs or database application packages to manipulate the information contained in the data files.

Integration of the most recent data with previous data contained in the files to present a comprehensive picture makes this an extremely effective technique. Intrauterine growth retardation is assessed by performing multiple examinations in which the head circumference and abdominal circumference are measured over a period of several weeks. Because the results from each examination are stored in a database management system, the computer can rapidly incorporate the most recent results with previous measurements to generate growth curves. The age determined by the first ultrasound examination now becomes the basis for the age determination on subsequent examination dates, and the rate of growth is evaluated easily.

A data file containing measured values for the head and abdominal circumferences for several examinations is shown in Table 10-3. Each record holds the results from one examination. For simplicity, only seven records are listed; in practice, the number of records can be several thousand. In addition, although only head circumference and abdominal circumference are included, the data associated with each record could be extended to contain multiple parameters. On command, the computer is able to examine the records in the data file to identify entries related to a search parameter (e.g., ID number). A request for information pertaining to C. Smith, ID number 123456, would result in record numbers 1, 3, and 6 being selected, as illustrated in Table 10-4. The first examination, conducted on October 5, 2002, establishes the fetal age as 15.2 weeks. This determination is used to project the fetal age for subsequent examinations conducted on November 25, 2002, and February 1, 2003, as 22.5 weeks and 32.1 weeks. An evaluation of both head circumference and abdominal circumference as a function of fetal age can now be performed to determine whether the rate of growth is within normal limits. For this fetus the head circumference increased from 10.8 cm at 15.2 weeks to 20 cm at 22.5 weeks and finally to 27.3 cm at 32.1 weeks. These values can be compared to several published studies that have shown normal growth curves.

SUMMARY

Digital manipulation of images has assumed a major role in ultrasound imaging. The digitization of scan data provides the advantage of quantitative manipulation and analysis of echo data in very rapid fashion. Many manufacturers have incorporated calculation options (e.g., fetal age based on measured parameters), as well as an array of preprocessing and postprocessing features into their scanners. The amount of information available from computerized ultrasound scanning has increased dramatically. The flexibility of user-selectable processing protocols further complicates the practice of sonography. Processing of information and images in a time-efficient manner to a form readily presentable for interpretation is the responsibility of the sonographer. Consequently, sonographers must acquire a fundamental knowledge of digital processing techniques.

REVIEW QUESTIONS

1. The processing technique to emphasize a change in signal level across an interface is called _____.
2. A magnification technique that is applied during data collection to restrict the field of view and enhance spatial detail is called _____.
3. How many different shades of gray may be represented if brightness levels are coded using 5 bits?
4. Which postprocessing technique is associated with a redistribution of gray scale to emphasize the difference in pixel values over a narrow range?
5. The postprocessing technique of frame averaging is applied to image data to reduce _____.
6. Which signal processing technique reduces the dynamic range?
7. Which digital filtering technique reduces noise in the filtered image?

BIBLIOGRAPHY

Hadlock FP et al: Fetal head circumference: relation to menstrual age, *AJR Am J Roentgenol* 138:649-653, 1982.

Hedrick WR, Hykes DL: Image and signal processing in diagnostic ultrasound imaging, *J Diagn Med Sonogr* 5:231-239, 1989.

Jeanty P: A simple reporting system for obstetrical ultrasonography, *J Ultrasound Med* 4:591-593, 1985.

Marateck SL: *BASIC,* ed 2, New York, 1982, Academic Press.

Ott WJ: The design and implementation of a computer-based ultrasound data system, *J Ultrasound Med* 5:25-32, 1986.

Pye SD, Wild SR, McDicken WN: Adaptive time gain compensation for ultrasonic imaging, *Ultrasound Med Biol* 18:205-212, 1992.

Robinson HP, Fleming JE: A critical evaluation of sonar crown–rump length measurements, *Br J Obstet Gynaecol* 82:702-710, 1975.

Whittingham TA: An overview of digital technology in ultrasonic imaging, *Eur Radiol* 9:S307-S311, 1999.

CHAPTER 11

Image Quality

Artifacts	Image contrast
Axial resolution	Lateral resolution
Clutter	Noise
Contrast resolution	Speckle
Geometric distortion	Temporal resolution

Image quality is a combination of many interrelated factors. The parameters that describe it include axial resolution, lateral resolution, sharpness, contrast resolution, artifacts, geometric distortion, noise, and temporal resolution. These parameters are interdependent, and as a consequence, improvement in one to enhance image quality often means another component is degraded. Also related to image quality is the concept of "dose," the amount of energy (power) transmitted into the patient in order to obtain the image. Since the potential for adverse biologic effect does exist, the image should be acquired with the lowest power setting that yields the appropriate diagnostic information.

Axial resolution and lateral resolution have been defined previously. Sharpness describes the ability of the scanner to reproduce tissue boundaries and, consequently, is closely related to spatial resolution. **Contrast resolution** is the minimum difference in signal strengths from adjacent structures that allows the observer to perceive the structures as separate entities. **Artifacts** are structures in the image that do not represent, with fidelity, the objects within the field of view (FOV). (See Chapter 12 for a more complete discussion of image artifacts.) **Geometric distortion** is a parameter describing the lack of adherence to original spatial relationships. Spurious signals, which do not correspond to the echo-induced signal, are generally classified as **noise.** Temporal resolution refers to the ability to accurately observe moving tissue along the path of motion.

AXIAL RESOLUTION

Axial resolution is determined primarily by the spatial pulse length, frequency, and the bandwidth of the transducer (Fig. 11-1). High frequency and broad bandwidth produce short transmission pulses, and the resultant short echo pulses can be faithfully converted into radiofrequency (RF) signals (good axial resolution). If the receiver bandwidth is less than that of the transmitted pulse, then the echo pulse length would be elongated, causing a loss of axial resolution. Generally, axial resolution is fairly constant with depth.

The finite spatial pulse length limits the axial resolution. By increasing transducer frequency or minimizing ringing, it is possible to shorten the spatial pulse length and improve axial resolution. The best possible axial resolution is the spatial pulse length divided by 2 (as discussed in Chapter 5).

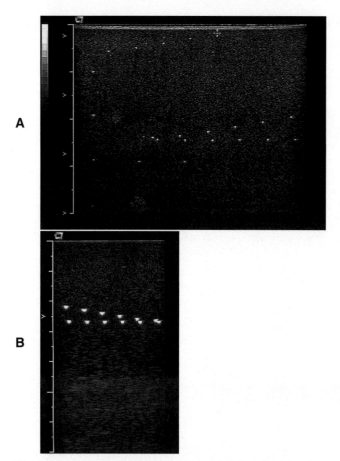

Fig. 11-1 Frequency dependence of axial resolution. Image of a tissue-mimicking phantom obtained with a frequency of **A,** 14 MHz and **B,** 4 MHz.

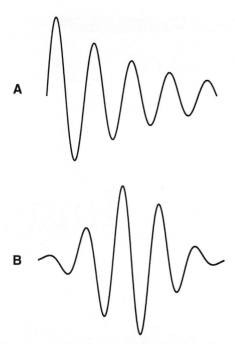

Fig. 11-2 Pulse shaping. **A,** Exponential pulse. **B,** Gaussian pulse.

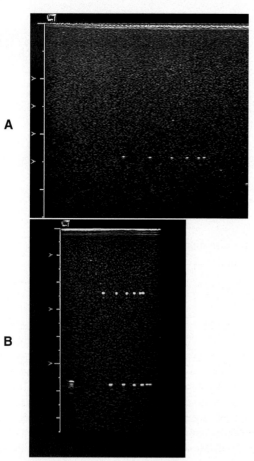

Fig. 11-3 Effect of frequency on lateral resolution. Sonograms of a phantom with nylon rods. **A,** 14 MHz. **B,** 4 MHz. Note that the lateral extent of the rods is greater at lower frequency.

Typical axial resolution of modern ultrasound systems is 0.5 to 2 mm. Objects smaller than this appear to be at least that size in the image (i.e., an object depicted with the incorrect size). Objects spaced closer together than the axial resolution merge together in the image (i.e., two objects appearing as one).

Broad bandwidth transducers require pulse shaping to maintain axial resolution throughout the scan range. As the pulse propagates through tissue, high-frequency components of a broad bandwidth spectrum are attenuated more rapidly than the low-frequency components. Consequently, the frequency composition of the detected echo shifts to lower frequency with a subsequent loss in resolution as the depth of the interface is increased. The Gaussian pulse shaping (Fig. 11-2) minimizes this frequency shift so that axial resolution remains nearly constant at all depths.

LATERAL RESOLUTION

Lateral resolution is improved by increasing the transmitted frequency (Fig. 11-3), aperture (see Fig. 8-23), and scan line density (Fig. 11-4) and by focusing the beam (Fig. 11-5). These parameters are determined by the type of transducer and by the beam former (both transmit and receive modes). The ability to detect small objects improves as the separation between scan lines decreases. The line density is controlled by the number of lines per frame, the width of the FOV, and the scan format. Frequency, aperture, and focusing affect beam width. Line density is limited by the number of elements in a linear array.

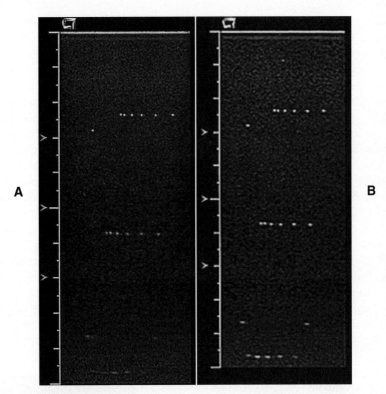

Fig. 11-4 Effect of line density on lateral resolution. Sonograms of a phantom with nylon rods. **A,** High line density. **B,** Reduced line density. Note that the definition of the rods is improved at high line density.

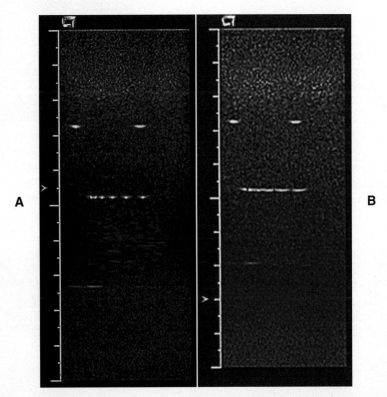

Fig. 11-5 Effect of transmit focusing on lateral resolution. Sonograms of a phantom with nylon rods at a depth of 5 cm. **A,** Transmit focal zone corresponds to the depth of the rods. **B,** Transmit focal zone moved to a different depth. Note that the definition of the rods is improved with focusing.

Consistent lateral resolution is desirable throughout the FOV. Multiple transmit zone focusing, dynamic receive focusing, and other methods to maintain constant beam width throughout the scan plane are necessary. Also, individual pixels and scan lines should not be discernible to the viewer. Interpolation deemphasizes the limited sampling within the FOV.

Unlike axial resolution that remains fairly constant with depth, the lateral resolution, which depends on beam width, changes with depth. For circular single-element crystals, annular arrays, and rectangular arrays, the beam shape is symmetrical (in-plane and out-of-plane dimensions equal) at a given depth. Linear arrays (phased or segmental) produce a beam pattern that is mechanically focused in the elevation direction and electronically focused in the in-plane direction. The in-plane and out-of-plane dimensions of the beam are not symmetrical. The beam width, and thus the lateral resolution, is best within the focal zone of the transducer. Two-dimensional imaging systems can achieve a lateral resolution of 1 to 3 mm if dynamic focusing is used. However, the same problem arises as with axial resolution: A small object appears larger than it really is, and two objects separated by less than the beam width appear as one on the display. The limitation in resolution contributes to an incorrect representation of the size and shape of reflectors and to missing interfaces. Objects as small as 0.5 to 1 mm in diameter can be resolved by modern real-time units.

CONTRAST RESOLUTION

Image contrast is the difference in luminance between regions of the displayed image. Often, the observer must make a decision as to whether or not a lesion (called the target) is present within a generalized background. Mathematically, image contrast is calculated by

11-1

$$C = \frac{B_t - B_b}{0.5\,(B_t + B_b)}$$

where B_t is the target brightness, and B_b is the background brightness. Brightness is difficult to measure, so signal level is often substituted for brightness in Equation 11-1. Low

contrast detectability (low contrast resolution) describes the ability to discern features with subtle differences in signal level. Fig. 11-6 demonstrates that smaller structures can be resolved as the relative signal levels between the target and background are increased.

Image contrast is composed of two components, intrinsic (detection) contrast and displayed contrast. Intrinsic contrast originates from physical differences between the detected interfaces (e.g., acoustic impedance mismatch), acquisition parameters (e.g., beam width, scan sequence, pulse shape), and processing (e.g., compression, edge enhancement). The stored pixel values in image memory represent intrinsic contrast. The displayed contrast translates pixel values to brightness levels on the monitor via the gray-scale map. Brightness also depends on the monitor phosphor and the monitor settings for contrast and brightness. Selection of the gray-scale map allows the operator to alter contrast in the displayed image.

The importance of matching the gray-scale map with the pixel values is illustrated by photographs of the Longaberger building in Newark, Ohio (Fig. 11-7). *Intrinsic contrast in*

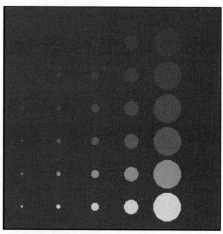

Fig. 11-6 Low contrast resolution. Disks of varying size and intrinsic contrast are displayed on a uniform background. As object size decreases, more intrinsic contrast is needed to detect the object. (Courtesy Mark Rzeszotarski, PhD, MetroHealth Medical Center, Cleveland, Ohio.)

A   B   C

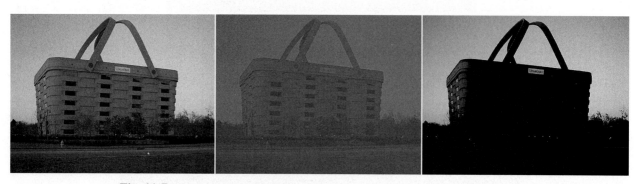

Fig. 11-7 Effect of gray map on image contrast. **A,** Gray scale distributed across all pixel values. **B,** All pixel values mapped to narrow range of gray levels. **C,** Pixel values mapped as either black or white.

the three photographs is unchanged, and the translation of pixel values to brightness levels alters the manner in which the data are displayed. Improper selection of displayed contrast degrades image quality.

Scan Sequence

Echoes originating from the previous transmitted pulse can contribute to the summed output obtained for the current

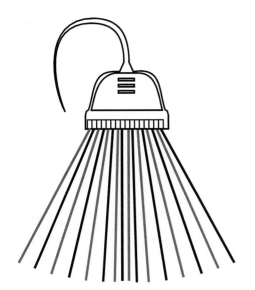

Fig. 11-8 Scan line sequence. Electronic steering allows the scan lines to be acquired in any order. Lines in black are obtained first, and then the lines in gray across the field of view. Interline interference is reduced by separating sequential scan lines.

scan line if it is adjacent to the preceding scan line. This results in a reduction in the signal-to-noise ratio. However, the sequence of sampling for an electronic array is not restricted to consecutive scan lines but rather can be performed in any order (Fig. 11-8). The time delays are adjusted to create large angle variation (linear phased array) or large separation (linear array) between consecutive transmit beams, thus reducing interline interference.

Partial Volume

The finite beam width can create a partial volume artifact related to slice thickness. When the beam includes both a cystic structure (low attenuation with weak echoes) and a solid structure (high attenuation with strong echoes), the scan line through that region is composed of echoes originating from both tissue types (Fig. 11-9). Thus the cyst would be misrepresented in the image as an object with immediate signal level. An accumulation of scan lines of this nature results in fill-in of hypoechogenic structures (Fig. 11-10). If the beam width were small compared with the dimensions of the cyst, then a more accurate portrayal would be possible.

NOISE

The variation in signal level contributed by noise causes brightness fluctuations in the image. A common example of the effect of noise is snow in the television picture received from a distant station (now virtually nonexistent with the advent of cable transmission). Similarly, a scan of a homogeneous object produces an image with variations

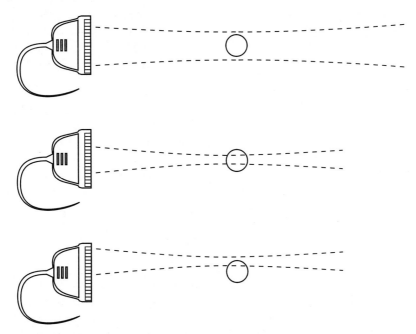

Fig. 11-9 Partial volume effect. **A,** A large beam width extends beyond the boundary of the cyst, allowing echoes from surrounding tissue to contribute to the scan line. **B,** Reducing the beam width limits the sampling to the cyst through the central portion of the cyst. **C,** When sampling occurs at the edge of the cyst, a narrow beam may include echoes from surrounding tissue. This leads to fill-in near the border of the cystic structure in the image.

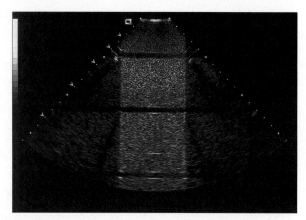

Fig. 11-10 Sonogram of simulated cysts within a tissue-mimicking phantom. Scan plane is along the long axis of the cylindrical structures. The simulated cyst within the elevation focal zone exhibits high contrast. The increased beam width outside the focal zone causes fill-in of the hypoechogenic structure.

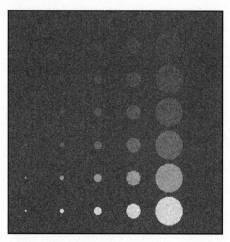

Fig. 11-11 Low contrast resolution in the presence of noise. The introduction of noise to the image in Fig. 11-6 inhibits our ability to discern low-contrast objects. (Courtesy Mark Rzeszotarski, PhD, MetroHealth Medical Center, Cleveland, Ohio.)

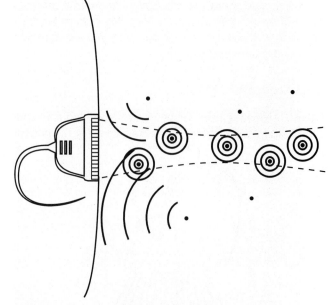

Fig. 11-12 Small reflectors in the beam scatter ultrasonic energy. Some of the energy is redirected toward the transducer by additional scatterers located outside the beam. The interference pattern produced by multiple path reflections is called speckle.

Clutter

The two-dimensional sonogram consists of multiple lines of sight acquired during a finite time interval. The data associated with a particular scan line, however, are not exclusively derived from structures located along that line of sight. Interactions originating outside the main beam path also contribute to the net induced signal. This modulation of scan line data precludes the totally faithful portrayal of anatomic structures.

Clutter is spurious signals arising from echoes induced by ultrasound transmission outside the main beam. Side lobes and grating lobes contribute to clutter. The inability to completely isolate each element to respond to pressure waves independently also creates spurious signals. Since clutter does not correspond to structures along the scan line, image contrast is degraded. Tissue harmonic imaging by tuning reception to twice the transmitted frequency improves image contrast by excluding clutter generated at the transmitted frequency.

Speckle

Numerous, small scattering centers within the volume of tissue interrogated by the ultrasound beam produce multiple scattered echoes over a wide range of angles. Nonspecular reflections within soft tissue, blood, and other fluids scatter ultrasound energy, which ultimately returns toward the transducer along different pathways. Multiple wavefronts from these scattering events strike the transducer simultaneously (Fig. 11-12). The mottled or grainy appearance observed in the image is a result of interference of these numerous scattered echoes detected by the transducer. The

in brightness. A true representation of the scanned material would exhibit uniform brightness throughout the image. Noise masks the signals from weak echoes and inhibits low contrast resolution (Fig. 11-11). A low-noise sonogram is one in which liquid-filled structures exhibit no signal. Noise originates from both electrical and acoustic sources.

The wide dynamic range of returning echoes results in the detection of very low voltage signals. These low signal amplitudes approach the noise level of the electronics, originating primarily from amplifiers and cabling. The pattern of the electronic noise is random but still is expressed as variation in brightness in uniform regions of the image. Methods to reduce random noise include reject control, frame averaging, and adaptive frame averaging.

Acoustic noise is defined as echo-induced signals that do not correspond to structures along the sampling path of the main beam. Clutter and speckle are types of acoustic noise.

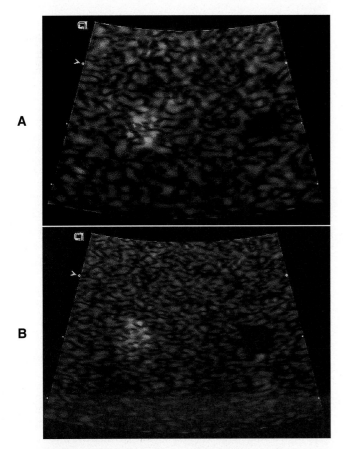

Fig. 11-13 Frequency dependence of speckle pattern. Sonograms of a tissue-mimicking phantom with a stimulated mass and cyst obtained with a frequency of **A,** 4 MHz and **B,** 2 MHz.

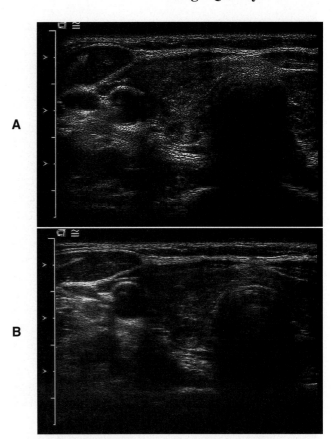

Fig. 11-14 Improvement of low contrast detectability. Sonograms of a thyroid with a nodule. **A,** No frequency compounding. **B,** Frequency compounding.

bright and dark variations in the image are responsible for the name **"speckle."**

Speckle appearance depends on transducer position, beam dimensions, direction of propagation, and frequency. For a particular scan plane the speckle pattern is constant with time. That is, if transducer position and other acquisition parameters are unchanged, then successive images yield the same speckle pattern. Scattering is frequency dependent and, consequently, the speckle pattern is altered if the transducer frequency is changed (Fig. 11-13).

Since speckle is a composite of numerous scattering events, the one-to-one correspondence between image brightness and physical structures is lost. Weak echoes from speckle are superimposed on other returning echoes. When echoes from specular reflectors are present, their signals dominate those from speckle and, consequently, speckle is masked in high-echogenic regions. Speckle is usually associated with regions devoid of strong reflectors (e.g., organ parenchyma).

Speckle Reduction

Speckle inhibits the detection of low contrast structures (i.e., objects with reflective properties similar to the surrounding tissue). Increasing ultrasound intensity does not suppress speckle. Spatial and frequency compounding enhances signals from tissue boundaries while suppressing speckle.

Multiple images of the same anatomic site are obtained under different conditions so that speckle patterns are not correlated. Speckle is partially cancelled out when the multiple images are added together. If the object is registered in the same location for each image, then speckle is reduced without blurring the object.

Frequency compounding acquires two images, each with a different frequency, and then sums these images. Since the speckle pattern is variable with frequency, speckle is diminished (Fig. 11-14). A similar effect is achieved by extended signal processing. The received broadband RF signal is divided into two more-narrow bandwidth subsignals with different center frequencies, which are subsequently processed in parallel before recombining to form one signal.

In spatial compounding, images are obtained with different beam angles and aperture locations and therefore exhibit different speckle patterns. The compound image has reduced speckle depending on the number of images added together and the independence of the sampling process. The improvement in contrast resolution by speckle reduction is illustrated in Fig. 11-15.

ARTIFACTS

An ultrasound image is the portrayal of anatomy probed by an ultrasonic beam. An **artifact** is any structure in that

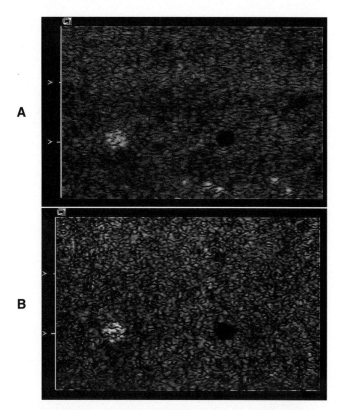

Fig. 11-15 Sonograms of a tissue-equivalent phantom with a stimulated mass and cyst. **A,** No spatial compounding. **B,** Spatial compounding. The borders of the objects are more clearly defined with spatial compounding. Also, the variability of the speckle pattern is reduced with spatial compounding.

image that does not correlate directly with actual tissue. Artifacts assume different forms—including perceived objects in the image that are not actually present, structures that should be represented in the image but are missing, and structures whose locations in the image are misregistered. These errors in acoustic presentation of the scanned subject are usually caused by technical limitations or anatomic factors, but occasionally equipment malfunction creates artifacts.

Miscalibration of ultrasound velocity, broken or deformed crystals, broken or improperly assembled backing or facing materials, faulty monitors, or defective recording devices can corrupt the imaging process. A defective recording device can introduce distortion, misrepresent the contrast scale, and cause a loss of image detail. An effective quality control program should identify malfunctions of the scanner and recording device.

Improper operation of equipment can also play a role in the production of artifacts. This is particularly true with poorly trained or inexperienced personnel. The sonographer may not properly set gain, time gain compensation (TGC), or other controls for sensitivity and uniformity. The wrong area may be scanned (not a true artifact), or the anatomy is scanned too rapidly.

The acoustic properties of tissues and the propagation of ultrasound waves through them can create imaging artifacts. In addition, certain assumptions are necessary for the mapping of returning echoes into a composite picture, and when these are erroneous, artifacts in the image result. A survey of image artifacts in real-time ultrasound is presented in Chapter 12.

GEOMETRIC DISTORTION

Size, shape, and relative positions of objects within the scan plane should be accurately portrayed by corresponding structures in the image. The inaccurate presentation of spatial relationships is called **geometric distortion.** Spatial mapping of the echo-induced signals depends on line density, beam width, number of sampling points, and interpolation during scan conversion. The acquisition parameter of pulse repetition frequency (PRF) and refraction may also affect the registration of the signals.

TEMPORAL RESOLUTION

Sampling must occur at frequent intervals during the movement of an interface to accurately depict the motion. Abrupt changes would be missed or blurred if the sampling rate is not adequate. Thus the frame rate required to visualize a moving object without blurring depends on the speed of the object. **Temporal resolution** describes the ability of a series of several frames acquired sequentially in time to discern the movement of structures.

Since frame rate, line density, and scan range are interdependent, an increase in frame rate is usually accompanied by a reduction in line density. Operator controls on some scanners allow adjustment of the tradeoff between frame rate and lateral resolution. Acquisition techniques such as multiple beam formers, which obtain multiple scan lines per transmitted pulse, enable high frame rates with little loss in lateral resolution.

REAL-TIME SYSTEM DESIGN

The following discussion is based on the published work of P.N.T. Wells and his colleagues. The reader is directed to the Bibliography at the end of this chapter for a more complete analysis.

Imaging performance is ultimately limited by technical considerations and the manner in which ultrasound is propagated through tissue. Physical properties of the tissue of concern include velocity, attenuation, scattering, inhomogeneity, nonlinearity, and motion. Based on the clinical application, system designers attempt to optimize imaging performance within the constraints imposed by these physical properties.

The first consideration is the scan range of the FOV. The time of travel to the maximum depth of penetration and return imposes a limit on the maximum PRF. The PRF establishes the number of lines of sight per second that can be acquired. Each frame consists of a certain number of lines of sight, which, once set, imposes a limit on the maximum frame rate. Recall that the PRF is equal to the product of the frame rate and the number of lines per frame.

Detectability of small objects improves as the separation between scan lines decreases. The line density is controlled by the number of lines per frame, the width of the FOV, and the scan format. The useful line density is restricted to what can be accommodated by the display monitor. Typically the tradeoff between frame rate and line density is balanced by selecting the lowest frame rate compatible with the clinical application so line density can be maximized. At a minimum, line density should be one line per millimeter in the linear format and one line per degree in the sector format. The velocity of ultrasound ultimately limits the lateral resolution and temporal resolution.

Axial resolution improves as frequency is increased. The rate of attenuation, however, increases in direct proportion to the frequency. Once the scanning range is established, the highest frequency compatible with that depth is used. The ability to detect weak echoes from deep-lying structures also depends on noise. Modern scanners can achieve a penetration depth of 17 cm at a frequency of 6 MHz. As a comparison, 10 years ago real-time scanners were capable of a penetration depth equal to 400 wavelengths (corresponding to a depth of 15 cm at 4 MHz).

Backscattering is responsible for the fine texture pattern in soft tissue and blood. This interaction is enhanced at high frequencies, but beyond an upper boundary of frequency, attenuation by intervening tissue decreases the returning echo intensity to an unacceptably low level. Again, the highest frequency compatible with the scanning depth should be used.

Physical properties of tissue are often anisotropic. Inhomogeneity refers to the dependence of velocity and attenuation on the direction of sound wave propagation in tissue. A different rate of travel during the positive-pressure half cycle from that during the negative-pressure half cycle is classified as nonlinear propagation. The sinusoidal waveform is converted to a sawtooth waveform, which experiences more rapid attenuation. Nonlinear propagation is likely to occur at high intensity levels. Increased acoustic output, neglecting safety considerations, does not have unlimited potential to improve sensitivity. Both inhomogeneity and nonlinearity distort the beam pattern, causing a loss in spatial resolution and contrast resolution. However, tissue harmonic imaging has developed as a new imaging technique based on nonlinear propagation.

TISSUE CHARACTERIZATION

Tissue characterization is the identification of tissue type by noninvasive means (e.g., by ultrasonic measurements or imaging). The goal is to obtain a specific pathologic diagnosis rather than the more general recognition that an abnormality exists. Three approaches in real-time imaging are possible. These include sonogram pattern recognition, signal processing of the RF signals, and statistics of the image data. Tissue characterization has been attempted for various organs including liver, spleen, kidney, breast, and eye.

Certain disease states produce an image with distinctive features. The most important clinical application of pattern recognition is the differentiation between cysts and solid masses. Cystic structures are categorized by having smooth, well-defined boundaries, low echogenicity of the liquid contents, no internal echoes, and low attenuation (indicated by signal enhancement distal to the cyst). Distinguishing benign and malignant solid mass lesions is less reliable. High echogenicity of organ parenchyma may be indicative of disease but is nonspecific.

The reflectivity of small particles is frequency dependent. Thus transducer frequency can affect contrast in the real-time image. Lesion detectability is sometimes improved by changing transducer frequency.

Another method assumes that the returning echoes contain information that, if correctly manipulated by signal processing, would indicate tissue parameters. Evaluation of various acoustic properties—including attenuation, speed of sound, and backscatter—has shown that none of these, however, is sufficiently dissimilar among different tissues to allow tissue characterization.

Quantitative analysis of textural features in the sonogram involves image statistics. In the first approach the frequency of pixel values within a region of interest is calculated. This yields the mean, variance, and symmetry of the distribution. The spatial relationship of pixel values can also be assessed. Gradient distribution corresponds to edge detection. Co-occurrence examines signal level combinations in spatially related pairs to determine the smoothness or coarseness of the texture pattern. In fractal feature analysis the two-dimensional image is expanded into the third dimension by assigning height based on each pixel value. Irregular surfaces are created and analyzed with respect to the size of the anatomic structures of interest. The fractal dimensions are evaluated over time for changes corresponding to different pathologic states.

SUMMARY

Axial resolution, lateral resolution, sharpness, contrast resolution, presence of artifacts, geometric distortion, noise, and temporal resolution each contribute to overall image quality. These factors are often interdependent. Adjustment in scan parameters to improve one of these factors causes degradation in another aspect. For example, increased scan line density improves lateral resolution, but more time is required to compose the image. By adjusting scan parameters, the sonographer must optimize image quality based on the study type and desired diagnostic information.

▬▬▬ REVIEW QUESTIONS ▬▬▬

1. Name four descriptors of image quality.
2. What term characterizes differences in brightness level or signal level between target and background?
3. In temporal compounding image noise can be reduced by _____ multiple frames together for display.
4. Acoustic noise is reduced by spatial and _____ compounding.
5. Name several factors that influence image contrast.
6. What is speckle?

BIBLIOGRAPHY

Allison JW et al: Understanding the process of quantitative ultrasonic tissue characterization, *Radiographics* 14:1099-1108, 1994.

Hall TJ et al: Ultrasound contrast-detail analysis: a comparison of low contrast detectability among scanhead designs, *Med Phys* 22:1117-1125, 1995.

Harris RA et al: Ultimate limits in ultrasonic imaging resolution, *Ultrasound Med Biol* 17:547-548, 1991.

Taylor KJW, Wells PNT: Tissue characterization, *Ultrasound Med Biol* 15:421-428, 1989.

Wells PNT, Harris RA, Halliwell M: The envelope that tissue imposes on achievable ultrasonic imaging, *J Ultrasound Med* 11:433-439, 1992.

Wells PNT, Ziskin MC, eds: *New techniques and instrumentation in ultrasonography,* 5, New York, 1980, Churchill Livingstone.

Image Artifacts

KEY TERMS

Comet tail
Defocusing
Enhancement
Ghost image
Mirror image
Misregistration

Partial volume
Reverberation
Shadowing
Velocity error (propagation
    error)

The complexity of ultrasound equipment makes it sometimes difficult to isolate and understand the causes of ultrasonic imaging artifacts. Limitations inherent in the ultrasound sampling process (i.e., the physical properties of ultrasound waves and their interactions with tissues) and improper functioning or operation of equipment can contribute to the presence of artifacts. This chapter describes artifacts that can occur in real-time imaging.

ASSUMPTIONS FOR TWO-DIMENSIONAL ECHO MAPPING

Certain assumptions are necessary for the mapping of returning echoes into a composite picture. When these assumptions are erroneous, artifacts in the image are produced.

- The transmitted wave travels along a straight-line path from the transducer to the object and back to the transducer.
- Attenuation of sound in tissue is uniform along the path.
- Beam dimensions are small in both section thickness and lateral directions.
- All detected echoes originate from the axis of the main beam only.
- All received echoes are derived from the most recently transmitted pulse.
- The ultrasound wave travels at the rate of 1540 m/s in tissue; thus the distance to the interface is determined from the time of flight (1 cm corresponds to 13 µs).
- Each reflector contributes a single echo when interrogated along a single scan line.
- The amplitude of the echo is derived from the object scanned alone and is directly related to the reflective properties of the object.

Violations of these assumptions produce artifacts in the image. The foregoing assumptions are fundamental for image composition purposes. Each scanning mode, however, may also be based on additional assumptions that can lead to artifactual image formation. Technical limitations (temporal pulse length, scan line density, beam width, and pulse repetition frequency [PRF]) restrict the fidelity of the overall imaging process.

TYPES OF IMAGE ARTIFACTS

Some artifacts (e.g., **enhancement** behind a cystic structure and **shadowing** behind a solid structure) aid in diagnosis. Other undesirable artifacts should be identified, because not recognizing them may result in a misdiagnosis. The object's size, shape, and location can be misrepresented. Its brightness on the display may not correspond with the strength of the reflector. The most difficult artifact to recognize is, however, the missing structure.

PARTIAL VOLUME

Finite beam width creates a **partial volume** artifact related to the simultaneous sampling of tissues with different acoustic properties. Recall that each pixel in the image is a depiction of three-dimensional volume encompassed by the ultrasound beam. Partial volume artifacts can occur in either the in-plane direction (lateral) or the out-of-plane direction (slice thickness or elevation).

For circular single-element transducers and annular arrays, the beam shape is symmetrical (lateral and elevation dimensions are equal) at a given depth. Linear arrays (phased or segmental) produce a beam pattern, which is mechanically focused in the elevation direction and electronically focused in the lateral direction. The in-plane and out-of-plane dimensions of the beam are not symmetrical. The beam width is most narrow within the focal zone of the transducer.

An accumulation of scan lines in which the beam width is greater than the lateral dimension of the structure produces fill-in and may lead to misdiagnoses, such as debris in the gallbladder or a mass in the urinary bladder (Fig. 12-1). Improper machine settings (high gain or time gain compensation [TGC]) increase the visibility of this artifact.

ATTENUATION

The most easily recognizable and useful artifacts are related to attenuation of the ultrasound beam as it propagates through tissue. The rate of intensity loss may vary greatly among different types of tissue. *Enhancement and shadowing affect the brightness of the displayed echoes obtained along weakly or strongly attenuated beam paths.*

Cysts and other liquid-filled structures are normally less attenuating and are hypoechoic compared with surrounding soft tissues. The region distal to them is interrogated with a beam having greater intensity than is obtained when the beam travels an equivalent distance in tissue. Thus the region behind a liquid-filled structure produces stronger echoes than are observed from adjacent tissues (Figs. 12-2, 12-3, and 12-4). For this reason the posterior wall of the bladder may appear thicker than the anterior wall.

Shadowing is the opposite effect; that is, calcifications, metal foreign bodies, and some solid masses are more attenuating compared with surrounding soft tissues. The area distal to these structures is interrogated with a beam of

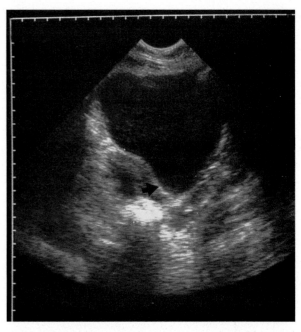

Fig. 12-1 Slice thickness artifact illustrated as debris at the base of the bladder *(arrow).*

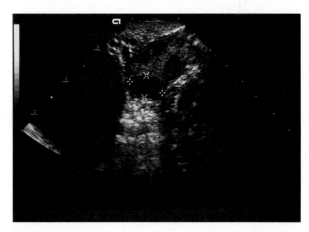

Fig. 12-2 Attenuation artifact. Transvaginal scan of ovarian follicle (designated by the cursors) showing enhancement.

decreased intensity, and thus the displayed signals appear to be reduced in brightness compared with the adjacent tissue (Figs. 12-5, 12-6, and 12-7).

Solid masses are generally more attenuating and often more echoic, demonstrating more internal structural detail than the surrounding soft tissues. The ability of ultrasound imaging to distinguish cystic and solid structures noninvasively has aided in its acceptance. However, hypoechoic masses that produce shadowing rather than enhancement do exist. Hyperechoic cysts must be distinguished from slice-section fill-ins and solid masses. Scanning from different directions and using different planes may aid in the diagnosis. These special cases also indicate the need for a further workup with computed tomography (CT) or magnetic resonance imaging (MRI).

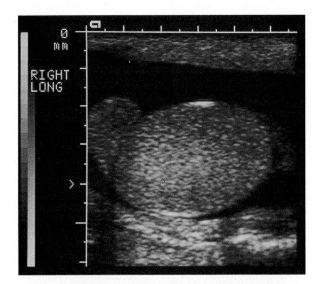

Fig. 12-3 Attenuation artifact. Enhancement distal to fluid surrounding a testicle.

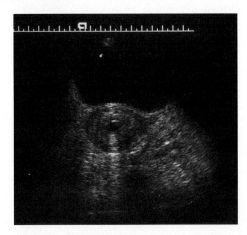

Fig. 12-4 Attenuation artifact. Enhancement distal to nabothian cyst.

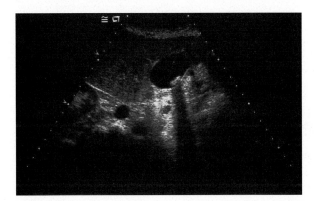

Fig. 12-5 Attenuation artifact. Shadowing behind stones in the gallbladder.

BANDING

Focusing characteristics of the transducer may create a banding artifact (Fig. 12-8), which is a region of increased brightness caused by greater intensity in the focal zone. This is particularly noticeable with real-time systems that have fixed transmit focusing and dynamic receive focusing.

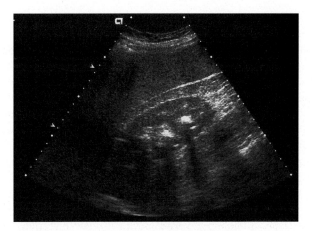

Fig. 12-6 Attenuation artifact. Shadowing distal to kidney stones.

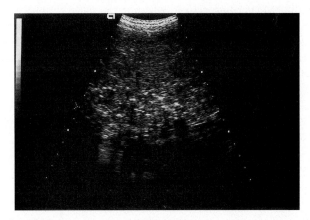

Fig. 12-7 Attenuation artifact. Sonogram of liver with multiple calcifications.

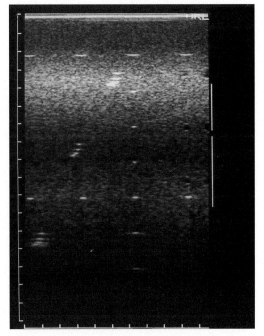

Fig. 12-8 Focal zone banding artifact (bright area on the image).

Images obtained with multiple transmit focal zones are subject to banding when the amplitude of signals from adjacent focal zones are mismatched. Banding can also be created by improper TGC settings.

REVERBERATION

When **reverberations** or multiple reflections from an interface are present, additional echoes from this interface are recorded in the image. The amount of sound energy reflected from an interface depends on the acoustic impedances of the two media. If the impedance mismatch is large (e.g., soft tissue–gas, fat–muscle, or fluid–gas) and the interface is oriented perpendicular to the direction of propagation, reverberations between the interface and the transducer can occur. A strong echo is created at the interface. On return to the transducer, some of its energy is redirected into the patient, where it can undergo a second reflection at the same interface. The second echo returns to the transducer, and the sequence is repeated. Since each succeeding echo is displaced in time, a series of bright bands of decreasing intensity and equidistant from each other is mapped in the image (Fig. 12-9). The fat–muscle interface near the skin surface is often the source of reverberation artifacts. Clinical examples of reverberation artifacts are shown in Figs. 12-10, 12-11, and 12-12.

The loss of intensity is caused by the multiple reflections that take place at the strong reflector and the transducer. A fraction of the incident energy is transmitted through an interface each time one is encountered. Attenuation by the elongated path is balanced by TGC.

Reverberations can also occur between two strong reflectors along the ultrasound beam path; and, similarly, progressively weaker bands are depicted in the image. The spacing between bands is equal to the separation of the reflectors.

Although anatomically related reverberation artifacts are commonly observed, defective equipment and improper technique can also produce them. Occasionally an air bubble will form within the fluid surrounding a mechanical sector crystal or be trapped in a fluid-filled condom encasing an endosonography probe. In either case a strongly reflecting interface located near the transducer inhibits proper sampling of the entire field of view.

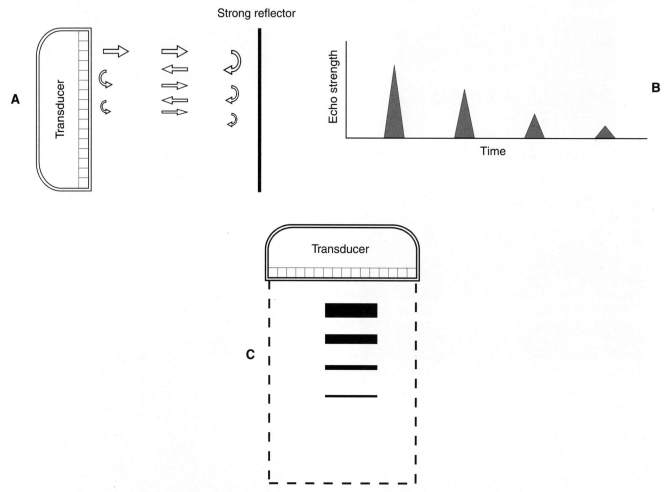

Fig. 12-9 Reverberation. **A,** For a single transmitted pulse, multiple reflections occur between a strong reflector and the transducer. **B,** The echoes along one line of sight are separated equally in time. **C,** Two-dimensional mapping of a reverberation artifact.

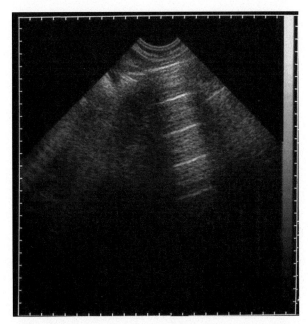

Fig. 12-10 Sonogram of the abdomen in which reverberation artifacts induced by bowel gas are present.

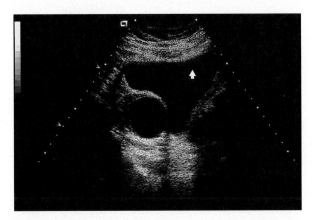

Fig. 12-11 Reverberation artifacts *(arrow)* in the bladder.

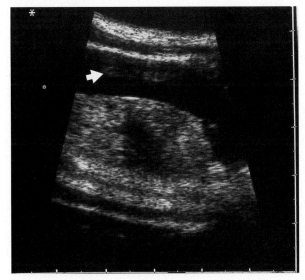

Fig. 12-12 Reverberation artifacts *(arrow)* and fill-in simulating a carotid plaque.

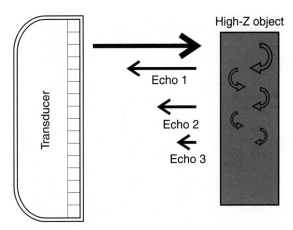

Fig. 12-13 Comet tail artifact. Internal reflections give rise to multiple echoes from an object.

COMET TAIL

Multiple internal reflections within a small but highly reflective object create a series of echoes. Compared with tissue, the object has high or low acoustic impedance. The acoustic impedance mismatch at the boundary of the object forms two highly reflective opposing interfaces that produce short-path reverberations (Fig. 12-13). The time delay between echoes is short, because the sound wave travels the distance across the object and back between echoes. The series of echoes is expressed as multiple small bands, called **comet tails,** in the image. Comet tails are usually seen in relatively echo-free regions. The trail of echoes is usually short, less than 2 cm in length.

Comet tail artifacts typically arise from the near wall or lumen of the gallbladder when crystalline deposits of cholesterol are present (Figs. 12-14 and 12-15). Banding is rarely observed from the deep wall, not because crystals are preferentially formed in the near wall, but because the hyperechoic background distal to the wall masks the comet tail.

The possibility of creating a comet tail is enhanced by the increasing difference in acoustic impedances. The complexity of a comet tail pattern depends on the shape, composition, and size of the object, as well as on the scan orientation and the distance from the transducer face. Metallic objects such as clips, staples, and sutures are susceptible to comet tail artifacts.

RESONANCE

A closely related phenomenon, called a ring-down artifact, occurs when a small gas bubble resonates, resulting in a continuous emission of ultrasound. Discrete banding associated with a comet tail is not seen. The track of ring-down artifacts is extensive, extending from the point of origin throughout the scan range (Figs. 12-16 and 12-17). Ring-down artifacts produce additional echoes in the image and mask other weaker echoes indicative of anatomic structures,

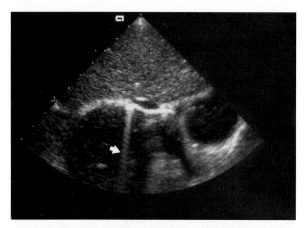

Fig. 12-14 Comet tail artifact *(arrow)* distal to a strong reflector. Note the bands in the comet tail.

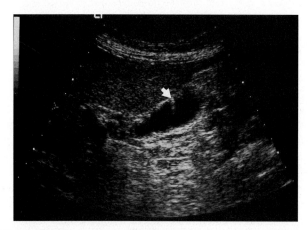

Fig. 12-15 Sonogram of gallbladder with adenomyomatosis showing comet tail artifact *(arrow)*.

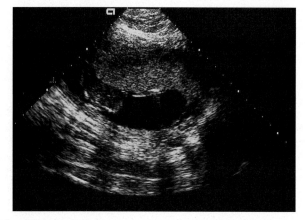

Fig. 12-16 Ring-down artifact from an air bubble introduced during amniocentesis. Note the lack of bands in the ring-down artifact.

MULTIPATH REFLECTIONS

Incorrect axial placement of an interface is caused by multipath reflections. The ultrasound beam strikes an interface at an angle and is subsequently reflected from a second (or third) interface before being reflected to the transducer. The detected echo does not travel in a straight-line path. Specular scatterers reflect the beam at an angle

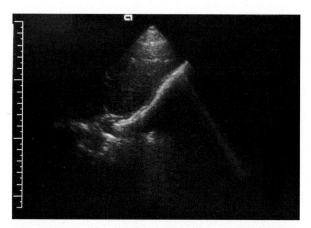

Fig. 12-17 Ring-down artifact caused by air in the stomach.

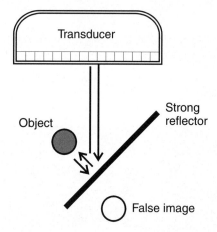

Fig. 12-18 Mirror image artifact. A strong reflector allows sampling of the object along lines of sight in which the sound beam does not follow a straight path.

that may not intercept the transducer, resulting in a "missing" interface in the image. Nonspecular reflectors scatter ultrasound in all directions, and therefore some ultrasonic energy is received from these reflectors. A special case of multipath reflection is the mirror image artifact.

MIRROR IMAGE

Mirror image artifacts are produced when an object is located directly in front of a highly reflective surface at which near-total reflection occurs. This artifact can also occur if the object is offset from a curved strong reflector, or the object and strong reflector are oriented at an angle. Examples of strong reflectors include the diaphragm, pleura, and bowel. Man-made objects placed in the patient can also act as strong reflectors.

Consider the illustrative example in Fig. 12-18. The object is imaged in the usual manner by scanning across it with multiple lines of sight. Along nearby lines (which normally would not interrogate the object), the ultrasound beam is reflected by the strong reflector toward the object. When the beam strikes the object, part of the energy is reflected back to the strong reflector, which then redirects the echo toward the transducer. The additional set of scan

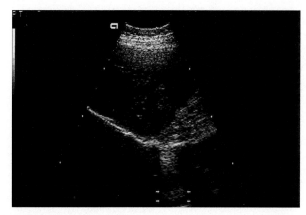

Fig. 12-19 Mirror image artifact of liver with a mass. The diaphragm acts as a strong reflector. The hemangioma is depicted improperly on each side of the diaphragm.

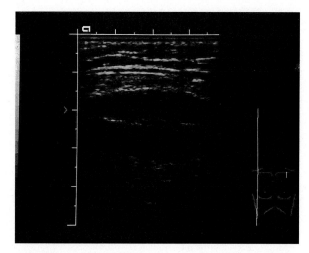

Fig. 12-21 Sonogram showing fluid collection in the left thorax.

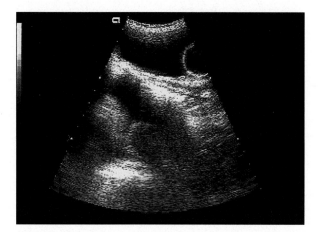

Fig. 12-20 Mirror image artifact of a Foley catheter placed in the bladder.

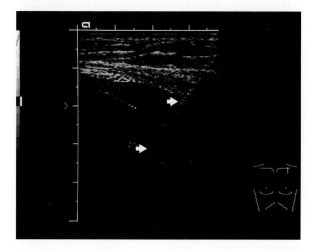

Fig. 12-22 Displacement of strong reflector (pacemaker wire) following needle insertion changes the presentation of the fluid collection. Arrows indicate needle path.

lines containing echoes from the object form a second image of the object located behind the strong reflector. The time required for the sound wave to travel between the strong reflector and the object creates the mirroring effect so that the true image and false image are equidistant, but on opposite sides, from the strong reflector (Figs. 12-19 and 12-20).

Clinical Example

An 85-year-old female presented with left thoracic pain following pacemaker insertion. Ultrasound examination with a 7 MHz linear array demonstrated a relatively large, subcutaneous, fluidlike structure in the anterior left thorax adjacent to the cardiac pacemaker (Fig. 12-21). The presence of a strong reflector and the symmetry of the echo pattern with respect to the strong reflector suggested that the distal portion of the fluid collection in the sonogram was a mirror image artifact.

Needle aspiration yielded a small quantity of blood, indicating that the mass was a hematoma. The introduction of the needle displaced the strong reflector and changed the presentation of the fluidlike structure in the sonogram (Fig. 12-22). The strong reflector was identified as a pacemaker wire.

The fluid structure is imaged in the usual manner by scanning across it with multiple lines of sight. For each line of sight in which the tissue-fluid interface is encountered, the following sequence of interactions occurs. When the ultrasound beam strikes the tissue-fluid interface, part of the energy is reflected back to the transducer (Fig. 12-23, *A*), and part of the energy is transmitted thorough the interface and strikes the pacemaker wire (Figs. 12-23, *B* and 12-23, *C*). The pacemaker wire reflects the sound energy back toward the transducer. At the tissue-fluid interface, part of the energy is transmitted to the transducer (see Fig. 12-23, *B*), and part is redirected toward the strong reflector where once again total reflection occurs, and the echo is then directed toward the transducer (see Fig. 12-23, *C*). Multiple path reflections from the tissue-fluid interface form a second image of the object located behind the strong reflector (Fig. 12-23, *D*). The additional time required for the sound wave to travel back and forth between the pacemaker wire and the tissue-fluid interface creates the mirroring effect so that the true image and false image are equidistant from the pacemaker wire.

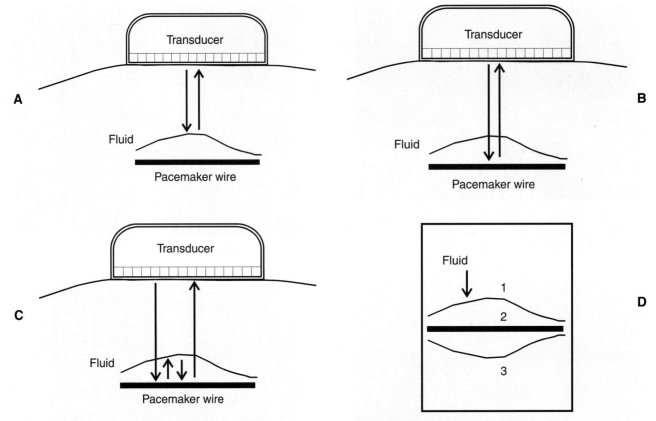

Fig. 12-23 Sampling of the tissue-fluid interface. The arrows are shown left to right to indicate the sequence of events. Only one line of sight is sampled for the events depicted. **A,** Proper placement of the tissue-fluid interface, labeled *1* in **D. B,** Proper placement of the strong reflector, labeled *2* in **D. C,** Improper placement of tissue/fluid interface by multiple path reflections, labeled *3* in **D. D,** Illustration of mirror image artifact.

REFRACTION

Refraction of the ultrasound beam at a boundary between two media with different velocities causes two types of artifacts, **misregistration** and **defocusing.** In addition to improper placement, misregistration may distort size and shape of the object. Defocusing in this connotation describes a loss of multiple beam coherence.

The formation of the image is predicated on the assumption that the ultrasound beam always travels in a straight line through tissue. In Fig. 12-24 an object appears at the wrong location in the image, because the assignment of position is based on the projected straight-line path of the beam, whereas the true location of the object is actually offset from the assumed path. A similar effect caused by the refraction of light is seen when an object under water is viewed from above. If one reaches for the object through the water, the misregistration becomes immediately apparent.

As predicted by Snell's law, the amount of deviation from the expected straight-line path changes with the angle of incidence and with the velocities in the associated media. This does not generally present any difficulty in diagnostic ultrasound, because the velocity of ultrasound in soft tissue is relatively constant. Although refraction is not a major problem in diagnostic ultrasound, under certain conditions the bending of the sound beam can cause artifacts.

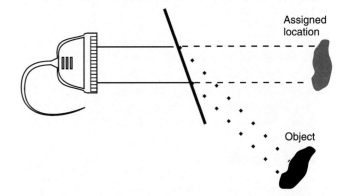

Fig. 12-24 Refraction along the beam path causes the object to be mispositioned in the image.

In Fig. 12-25 the fat layer surrounding the liver bends the beam from the straight-line path (velocity in fat is less than the velocity in soft tissue). This causes the pole of the kidney located laterally to the assumed direction of sampling to be placed incorrectly along the scan line. The kidney is properly represented by other beam paths that do not traverse the liver. Consequently, the kidney appears elongated, since the pole of the kidney is duplicated in the image (Fig. 12-26). This artifact is avoided by scanning with a posterior approach or along a pathway that is completely covered by the liver.

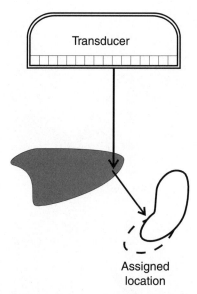

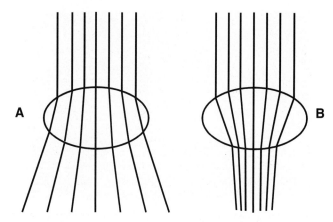

Fig. 12-27 Loss of beam coherence. **A,** Velocity of curved structure is less than surrounding soft tissue. **B,** Velocity of curved structure is greater than surrounding soft tissue.

Fig. 12-25 Refraction. Bending of the sound beam by the liver *(shaded area)* causes the spatial assignment for the pole of the kidney *(dashed line)* to be in error.

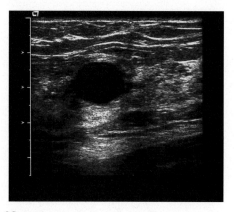

Fig. 12-28 Refraction (defocusing) artifact at the edge of a cystic structure illustrating shadowing.

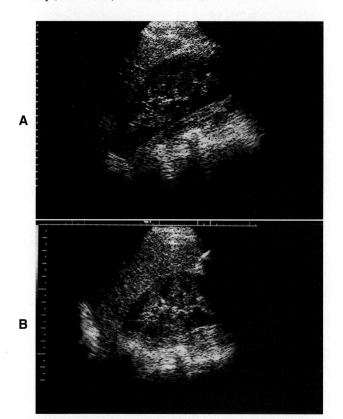

Fig. 12-26 Distortion of kidney size caused by refraction. **A,** Partial coverage by liver. **B,** Complete coverage by liver.

Defocusing

Refraction also produces shadowing at the edges of large (compared with the width of the ultrasound beam), curved structures. The amount of bending varies along the curve surface, resulting in a loss of scan line coherence. After passing through such structures, the beams from multiple scan lines diverge or converge depending on the velocity within the structure (Fig. 12-27). For a cyst the velocity is

typically lower than in the surrounding tissue, and a narrow-angle shadow projection is created (Fig. 12-28). A wide-angle shadow projection occurs when a relatively high-velocity structure, such as bone, is encountered (Fig. 12-29). The shadowing is, in part, caused by the increased attenuation as the beam is bent along the walls of these structures (effectively creating a longer path through the wall).

GHOST IMAGE

A special case of refraction artifact, called the **ghost image,** is caused by altered paths of the sound beam as it passes through the overlying rectus muscles. The rectus muscles (recti abdominis) act as lenses, causing refraction of the ultrasound beam that leads to duplication of a small object distal to the muscles (Fig. 12-30). The multiple sampling of small objects by the redirected sound beams results in the duplication or triplication of these objects. The recognition of this artifact is critical, since a single gestational sac may appear multiple times (Fig. 12-31). One common indication of ghost imaging is when the movement in unison of the displayed fetuses actually turns out to be motion of one mirrored. The ghosting can be removed by scanning from different angles or directions. Changing to an endosonography probe eliminates the artifact.

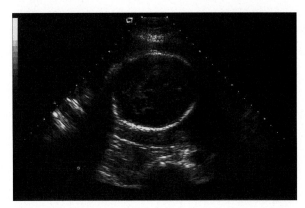

Fig. 12-29 Sonogram of fetal head illustrating the defocusing artifact.

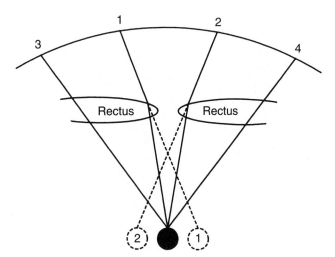

Fig. 12-30 Ghost image artifact. Refraction at the edges of a strong reflector (the recti) causes misplacement of the gestational sac (sampling positions *1* and *2*). At sampling positions 3 and 4 the gestational sac is correctly registered in the image. (Adapted from Buttery B, Davison G: *J Ultrasound Med* 3:49-52, 1984.)

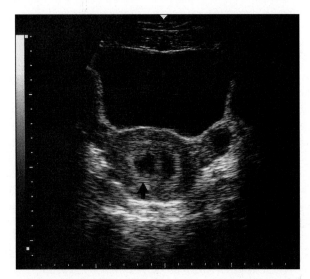

Fig. 12-31 Ghost image artifact in which a single gestational sac *(arrow)* is duplicated in the image.

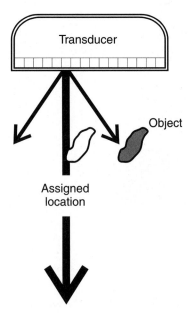

Fig. 12-32 Side lobe artifact. A highly reflective object along the path of a secondary lobe *(small arrows)* produces an echo that is incorrectly assigned a location in the direction of the main beam *(large arrow)*.

SIDE LOBES

Side lobes, which are present with all transducers, result from interference phenomena attributed to nonthickness mode vibrations and multiple source beam formation. The regular periodic spacing of elements within a multiple element array causes one type, the grating lobe. Side lobes are typically of low intensity compared with the main beam (<10% of the main beam intensity) and are generated at various angles with respect to the main beam.

Side lobes and grating lobes induce positioning or range artifacts and false interfaces. These off-axis lobes interrogate structures outside the main beam. If a highly reflective interface is encountered, it will be incorrectly positioned in the image along the path of the main beam (Fig. 12-32). This artifact is often observed during needle biopsy with ultrasound guidance (Fig. 12-33). Gas in the bowel can contribute a side lobe artifact in the scan of the gallbladder (Fig. 12-34). Another example of off-axis lobe artifacts is shown in Fig. 12-35.

The highly reflective structure may lie outside the scan plane and may not be readily identified as a source of additional echoes. In this case reorientation of the scan plane is required. High-frequency linear arrays and curvilinear arrays are most likely to produce off-axis lobe artifacts.

RANGE AMBIGUITY

When the area of interest is limited in depth by high PRFs (e.g., in endosonography, small parts sonography, and echocardiography), structures beyond the indicated range may be depicted in the image. This ambiguity in depth placement occurs, because the time between the transmitted pulse and the detected echo is not measured properly. Real-

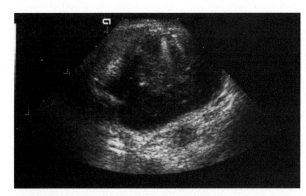

Fig. 12-33 Sonogram of a thyroid during needle biopsy. The misregistered image of the needle is on the left.

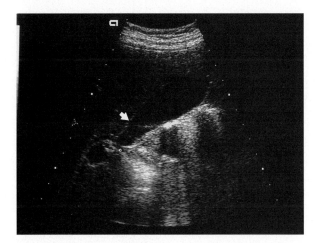

Fig. 12-34 Sonogram of a gallbladder. Gas in the duodenum located outside the scan plane produces a side lobe artifact.

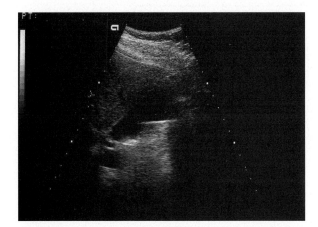

Fig. 12-35 Off-axis lobe artifacts. Sonogram of the pelvis in which structures are misregistered in the anechoic region of the bladder *(arrow)*.

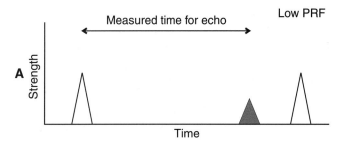

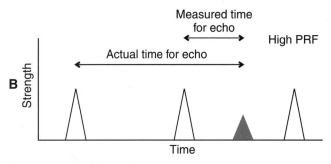

Fig. 12-36 Timing between the transmitted pulse *(clear area)* and the echo *(shaded area)*. **A,** At low pulse repetition frequencies (PRFs) the measured time for the echo is proper. **B,** At high PRFs the time between the most recently transmitted pulse and the echo does not correspond to the actual depth.

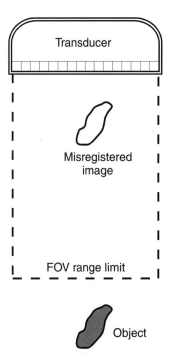

Fig. 12-37 Depth assignment ambiguity. When the range of scanning is limited by a high pulse repetition frequency, deep-lying structures are incorrectly placed near the transducer in the image.

time image formation assumes that all received echoes are formed from the most recent transmitted pulse. Normally a short pulse of ultrasound is sent out from the transducer, and the transducer is silent for a time to listen for returning echoes. All echoes received during this sampling period are assigned a depth based on the time interval between the transmitted pulse and the detected echo. A second pulse is then sent out, and the transducer again is silent to listen for returning echoes. At high PRFs echoes from deep structures interrogated by the first pulse arrive at the transducer after the second pulse has been transmitted. These echoes are interpreted as having originated from the most recent (second) transmitted pulse and are incorrectly placed near the transducer in the image (Figs. 12-36 and 12-37).

VELOCITY ERROR

Registration of interfaces in the image is based on the echo-ranging principle, in which the velocity of ultrasound is assumed to be 1540 m/s. Errors in calibration of the velocity or scanning through tissues (bone, lens of the eye, cartilage, fluid, silicone, and fat) that have different velocities of sound can cause an artifact called a **velocity error,** or **propagation error.** This artifact depends on the actual speed of ultrasound in the medium compared with the calibrated velocity.

Propagation speed error causes a displacement of the interface in the image. If a low acoustic velocity structure is encountered along the scan line path to a more distant object, then the echo is delayed in time, and the object is misrepresented at an increased depth. If a high acoustic velocity structure is encountered along the scan line path to a more distant object, then the elapsed time for echo detection is reduced, and the object is misrepresented at a more shallow depth (Figs. 12-38, 12-39, and 12-40).

Measurements of distances, areas, and volumes are of particular importance in diagnostic ultrasound. For small objects, a large velocity difference is necessary to observe a significant error. For large objects, however, a small deviation in velocity can introduce a large error in distance calculations, leading to the incorrect depth assignment of objects.

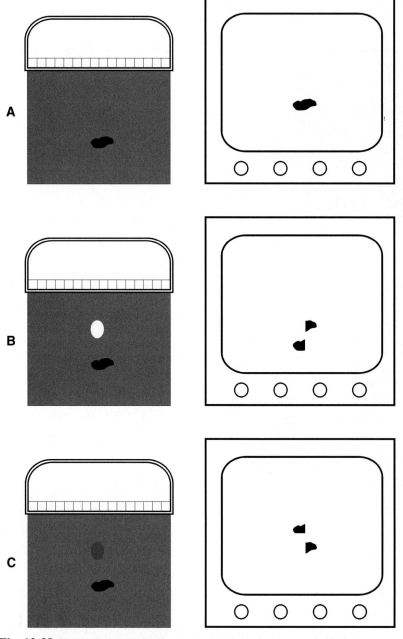

Fig. 12-38 Velocity error. **A,** Uniform velocity along the beam path. **B,** Low velocity structure along the beam path causes the interface to be displaced distal to the true location. **C,** High velocity structure along the beam path causes the interface to be displaced proximal to the true location.

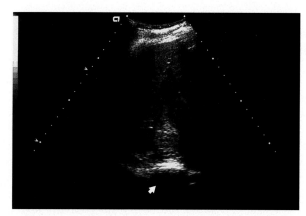

Fig. 12-39 Velocity error artifact. Sonogram of the liver with a hyperechoic mass that causes a disjointed image of the diaphragm *(arrow)*.

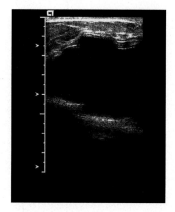

Fig. 12-40 Velocity error artifact. Sonogram of the breast with a silicon implant that causes a disjointed image of the fibrous capsule surrounding the implant.

An interface is displaced toward the transducer, and the size of the object is reduced if the actual speed is greater than the calibrated velocity. For example, consider a 10-cm diameter mass, in which the front face is 5 cm deep in tissue, and the velocity of ultrasound is 2000 m/s. The front interface of the mass is properly located in the image, because the velocity in the overlying tissue is correct; however, the back of the mass is displayed at a depth of 12.7 cm (rather than the actual 15 cm). The calculation is illustrated in Example 12-1.

■ **Example 12-1**

Using $z = ct$, first convert the distance through the 10-cm mass to time (actual distance is 20 cm or 0.2 m because of the 10 cm down and 10 cm back).

$$0.2 \text{ m} = (2000 \text{ m/s}) (t)$$
$$t = \frac{0.2 \text{ m}}{2000 \text{ m/s}}$$
$$t = 1 \times 10^{-4} \text{ s}$$

Convert this time to the depth in tissue, assuming the unit is calibrated for 1540 m/s.

$$z = ct = (1540 \text{ m/s}) (1 \times 10^{-4} \text{ s})$$
$$z = 0.154 \text{ m or } 15.4 \text{ cm}$$

The actual diameter displayed is half this value, or 7.7 cm, rather than the true 10 cm.

Of course, the opposite effect (reflector position depicted farther away from the transducer and the object magnified) occurs if the actual velocity is less than the calibrated velocity. Another scenario that produces similar results is when the actual velocity in tissue is 1540 m/s, but the unit is calibrated for a different value.

DISTANCE MEASUREMENT

The measurement of distance is usually more accurate along the direction of propagation than along the direction perpendicular to the beam path. Axial mapping, even with the changes in velocity for different types of soft tissue, has a misregistration error less than the lateral smearing of objects caused by beam width.

TEMPORAL RESOLUTION

To adequately depict the movement of tissue, sampling must occur at frequent intervals during the motion. Frame rate determines the temporal resolution. Fast-moving structures (e.g., the fetal heart) require high frame rates (50 frames per second). Abdominal imaging may be satisfactory at a frame rate as low as 4 per second. At low frame rates scan data are placed in a buffer that continuously refreshes the display monitor to prevent flicker.

Limits of human visual perception cause the appearance of structural boundaries on real-time images, but the same boundaries disappear on static freeze-frame images.

ENVIRONMENTAL INTERFERENCE

Instrument noise caused by environmental electrical or radiofrequency interference from other electronic devices in the vicinity also can create artifacts in the image. Normally, though not always, a repetitive pattern of stripes or flashes occurs across the face of the display monitor. Although these artifacts usually are easily recognizable, their actual source may be difficult to determine. If severe enough, they can cause the unit to be unusable where they are present. Manufacturers have improved the shielding design to reduce the effects of environmental interference; thus these site-specific problems are not encountered frequently.

SUMMARY

Sonographers and physicians must be aware that artifacts can lead to misdiagnosis. In addition to operator error and machine malfunction, violations of the assumptions with regard to image formation create potential artifacts. Propagation properties of ultrasound in tissues, side lobes, high PRFs, and finite beam size can contribute to the improper

■ **Table 12-1** Classification of Artifacts

Type	Effect	Cause
Partial volume	Fill-in	Beam width extends over different tissue types
Attenuation	Shadowing	Absorption greater than adjacent paths
Attenuation	Enhancement	Absorption less than adjacent paths
Reverberation	Equally spaced banding	Multiple echoes from single reflector
Comet tail	Closely spaced bands	Multiple internal echoes from single reflector
Ring-down	Continuous band extending through field of view	Gas bubble resonance
Mirror image	Structures duplicated	Presence of strong reflector near the object
Side lobe	Misregistration	Strong reflector interrogated by a secondary lobe
Refraction	Misregistration	Bending of the sound waves along the beam path
Refraction (defocusing)	Shadowing	Bending of the sound waves by a curved surface
Range ambiguity	Misregistration	Echo not generated by most recent transmitted pulse
Velocity error	Misregistration	Velocity not constant along beam path

spatial mapping of detected echoes. This can result in missing interfaces, wrongly placed interfaces, interfaces with misrepresented size or shape, interfaces with improper brightness, and false interfaces. A summary of different types of artifacts, including cause and effect, is presented in Table 12-1.

Artifacts are inherent in the imaging process and cannot be totally eliminated. To interpret the study accurately, the diagnostician must be able to recognize image artifacts and, if appropriate, modify the examination accordingly.

■ **REVIEW QUESTIONS** ■

1. What assumptions are necessary for the spatial mapping of detected echoes?
2. Lateral displacement of a single object in the image from its true position is most likely caused by _____.
3. Name three types of artifacts that are associated with multiple reflections along the beam path.
4. Depth range ambiguity is caused by high _____.
5. The _____ artifact produces a true image and false image of the object equidistant from a strongly reflective interface.
6. Propagation speed errors are caused by improper velocity calibration of equipment and when the _____ is different than calibration velocity.
7. Assume that the front of a cystic structure rests 3 cm from the face of the transducer and is 10 cm in diameter. If the

velocity of ultrasound in the cyst is 1000 m/s, what is the actual size of the displayed cyst? Assume the calibration velocity is 1540 m/s.
8. Referring to Question 7, the position of _____ interface would be properly represented in the image.

■ **BIBLIOGRAPHY** ■

Avruch L, Cooperberg PL: The ring-down artifact, *J Ultrasound Med* 4:21-28, 1985.

Buttery B, Davison G: The ghost artifact, *J Ultrasound Med* 3:49-52, 1984.

Hedrick WR, Milligan CL: Mirror image artifact produced by cardiac pacemaker, *J Diagn Med Sonogr* 16:26-28, 2000.

Hedrick WR, Peterson CL: Image artifacts in real-time ultrasound, *J Diagn Med Sonogr* 11:300-308, 1995.

Kremkau FW, Taylor KJW: Artifacts in ultrasound imaging: a review, *J Ultrasound Med* 5:227-237, 1986.

Laing FC, Kurtz AB: The importance of ultrasonic side-lobe artifacts, *Radiology* 145:763-768, 1982.

Nilsson A: Artefacts in sonography and Doppler, *Eur Radiol* 11:1308-1315, 2001.

Scanlan KA: Sonographic artifacts and their origins, *AJR Am J Roentgenol* 156:1267-1272, 1991.

Thickman DI et al: Clinical manifestations of the comet tail artifact, *J Ultrasound Med* 2:225-230, 1983.

Ziskin MC et al: The comet tail artifact, *J Ultrasound Med* 1:1-7, 1982.

CHAPTER 13

Hemodynamics

Bernoulli's principle
Eddy flow
Hydrostatic pressure
Inertia loss
Laminar flow
Poiseuille's equation

Pressure difference
Turbulence
Velocity profile
Viscosity
Volume flow rate

Doppler ultrasound detects blood flow in vessels. Flow patterns in normal vessels are extremely complex and vary with anatomic location, time within the heart cycle, and exercise. Pathologic conditions create even more diversity in flow patterns. The basic concepts of hemodynamics are introduced here, before Doppler physics and instrumentation are discussed in Chapter 14.

Hemodynamics is the study of the physical principles of blood circulation. Blood is a viscous fluid consisting of cells and plasma. **Viscosity** is the physical parameter that characterizes a fluid's ability to resist a change in its shape. For a viscous fluid to be deformed, strong intermolecular attractions must be overcome. When pressure is applied to blood in a vessel, the blood is propelled through the vessel by a pressure drop along its path. Resistance to flow depends on the viscosity of the blood and the radius of the vessel lumen. Frictional forces caused by the viscosity of the blood produce variations in velocity across the vessel lumen.

The major cellular component of blood is the erythrocyte or red blood cell (RBC). Normal RBCs are biconcave disks with a diameter of approximately 7 μm and a thickness ranging from 2 μm at the edge to 1 μm in the center. The viscosity of blood at normal hematocrit is 0.03 poise or dynes-seconds per cm^2, a value approximately four times the viscosity of water. With an increased concentration of RBCs, the viscosity becomes greater.

VELOCITY PROFILE

The velocity of blood movement is not uniform across the vessel lumen. When a fluid moves through a long, smooth cylindrical tube at a steady rate, concentric layers of fluid flow are formed within the tube. Each layer remains a fixed distance from the tube wall and does not mix with adjacent layers. Friction between the layers alters the velocity. The velocity is not the same in every layer but progressively increases as the distance from the wall increases. The distribution of flow velocities into layers is called **laminar flow.** Blood often exhibits laminar flow in vessels that are straight and smooth.

Viscous friction between blood and vessel wall causes the lowest velocities to occur along the wall. The highest velocities are in the central portion of the vessel. Fig. 13-1

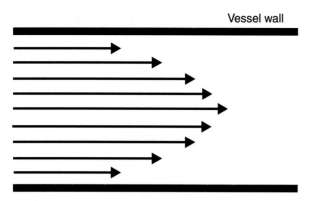

Vessel wall

Fig. 13-1 Velocity profile of blood exhibiting laminar flow in a vessel.

depicts the velocity as a function of position through the cross section of a vessel with laminar flow. If the velocity distribution exhibits a wall distance–squared dependence, the **velocity profile** is described as parabolic. For a parabolic velocity profile the average velocity throughout the lumen is equal to half the maximum velocity.

PRESSURE/FLOW RELATIONSHIP

Poiseuille's Equation

Volume flow rate (Q) is the quantity of blood moving through the vessel per unit of time, usually expressed in cubic centimeters per second. The viscosity of the fluid, the geometry of the vessel, and the pressure influence the volume flow rate. **Poiseuille's equation** predicts volume flow rate in a cylindrical vessel:

13-1

$$Q = \frac{\pi p r^4}{8 \, l\eta}$$

where l is the length of the vessel, η the viscosity, p the **pressure difference** between the ends of the vessel, r the radius of the vessel, and π a constant (value 3.14). Typically the lengths of vessels in the cardiovascular system do not vary. As flow rate slows, the stronger cell-to-cell and cell-to-protein adhesion causes the viscosity of blood to increase. Flow is regulated primarily by changes in the pressure difference or radius. The dependence of flow on the fourth power of the radius makes small vessels highly resistant to flow. For a small lumen with a radius less than 1 mm, blood no longer acts as a liquid, and Poiseuille's equation is not applicable.

Blood pressure is usually measured in millimeters of mercury (mm Hg). The units for pressure in the centimeter-gram-second (CGS) and meter-kilogram-second (MKS) systems are dynes/cm^2 and newtons/m^2, respectively. The conversion factors between these pressure units are

$$1 \text{ mm Hg} = 1333 \text{ dynes/cm}^2$$
$$1 \text{ mm Hg} = 133.3 \text{ newtons/m}^2$$

The unit of viscosity is the poise, which equals force times distance divided by the product of area and velocity. In the CGS system, poise is equivalent to dynes-s/cm^2.

▪ **Example 13-1**

Calculate the volume flow rate in cm^3/s through a vessel in which the pressure differential is 20 mm Hg (2.67×10^4 dynes/cm^2). The length of the vessel is 10 cm, and the radius of the lumen 0.25 cm. The viscosity of blood is 0.03 poise.

Using Equation 13-1

$$Q = \frac{\pi p r^4}{8 \, l\eta}$$

$$Q = \frac{(3.14)\,(2.67 \times 10^4 \text{ dynes/cm}^2)\,(0.25 \text{ cm})^4}{8(10 \text{ cm})\,(0.03 \text{ poise})}$$

$$Q = 136 \text{ cm}^3/\text{s}$$

Intravascular Pressure

Pressure produced by contraction of the heart, static filling pressure, and **hydrostatic pressure** each contribute to the overall intravascular pressure. Elastic vascular walls allow the lumen to expand and accommodate a higher volume of blood. Filling of the vessel causes additional force, and hence pressure, to be applied to the blood within the vessel by the elastic walls. Just as when a rubber band is stretched it exerts more force in attempting to return to a less distended state, so the elastic walls of a vessel act to exert pressure on the blood. This is called static filling pressure. Static filling pressure is typically much lower (about 7 mm Hg) than hydrostatic pressure and the pressure from heart contractions.

Hydrostatic pressure (p) is generated when a fluid is positioned vertically in a gravitational field. The weight of each overlying layer is transmitted to the bottom layer. More pressure is applied as the height is increased. Hydrostatic pressure is given by

13-2

$$p = -\rho g h$$

where ρ is the density of blood, g the acceleration due to gravity (980 cm/s^2), and h the height of the blood. Since the calculation of hydrostatic pressure yields a relative value, height is expressed as the distance from a reference point.

For the general circulation the right atrium is considered the reference point. Blood at the same elevation as the right atrium has zero hydrostatic pressure. That below the right atrium experiences a positive hydrostatic pressure, and that above the right atrium a negative pressure. Hydrostatic pressure can be large, comparable to the pressure from heart contractions. In an upright man it causes the intravascular pressure in an artery of the ankle to be approximately 90 mm Hg greater than the hydrostatic pressure in the aortic arch.

▪ **Example 13-2**

Calculate the pressure in the ankle when it is located 120 cm below the right atrium. The density of blood is 1.06 g/cm^3.

Using Equation 13-2

$$p = -\rho g h = -(1.06 \text{ g/cm}^3)\,(980 \text{ cm/s}^2)\,(-120 \text{ cm})$$

$$p = 1.25 \times 10^5 \text{ dynes/cm}^2$$

The height has a negative sign to indicate that the ankle is at a lower elevation than the reference point.

Convert the pressure to units of mm Hg:

$$p = \frac{1.25 \times 10^5 \text{ dynes/cm}^2}{1333 \text{ dynes/cm}^2/\text{mm Hg}}$$

$$p = 94 \text{ mm Hg}$$

BERNOULLI'S PRINCIPLE

The movement of blood in the circulation is determined primarily by intravascular pressure. Other factors can influence blood flow, however, even to the extent of causing the blood to move against a pressure gradient. The description of fluid dynamics requires an analysis of fluid energy.

Types of Fluid Energy

Total fluid energy consists of kinetic energy from the blood's moving at a certain velocity, potential energy due to its elevation in a gravitational field, and the work done when pressure (force) is applied to move it. When a nonviscous liquid flows at a steady rate, the total energy content does not change. At any location along the vessel the sum of the work done, the potential energy, and the kinetic energy is the same as that obtained at any other point. The condition mentioned previously is a statement of **Bernoulli's principle.** Mathematically, Bernoulli's equation expresses this energy relationship as

$$p + \rho gh + \tfrac{1}{2}\rho v^2 = \text{Constant} \qquad \textbf{13-3}$$

Some rearrangement of factors has been performed to present this equation in the most common form. It is the fundamental equation of fluid mechanics.

A comparison between any two points can be obtained by rewriting Equation 13-3 as

$$p_1 + \rho gh_1 + \tfrac{1}{2}\rho v_1^2 = p_2 + \rho gh_2 + \tfrac{1}{2}\rho v_2^2 \qquad \textbf{13-4}$$

where the subscripts denote the respective locations.

Energy Conversion

An important consequence of Bernoulli's principle is the conversion of potential energy to kinetic energy or increased pressure. Water at the top of a waterfall certainly gains momentum as it falls to a lower elevation. Potential energy, by virtue of the water's position in a gravitational field, is changed to kinetic energy.

■ **Example 13-3**

A fluid flows through a vertical tube at constant pressure and falls a distance of 10 cm. Velocity at the top of the tube is 20 cm/s. Calculate the velocity at the exit. Assume the total fluid energy is unchanged.

Using Equation 13-4

$$p_1 + \rho gh_1 + \tfrac{1}{2}\rho v_1^2 = p_2 + \rho gh_2 + \tfrac{1}{2}\rho v_2^2$$

Since pressure is constant, $p_1 = p_2$

$$\tfrac{1}{2}v_2^2 = \tfrac{1}{2}v_1^2 + g(h_1 - h_2)$$

$$\tfrac{1}{2}v_2^2 = \tfrac{1}{2}(20 \text{ cm/s})^2 + (980 \text{ cm/s}^2)(10 \text{ cm})$$

$$\tfrac{1}{2}v_2^2 = 10{,}000 \text{ cm}^2/\text{s}^2$$

$$v_2 = 141 \text{ cm/s}$$

■ **Example 13-4**

A fluid flows through an inclined tube at constant velocity and falls a distance of 10 cm. The pressure at the top of the tube is 50 mm Hg. Calculate the pressure at the bottom. Assume the total fluid energy to be unchanged.

Using Equation 13-4

$$p_1 + \rho gh_1 + \tfrac{1}{2}\rho v_1^2 = p_2 + \rho gh_2 + \tfrac{1}{2}\rho v_2^2$$

Since velocity is constant, $v_1 = v_2$

$$p_2 = p_1 + \rho g(h_1 - h_2)$$

$$p_2 = 50 \text{ mm Hg} + \frac{(1.06 \text{ g/cm}^3)(980 \text{ cm/s}^2)(10 \text{ cm})}{1333 \text{ dynes/cm}^2/\text{mm Hg}}$$

$$p_2 = 57.8 \text{ mm Hg}$$

Energy Losses

Equations 13-3 and 13-4 are valid for a frictionless fluid system. Since blood is a viscous fluid, however, energy losses occur as it moves through the circulation. The dissipated energy appears in the form of heat. Equation 13-4 must be modified to include a term for the frictional losses:

$$p_1 + \rho gh_1 + \tfrac{1}{2}\rho v_1^2 = p_2 + \rho gh_2 + \tfrac{1}{2}\rho v_2^2 + \text{Heat} \qquad \textbf{13-5}$$

Kinetic energy depends on the flow velocity squared. A decrease lowers the kinetic energy content—this is described as an **inertia loss.** Since inertia losses are dictated by velocity, they exhibit a strong dependence on luminal size (inversely proportional to the fourth power of the radius). Pulsatile flow, vessel curvature, branching, and vessel dilation can induce a velocity change and cause inertia loss.

The total fluid energy content of blood decreases as it moves through the circulation. Blood ejected into the aorta is at high velocity and high pressure, but on return through the veins it moves more slowly and is at lower pressure. The energy supplied by contractions of the heart is dissipated by frictional losses. An energy gradient is created along the pathway: left ventricle, aorta, arteries, capillaries, veins, and right atrium.

ARTERIAL HEMODYNAMICS

Cardiac Output

The heart rhythmically ejects blood into the aorta. The volume of blood per minute pumped is the cardiac output. The normal cardiac output for a healthy adult man is about 5 liters per minute. Women have, on average, 10% less cardiac output than men of the same body size. Exercise can increase cardiac output five to six times in a well-conditioned athlete.

Arterial Pressure

High but fluctuating arterial pressure is maintained by the pumping heart. Peak pressure, usually about 120 mm Hg, occurs during systole. Each pressure pulse is transmitted along the aorta to more distant vessels. Pressure progressively decreases from the arterial to venous circulation. Pulsatile pressure fluctuations are damped out by the arteries. Fig. 13-2 shows the pressure variations throughout the circulatory system caused by heart contractions.

Large arteries have low frictional losses and provide little resistance to flow. They act as distributors of blood to the remainder of the arterial tree. Flow in them is altered by changes in the peripheral resistance.

Compliance

Arterial vessel walls are strongly elastic, which allows luminal size to increase when additional pressure is applied. As blood is ejected from the heart, the arteries become distended and store large quantities of blood. This property is called compliance. The arteries act as reservoirs that provide continuous flow to peripheral vessels during diastole. The effect of pulsatile action of the heart is diminished by compliant arteries; pressure fluctuations are reduced in magnitude as distance of transmission of the pressure wave is increased.

Pulsatile Flow

Arterial pressure oscillation is a complex combination of several factors, including stroke volume, time course of ventricular ejection, peripheral resistance, and vascular compliance. The pressure fluctuations give rise to pulsatile flow in the arteries. In normal peripheral arteries the flow velocity increases rapidly to a peak during early systole, followed by an end-systolic flow reversal of short duration, and then a resumption of forward flow at lower velocity during diastole (Fig. 13-3).

The changes in velocity within the heart cycle are sometimes characterized by descriptive indices, such as the pulsatility index (PI). Large differences in flow velocity between systole and diastole yield high PI values. Conversely, small differences in flow velocity between systole and diastole yield low PI values.

The velocity pattern is highly variable depending on anatomic location and exercise. Exercise causes vasodilation of lower limb arteries, which decreases the resistance to flow. Antegrade flow is present during both systole and diastole and produces a low pulsatile flow pattern.

Pathologic conditions including obstruction, aneurysm, arteriovenous fistulae, and vasospasm may alter the velocity pattern dramatically. Flow patterns associated with an obstruction are of particular interest and are discussed later in this chapter.

VENOUS HEMODYNAMICS

Venous Function

The major function of veins is to act as a conduit for the flow of blood back to the heart, but the venous system also participates in regulation of the circulation. Veins can

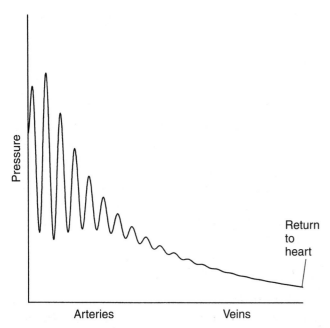

Fig. 13-2 Pressure variations throughout the circulation caused by contractions of the heart.

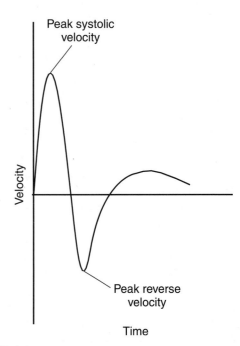

Fig. 13-3 Time course of flow in an artery during one heart cycle.

constrict or enlarge to change peripheral resistance and alter flow. The walls of veins are not as strongly elastic as those of arteries; for a similar increase in pressure a vein can contain 6 to 10 times the volume of blood as an artery of comparable size. Large quantities of blood can be stored in veins until needed (veins also exhibit compliance).

Venous return tends to increase when blood volume is increased, peripheral venous pressure is increased, or small vessels are dilated. The primary regulatory control on cardiac output is the peripheral resistance. As more vessels dilate in the peripheral circulation, resistance is decreased, and cardiac output becomes greater.

Venous Pressure

The pressure pulses in the arteries are damped out before they reach the veins, as illustrated in Fig. 13-2. The constant pressure difference along the vessel tends to give rise to continuous flow. Laminar flow is established at low velocities and the velocity flow profile is parabolic.

When distended, large veins have little resistance to flow. Veins are compressed by sharp angulations over bone, however, as well as by outside atmospheric pressure (on superficial vessels) and by the bulk of abdominal organs. With the compression, resistance is increased, and flow reduced. Veins inside the thorax are normally distended, because the surrounding air pressure is low.

When a person is standing upright, the weight of blood in the vessels creates a hydrostatic pressure that inhibits flow to the heart. Blood tends to accumulate at points of high hydrostatic pressure. The effect is most pronounced the farther it is from the heart, such as in the lower legs and feet. A venous pump counteracts this action of the hydrostatic pressure. Veins contain a series of valves that allow flow only toward the heart. Leg muscular movement compresses the distended veins and propels the blood toward the heart. The valves then block reverse flow as blood accumulates in the next section of the vessel.

Control of Flow

Constriction of the veins increases the peripheral resistance and raises arterial pressure. Also, stored blood in the veins is released to increase the blood volume and enhance venous return. Under conditions of extreme cold, the constriction of superficial vessels reduces blood volume flow to conserve body heat.

Severe arterial obstruction can decrease the flow in veins by inhibiting the transport of blood to the capillary bed. Chronic venous obstruction results in edema. Acute venous obstruction is generally associated with the formation of a thrombus, which can lead to pulmonary embolism.

PEAK VELOCITY

Peak velocity is the maximum velocity within the lumen of the vessel. It varies with anatomic location, being highest in vessels near the heart. Peak velocities tend to decrease distal

to the heart, because the total cross-sectional area of all vessels increases. Table 13-1 lists the normal range of peak velocity for various arteries. Exercise and pathologic conditions can alter these values.

MODIFICATIONS OF VELOCITY PROFILE

Velocity profile can be affected by accelerated flow, curvature of a vessel, branching to smaller vessels, obstruction in a vessel, and diverging cross section. Velocity components across the lumen also exhibit time-dependent behavior during the heart cycle.

Laminar flow in an artery is converted to a more uniform distribution of flow velocities across the lumen when blood is accelerated or propelled through a narrowed opening (Figs. 13-4 and 13-5). This nonlaminar flow is called blunt flow or plug flow and commonly occurs in the thoracic aorta where the blood experiences large accelerations by the pumping heart.

The passageway for blood flow is reduced at an obstruction and when a large artery branches to a small one. The inlet effect describes the conversion from laminar flow to a flat velocity profile at the origin of the small artery. The uniform flow gradually reverts to laminar flow after moving a short distance in the small artery.

Laminar flow entering the bend of a tortuous vessel is skewed; thus high-velocity components occur at the outer

■ **Table 13-1** Peak Velocities in Arteries (m/s)

Artery	Systolic	Reverse
Common femoral	0.9-1.4	0.3-0.5
Superficial femoral	0.7-1.1	0.25-0.45
Popliteal	0.5-0.8	0.2-0.4
Internal carotid	0.6-1	*
External carotid	0.6-1.2	*
Common carotid	0.4-1.2	*

Modified from Polak JF: *Peripheral vascular sonography: a practical guide,* Baltimore, 1992, Williams & Wilkins. (Also based on our clinical observations.)
*Reverse flow is weak or not commonly present.

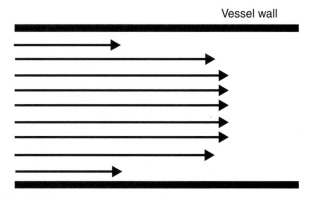

Fig. 13-4 Laminar flow is changed to plug flow when blood undergoes acceleration.

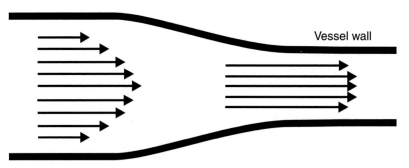

Fig. 13-5 A narrowed lumen alters laminar flow to a flat velocity profile.

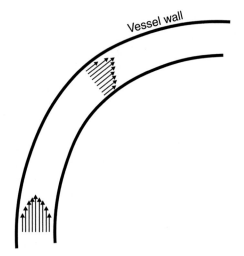

Fig. 13-6 Vessel curvature skews the blood flow velocities so higher velocity components are present at the outer edge of the vessel.

curve of the vessel (Fig. 13-6). Diverging cross section refers to a widening of the lumen; it can create regions with multiple flow patterns including uniform high-velocity flow, stagnant flow, and eddy flow (Fig. 13-7).

EDDY FLOW

Eddy flow is the localized slow rotation of concentric blood layers. The rotation creates regions of reversed flow. A zone of stagnant flow, called flow separation, divides the circular motion of eddy flow from the central region of high-velocity flow. Eddy flow occurs at arterial bifurcations, within vessels undergoing rapid expansion of luminal diameter, and distal to an obstruction.

Regional flow patterns at a bifurcation are extremely complex. The laminar flow incident on the bifurcation is disrupted by the vessel wall. Blood striking the wall is redirected across the vessel lumen, creating flow counter to the prevailing direction. Flow becomes disjointed. Regions of slow and reversed flow are created near the outer vessel wall. Zones of stagnation are also present. A large rock placed in the middle of a gently flowing stream has a similar effect. Water no longer can continue along the projected path but is directed around the rock. Cross currents, flow eddies, and zones of stagnation form as it circumvents the obstacle. The regional flow patterns for the carotid bifurcation are shown in Fig. 13-8.

TURBULENCE

Turbulence is chaotic flow in which the coherence of flow velocities across the vessel lumen is lost. Flow is no longer directed along the length of the vessel but occurs crosswise. Velocity components become varied and fluctuate randomly.

Turbulence is more likely to occur at high velocities within large vessels, distal to an obstruction, along a rough surface, and within the sharp turn of a vessel. Vessels typi-

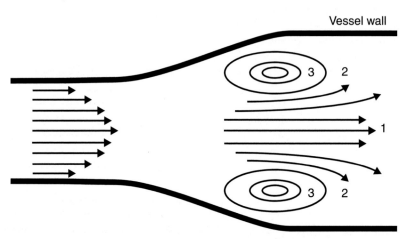

Fig. 13-7 A sudden increase in vessel diameter creates multiple flow patterns. Region 1, uniform high velocity flow; Region 2, stagnant flow; Region 3, eddy flow.

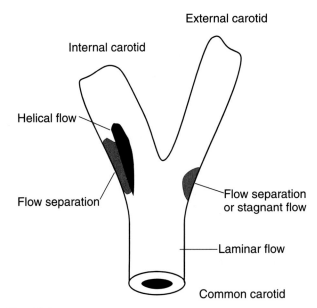

Fig. 13-8 Regional flow patterns at the carotid bifurcation.

cally exhibit laminar flow at normal blood flow velocities. When velocity exceeds a critical threshold, turbulence is induced.

Reynolds' Number

The likelihood of turbulence is expressed in terms of the Reynolds' number (Re):

13-6

$$Re = \frac{\rho v d}{\eta}$$

where v is the velocity (cm/s), ρ is the density of blood (g/cm^3), d the diameter of the vessel (cm), and η the viscosity (poise). Vessels with comparable Reynolds' numbers exhibit similar flow characteristics. A high Re (above 2000) in straight, smooth vessels indicates turbulent blood flow. If the Re is less than 2000, blood is constrained to remain in layers by the viscous forces. Local disturbances are suppressed and do not spread through the vessel to disrupt flow in nearby layers. At branches of large arteries a much lower value for the Re (above 200) may be sufficient to cause turbulent flow. After branching, laminar flow is reestablished in the smooth portion of the vessel.

■ **Example 13-5**

Calculate the Reynolds' number for a 2-cm diameter vessel in which the flow velocity is 80 cm/s.
  Using Equation 13-6

$$Re = \frac{\rho v d}{\eta}$$

where ρ is 1.06 g/cm^3, v is 80 cm/s, d is 2 cm, and η is 0.03 poise.

$$Re = \frac{(1.06 \text{ g/cm}^3)\,(80 \text{ cm/s})\,(2 \text{ cm})}{0.03 \text{ poise}}$$

$$Re = 5653$$

■ **Example 13-6**

Calculate the Reynolds' number for a 0.5-cm diameter vessel in which the flow velocity is 80 cm/s.
  Using Equation 13-6

$$Re = \frac{\rho v d}{\eta}$$

where ρ is 1.06 g/cm^3, v is 80 cm/s, d is 0.5 cm, and η is 0.03 poise.

$$Re = \frac{(1.06 \text{ g/cm}^3)\,(80 \text{ cm/s})\,(0.5 \text{ cm})}{0.03 \text{ poise}}$$

$$Re = 1413$$

The Reynolds' number in small vessels is not likely to be high enough to cause turbulent flow.

OBSTRUCTION

Arterial obstruction is usually in the form of a plaque. Plaques are associated with degenerative changes in the arterial wall accompanied by lipid deposits and, often, calcium deposits as well. When a plaque protrudes into the vessel lumen, flow is disrupted. A high proportion of the artery must be blocked, however, before the flow volume rate is affected.

Certain locations are predisposed to the formation of plaques. Areas of relative stagnation appear more susceptible. A notable site is the carotid bifurcation (in the carotid bulb near the origin of the internal carotid artery).

An obstruction in the flow path reduces the cross-sectional area; thus if volumetric flow rate is to be maintained, flow velocity must increase across the narrowed lumen. The high-velocity jet at the site of a stenosis has relatively uniform velocity components (flat velocity profile).

As the jet of blood exits the stenotic region, the lumen widens to its normal diameter. The expanded area causes the high-velocity jet to slow and to disperse flow velocities. A zone of flow reversal is formed immediately beyond the narrowed lumen. Distal to the stenosis, flow reversal disappears, and a region of flow turbulence develops before laminar flow is reestablished (Fig. 13-9). Five distinct velocity profiles are observed in the vicinity of the stenosis. These velocity profiles are summarized in Table 13-2.

If the narrowing of the lumen is severe, pressure and flow distal to the stenosis are reduced. For iliac, femoral, renal, and carotid arteries, 70% to 90% of the lumen must be occluded before flow will be significantly impaired. This is classified as critical stenosis. When critical stenosis is reached, small additional narrowing of the lumen causes a rapid decrease in flow and pressure distal to the restriction.

The major consideration is the size of the restricted opening, although many other factors influence the disturbed flow pattern. These include length of the narrowed segment, roughness of the endothelial surface, irregularity of the opening, peripheral resistance, volume flow rate, and pressure differential.

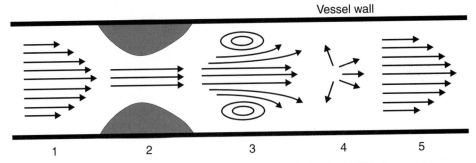

Fig. 13-9 Disruption of flow caused by stenosis *(shaded regions).* Velocity profiles include *(1)* laminar, *(2)* jet, *(3)* flow reversal, *(4)* turbulence, and *(5)* laminar.

■ **Table 13-2** Velocity Profiles in the Vicinity of a Stenosis

Location	Features
Proximal	Laminar
Coincident	Jet, high velocity, uniform velocity components
Immediately distal	Broadened velocity components, reduced peak velocity from jet
Distal	Turbulence
More distal	Laminar

SUMMARY

Arterial and venous flow dynamics is extremely complex. Volume flow rate is regulated primarily by changes in the resistance and pressure differential along the length of a vessel. Friction caused by the viscosity of blood produces velocity variations across the lumen. The velocity profile at a specific location is time dependent and affected by the physical properties of the vessel including curvature, lumen diameter, and branching.

Disease can modify the normal patterns of flow dynamics. For example, severe stenosis creates high-speed jets, eddy currents, and turbulent flow. Volume flow rate may decrease.

An understanding of hemodynamics and a knowledge of normal flow patterns provide the basis for the interpretation of a clinical examination performed with Doppler instrumentation.

REVIEW QUESTIONS

1. What are the features of laminar flow?
2. Volume flow rate through a vessel is regulated primarily by _____ and _____ .
3. Name the type of pressure produced by the position of blood in a gravitational field.
4. Name the fundamental equation of fluid mechanics. What is the principle of this equation?
5. The total fluid energy content decreases as the blood moves through the circulation. What causes this energy loss? The energy is converted into _____ .
6. A decrease in fluid kinetic energy is called an _____ loss.
7. What factors can modify the velocity profile?
8. Characterize the velocity profile of plug flow.
9. What is eddy flow?
10. What are the features of turbulent flow?
11. Calculate the Reynolds' number for a 1.5-cm diameter, straight, smooth vessel in which the flow velocity is 50 cm/s. Is turbulence likely to occur?
12. How is laminar flow altered by a stenosis?

BIBLIOGRAPHY

Burns PN: Hemodynamics. In Taylor KJW, Burns PN, Wells PNT, eds: *Clinical applications of Doppler ultrasound,* New York, 1988, Raven Press.

Carter SA: Hemodynamic considerations in peripheral and cerebrovascular disease. In Zwiebel WJ, ed: *Introduction to vascular ultrasonography,* ed 2, Orlando, Fla, 1986, Grune & Stratton.

Guyton AC: *Textbook of medical physiology,* ed 8, Philadelphia, 1991, WB Saunders.

Hatle L, Angelsen B: *Doppler ultrasound in cardiology: physical principles and clinical applications,* ed 2, Philadelphia, 1985, Lea & Febiger.

Polak JF: *Peripheral vascular sonography: a practical guide,* Baltimore, 1992, Williams & Wilkins.

Sumner DS: Hemodynamics and pathophysiology of venous disease. In Rutherford RB, ed: *Vascular surgery,* ed 2, Philadelphia, 1984, WB Saunders.

CHAPTER 14

Doppler Physics and Instrumentation

Aliasing	Frequency domain processing
Beat frequency	High-pass filter
Doppler angle	Low-pass filter
Doppler effect	Nyquist limit
Doppler shift	Quadrature phase detector

Doppler ultrasound can detect the presence, direction, velocity, and properties of blood flow in vessels. During the past few years Doppler ultrasound has experienced considerable growth in both the number and the diversity of examinations performed. This increase has come about because of the need to evaluate the vascular system noninvasively and the greater sophistication of Doppler instrumentation. Several types of Doppler scanners are available. Although each uses the Doppler principle to detect motion, the manner in which it acquires, processes, and displays signals distinguishes one type of instrument from another. An introduction to continuous wave and pulsed wave Doppler scanners is presented in this chapter.

Doppler instruments often quantify the rate of movement or speed of the moving interfaces within the sound beam. From a physics viewpoint the term *speed* is proper because the magnitude of the movement (a scalar quantity), and not the absolute direction of movement, is of interest. Nevertheless, the term *velocity* has been used traditionally in Doppler ultrasound applications.

DOPPLER EFFECT

The **Doppler effect** is a phenomenon in which an apparent change in the frequency of sound is observed if there is relative motion between the source of the sound and the receiver. An analogy involving waves striking a boat on the water illustrates the Doppler effect. Assume that the wind is blowing at a constant rate from the west and that the waves all have the same distance between peaks (same wavelength). By remaining stationary in the water, the boat encounters the same number of wave crests each second (constant frequency) as are produced by the source. If the boat travels westward, the wave crests come more frequently. A person standing on board sees an increase in the wave frequency, although the waves are actually created at the same rate. If the boat reverses its direction and travels eastward (away from the source of the waves), fewer crests are encountered. The observed frequency decreases. As the boat moves faster in either direction, the difference between the actual and observed frequencies becomes more pronounced. The only circumstance in which the actual and observed frequencies coincide is when the boat is stationary.

DOPPLER SHIFT

A sound source produces a series of concentric pressure wavefronts moving out and away from it. The same effect (in two dimensions) is seen when a stone is dropped into a pond. Concentric rings form, the most peripheral being the oldest and the most central being the newest. The source determines the frequency of the waves, and the medium determines their speed of propagation. The frequency and speed of propagation together define the wavelength (or space between the wavefronts radiating from the source).

A stationary receiver views the same number of pressure waves as are emitted by the stationary source (Fig. 14-1). The motion of the source distorts the pattern of symmetric wavefronts. The observed frequency is influenced by the rate of movement of the source or the receiver either toward or away from the other. More or less pressure waves per unit of time strike the receiver and cause a higher or lower pitch to be heard. This is the Doppler effect and the change in frequency between the transmitted frequency and the received frequency is the **Doppler shift frequency** (often abbreviated as the Doppler shift).

The Doppler effect is experienced in daily life when an ambulance approaches with its siren sounding (the siren produces sound of constant frequency) and the sound appears to increase in pitch. As the ambulance moves past the listener, an apparent decrease in pitch is heard, although the siren is still producing the same constant frequency sound. Police radar systems use microwaves instead of sound waves to monitor the speed of automobiles. The microwaves operate via this same phenomenon.

The difference between transmitted and observed frequencies, or the Doppler shift (Fig. 14-2), depends on how rapidly the sound source, receiver, or both are moving; that is, an increase in the relative velocity between source and receiver causes a greater change in the observed frequency. The Doppler shift is also affected by the velocity of sound in the medium and by the transmitted frequency.

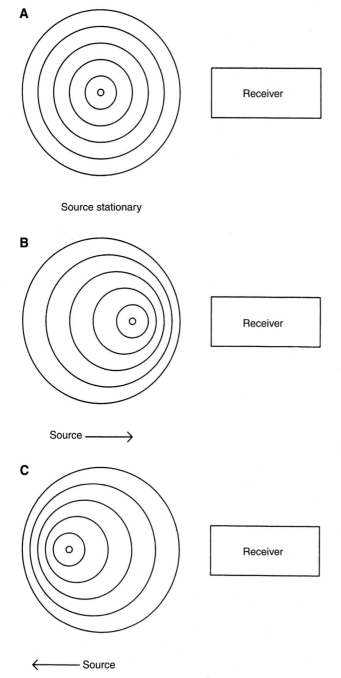

Fig. 14-1 The Doppler effect. **A,** Stationary sound source and receiver, showing a constant observed frequency equal to the frequency of the sound source. **B,** Sound source moving toward the receiver, showing an increase in the observed frequency compared with the actual frequency emitted by the sound source. **C,** Sound source moving away from the receiver, showing a decrease in the observed frequency compared with the actual frequency emitted by the sound source.

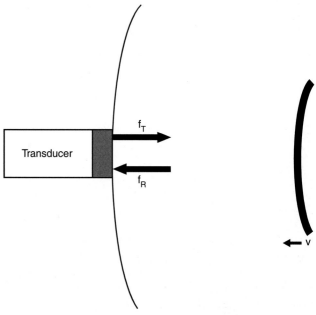

Fig. 14-2 The frequency of a detected echo (f_R) is not the same as the transmitted frequency (f_T) when the reflector is moving toward the transducer. The symbol v indicates the velocity of the interface.

Doppler Shift Equation

The Doppler shift (f_D) produced by scanning an interface moving along the direction of propagation is calculated from the following equation:

14-1

$$f_D = \frac{2\,vf}{c}$$

where c is the velocity of sound in tissue, v the velocity of the interface, and f the frequency of the transducer.

Equation 14-1 is, in reality, an approximation based on the assumption that the speed of the interfaces for biological systems is relatively small (0.5 to 200 cm/s) compared to the velocity of sound in tissue (1540 m/s). As a numerical example, consider an object moving toward a 5 MHz transducer at a velocity of 15 cm/s. The observed frequency of 5,000,974 Hz is 974 Hz above the original transmitted frequency of 5 MHz. The calculation of this frequency shift is as follows:

$$f_D = \frac{2(0.15 \text{ m/s})\,(5 \times 10^6 \text{ Hz})}{1540 \text{ m/s}}$$
$$f_D = 974 \text{ Hz}$$

If the object is moving away from the transducer at 15 cm/s, the observed frequency will be 4,999,026 Hz or 974 Hz below the original transmitted frequency.

Remember: The velocity of the sound wave remains constant. (It is a function of the medium being scanned.) The observed change in frequency occurs because relative motion is present between the source and the detector. The above formula predicts that an increase in velocity of the interface results in a greater Doppler shift. *If the frequency shift can be measured, the velocity of the moving interfaces (e.g., red blood cells in vessels) can be determined.*

Equation 14-1 is valid only if the direction of motion between the sound source and the moving reflector is parallel to the direction of sound wave propagation. If the sound beam is incident at an angle other than 0 degrees with

respect to the motion of the reflecting interface (Fig. 14-3), the above equation must be modified by including the cosine of this insonification angle φ (referred to as the **Doppler angle**):

14-2

$$f_D = \frac{2\,vf \cos\varphi}{c}$$

The combination of v and cos φ gives the component of the velocity along the direction of propagation for the ultrasound beam. If the Doppler angle is increased from 0 to 45 degrees, the Doppler shift is found to be 689 Hz instead of the 974 Hz obtained for parallel incidence (974 Hz × cos 45 degrees = 974 Hz × 0.707 = 689 Hz). For a given reflector velocity the detected Doppler shift decreases as the Doppler angle is increased. Doppler shifts as a function of transducer frequency, reflector velocity, and Doppler angle are listed in Table 14-1.

■ **Table 14-1** Dependence of Doppler Shift on Transducer Frequency, Velocity of the Moving Reflector, and Doppler Angle

Doppler Shift (kHz)	Frequency (MHz)	Velocity (cm/s)	Doppler Angle (Degrees)
260	2	10	0
225	2	10	30
184	2	10	45
130	2	10	60
649	2	25	0
562	2	25	30
459	2	25	45
325	2	25	60
2597	2	100	0
2250	2	100	30
1837	2	100	45
1299	2	100	60
649	5	10	0
562	5	10	30
459	5	10	45
325	5	10	60
1623	5	25	0
1406	5	25	30
1148	5	25	45
812	5	25	60
6494	5	100	0
5624	5	100	30
4592	5	100	45
3248	5	100	60
974	7.5	10	0
844	7.5	10	30
689	7.5	10	45
487	7.5	10	60
2435	7.5	25	0
2109	7.5	25	30
1722	7.5	25	45
1218	7.5	25	60
9740	7.5	100	0
8436	7.5	100	30
6888	7.5	100	45
4872	7.5	100	60

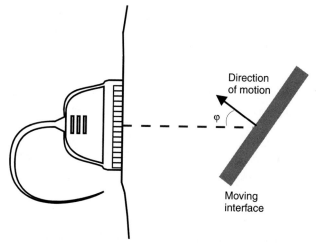

Fig. 14-3 Motion of an interface not parallel with the direction of travel of the sound beam. The angle φ is used in the Doppler shift equation.

■ Example 14-1

Calculate the Doppler shift (f_D) produced by scanning an interface moving at a velocity of 50 cm/s if the angle of insonation is 30 degrees. The center frequency of the transducer is 3.5 MHz.

Using Equation 14-2

$$f_D = \frac{2\,vf\cos\varphi}{c}$$

$$f_D = \frac{2\,(50\text{ cm/s})\,(3.5 \times 10^6\text{ Hz})\cos 30°}{154,000\text{ cm/s}}$$

$$f_D = 1968\text{ Hz}$$

Actual determination of the Doppler angle may be difficult. Minimum shift should occur at a 90-degree angle of incidence, because the cosine of 90 degrees is 0. In practice, the signal never goes to 0, because there is always some portion of the beam that is not perpendicular to the motion as a result of divergence.

Velocity Determination

The velocity of a moving interface is calculated from measurements of the Doppler shift and Doppler angle by rearranging Equation 14-2.

14-3

$$v = \frac{c\,f_D}{2\,f\cos\varphi}$$

The absolute determination of reflector velocity requires that the Doppler angle be included in this calculation. Ignoring the contribution of the Doppler angle causes an underestimation of the true velocity.

■ Example 14-2

Calculate the velocity (v) of a moving reflector if a Doppler shift of 1000 Hz is observed. The angle of insonation is 60 degrees. The center frequency of the transducer is 5 MHz.

Using Equation 14-3

$$v = \frac{c\,f_D}{2\,f\cos\varphi}$$

$$v = \frac{(154,000\text{ cm/s})\,(1000\text{ Hz})}{2\,(5 \times 10^6\text{ Hz})\cos 60°}$$

$$v = 31\text{ cm/s}$$

Uncertainty in measuring the Doppler angle, particularly at large angles, introduces error in the velocity computation. A 5-degree error for a 70-degree Doppler angle causes the velocity estimation to deviate by 24%. A decrease in the Doppler angle to 40 degrees reduces this deviation to 8% for the same uncertainty of 5 degrees in angle measurement (Table 14-2). A greater uncertainty in the Doppler angle further increases the error in velocity computation. As a general guideline, Doppler signals from superficial blood vessels (e.g., the carotids) should be acquired at angles between 30 and 60 degrees. The lower angular limit is recommended, because total internal reflection occurs at the vessel wall–blood boundary for small angles, and the sound

■ **Table 14-2** Percent Error in Velocity Measurements for a 5-degree Angle Error

True Angle (Degrees)	Percent Error
30	5
40	8
50	10
60	15
70	24
80	50

beam does not reach the moving blood. The higher angular limit avoids large errors in the velocity estimate from inaccuracy in the Doppler angle.

Accurate determination of the Doppler angle is difficult for tortuous vessels that radically change direction. If demonstration of the presence of flow in a vessel is sufficient, however, accurate measurement of the Doppler angle is not required. Most Doppler instruments allow the operator to specify the direction of flow on an image and then automatically calculate the Doppler angle based on beam direction.

Clinical Considerations

Doppler units are designed to extract the Doppler shift(s) from received signals. This change in frequency (as illustrated by the discussion following Equation 14-1) is in the audible range (typically between 200 and 15,000 Hz), which enables audioamplifiers with earphones or loudspeakers to be used as output devices. The display system in this case is very different from the cathode ray tube in A-mode scanners or the scan converter in B-mode scanners. A strip chart recorder may be used to generate a hard copy printout of the Doppler shifts. The frequency spectrum depicting multiple Doppler shifts may also be presented on a video display. The preferred format is to convert the measured Doppler shift to an absolute velocity, which is independent of instrument parameters. Doppler shifts expressed in kilohertz from repeated examinations, different instruments, or various hospitals are not readily comparable unless the transducer frequencies and Doppler angles are given.

For monitoring flow in vessels, red blood cells (RBCs) act as scattering centers. Because the RBC, with a diameter of 7 μm, is much smaller than the wavelength of the sound wave (usually 0.2 to 0.5 mm), Rayleigh scattering occurs. Scattering from many small moving targets creates multiple wavefronts that form a fluctuating interference echo pattern in time and space. This varying echo pattern is responsible for the noiselike appearance of the Doppler signal.

The intensity of the scattered sound is proportional to the number of RBCs and thus indicates the quantity of blood in the sample volume. The nonspecular reflection from RBCs, however, is small compared to echoes produced by soft tissue interfaces. The echo-free appearance of blood-filled structures on B-mode images demonstrates this relatively weak scattering from RBCs. The intensity of the scattered sound is also proportional to the fourth power of the frequency. To produce a strong echo, a high-frequency transducer should be used, but as the frequency is increased, the rate of absorption of the sound beam by the intervening tissues also increases. These two effects must be balanced in Doppler scanning by matching the transducer frequency with the depth of the region of interest. The optimum frequency (f_o) in megahertz for a Doppler examination is given by

14-4

$$f_o = \frac{90}{R \ (mm)}$$

where R is the soft tissue distance to the region of interest in millimeters. In general the optimal Doppler frequency is lower than the frequency used for imaging. For a depth of 60 mm, imaging is optimized at a transducer frequency of 5 MHz, although Equation 14-4 indicates that a frequency of 1.5 MHz is more appropriate for obtaining Doppler information. Doppler probes usually operate in the frequency range of 2 to 10 MHz, because other constraints are placed on the system: a single transducer with dual imaging and Doppler functions, a desired frequency range for Doppler shifts, and the problem of aliasing (discussed later in this chapter). High frequencies, typically 5 to 7 MHz, are employed for peripheral vascular Doppler examinations, whereas examinations of deep-seated vessels are performed at frequencies near 2 MHz.

CONTINUOUS WAVE DOPPLER

Continuous wave (CW) Doppler units use two crystals in the transducer: one to transmit the sound waves of constant frequency continuously and one to receive the reflected echoes continuously (Fig. 14-4). One crystal cannot send and receive at the same time, because an ultrahigh dynamic range receiver circuit would be required to detect the small echo signals superimposed on the transmitting signal. Since the transmitted sound wave is not pulsed, broad bandwidth transducers are not used or even appropriate (wide frequency range yields multiple Doppler shifts for a single

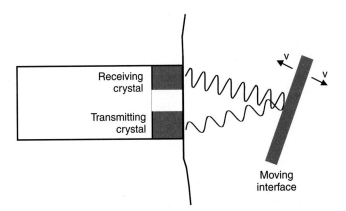

Fig. 14-4 Continuous wave Doppler transducer. One crystal acts as the transmitter, the other as the receiver. The continuous sound wave is reflected from the moving interface.

reflector). A backing layer is not required, but a matching layer improves transmission of ultrasound energy into the patient.

The sampling region is positioned by geometric arrangement of the crystals. The two elements are angled slightly to allow overlap between their respective lines of sight (transmission and reception). For a moving reflector to be detected it must be located along the path of the transmitted beam, and the resulting echo must strike the receiving crystal. The sensitivity or focal volume is defined by the intersection of the ultrasound field and the reception zone. In essence, each transducer is focused to a particular depth. Depending on the clinical application, the sonographer selects a CW transducer with the appropriate operating frequency and depth of focus.

For an operating frequency below 7 MHz, the transducer consists of two D-shaped elements obtained by cutting a piezoelectric disk in half. The elements are placed as close together as possible within the transducer housing but are electrically and mechanically isolated. They are often angled slightly to maximize the overlap between transmitted beam and reflected echoes. Separate rectangular crystals with dimensions on the order of 1 mm are mounted side by side in a high-frequency CW transducer.

Doppler Shift

The transmitted sound wave interacts with various interfaces, some of which are stationary and others moving. A fraction of the sound wave is reflected at the various interfaces. If the interfaces are stationary, the frequency of the reflected sound wave is the same as the transmitted frequency, and consequently no Doppler shift is observed. Moving interfaces initially act as "receivers" of the ultrasound beam and cause the frequency of the reflected beam to shift up or down depending on whether they are moving toward or away from the sound source. The second crystal in the transducer acts as a receiver for the returning echoes. Although the receiving crystal is stationary, another change in frequency occurs, because the moving interfaces are now acting as a sound source. These two shifts in frequency are responsible for factor 2 in the Doppler shift equation.

Beat Frequency

The method used to measure a Doppler shift is based on the principle of wave interference. The reflected wave received from a moving interface varies slightly in frequency from the original transmitted wave because of the Doppler phenomenon. Waves of different frequencies algebraically add together, giving a resulting frequency called the **beat frequency** (Fig. 14-5). The beat frequency corresponds to the Doppler shift.

Fig. 14-6 illustrates the steps necessary to generate a Doppler signal. An oscillator regulates the transmitter to emit a continuous single-frequency sound wave. The returning echo incident on the receiving crystal is converted to a radiofrequency (RF) signal. An RF amplifier increases the

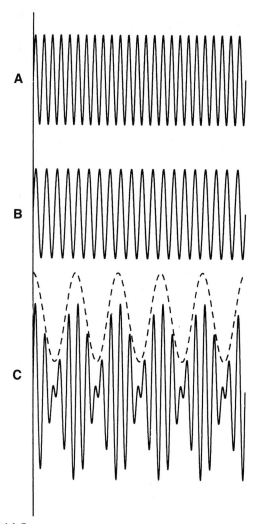

A

B

C

Fig. 14-5 Beat frequency. **A,** Continuous transmitted wave of constant frequency (25 cycles are shown). **B,** Continuous reflected wave of constant frequency (20 cycles are shown). **C,** Addition of the transmitted and received sound waves in **A** and **B** produces a complex waveform. The beat frequency (five cycles are shown) is illustrated as the outer envelope *(dotted line)* of this complex waveform.

RF signal level. The reference signal from the oscillator (mimicking the transmitted wave) is combined with the received signal, which creates a complex resultant wave by wave interference. This wave is demodulated to remove all but the beat frequency. Isolation of the beat frequency forms the Doppler signal, which has a frequency equal to the Doppler shift.

Complex Doppler Signal

The signal processing in Fig. 14-6 yielded a single beat frequency, which denoted reflectors moving at a single, constant velocity. RBCs within a vessel, depending on the flow pattern, have a range of velocities. Each velocity associated with moving reflectors corresponds to a characteristic beat frequency upon echo detection and processing. Multiple beat frequencies representing all detected motion comprise the Doppler signal. This produces a complex

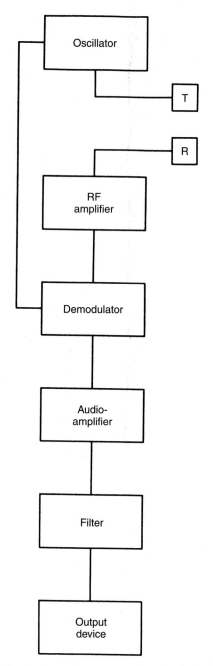

Fig. 14-6 Continuous wave Doppler unit. *T,* Transmitter; *R,* receiver.

Doppler signal by interference of all the Doppler shifts present after demodulation.

Instrument Design

The Doppler signal is sent to an audioamplifier, filtered to remove unwanted components, and routed to a loudspeaker or earphones for audible "display." Large, slow-moving specular reflectors in the body (e.g., vessel walls) generate strong echoes with low-frequency Doppler shifts. The distracting thumping sound produced in the unfiltered output is called "wall thump." High-pass filtering removes these low frequencies, which are normally not of major interest and could mask other signals. A **high-pass filter** accepts all frequencies above a threshold value and rejects all frequencies below the threshold value. The threshold is usually set to remove frequencies below 100 Hz, although on some units the cutoff frequency is adjustable to between 40 and 1000 Hz. Other units automatically set the threshold value based on study type. Because the high-pass filter removes all frequencies below the cutoff value, Doppler shifts from slow-moving RBCs may be eliminated from the final output. The high-pass filter should be set at the lowest possible value to remove wall thump while not distorting the blood-flow components of the Doppler signal.

A **low-pass filter** eliminates high-frequency noise, but its application imposes an upper limit for velocity measurement. The pitch of the audio output corresponds to the frequency shift between the transmitted and received sound waves and indicates the speed of flow within the vessel. As the speed of flow becomes greater, a higher pitch is heard.

CW Doppler has high sensitivity to detect slow flow with small frequency shifts and, further, can discriminate small differences in flow velocity (Fig. 14-7). The CW Doppler unit as described in Fig. 14-6 detects only speed of movement. It must be modified to determine the actual direction of movement (i.e., whether toward or away from the transducer) such as in blood flow. (Various directional methods are discussed later.)

Because the Doppler shift corresponding to motion along the direction of sound propagation within a reception zone is detected, no scanning arm is necessary to denote the position of the transducer. The observed Doppler signal can be extremely complex, however, because the sum of Doppler shifts generated by all the moving interfaces within the focal volume is represented. If the sampling volume includes multiple vessels, the superposition of resulting Doppler shifts becomes especially problematic.

Furthermore, extensive flow volumes (e.g., those encountered in the left ventricle) cannot be accurately assessed with CW Doppler methods. *CW Doppler units operate at low acoustic power levels but provide no depth*

information, and since the time between transmitted sound wave and detected echo is unknown, time gain compensation cannot be applied. Consequently, provided that they are of similar acoustic properties, superficial moving structures produce stronger signals than deep moving structures do. Depth discrimination is achieved by pulsing the transmitted ultrasound wave.

Operator Controls

Most CW Doppler units have operator controls for power, gain, volume, and wall filter (the latter discussed in the previous section). Transmit power control adjusts the intensity of the ultrasound beam transmitted into the patient. Increased intensity enhances sensitivity (detection of low number of RBCs moving with a specific velocity). Receiver gain modifies the amplification of echo-induced signals before demodulation. This also can affect the sensitivity. The volume control for the audio amplifier regulates loudness for Doppler signal output to speakers.

PULSED WAVE DOPPLER

Pulsed wave (PW) Doppler units use the echo-ranging principle to provide quantitative depth information of the Doppler shift. The transducer is electrically stimulated to produce a short burst of ultrasound and then is silent to listen for echoes before another burst is generated. Beat frequency determination requires a longer pulse duration (minimum of four cycles) than is used in B-mode imaging (Fig. 14-8). The necessity for increased pulse duration lies in the desire to detect received frequencies associated with slow flow that are almost the same as the transmitted frequency. Imagine that the sampling was confined to the first four cycles in Fig. 14-7. Certainly, the ability to distinguish small changes compared with the transmitted frequency is reduced as sampling time is decreased.

The received signals are electronically gated for processing so only the echoes that are detected in a narrow time interval after transmission, corresponding to a specific depth, contribute to the Doppler signal. Some authors refer to this scanning method as C-mode. The delay time before the gate is turned on determines the axial location of the sensitive volume; the amount of time the gate is activated establishes the axial length of the sample volume (Fig. 14-9). Gate parameters are selectable by the sonographer; thus the depth and length of the sensitive volume can be adjusted. The sample length is usually between 1 and 15 mm. The remaining dimensions of the sampling volume are dictated by the beam width in the in-plane direction and beam width in elevation direction, which are influenced by the transducer frequency and focusing characteristics.

Multiple echoes from a moving reflector separated in time must be accrued to detect the motion. In order to achieve this, transmitted pulses are repeatedly directed along the same scan line to interrogate the sampling volume. Suppose Ansel Adams took a single stop-action photograph (with an extremely short shutter time) of a car traveling

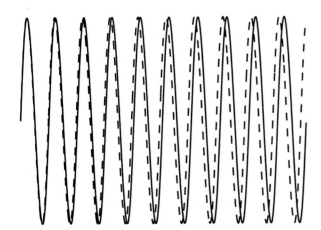

Fig. 14-7 Sensitivity of continuous wave Doppler. The received frequency from a slow-moving reflector *(dotted line)* is only perceived as different from the transmitted frequency *(solid line)* after the buildup of several cycles.

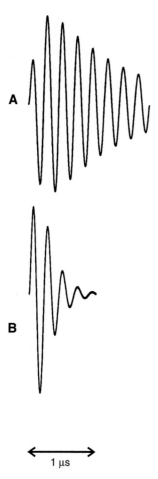

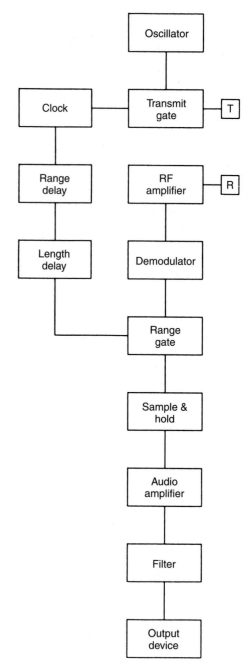

Fig. 14-8 Doppler pulse duration, **A,** compared with real-time pulse duration, **B.**

Fig. 14-10 Pulsed wave Doppler unit.

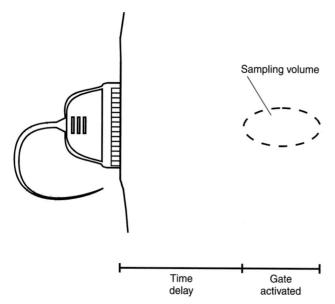

Fig. 14-9 In pulsed wave Doppler, activation of the gate determines the depth and axial length of the sampling volume.

west at 60 miles per hour on Highway 66. If you were shown that photograph, you would be unable to tell if the car was moving or not. And certainly, the direction of travel and speed would be indiscernible. However, if a series of stop-

action photographs were acquired and then shown rapidly one after the other, the motion would be clearly depicted.

Instrument Design

In PW Doppler the basic CW design is modified to accommodate gating and to collect successive processed echoes in a sample-and-hold circuit (Fig. 14-10). The clock functions as a master synchronizer for timing purposes (pulse repetition frequency [PRF] and gating). Some units allow the sonographer to adjust the PRF manually, whereas others vary the PRF automatically in response to the sampling depth. A single gate limits the interrogation to one depth along the line of sight. Doppler shifts can be acquired simultaneously from multiple separate sample volumes along the direction of propagation by incorporating parallel receiver channels, each with a gate set with a different time delay. Multigate PW systems typically contain 6 to 32 gates, with a minimum axial length of 1 mm for each sample volume. No sacrifice is made with respect to PRF or processing time; the parallel receiver channels act independently during each pulse repetition cycle to process the information from designated sampling regions. Headphones and a spectrum analyzer are typical output devices.

Signal Processing

The received echo must be evaluated to determine whether the reflector is moving. This is accomplished by comparing the phase of the echo with a reference signal for which phase is synchronized with the transmitted pulse. Two waves are described as being in phase if their maximum, minimum, and zero points occur concurrently. The echo from a stationary reflector has the same phase as the reference signal, whereas the echo from a moving structure undergoes a phase shift via the Doppler effect. The phase relation between detected echoes and the reference signal is depicted in Fig. 14-11.

The echoes from different reflectors, one moving and the other stationary, are received after different time intervals (time 1 and time 2) following the transmitted pulse. The reference signal has the same frequency and phase as the transmitted pulse but is extended over time so the received signals can be compared with the original transmitted

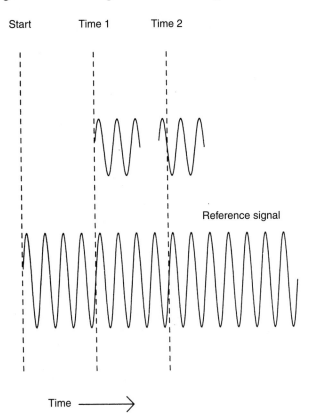

Start　　　Time 1　　　Time 2

Reference signal

Time ⟶

Fig. 14-11 The echo from a stationary reflector received at time 1 is in phase with the reference signal. The echo from a moving reflector received at time 2 is not.

waveform. The dotted lines in Fig. 14-11 place the detected echoes on the same time scale as the reference signal. The phase is unchanged for the stationary reflector, whose echo is received at time 1. The shift in phase at time 2 indicates that the reflector at a specific depth is moving.

Sample and Hold

For a single reflector moving at constant velocity within the sampling volume, a series of echoes from successive transmitted pulses are obtained over time in a sample-and-hold circuit. The depth-specific echo from each transmitted pulse when processed provides one instantaneous value of the Doppler signal. The sample-and-hold circuit assembles the measured values obtained from multiple transmitted pulses to form the beat frequency. In essence, the PRF indicates how often the beat frequency is sampled. Typically, a sequence of 64 to 128 pulses is transmitted along the scan line to interrogate the sample volume. The total observation time is usually 10 ms or less.

A description of the sample-and-hold circuit function follows. Each echo-induced signal is combined with the reference signal (same frequency as the transmitted pulse) to generate one point in the sample-and-hold data set. The relative phase between the echo signal and the reference signal determines the magnitude of the sample-and-hold signal. The magnitude is plotted as a function of time. The time axis is defined by the time during which the sequence of transmission pulses is directed along the line of sight to the sampling volume. Multiple measurements create a pattern from which the beat frequency can be inferred (Fig. 14-12).

The beat pattern is not as well defined as with CW Doppler, because the pulsed echoes are equivalent to sampling the CW signal at discrete intervals (Fig. 14-13). The beat pattern can be more clearly delineated if more pulses per unit time are used, which would require an increase in the PRF. Multiple reflectors moving with a range of velocities within the sample volume would give rise to a complex Doppler signal consisting of many different beat frequencies.

Velocity Detection Limit

At a minimum, two pulses are required per beat cycle to define the beat frequency unambiguously. This creates a very important limitation in PW Doppler scanning. The maximum Doppler shift, $f_D(max)$, that can be detected is related to the sampling rate or PRF:

14-5

$$f_D(max) = \frac{PRF}{2}$$

To measure reflectors moving with high velocity and producing large Doppler shifts, a high PRF is necessary; however, a high PRF limits the depth that can be sampled, because a certain time is required to collect the echoes arising from that depth before the next pulse is sent out. The

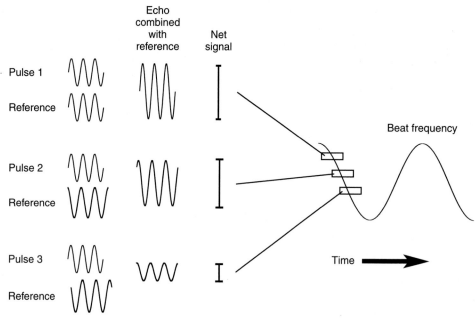

Fig. 14-12 Sample and hold. The echo from a moving reflector within the range gate undergoes a phase shift, which in combination with the reference signal yields the net signal. Multiple echoes are acquired from the same reflector at a time interval equal to the pulse repetition period. Successive echoes from the moving reflector have varying phase shifts. The net signal is reduced in magnitude as the phase shift is increased. The beat frequency is formed by plotting the net signal from the series of echoes as a function of time.

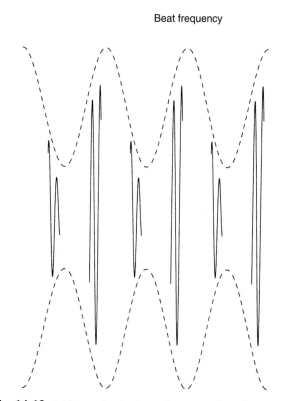

Fig. 14-13 Addition of pulsed sound waves to the reference signal yields the interpreted beat frequency *(dotted line)*.

problem becomes more complex when it is realized that the Doppler shift depends on transducer frequency. Nevertheless, the relation between depth of interest *(R)*, transducer frequency *(f)*, Doppler angle *(φ)*, velocity of sound in tissue *(c)*, and maximum reflector velocity *(V_{max})* is described by a single equation:

14-6

$$V_{max} = \frac{c^2}{8\,fR\cos\varphi}$$

The maximum velocity as a function of depth and transducer frequency for a Doppler angle of 0 degrees is listed in Table 14-3. If the Doppler angle is not 0 degrees, the maximum velocity is increased by the factor $1/\cos\varphi$.

■ **Table 14-3** Dependence of Maximum Velocity Limit on Transducer Frequency and Depth of the Moving Reflector in Pulsed-Wave Doppler

	Maximum Velocity Limit* (cm/s)		
Depth (cm)	2 MHz	5 MHz	10 MHz
1	1480	590	295
5	295	120	60
10	150	60	30
15	100	40	20
20	75	30	15

*The Doppler angle is 0 degrees.

The ramifications from Equation 14-6 are threefold. First, if the depth of interest is increased, the maximum reflector velocity that can be measured is decreased. Second, a low-frequency transducer allows greater velocities to be detected. Third, an increase in Doppler angle extends the maximum velocity limit. These limitations occur, because the motion of the reflector is sampled at discrete intervals and not continuously, as in CW units. Unless low-pass filtering is applied, there is no maximum reflector velocity limit for CW scanners.

The following numerical examples illustrate the maximum velocities measurable in the clinical environment. The maximum PRF for a 10 cm depth is approximately 7700 pulses per second. (A 130 μs time delay is required between transmission of the pulse and the reception of the returning echo.) With a 3.5-MHz transducer and a Doppler angle of 30 degrees, the Doppler shift is limited to 3850 Hz, which corresponds to a maximum velocity for a moving reflector of 98 cm/s.

$$V_{max} = \frac{(154{,}000 \text{ cm/s})^2}{8 \ (3.5 \times 10^6 \text{ Hz}) \ (10 \text{ cm}) \cos 30°}$$
$$V_{max} = 98 \text{ cm/s}$$

By decreasing the transducer frequency to 2 MHz, it is possible to increase the maximum velocity detectable to 171 cm/s. Changing the depth of interest to 15 cm while maintaining the transducer frequency at 2 MHz lowers the measurable maximum velocity to 114 cm/s. Fortunately, these conditions are such that the physiologic velocities of moving structures (except the heart) usually occur within the detectable range of PW Doppler units.

Aliasing

If the sampling rate is not adequate for high-frequency Doppler shifts, artifactual lower-frequency Doppler shifts are displayed. Because beat frequency is sampled intermittently, it must be inferred from the limited data available. When the sampling occurs less than twice during a beat cycle, the data are misinterpreted as being at a lower frequency than the actual beat frequency. The requirement that the sampling rate must be at least twice the maximum frequency present in the Doppler signal is referred to as the Nyquist criterion. One half of the pulse repetition frequency is the **Nyquist limit** as defined by Equation 14-5; Doppler shifts above the Nyquist limit are falsely depicted as low-frequency shifts corresponding to slow-moving reflectors. Imagine that a measurement is taken of the amplitude of the beat frequency at various points and that a new waveform is constructed from this collection of amplitude measurements (Fig. 14-14). The actual beat frequency is misinterpreted as a waveform with a lower frequency, because sampling occurred only five times over four cycles. This is called **aliasing,** and it also is not present in CW units.

The motion picture industry provides a visual example of aliasing. In movies of the old West, a buckboard is often pulled across the prairie by a team of horses. You undoubtedly recall how the wheels on the buckboard appeared to be

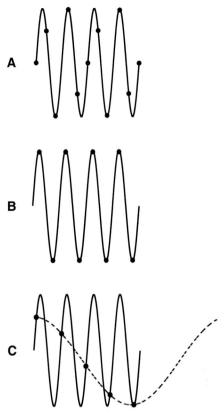

Fig. 14-14 Intermittent sampling of the beat frequency (*solid line*). **A,** Multiple measurements during four cycles allow accurate assessment of the beat frequency. **B,** A minimum of two measurements per cycle also provides accurate interpretation of the beat frequency. **C,** When the sampling rate is not adequate, the true beat frequency (*solid line*) is interpreted incorrectly as a lower frequency (*dotted line*).

going backward, which was visually inconsistent with the movement of other objects depicted in the scene. In making the movie, a series of stop-action photographs was taken and shown one after another to give the appearance of motion. There was a time delay between frames, however, which meant that the recording system was sampling the motion at discrete intervals. If the motion became very rapid, as with the rotating wheel on the buckboard, the sampling could not properly represent the motion. (The spokes of the wheel move too large a distance between successive photographs.) To solve this problem, the time between frames could be decreased (i.e., more photos taken) so the wheel moved a shorter distance between photographs. More frequent sampling allows the recording system to reproduce the motion accurately. Note that in the movie, only objects moving at high velocity were affected by the noncontinuous sampling; the motion of slower-moving objects was correctly reproduced. In ultrasound the boundary for the correct interpretation of object velocity is given by the Nyquist limit, which depends on the PRF.

■ **Example 14-3**

Calculate the minimum PRF necessary to prevent aliasing if the velocity of the moving reflector is 15 cm/s. The angle of insonation is 40 degrees, and the transducer frequency is 2 MHz.

Using Equation 14-2

$$f_D = \frac{2\,vf\cos\varphi}{c}$$

$$f_D = \frac{2\,(15\text{ cm/s})\,(2\times10^6\text{ Hz})\cos40°}{154{,}000\text{ cm/s}}$$

$$f_D = 298\text{ Hz}$$

The minimum PRF is equal to two times the Doppler shift.

$$PRF = 2\,f_D = 2\,(298\text{ Hz}) = 596\text{ Hz}$$

If reflectors are moving at velocities above those imposed by the Nyquist limit, the sonographer has several options to remove the aliasing artifact:

1. An increase in the PRF raises the Nyquist limit, possibly to a level that is sufficient to measure reflector velocity accurately. The maximum PRF is usually set by the pulse transit time to the depth of interest. If a PRF corresponding to this transit time limit does not remove the aliasing artifact, then adjusting the PRF even higher may do so. An ambiguity in sampling location, however, is created by ignoring the transit time limitation. In effect, echoes are now obtained simultaneously from two sampling volumes. Strategic positioning of one sampling location where no flow is present removes the ambiguity.
2. If reverse flow is not of concern, the baseline can be adjusted to devote the entire range of velocity detection to forward flow. This technique doubles the maximum velocity that can be measured without aliasing but assumes that no flow in the opposite direction is present.
3. Examination of Equation 14-6 reveals that the Doppler angle and transducer frequency also affect the Nyquist limit. By increasing the Doppler angle or lowering the transducer frequency, the sonographer can eliminate aliasing.
4. Finally, switching from PW to CW modes enables the fastest motion to be observed without an aliasing artifact (although depth information is then sacrificed in the CW mode).

Pulsed Wave Bandwidth

The transducer in a PW Doppler unit does not produce a single-frequency sound wave. Because the ultrasound beam is on for only a short time, each sound pulse consists of a range of frequencies characterized by the bandwidth. As with imaging transducers, a very short pulse creates a spectral distribution of frequencies with a wide bandwidth. Hence frequencies are already present at transmission that are expected in the returning echoes from moving reflectors. In addition, the multiple frequency components cause frequency variations in the observed Doppler shifts and a reduction in the signal-to-noise ratio (SNR). Decreasing the bandwidth by lengthening the pulse improves the system's ability to detect slow flow (small Doppler shifts) and small differences in flow velocity, but longer spatial pulse length degrades the spatial resolution. PW Doppler units require

pulses that consist of at least four to five cycles. Note that several cycles were required in Fig. 14-7 to observe a difference between the transmitted wave and the received wave. The same principle applies in PW Doppler. The reflectivity of blood is 40 dB to 60 dB less than soft tissue and results in a detected Doppler signal with a low signal-to-noise level (about 10 dB). Manufacturers compensate for the poor SNR by increasing the acoustic power.

The spectral distribution of frequencies poses two additional problems. First, the preferential attenuation of high-frequency components as the beam traverses tissue causes a downward distortion in the frequency distribution, which is interpreted incorrectly as a Doppler shift. This attenuation effect varies with the depth of the moving reflectors. Second, the frequency dependence of scattering enhances the high-frequency components in the echo and thus tends to counteract the effect of attenuation.

DIRECTIONAL METHODS

The received echo from a moving reflector is shifted in frequency above or below the reference signal depending on whether the motion is toward or away from the transducer. This process of demodulating the signal indicates that a shift has occurred, but it cannot identify whether the shift is positive or negative. Three processing methods—including single sideband, heterodyne, and quadrature phase detection—have been developed to distinguish between motion toward and motion away from the transducer.

Single-Sideband Detector

The operation of a single-sideband detector system is shown in Fig. 14-15. The received signal consists of reflected echoes from both stationary and moving structures. The reflections from stationary structures are equal in frequency to the transmitted beam, whereas those from moving structures are offset in frequency.

The signal from the radiofrequency amplifier is split into two components and then filtered. One filter is designed to pass all frequencies above the reference signal (forward motion), and the other all frequencies below the reference signal (reverse motion). The output of each filter is mixed with the reference signal and then filtered by a sideband filter in which all components except the shifted signals are removed. This results in two separate signals corresponding to the forward and reverse motions.

Heterodyne Detector

In a heterodyne detector the offset signal combines with the reference signal before being added to the received signal to obtain the Doppler shift. This technique displaces the Doppler shift to a new frequency range. Forward and reverse motions are differentiated by the magnitude of the Doppler shift compared with the offset frequency. For example, if the offset frequency is 5 kHz, the Doppler shift (f_D) is given as

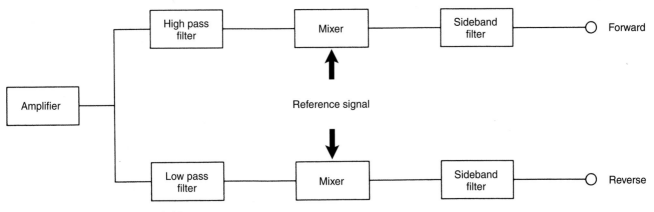

Fig. 14-15 Single sideband Doppler unit.

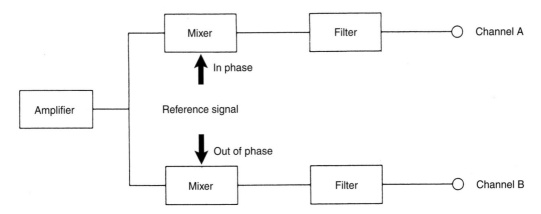

Fig. 14-16 Quadrature phase detection divides the received signal into two components and then mixes these with a varying phase reference signal.

14-7

$$f_D = f_R - (f_T - 5 \text{ kHz})$$

where f_R is the frequency of the received signal and f_T the transmitted frequency.

Note that Equation 14-7 reduces to the usual definition of Doppler shift (the difference in frequency between received and transmitted signals) if the offset signal is set to zero. The offset signal, however, allows reverse motion ($f_R < f_T$) to be displayed as frequencies below 5 kHz and forward motion ($f_R > f_T$) to be displayed as frequencies above 5 kHz (usually up to 15 kHz).

Quadrature Phase Detector

Fig. 14-16 illustrates quadrature phase detection, the most commonly used directional technique. The signal from the radiofrequency (RF) amplifier is split into two components, and each is mixed with the reference signal (one channel 90 degrees out of phase with the other or one quarter of the period, hence the name quadrature). After filtering, the output from each channel contains a mixture of forward and reverse flow signals. In time domain processing the presence of flow in one direction only causes each channel to exhibit the same voltage variation as a function of time, although the pattern is shifted in time. If flow is in the forward

direction, the output from channel A shows the leading edge of the pattern first. Flow in the opposite direction causes the output from channel B to precede the output from channel A. The outputs from both channels are analyzed simultaneously by comparing their relative phase to determine whether flow is in the forward or reverse directions. This detection system does not work properly, however, if forward and reverse flow signals occur concurrently. The method also is susceptible to switching flow artifacts if high noise levels or strong low-frequency signals are present.

A technique called **frequency domain processing** is applied after quadrature phase detection to generate two output signals, each associated with a particular direction of flow. These signals can be routed to headphones in which the sounds in one ear represent motion toward the transducer, and those in the other ear correspond to motion away from the transducer. Fig. 14-17 demonstrates the operation of the frequency domain detector. A pilot signal within the audible frequency range is mixed with the channel output signals from the **quadrature phase detector** (channels A and B). The mixed signal from channel A is added with the unmixed quadrature signal from channel B to produce the reverse flow channel. Similarly, the mixed signal from channel B is added with the unmixed quadrature signal from channel A to produce the forward flow channel.

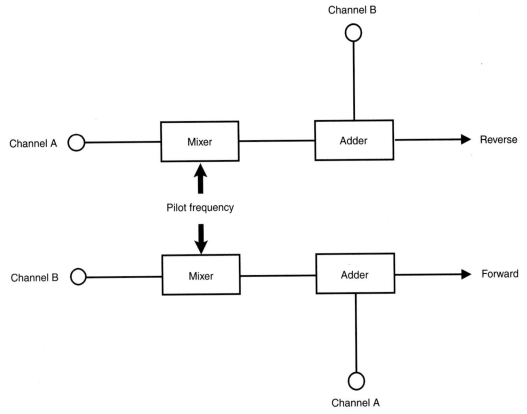

Fig. 14-17 Frequency domain processing. A pilot signal is applied to each channel output from a quadrature phase detector. Each mixed signal is then added with the unmixed opposite quadrature channel output, and the frequency components of the output are separated into the forward and reverse flow signals.

DUPLEX SCANNERS

Duplex Doppler units combine real-time imaging with CW or PW Doppler detection. The B-mode image depicts stationary reflectors (e.g., plaques inside the vessel and other anatomic structures), whereas the Doppler mode provides flow information for a selected region. The display of anatomic structures aids in selecting the line of sight for CW Doppler or placement of the sample volume for PW Doppler. Markers for the sampling region are superimposed on the real-time image. The Doppler angle can be ascertained from the B-mode image. The assessment of angle assumes that flow is parallel to the vessel wall, and the vessel does not curve within the scan plane. While these assumptions may not be entirely correct, the errors introduced are generally small so that reasonable estimates of velocity can be obtained. Visualization of the physical size and shape of plaque with real-time scanning is an important factor in the diagnosis of vascular disease.

The duplex scanner must perform both imaging and Doppler functions (Fig. 14-18). Because the optimal design specifications for each of these functions are not the same, various transducer configurations have been developed. Mechanical sector, annular phased array, linear phased array, and linear array transducers have been used for real-time imaging and then switched to operate in the Doppler mode. Real-time imaging is interrupted while the flow

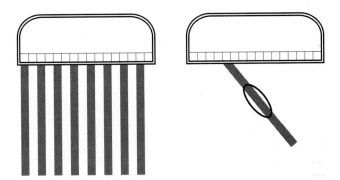

Fig. 14-18 Duplex scanning with a linear array transducer. B-mode image is obtained with parallel scan lines across the length of the array. The beam is then electronically steered along the line of sight designated for Doppler acquisition. Gating the signals from received echoes from this line of sight establishes the sampling volume *(ellipse)*.

information is acquired, usually over a period of several milliseconds.

The ultrasound beam must be repeatedly directed along one line of sight in the Doppler mode. Multiple echoes from the same reflector are necessary for determining the beat frequency. The rotational inertia of mechanically steered transducers prohibits rapid switching between imaging and Doppler modes. The electronic interleaving of Doppler pulses between imaging pulses in simultaneous duplex scanning permits real-time imaging, though at a reduced frame rate. Some systems use a separate transducer operating at a different frequency for the Doppler mode. A linear array with an offset Doppler transducer is one example. The offset transducer also provides a more appropriate Doppler angle, but good coupling between the probe and skin is difficult.

A single broadband transducer operating at low frequency in the Doppler mode and high frequency in the imaging mode is also feasible. An annular phased array that obtains the image data at 5 MHz and then activates the central disk only for Doppler detection at 3 MHz has been developed.

In duplex scanning, the flow information is acquired for a highly restricted region and displayed in real time. *The pattern of flow must be ascertained by sampling multiple regions one after the other throughout the field of view.* Isolated flow disturbances may go undetected. The characteristics of duplex scanning are presented in Box 14-1.

SUMMARY

Doppler instrumentation detects the presence, direction, velocity, and characteristics of blood flow. The Doppler shift is extracted by combining the detected echoes with the reference signal followed by demodulation to produce the beat frequency. PW Doppler allows the depth of the moving reflector to be determined, but a maximum velocity detection limit is imposed by the intermittent sampling. Aliasing occurs if reflector velocity exceeds this limit. CW Doppler eliminates aliasing artifacts, although spatial information is also lost. A comparison of CW and PW Doppler instruments is shown in Table 14-4.

REVIEW QUESTIONS

1. What is the Doppler effect?
2. The magnitude of the Doppler shift depends on the relative _____ between the source and receiver.
3. The maximum Doppler shift occurs when the motion of the interface is _____ with respect to beam propagation.
4. Assuming that a 4 MHz transducer is directed at an interface moving toward the transducer with a velocity of 15 cm/s, what is the Doppler shift? The angle of incidence is 0 degrees.
5. For Question 4, what is the Doppler shift if the Doppler angle is increased to 60 degrees?
6. Calculate the velocity of the moving reflector if a Doppler shift of 800 Hz is observed. The angle of insonation is 45 degrees. The center frequency of the transducer is 3 MHz.
7. Calculate the minimum PRF in pulses per second to prevent aliasing if the velocity of the moving reflector is 25 cm/s. The angle of insonation is 60 degrees, and the transducer frequency is 5 MHz.
8. What is the beat frequency?
9. What is the purpose of the high-pass filter in a CW Doppler scanner?
10. The CW Doppler unit provides depth discrimination. (True/False)

Box 14-1 Duplex Scanning

Advantages	Disadvantages
Simultaneous display of B-mode and Doppler	Small sample volume
Ability to define Doppler angle	No global presentation of flow
Measurement of flow velocity	Manual adjustment of Doppler angle
Identification of complex flow components	Reduced frame rates
Real-time flow information	

■ **Table 14-4** Comparison of Doppler Instruments

Continuous Wave Doppler	Pulsed Wave Doppler
No range resolution	Depth information
Narrow bandwidth	Wide bandwidth
No velocity limit	Maximum velocity limit
High sensitivity to slow flow	Low sensitivity to slow flow
No aliasing	Aliasing

11. In PW Doppler the axial dimension of the sampling volume is defined by _____.
12. An artifactual display of low-frequency components caused by an inadequate sampling rate of high-frequency Doppler shifts is called _____.

■ BIBLIOGRAPHY ■

Boote EJ: Doppler ultrasound techniques: concepts of blood flow detection and flow dynamics, *Radiographics* 23:1315-1327, 2003.

Forsberg F: Principles of Doppler imaging. In Goldman LW, Fowlkes JB, eds: *Categorical course in diagnostic radiology physics: CT and US cross-sectional imaging*, Oak Brook, Ill, 2000, Radiological Society of North America.

Hedrick WR, Hykes DL: Doppler physics and instrumentation: a review, *J Diagn Med Sonogr* 4:109-120, 1988.

Kremkau FW: Doppler principles, *Semin Roentgenol* 27:6-16, 1992.

Merritt CRB: Doppler US: the basics, *Radiographics* 11:109-119, 1991.

Nelson TR, Pretorius DH: The Doppler signal: where does it come from and what does it mean? *AJR Am J Roentgenol* 151:439-447, 1988.

Rubin JM: Spectral Doppler US, *Radiographics* 14:139-150, 1994.

Smith H, Zagzebski J: *Basic Doppler physics*, Madison, Wisc, 1991, Medical Physics Publishing.

Taylor KJW, Holland S: Doppler ultrasound, I, basic principles, instrumentation, and pitfalls, *Radiology* 174:297-307, 1990.

Wells PNT: Ultrasonic Doppler equipment. In Fullerton GD, Zagzebski JA, eds: *Medical physics of CT and ultrasound-tissue imaging and characterization*, New York, 1980, American Institute of Physics.

Zagzebski JA: Physics and instrumentation in Doppler and B-mode ultrasonography. In Zweibel WJ, ed: *Introduction to vascular ultrasonography*, ed 2, Orlando, Fla, 1986, Grune & Stratton.

Doppler Spectral Analysis

Doppler spectral waveform
Fast Fourier transform
Maximum Doppler shift
Maximum velocity waveform
Mean frequency
Power spectrum

Pulsatility index
Resistive index
Spectral analysis
Stenosis
Transit time broadening
Volume flow rate

In the cross section of a vessel, red blood cells (RBCs) at various radii from the center are moving at different velocities, resulting in a Doppler signal that is a combination of all the frequency shifts. The process of determining the individual Doppler shifts that are present in this complex Doppler signal and the relative importance of each is called **spectral analysis.** Spectral analysis, when repeated rapidly in time, characterizes the flow in vessels.

FAST FOURIER TRANSFORM

The analysis of complex Doppler signals is usually accomplished with a mathematical algorithm called the **fast Fourier transform (FFT).** Fourier analysis is the process of separating a waveform into a series of single-frequency sine-wave components. When algebraically combined, these components yield the original waveform. A more complete

description of Fourier analysis is presented in Appendix B. Other methods (e.g., the parallel filter bank and time compression) have also been used to quantify individual frequency components in the Doppler signal. However, computer speed and cost effectiveness have made FFT the preferred method. Several examples follow to illustrate the principle of spectral analysis.

Fig. 15-1 is a cross-sectional view of a vessel lumen. In regions 1, 2, and 3, RBCs move at different velocities ($v_3 > v_2 > v_1$) through the vessel. For simplicity, the same total number of RBCs is assumed to pass through each region and to flow at a continuous (nonpulsatile) rate. If the ultrasound beam is made very small so that each of these regions is sampled individually, a characteristic Doppler shift is obtained for each region (Fig. 15-2). Three frequency shifts are observed (f_1, f_2, and f_3). The Doppler shift is largest for region 3, because RBCs in this region are moving at the greatest velocity. Because an equal number of RBCs is present in each region, the amplitude of the individual frequency shifts is the same. This is represented by the heights of the individual waveforms in Fig. 15-2, which are identical.

If all three regions are sampled simultaneously by the ultrasound beam, a complex Doppler signal will be obtained, as shown in Fig. 15-3, which is an algebraic sum of the three waveforms in Fig. 15-2. This detected Doppler signal must be simplified to associate groups of RBCs with individual frequency shifts and thus with rates of movement.

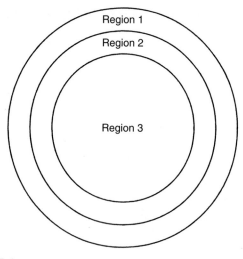

Fig. 15-1 Regions of red blood cell velocity across a vessel lumen.

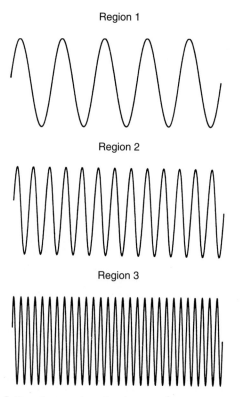

Fig. 15-2 Beat frequencies of regions 1, 2, and 3 in Fig. 15-1. Note that they increase with increasing velocity of the red blood cells.

Spectral analysis separates the complex signal into its individual frequency components and determines the relative importance of each; that is, the waveform in Fig. 15-3, the detected signal, is mathematically converted into the various individual frequency shifts shown in Fig. 15-2. *The determination of the frequency shifts present in the Doppler signal is performed without prior knowledge of these frequency components.* All frequency shifts that occur in the Doppler signal are isolated by spectral analysis.

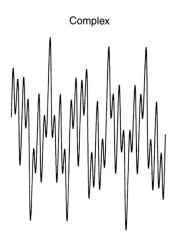

Fig. 15-3 This complex Doppler signal is the sum of the waves in Fig. 15-2.

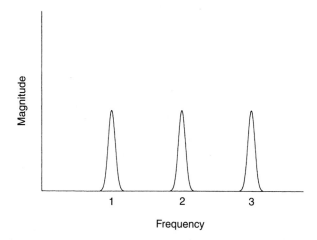

Fig. 15-4 Power spectrum of the complex Doppler signal in Fig. 15-3. Each flow velocity is depicted as a peak. The three flow velocity peaks corresponding to different regions are the same height.

POWER SPECTRUM

An alternative, but informational equivalent, way to display the spectral analysis is in the form of a **power spectrum** in which the magnitude of individual frequency components is plotted against the frequency (Fig. 15-4). This converts the complex Doppler signal from the time domain into the frequency domain. The power spectrum is an extremely useful analysis technique, because it displays the desired flow information, the distribution of Doppler shifts, directly. The magnitude is determined by the amplitude of the respective waveform corresponding to a particular frequency and represents the relative importance of each frequency (i.e., the number of RBCs moving at the velocity given by the frequency shift). In this case the height for each observed frequency is the same since the initial assumption was that an equal number of RBCs is flowing through each region.

Suppose, for example, that the number of RBCs moving through region 1 is doubled. The amplitude of the beat frequency corresponding to this region also doubles and results in an altered complex Doppler signal, as shown in

Fig. 15-5. The frequency of the Doppler shift for region 1 remains the same, because the velocity of the RBCs has not changed. The spectral analysis presented by the power spectrum in Fig. 15-6 depicts the increased importance of the lowest frequency by the increased height of the peak corresponding to this frequency. The display of the complex Doppler signal as a function of time does not allow the sonographer readily to ascertain this increase in flow through region 1, but it can be easily interpreted from the power spectrum.

The relationship between the frequency domain display and the velocity of RBCs is further illustrated by the power spectrum associated with plug flow. Plug flow is blood moving at a single velocity. Suppose that all the RBCs throughout the vessel are moving slowly at a constant velocity; the power spectrum contains a single peak at low frequency (Fig. 15-7). If the velocity of the RBCs increases, the power spectrum once again shows a single peak but at a higher frequency (Fig. 15-8).

In reality, blood does not typically flow in discrete velocities; rather, it exhibits a wide range of velocities. A sample velocity distribution of RBCs is depicted in Fig. 15-9. The fullness of each bin indicates the number of RBCs within the corresponding velocity range. Note that all velocity ranges are not equally represented. The power spectrum reflects this variation in the number of RBCs moving at different velocities by assigning a specific magnitude for each velocity.

Laminar flow consisting of many components is often encountered in the vascular system. Laminar flow with a velocity profile ranging from zero near the vessel wall to a maximum in the central portion of the vessel yields a continuous power spectrum, as shown in Fig. 15-10. The power spectra associated with other velocity profiles are presented in Figs. 15-11 and 15-12.

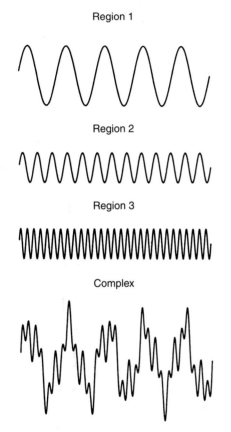

Fig. 15-5 Beat frequencies for regions 1, 2, and 3. Region 1 contains twice as many red blood cells (RBCs) as the other regions, and changes in the complex Doppler signal occur from doubling the number of RBCs in that region.

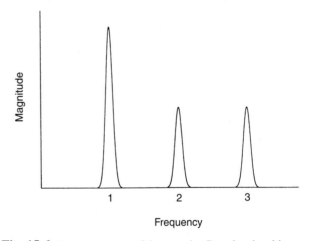

Fig. 15-6 Power spectrum of the complex Doppler signal in Fig. 15-5.

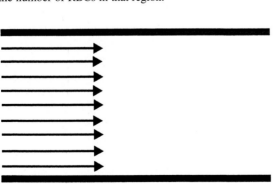

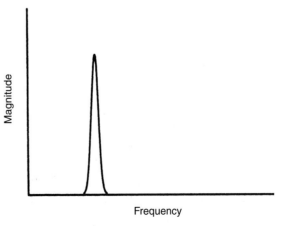

Fig. 15-7 Power spectrum of red blood cells moving uniformly at a low velocity.

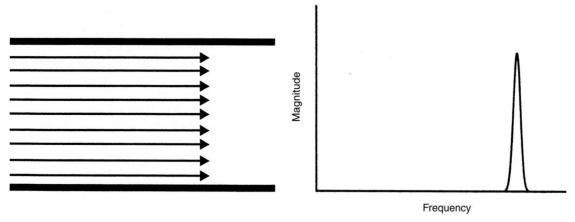

Fig. 15-8 Power spectrum of red blood cells moving uniformly at a high velocity.

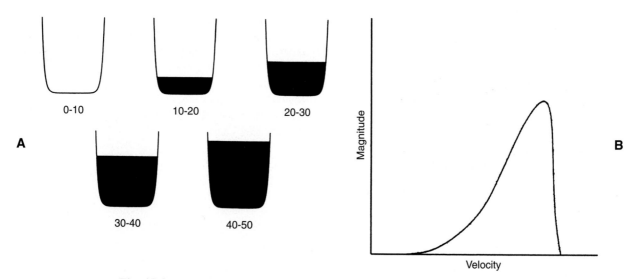

Fig. 15-9 Distribution of red blood cells (RBCs) moving with different velocities across the vessel lumen. **A,** The fullness of each bin indicates the number of RBCs within that velocity range. All velocities are not equally represented. **B,** Power spectrum of the different velocity components represented.

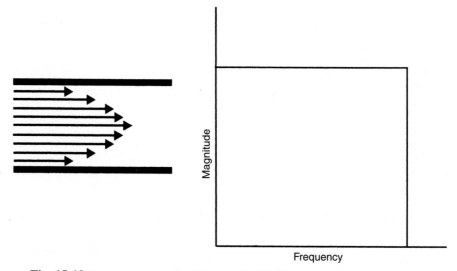

Fig. 15-10 Power spectrum of red blood cells (RBCs) moving with varying velocities. The number of RBCs at each velocity is the same.

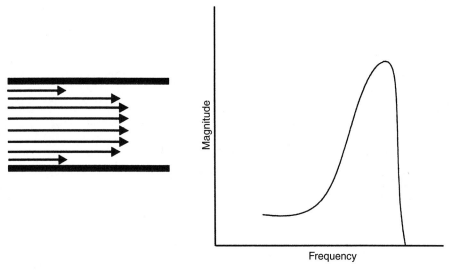

Fig. 15-11 Power spectrum obtained when the velocity profile is dominated by high-velocity components.

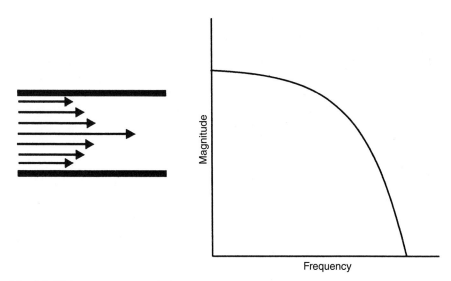

Fig. 15-12 Power spectrum obtained when the velocity profile is dominated by low-velocity components.

Stenosis creates disturbed flow, which is characterized by fast jets, slowly moving elements, and circulating eddies. The power spectrum demonstrates a broad range of frequency components, including negative values (which indicate reverse flow) (Fig. 15-13).

INFLUENCE OF BEAM SHAPE

In the previous examples of power spectra associated with different velocity distributions, the magnitude of the frequency component indicated the volume of blood moving at the velocity given by that particular frequency. The ultrasound beam is assumed to be large enough to insonate all RBCs within the vessel uniformly. Pulsed wave (PW) Doppler scanners are designed to generate highly directional beams that restrict sampling to small volumes. Beam shape,

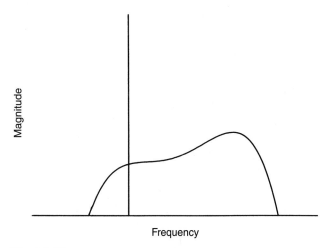

Fig. 15-13 Power spectrum produced by turbulent flow.

as characterized by cross-sectional uniformity and sample axial length, has a major effect on the detected Doppler signal. This beam-shape dependence becomes particularly problematical in the quantitative measurement of blood volume flow rate.

Consider once more the situation of laminar flow in which the velocity profile varies from zero near the vessel wall to a maximum in the central portion of the vessel. The effect of ultrasound beam shape on the power spectrum is shown in Fig. 15-14 for three different sampling volumes. If the ultrasound beam encompasses the entire vessel uniformly, an accurate power spectrum depicting the various velocities is obtained. When the vessel is insonated nonuniformly, the contribution to the power spectrum by the slowly flowing RBCs near the wall is diminished. If the beam were restricted to the central portion of the vessel, only the most rapidly moving RBCs would contribute to the Doppler signal, and the power spectrum would then become distorted. In each case the conditions of blood flow would not change, but the measurement process would yield very different results depending on the relative dimensions of the vessel and the ultrasound beam.

The actual Doppler sampling volume may not correspond to the region selected by the sonographer. Refraction by soft tissue interfaces sometimes causes the sound beam to deviate from the anticipated straight-line path. If the ultrasound beam partially intercepts the vessel, the Doppler spectrum will not accurately portray flow velocities throughout the vessel.

TIME DISPLAY OF THE POWER SPECTRUM

In vessels the velocity distribution is not constant with time; rather, cyclic pressure changes give rise to pulsatile flow. Consequently, it is desirous to display the changing flow patterns depicted by the power spectrum as a function of time (called **Doppler spectral waveform**). Three variables (frequency, magnitude, and time) must be included in this two-dimensional display. The magnitude in the power spectrum is now represented by varying the brightness level to indicate the relative importance of each frequency. Consider the power spectrum in Fig. 15-15, *A*, in which the high-velocity group of RBCs produces twice the signal as the middle-velocity group, which in turn produces twice the signal as the low-velocity group. This information is converted to points of varying brightness along a straight line, representing the frequency axis (Fig. 15-15, *B*). Increased distance along the axis corresponds to higher frequency. Note that, in this example, the high frequency is brighter than the middle frequency, which is brighter than the low frequency.

Flow hemodynamics is not constant throughout the cardiac cycle. Peak flow velocities typically occur at peak systole. Good temporal resolution is necessary for the interpretation of flow patterns. The dimension of time is obtained by sampling the Doppler signal repeatedly in small increments of a few milliseconds. An FFT frequency analysis is then applied to each short time segment of the

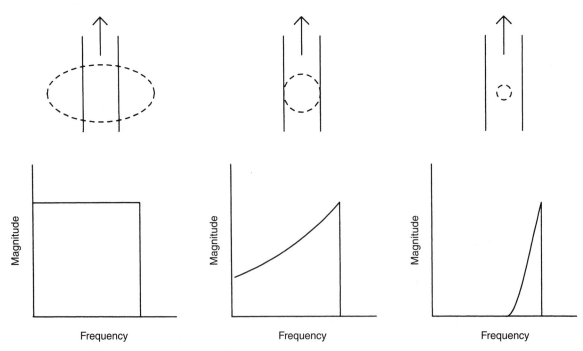

Fig. 15-14 Effect of beam shape on the laminar flow power spectrum. The dotted line indicates the sampled region in each case. On the left, sampling of the entire vessel lumen with uniform intensity. In the middle, sampling with decreased intensity at the vessel wall. On the right, sampling restricted to the central portion of the lumen.

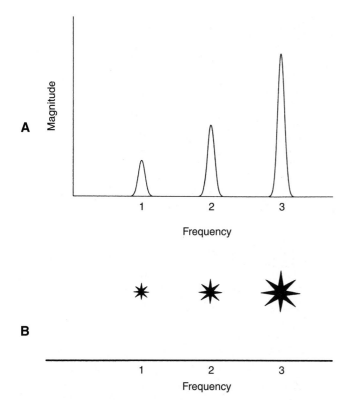

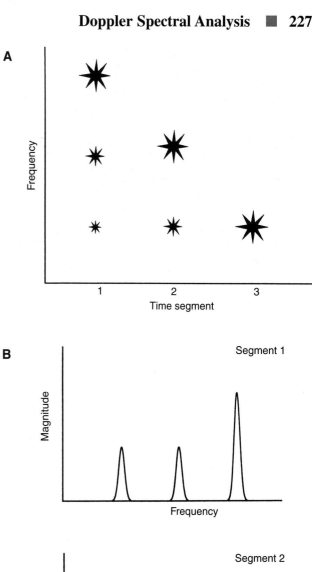

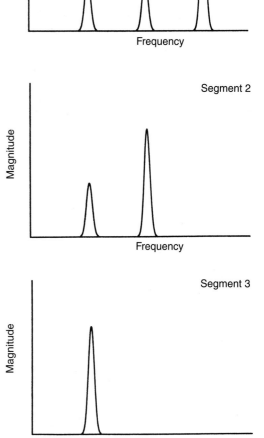

Fig. 15-15 A, Power spectrum depicting three discrete groups of red blood cells in which the signal decreases in importance from high frequency to low frequency. **B,** Brightness-modulated power spectrum, which has the same information content as **A.**

Doppler signal. High-speed digital–integrated circuits perform the necessary calculations on the most recently collected data while the Doppler signal for the following time segment is being acquired. The FFT processing allows a series of power spectra to be analyzed in real time. The display of these multiple analyses consists of a vertical axis corresponding to frequency with varying brightness levels representing magnitude of each frequency and a horizontal axis corresponding to time. Each analysis of a short time segment of the Doppler signal is presented as a single vertical line. By placing succeeding frequency analyses side by side, a fixed distance apart, the vertical lines scroll left to right with time to build up a pattern (Fig. 15-16).

A more useful presentation is to convert the frequency distribution to a velocity distribution using the Doppler shift equation with values for transmitted frequency, acoustic velocity in tissue, and Doppler angle. The ability to display quickly changing velocities within the vessel is thereby achieved (Fig. 15-17). The frequency or velocity scale of the spectrum analyzer is adjusted by changing the pulse repetition frequency (PRF). Time-varying physiologic signals (e.g., an electrocardiogram) can be displayed in conjunction with the brightness-modulated power spectra.

A high-pass filter, applied to the Doppler signal to eliminate the distracting low-frequency wall thump, may remove low-velocity blood flow components in the power spectrum. Under these conditions the velocity distribution becomes distorted by the application of a filter. Operator-

Fig. 15-16 A, Time sequence of the brightness-modulated power spectra shown in **B. B,** Power spectra corresponding to the three time segments in **A.**

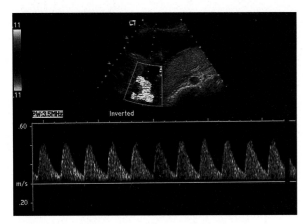

Fig. 15-17 Doppler spectral waveform obtained for the umbilical cord.

controlled amplifier gain may also influence the Doppler spectral waveform. High gain broadens the velocity components that are displayed. Flow information can be lost at low gain settings, however.

ALIASING

Aliasing is characterized by wraparound, whereby the high-velocity components above the Nyquist limit appear below the baseline (Fig. 15-18, *A*). The aliasing artifact is removed by changing the velocity scale (Fig. 15-18, *B*) or adjusting the baseline (Fig. 15-18, *C*). An increase in the PRF extends the maximum velocity according to the Nyquist criterion, which is expressed as the upper range limit on the velocity scale. The velocity range for reverse flow can be set to a lower value than that for forward flow (zero if reverse flow is not a concern). Baseline control can double the maximum velocity in one direction, but directional discrimination is lost. Other techniques to eliminate the aliasing artifact are to increase the angle of insonation (Fig. 15-19), decrease the depth to the sample volume by rocking the transducer heel to toe, or switch to a lower transmitted frequency. In summary, aliasing can be eliminated by the following techniques:
- Increase velocity scale (PRF)
- Adjust baseline
- Increase angle of insonation
- Decrease depth to sample volume
- Switch to lower transmitted frequency

SPECTRAL MIRROR ARTIFACT

Another improper presentation of the power spectra, called the mirror image artifact or preferably spectral mirror artifact, occurs when weak Doppler signals are detected with high gain settings (Fig. 15-20). The large amount of clutter from stationary scatterers prevents the receiver from processing all incoming Doppler signals. The quadrature phase detector becomes saturated, resulting in a loss of directional discrimination. Forward and reverse spectra emulate each other.

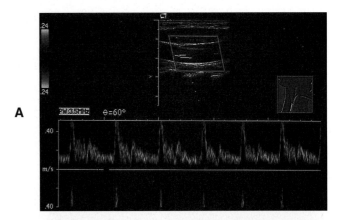

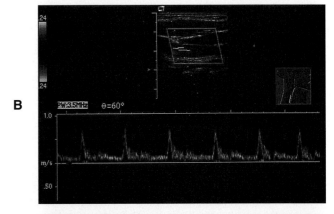

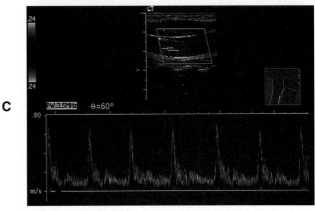

Fig. 15-18 A, Aliasing artifact in which high-velocity components demonstrate wraparound. The velocity range on the vertical scale is –0.4 to 0.5 m/s. **B,** Increasing the velocity limit to remove the aliasing artifact. The velocity range is –0.5 to 1 m/s. **C,** Adjusting the baseline to remove the aliasing artifact. The velocity range is 0 to 0.8 m/s in the forward direction only.

LIMITATIONS OF FAST FOURIER TRANSFORM ANALYSIS

The FFT is applied to a block of data that have been collected previously. For the spectral display to respond to rapid changes in the velocity distribution, short sampling times are desirable. The duration of the analyzed segment, however, determines the frequency resolution. Each brightness-modulated dot in the power spectrum represents a range of shift frequencies equal to the inverse of the sampling time. A time segment of 5 ms yields a frequency

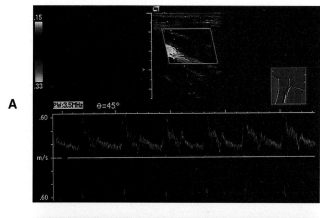

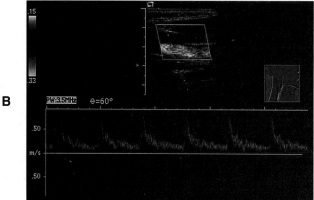

Fig. 15-19 **A,** Aliasing artifact in which high-velocity components demonstrate wraparound. The insonation angle is 45 degrees. **B,** Increasing the insonation angle to 60 degrees to remove the aliasing artifact.

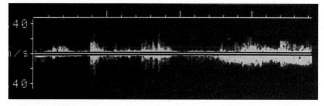

Fig. 15-20 Pulsed wave Doppler spectral waveform showing spectral mirror artifact.

resolution of 200 Hz; a longer time segment, 10 ms, improves the frequency resolution to 100 Hz.

Because the Doppler signal is a changing entity, statistical variations are introduced into the FFT analysis. To reduce these inaccuracies, several FFTs are performed within each observation time, and the results averaged to generate the final spectrum. For example, an FFT calculated every 3 ms within an observation time of 12 ms provides a redundancy of four analyses. Note that the frequency resolution, which in this case is 330 Hz, is now controlled by the segment analyzing time.

SPECTRAL BROADENING

A single-frequency Doppler shift for a reflector moving at constant velocity is obtained only for a very large-plane

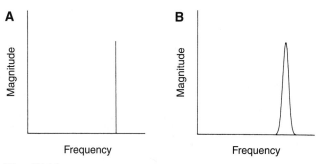

Fig. 15-21 **A,** Idealized power spectrum for a constant-velocity reflector. **B,** The effect of transit-time broadening on this power spectrum.

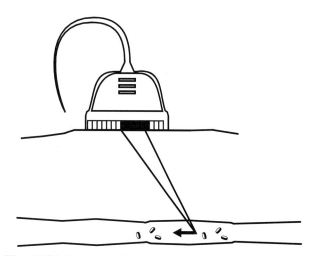

Fig. 15-22 The physical dimensions of the active aperture create multiple insonation angles for a steered beam.

target insonated by a large acoustic field. The reflector only contributes to the backscattered signal as it moves across a finite-width beam. The fluctuation of the detected signal as RBCs move in and out of the sampling volume causes the beat frequency to vary in amplitude, which is interpreted as additional frequency components above and below the idealized Doppler shift (Fig. 15-21). The broadening of the spectrum is called **transit time broadening** and creates difficulties in spectral interpretation. The spectrum produced by scatterers moving at different velocities is the same as that observed when scatterers are moving at constant velocity with transit time broadening. The overall effect of transit time broadening is to smear the magnitude of a frequency component over a wider range of frequencies. Transit time broadening that is 7% of the Doppler shift is considered acceptable but can be much higher (33%).

Narrowing the beam width and shortening the receiver gate in PW mode accentuate the broadening effect. The simultaneous measurement of reflector position and velocity in PW Doppler limits the ability of these systems to determine high-velocity flow in small localized regions. Longer pulse lengths with a corresponding loss in positional information are necessary to assess high-velocity jets accurately.

The transmitted pulse consists of multiple frequencies, which introduces variations into the received frequency and

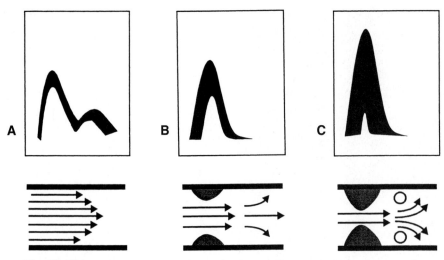

Fig. 15-23 Doppler spectral waveforms. **A,** Normal. **B,** Partially blocked lumen. **C,** Severe stenosis.

contributes to spectral broadening. Also, the physical size of the beam aperture creates a range of angles that intercept the vessel (Fig. 15-22). Even if all RBCs were moving at the same velocity, a range of Doppler shifts would be detected, because the angle of insonation is not uniform across the beam width. This effect may be mitigated by using a small Doppler angle of near 30 degrees.

DISTURBED FLOW POWER SPECTRA

For a vessel with a nearly uniform velocity distribution, the spectral display, particularly during systole, shows a characteristic window appearance (Fig. 15-23, *A*). The window is an area between the high-velocity components and the baseline that is relatively signal free. Doppler shifts are confined to a relatively narrow velocity range. Partial blockage of a vessel causes flow disturbance, which extends the velocity distribution over a wider range. The increased variation in Doppler shifts is evidenced by a broadening of the spectral display (Fig. 15-23, *B*). The window is reduced and is not as distinct. A nearly blocked lumen creates high-speed jets with rotating flow elements (Fig. 15-23, *C*). Arterial regions with eddy flow exhibit time-dependent behavior in which the velocity distribution reverts to laminar flow during periods of reduced pressure. The spectral display changes shape to reflect a loss in pulsatility. In summary: The four features of disturbed flow immediately distal to the obstruction include increased peak velocity, spectral broadening, altered flow direction, and less pulsatile shape. *The peak velocity, in particular, increases as luminal size decreases and is used as an indicator of severity of the stenosis.*

POWER SPECTRUM DESCRIPTORS

Maximum frequency, mean frequency, median frequency, and mode frequency are descriptors of the power spectrum that help characterize vascular Doppler signals. Various

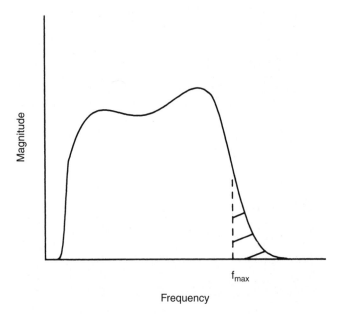

Fig. 15-24 Maximum frequency derived from the power spectrum with a cutoff limit of 5%.

signal-processing techniques are incorporated within the Doppler unit to generate these descriptors.

Maximum Frequency

The **maximum Doppler shift** (f_{max}) corresponds to the fastest-moving RBCs within the sample volume at the time of measurement. Each FFT segment is analyzed for the maximum frequency shift, which is then presented as a time-varying trace on the display. Usually a 1% to 5% upper cutoff limit is applied to prevent the maximum Doppler shift from being associated with high-frequency noise. The cutoff limit indicates the portion of the power spectrum that is above the calculated maximum frequency. Perhaps the alternative description is easier to conceptualize: 100 minus the cutoff limit gives the percentage of total Doppler signal

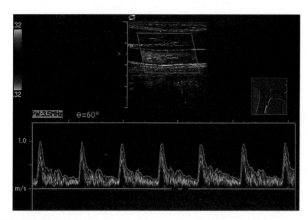

Fig. 15-25 Maximum velocity waveform.

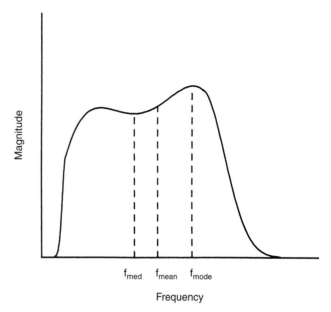

Fig. 15-26 Median, mean, and mode frequencies in a power spectrum.

that lies below the calculated maximum frequency. Fig. 15-24 illustrates the relation between FFT analysis and maximum frequency. If the power spectrum demonstrates a relatively steep falloff in magnitude for the high-frequency components, f_{max} is a good approximation of the true maximum frequency.

Often the maximum Doppler shift in each time segment is converted to velocity using transducer frequency and Doppler angle. This trace is referred to as the **maximum velocity waveform** (Fig. 15-25). An ECG tracing may be included in the display to associate events with the cardiac cycle. Many units are designed to provide an automatic derivation of the velocity waveform.

Mean, Median, and Mode Frequencies

The **mean frequency** (f_{mean}) is calculated from the weighted sum of all frequencies in the power spectrum, in a manner similar to finding the statistical mean for a set of measurements. It can also be presented as a time-varying trace on the display. If insonation is uniform throughout the vessel, the average Doppler shift will correspond to the average velocity within the sample volume. Estimation of volume flow rate is commonly based on measurement of the average velocity. The preferential absorption of high-frequency components by tissue causes a downward shift of the mean frequency, which is dependent on ultrasound path length. The application of a filter can also alter f_{mean} by removing low-frequency components.

The Doppler shifts of all reflectors are equally divided above and below the median frequency. The mode frequency indicates the prevalent Doppler shift in the power spectrum (the frequency at which the peak occurs). The relation of these three descriptors is illustrated in Fig. 15-26.

TIME-COMPRESSED SPECTRAL ANALYSIS

In time compression the complex Doppler signal is sampled for a short time (8 ms) and then stored in digital memory. Once stored, it can be played back at an accelerated rate (250 times normal speed). The time-compressed signal is analyzed during the time that the next Doppler signal is being collected for analysis. A filter with a bandwidth of 150 Hz is swept through a wide frequency range (200 Hz to 15 kHz). In other words, the filter is initially set at a baseline of 200 Hz with a window of 150 Hz, and the Doppler signal is examined for frequency components in this range. The baseline is then incremented by 150 Hz, and the Doppler signal is reexamined for frequency components in this new range. The process is repeated several times until the Doppler signal is analyzed throughout its entire frequency range. The accelerated rate of playback is necessary to complete the analysis of multiple frequency windows in real time.

ZERO CROSSING DETECTORS

Zero crossing detectors are designed to monitor how rapidly the complex Doppler signal is oscillating between maximum and minimum. This provides an indicator of the frequency shifts that make up the Doppler signal.

Each time the Doppler signal crosses zero in one direction (e.g., moving from below zero to above zero), a trigger pulse is generated. To reduce the influence of electronic noise, the signal must exceed a threshold value above zero for a trigger pulse to be produced. The number of pulses per second gives rise to the zero crossing frequency, which represents an averaging of all the frequencies in the Doppler signal. This spectral average is described as the root mean square of the instantaneous frequency distribution, which approximates the mean frequency waveform. The zero crossing frequency is similarly dependent on the velocity components of the flowing blood; that is, it increases if the velocity of flow becomes faster. It is susceptible to error when broad frequency spectra are encountered, however, and consequently FFT methods are generally preferred for the evaluation of flow.

PULSATILITY INDEX AND RESISTIVITY INDEX

Several indices have been formulated to characterize the time-varying Doppler spectrum. **Pulsatility index (PI)** is commonly used to quantify impedance or resistance to flow. This index is calculated from the maximum velocity (v_{max}), the minimum velocity (v_{min}), and the mean velocity (v_{mean}) throughout one cardiac cycle as illustrated in Fig. 15-27:

15-1

$$PI = \frac{v_{max} - v_{min}}{v_{mean}}$$

Sometimes the pulsatility index is defined in terms of the systolic velocity (S) and diastolic velocity (D) instead of the maximum and minimum velocities:

15-2

$$PI = \frac{S - D}{v_{mean}}$$

Many ultrasound scanners automatically calculate the mean velocity, and the operator must indicate the maximum and minimum points using a cursor on the spectral display to generate the pulsatility index.

Higher values of the PI are obtained as flow is impeded by a stenosis. Advantages of this index include the following: (1) the Doppler angle and vessel size do not need to be known; (2) computation is internally consistent within the Doppler spectrum (instrument parameters and Doppler angle are unchanged); (3) abnormal waveforms are identified with high sensitivity; and (4) vessels too small or too tortuous to image can be evaluated. The PI should be calculated for each of several cardiac cycles, and the values averaged to obtain the final result.

Two other parameters, the **resistive index** and the systolic/diastolic ratio, are commonly used clinically:

15-3

$$RI = \frac{v_{max} - v_{min}}{v_{max}}$$

15-4

$$Systolic\text{-}to\text{-}diastolic\ ratio = \frac{S}{D}$$

With these indices computation is easier, because the mean velocity does not need to be determined. The resistive index has been used to assess vascular rejection of renal transplants. In obstetric sonography, waveforms from the umbilical cord and uteroplacental arteries have been characterized with the systolic/diastolic ratio. Intrauterine growth retardation is evaluated by measuring placental impedance.

Pressure gradients are sometimes estimated using peak values in the maximum velocity waveform. The derivative of this waveform yields flow acceleration. To depict acceleration with reasonable precision, time segments must be short. Mean or median velocity, when normalized to maximum velocity, tends to decrease as spectral broadening occurs.

VOLUME FLOW RATE MEASUREMENTS

Volume flow rate delineates the amount of blood moving through the vessel per unit of time. Its estimation is commonly derived from measurements of the velocity distribution and the cross-sectional area of the vessel. The velocity distribution is analyzed to obtain the mean velocity. The product of the mean velocity and the cross-sectional area yields the volume flow rate (Q):

15-5

$$Q\ (cm^3/s) = Mean\ velocity\ (cm/s) \times Area\ (cm^2)$$

For an accurate assessment of volume flow rate to be obtained, all velocity components must be included in the

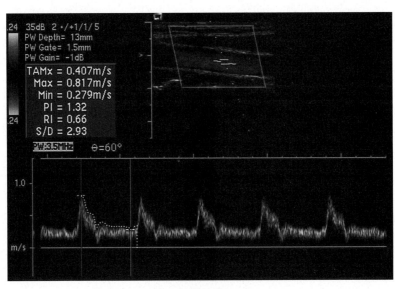

Fig. 15-27 Determination of pulsatility index.

calculation of mean velocity. Several methods have been developed to quantify volume flow rate.

Velocity Profile Method

A PW Doppler system with a small sample volume is used to evaluate the mean velocity at multiple locations across the vessel lumen. At each measurement point the mean velocity is followed throughout the cardiac cycle to obtain a time average. A profile of velocities across the lumen is thus generated. Provided that the lumen is circular, total flow is determined by adding the product of the velocity and the corresponding semiannular area at each point in the profile. A multigate Doppler system containing 16 or 32 gates (each ≈1 mm in axial length) provides instantaneous presentation of the velocity profile. Volume flow rate can be assessed during a single cardiac cycle, which is less susceptible to beat-to-beat variations. This method is most suitable for large and easily accessible vessels (e.g., the aorta and common carotid arteries), which allow a high-frequency transducer to be placed directly over the vessel.

Even Insonation Method

The mean velocity is determined for the entire vessel, which is insonated with a uniform beam. This is multiplied by the cross-sectional area of the lumen to yield the instantaneous volume flow rate. Averaging the instantaneous value over the cardiac cycle results in the time-averaged flow rate. The cross-sectional area fluctuates during the cardiac cycle. Therefore the instantaneous mean velocity and cross-sectional area should be determined simultaneously. In practice, this cannot be achieved, because imaging of the luminal diameter should be conducted with the beam positioned perpendicular to the direction of flow, and the Doppler signal should be obtained with the beam oriented along the direction of flow. As an alternative, the mean velocity and cross-sectional area are measured separately, individually averaged over time, and combined to estimate the volume flow rate.

The even insonation method is subject to a wide variety of additional problems. The cross-sectional area is often calculated from the luminal diameter. The dependence of the area on the square of the diameter necessitates that the diameter be determined accurately. A nonuniform intensity throughout the vessel deemphasizes the low-velocity components near the vessel wall, causing an upward shift in the spectral distribution and an overestimation of the mean velocity. A high-pass filter has a similar effect. Transit-time broadening, clutter, and noise all distort the mean velocity measurement. Frequency-dependent attenuation by intervening tissue lowers the observed mean velocity. The response of the receiver is not time and frequency independent. The flow is assumed to be parallel to the vessel wall. The intensity of the scattered sound beam is altered if turbulence is present. Consequently, this method cannot be used to assess turbulent flow.

Assumed Velocity Profile Method

The velocity profile is determined at one segment of a vessel, and this profile is assumed to exist at different locations in the vessel. For vessels exhibiting plug flow (in which the velocity profile is nearly uniform), the mean velocity is equated to the maximum velocity, an easily measured parameter. This method has limited validity, because velocity profiles are known to change during the cardiac cycle and along various segments of a vessel.

Attenuation-Compensated Flow Volume Ratemeter

A device called an attenuation-compensated flow volume ratemeter has been developed to overcome the difficulty of path-dependent attenuation on velocity measurements. An annular array transducer alternately generates a wide, then narrow, beam. The wide beam encompasses the entire vessel with a uniform ultrasonic intensity. The narrow beam samples the central portion of the vessel only. Because both beams traverse the same ultrasonic path, the effect of attenuation is identical, and any difference in received signal strengths is attributed to the increased amount of blood in the large sample volume. The spectral distribution from the broad beam is also analyzed for mean frequency. A calibration factor is required to convert the measured parameters of mean frequency, broad-beam signal strength, and narrow-beam signal strength into volume flow rate. However, the Doppler angle and luminal cross-sectional area need not be known for this estimation of volume flow rate.

Time Domain Velocity Profile Method

The time domain Doppler detection technique measures displacement of the acoustic speckle pattern associated with a group of RBCs. Since the time interval between measurements is known, the velocity of the RBCs can be determined. Time domain processing uses a wide bandwidth, which allows accurate presentation of spatial information.

The velocity profile is measured along a single line of sight. Good temporal resolution is achieved by sampling at high PRFs. The spatial extent of the velocity profile indicates the size of the lumen. By assuming circular symmetry of the lumen, it is possible to calculate the volume flow rate. The angle of incidence with respect to the direction of flow must be known, however.

CLINICAL EXAMPLES

B-mode images and Doppler spectral waveforms must be interpreted based on a knowledge of anatomy, hemodynamics, disease processes, instrumentation, and physics. Time-varying Doppler spectral analysis yields waveforms that are characteristic of flow within the respective arteries.

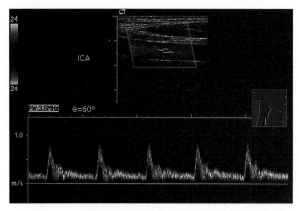

Fig. 15-28 Normal Doppler spectral waveform for the internal carotid artery.

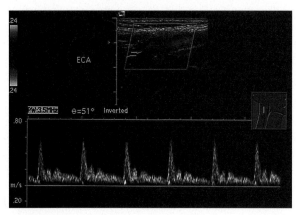

Fig. 15-29 Normal Doppler spectral waveform for the external carotid artery.

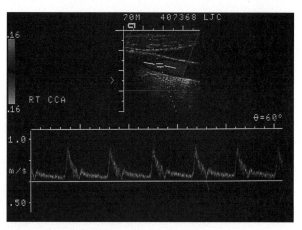

Fig. 15-30 Normal Doppler spectral waveform for the common carotid artery.

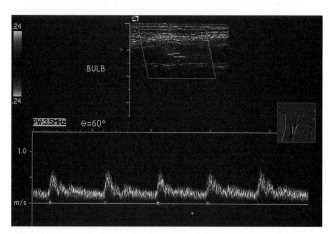

Fig. 15-31 Normal Doppler spectral waveform for the carotid bulb.

Carotid Arteries

The normal internal carotid artery Doppler spectral waveform (Fig. 15-28) demonstrates a maximum peak velocity during systole with a narrow distribution of velocities. This provides the window appearance of the waveform during systole. The low resistance of downstream vessels in the brain allows antegrade flow during diastole. The normal external carotid artery waveform (Fig. 15-29) demonstrates a relatively sharp maximum velocity peak during systole with possible flow reversal in early diastole. The high resistance of downstream vessels in muscle hinders antegrade flow during diastole. The normal common carotid artery waveform (Fig. 15-30) is a composite of the internal carotid artery and external carotid artery waveforms. In the carotid bulb multiple velocity components, including reverse flow, are expected (Fig. 15-31). Typically, peak velocities in the carotid arteries are between 60 and 100 cm/s. The external carotid artery may have slightly lower peak velocity than the internal carotid artery and common carotid artery. Flow is symmetrical on the left and right.

Stenosis, which causes a 75% reduction in cross-sectional area (or, equivalently, a 50% reduction in luminal diameter), disrupts the normal flow patterns. High-velocity jets are formed in the region of maximum narrowing. Sampling within the stenotic jet produces high-velocity,

uniform flow with a clear spectral window (Fig. 15-32). However, at extremely high velocities created by severe stenosis, spectral transit time broadening causes a fill-in of the spectral window (Fig. 15-33). Immediately distal to the stenosis the flow velocities become less uniform and are distributed over a wider range. Spectral analysis detects this change as a continued high velocity peak (although usually less than the stenotic jet) and a fill-in of the window (Fig. 15-34). Turbulence is often observed distal to the stenosis before the normal flow pattern is reestablished (Fig. 15-35).

Multiple velocity measurements or ratios have been used as predictors of stenosis. These include the internal carotid artery (ICA) peak systolic velocity, ICA/common carotid artery (CCA) systolic velocity ratio, ICA end-diastolic velocity, ICA peak diastolic velocity, and ICA/CCA diastolic velocity ratio. Criteria for three of these parameters are presented in Table 15-1. The ICA peak systolic velocity, as a single index, appears to be a good predictor of stenotic disease and is easy to measure. Stenosis classification may be improved by the use of additional velocity parameters. The sonographic appearance of the plaque does not predict progression of disease.

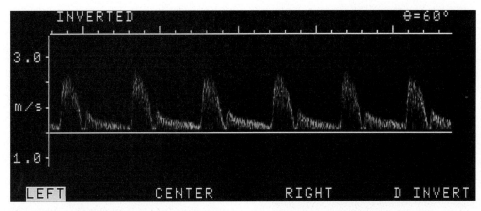

Fig. 15-32 Doppler spectral waveform for the internal carotid artery with stenosis acquired in the region of flow restriction.

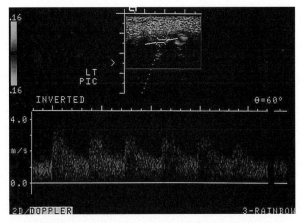

Fig. 15-33 Doppler spectral waveform for the internal carotid artery with severe stenosis.

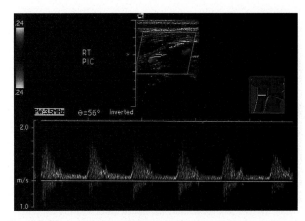

Fig. 15-35 Doppler spectral waveform for the internal carotid artery in which turbulence is present.

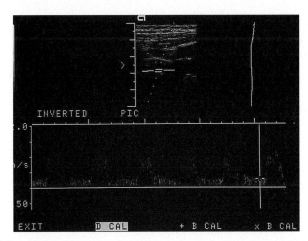

Fig. 15-34 Doppler spectral waveform for the internal carotid artery immediately distal to stenosis.

■ **Table 15-1** Diagnostic Criteria for ICA Stenosis

	Reduction in Luminal Area			
	50%	75%	90%	>98%
Peak systolic velocity (cm/s)	155	325	525	<210
End diastolic velocity (cm/s)	49	60	200	*
ICA/CCA ratio	1.8	4.5	7.5	*

ICA, Internal carotid artery; *CCA*, common carotid artery.
*Limited data.

Peripheral Arteries

Peripheral arterial ultrasonography is most often concerned with possible stenosis in the femoral and popliteal arteries. Normal Doppler spectral waveforms for these arteries are shown in Figs. 15-36 and 15-37. Applications also include assessment of arterial graft patency after surgery; monitoring the effectiveness of peripheral vascular angioplasty; evaluation of dialysis shunt patency; and detection of aneurysm, pseudoaneurysm, and vascular malformation.

An arteriovenous fistula is a congenital malformation in which abnormal shunting between an artery and a vein causes high-velocity, possibly pulsatile, flow in the vein. It may also be induced by trauma.

Although ultrasonographic examination of the carotids has become a well-accepted clinical diagnostic procedure, limitations do exist. Improper Doppler angle or incorrect placement of the cursor (not parallel to the direction of flow) introduces error in the Doppler measurements. Attenuation artifacts from calcifications may obscure a segment of the vessel. Stenosis at the origin of the CCA or within the intracranial ICA is difficult to detect.

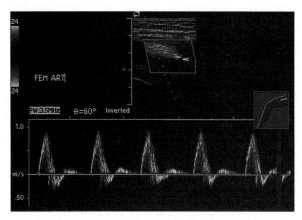

Fig. 15-36 Normal Doppler spectral waveform for the femoral artery.

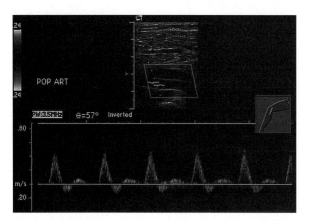

Fig. 15-37 Normal Doppler spectral waveform for the popliteal artery.

Pseudoaneurysm usually presents as a hypoechoic mass in which blood flows into the cavity during systole and exhibits a swirling pattern. These features allow differentiation between the pseudoaneurysm and a postangiographic hematoma or arteriovenous fistula.

The normal maximum velocity waveform of the femoral artery exhibits multiphasic (specifically, triphasic) behavior. Maximum forward flow occurs during systole, followed by reverse flow in early diastole, and then slow forward flow in late diastole. Flow reversal is caused by arterial pressure wave reflection from the distal muscle arterioles, which have high resistance. Arterial compliance is responsible for reestablishing the forward flow in late diastole. This late phase may be lost or greatly reduced in elderly patients. The normal maximum velocity waveform of the popliteal artery is also triphasic and similar to that from the femoral artery, the major difference being that forward flow in late diastole is low or nonexistent.

A gradual reduction in peak systolic velocity is observed in arteries more distal to the heart. For example, maximum velocity in the common femoral and popliteal arteries is 90 cm/s and 59 cm/s, respectively.

Monophasic waveform, increased maximum velocity, and broadening of velocity components are characteristics

of the Doppler spectrum when significant stenosis is present (i.e., greater than 75% reduction). The maximum velocity may change by a factor of 4 to 7 above the normal value. The peak velocity provides an indirect measure of the pressure gradient in a vessel segment.

Abdominal and Pelvic Vascular Ultrasonography

Vascular ultrasonographic applications in the abdomen and pelvis include determination of vessel patency, detection of aortic aneurysms, pseudoaneurysms, arteriovenous fistulas, and other vascular malformations; visualization of large vessels supplying neoplastic tumors; and evaluation of suspected thrombosis.

The renal hilum, splenic hilum, and porta hepatis can be evaluated for thrombosis. Cirrhosis and portal hypertension may affect the patency of the portal vein, and these are detectable by ultrasonography. The bile ducts are readily distinguished from the hepatic artery and portal vein by means of Doppler techniques. Obesity, massive ascites, bowel gas, high attenuation rate of a diseased liver, and the inability to achieve an appropriate Doppler angle may all compromise examination of the liver. Overlying bowel gas obstructs insonation of the inferior vena cava and the iliac and pelvic veins.

SUMMARY

The Doppler signal obtained from RBCs is analyzed for frequency (and hence velocity) components using the FFT. The power spectrum shows the relative contribution of each velocity component. Velocity profile across the vessel lumen and sampling conditions affect the power spectrum. Time-dependent flow velocities within a vessel are depicted by brightness-modulated power spectra acquired successively in short time segments.

Doppler methods are necessary for the investigation of blood flow dynamics. The presence of flow, its direction, and other physiologic aspects of flow (pulsatility, resistivity, high-velocity jets, and turbulence) are assessed with Doppler techniques.

The information content of the brightness-modulated power spectra is simplified by displaying the maximum velocity waveform. This time-varying trace corresponds to the maximum Doppler shift and thus the fastest-moving RBCs within each FFT segment.

B-mode imaging and PW Doppler spectral analysis are both necessary for evaluations of the vascular system. Vessel size and surrounding anatomy are shown in the gray-scale image, and clots and plaques, when present, are often visualized. Hemodynamic information is acquired via Doppler techniques. The B-mode image acts as a roadmap for placement of the sampling volume for PW spectral Doppler. The time-dependent spectral Doppler spectral waveform indicates the velocity components in a small segment of the vessel. However, multiple samplings from different locations must be obtained before a composite representation of regional flow can be formed.

REVIEW QUESTIONS

1. Why is the vessel lumen depicted as a signal void in real-time imaging?

2. The fast Fourier transform (FFT) analysis of the complex Doppler signal is displayed by the power spectrum. What two aspects of blood flow are included in the power spectrum?

3. Multiple FFT analyses of the complex Doppler signal are performed sequentially at short time intervals to form the Doppler spectral waveform. What three aspects of blood flow are represented in the Doppler spectral waveform?

4. What features of disturbed flow immediately distal to an obstruction are presented on a Doppler spectral display?

5. What is the maximum velocity waveform?

6. If pulsed wave (PW) Doppler sampling volume is reduced, how is spectral broadening affected?

7. Why is short acquisition time of the complex Doppler signal for FFT analysis desirable?

8. What is the advantage of longer sampling time of the complex Doppler signal before FFT analysis?

9. If the PW Doppler sampling volume is displaced from the indicated position on the B-mode image such that only blood flow near the vessel wall is examined, what is the effect on the maximum velocity waveform? Assume laminar flow is present in the vessel.

10. If Doppler angle is changed from 30 degrees to 60 degrees, what change occurs in the pulsatility index?

BIBLIOGRAPHY

Boote EJ: Doppler ultrasound techniques: concepts of blood flow detection and flow dynamics, *Radiographics* 23:1315-1327, 2003.

Burns PN: The physical principles of Doppler and spectral analysis, *J Clin Ultrasound* 15:567-590, 1987.

Burns PN, Jaffe CC: Quantitative flow measurements with Doppler ultrasound: techniques, accuracy, and limitations, *Radiol Clin North Am* 23:641-657, 1985.

Forsberg F: Principles of Doppler imaging. In Goldman LW, Fowlkes JB, eds: *Categorical course in diagnostic radiology physics: CT and US cross-sectional imaging,* Oak Brook, Ill, 2000, Radiological Society of North America.

Hedrick WR, Hykes DL: Doppler physics and instrumentation: a review, *J Diagn Med Sonogr* 4:109-120, 1988.

Kremkau FW: Doppler principles, *Semin Roentgenol* 27:6-16, 1992.

Merritt CRB: Doppler US: the basics, *Radiographics* 11:109-119, 1991.

Polak JF: Carotid ultrasound, *Radiol Clin North Am* 39:569-589, 2001.

Rubin JM: Spectral Doppler US, *Radiographics* 14:139-150, 1994.

Smith H, Zagzebski J: *Basic Doppler physics,* Madison, Wisc, 1991, Medical Physics Publishing.

Taylor KJW, Holland S: Doppler ultrasound, I, basic principles, instrumentation, and pitfalls, *Radiology* 174:297-307, 1990.

Doppler Imaging

Doppler imaging (also called color flow imaging, color flow Doppler, color Doppler [CD], color velocity imaging, energy Doppler, and power Doppler) is a scanning mode that combines gray-scale imaging with two-dimensional (2D) mapping of flow information in real time. Frame rates (FRs) are slower than those achieved by real-time B-mode scanning (considerably more computational analysis is required), although 4 to 32 frames per second (fps) are possible. A frame rate of 10 fps is common for Doppler imaging. The gray-scale component of the image is designated as real-time, gray-scale, 2D, or B-mode. Motion is depicted throughout the scan plane by superimposing

different colors on the 2D gray-scale image. Color encoding is based on a single parameter related to velocity or the quantity of blood flow.

COLOR DOPPLER IMAGING

The first type of color flow instrument processed Doppler shift signals to obtain 2D velocity information and hence was called **CD imaging.** A time domain correlation method to measure reflector velocity directly has also been developed as an alternative to frequency shift signal processing, and the term *CD* has been retained to describe this imaging technique.

Both stationary and moving structures are detected by analyzing the received echoes with respect to amplitude, phase, and frequency in the Doppler-signal method or with respect to spatial origin in the direct velocity measurement method (Fig. 16-1). Stationary structures are assigned a gray-scale level based on signal strength as previously shown for B-mode scanners. Moving reflectors cause a phase shift or time shift in the received echo signals that indicates the presence and direction of motion. For Doppler signal processing, the magnitude of the frequency shift gives the relative velocity of the moving reflector via the Doppler-shift equation (not corrected for Doppler angle). When flow determination is made by time domain correlation, reflector velocity is directly proportional to the measured change in

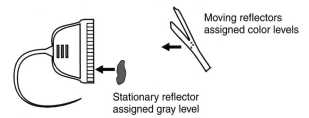

Fig. 16-1 Doppler imaging. Echoes from stationary and moving reflectors are detected and processed to depict flow and anatomy.

spatial origin in the series of received echoes from the moving reflector. *A single representative velocity (usually the mean) at each sampling site where motion is detected is color encoded by hue, saturation, or brightness and superimposed on the gray-scale image.*

COLOR ENCODING

A **color map** assigns various shades or brightness of color to represent different velocities while maintaining directional information (either toward the transducer or away from the transducer). For example, flow at 10 cm/s toward the transducer could be displayed in dark red, and flow at 10 cm/s away from the transducer could be displayed in dark blue.

Hue color coding varies the light frequency to represent colors of the rainbow (violet, blue, green, yellow, orange, and red). Each color signifies a specific velocity range (Fig. 16-2). Multiple color schemes from different manufacturers are used.

Color coding with saturation adds white light to a color to decrease the purity of the light. Typically, red indicates motion in one direction, and blue indicates motion in the opposite direction. Regions with high-velocity flow are displayed by increased color saturation (increased whiteness). Fast-moving reflectors are represented in light shades of red or blue, and slow-moving reflectors in dark shades (Color Plates 4 and 5).

The final method of color coding changes the intensity or brightness of the displayed color. Fast-moving reflectors are represented in high brightness levels of red or blue, and slow-moving reflectors in low brightness levels. This type of color encoding is seldom used, because velocity changes are not readily apparent to the observer.

VELOCITY DISPLAY

The range of displayed velocities is set by the sonographer. For arterial work a high velocity range is appropriate, but for venous flow a low velocity range is necessary. If the phase shift is positive, the reflector is moving toward the transducer and is depicted in red (with the saturation method). If the phase shift is negative, the reflector is moving away from the transducer and is depicted in blue. The association of color with a particular direction of flow is interchangeable, however. The importance of the two-color scheme is not to code for arterial and venous flow but rather to depict simultaneous flow in opposite directions on

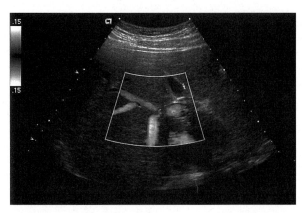

Fig. 16-2 Doppler imaging of the portal vein. Flow in the anterior right portal vein and the posterior right portal vein is shown using a rainbow color map. (See Color Plate 3.) Color Plates 4 and 5 show a color map depicting flow toward the transducer in red and blue, respectively.

the real-time image. Rainbow color maps, which employ two different color sets to code the directional flow, also allow simultaneous imaging of flow in opposite directions. Compare Color Plates 3, 4, and 5 (see Fig. 16-2), which use three different color maps to display the same flow data. The information content is the same, although the translation from velocity to color is different. The highest priority in color-flow imaging is the observation of motion. If certain criteria are met, the assignment of color always takes precedence over gray-scale imaging.

SPATIAL FLOW PATTERNS

The major disadvantage of duplex scanning is that flow is not evaluated simultaneously throughout the field of view (FOV) but rather is sampled at a particular location as selected by the sonographer. To establish the regional flow pattern, the fast Fourier transform (FFT) analysis must be performed at multiple sites throughout the vessel, which requires precise positioning of the sampling volume. Focal regions of abnormal flow are sometimes overlooked. Also, the repetition of sampling is a time-consuming process. *By displaying the 2D spatial distribution of the velocities and the temporal changes in these velocity patterns, real-time CD imaging overcomes these difficulties and enables regions of flow disturbance to be more easily visualized.*

VELOCITY DETECTION

To assess motion, multiple echoes from the same reflector must be collected using a series of transmitted pulses. Recall the analogy in which a series of stop-action photographs of a moving car allows its velocity to be determined, but a single photograph in the series does not indicate whether it is moving or not. Color-flow imaging requires positional information as well as velocity of the moving reflector. Spatial origin of the echoes is obtained by the principle of echo ranging in which the induced signals from echoes are time gated.

Pulsed Wave Doppler Fast Fourier Transform

Velocity information must be obtained for a large number of sample volumes throughout the FOV in a very limited amount of time. Range-gated pulsed wave (PW) Doppler spectral analysis requires a relatively long sampling time for each line of sight (typically about 10 milliseconds [ms]). The sampling time or **dwell time** is the product of the pulse repetition period (PRP) and the number of pulses used to interrogate the moving reflectors along one line of sight. Parallel processing of a multigated system allows several locations along the line of sight to be examined with no increase in sampling time. The gates are activated sequentially following the excitation pulse. Each gate corresponds to one pixel. Hundreds of gates, to acquire the Doppler signals partitioned by depth along the entire scan line, are necessary.

The most important consideration is the time constraint imposed by the requirement that the image must be updated every 0.05 to 0.1 second (corresponding to a frame rate of 10 to 20 images per second). Range-gated PW Doppler spectral detection does not satisfy this condition, because the time necessary to form an image of the Doppler signals is on the order of seconds. Each image consists of 100 to 200 scan lines, and each scan line requires a dwell time of 10 ms. A faster method to detect Doppler signals is needed.

AUTOCORRELATION

Spectral analysis has a high informational content in that the individual frequency components of the Doppler signal are identified. By characterizing the Doppler signal with a single parameter (usually the mean frequency), informational content (spectral analysis of the Doppler shifts) is sacrificed, but the sampling time can be shortened considerably. The rapid acquisition and analysis of flow data are achieved with **autocorrelation** detection. Fewer transmitted pulses are applied along the scan line compared with PW spectral analysis, and consequently autocorrelation is less sensitive to slow flow and flow in small vessels.

Quadrature Detection

Doppler signal processing is initiated with a quadrature detection (QD) circuit (Fig. 16-3). Two output signals labeled

in-phase QD and out-of-phase QD are generated. For reflectors interrogated with a continuous wave (CW) sound beam as illustrated in Fig. 16-4, the QD signals are continuous waveforms during the observation time. The PW technique is necessary to obtain positional information, which necessitates discrete sampling of these QD signals during the observation time (Fig. 16-5). Observation time is time during which Doppler information is acquired along one scan line (usually about 1 ms).

A succession of echoes from the same reflector is collected by sequential transmitted pulses, processed through the QD circuit, segmented by depth, and placed in depth-specific hold circuit. In the time following a transmitted pulse the output from each QD channel is segmented into different depths by echo ranging. Each PRP contributes one data point to the composite in-phase QD signal and the composite out-of-phase QD signal at each depth. Multiple transmitted pulses allow the buildup of time-dependent QD signals as illustrated in Fig. 16-5. The time between data points is equal to the PRP. This scheme allows QD signals

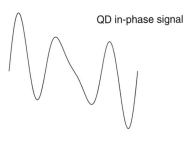

QD in-phase signal

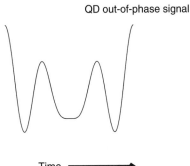

QD out-of-phase signal

Time ⟶

Fig. 16-4 Output signals from the quadrature detection (QD) circuit. The in-phase QD signal and out-of-phase QD signal are not the same but are mathematically related.

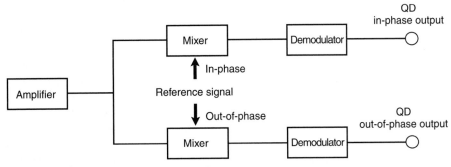

Fig. 16-3 Quadrature detection circuit.

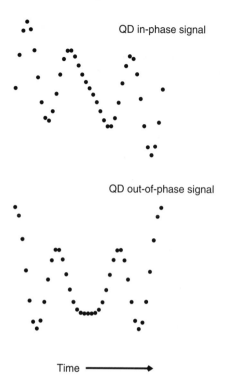

QD in-phase signal

QD out-of-phase signal

Time ⟶

Fig. 16-5 Intermittent sampling depicts the in-phase quadrature detection (QD) and out-of-phase QD signals in Fig. 16-4 as a series of points.

to be generated from many depth segments during the dwell time for the line of sight. The depth sampling interval can be made 0.5 mm or smaller.

Signal Processing

In QD the time-varying output from each channel is a complex function of amplitude and phase of the echo signals. Both stationary and moving reflectors contribute to the QD waveform. The phase of the received signal from a stationary reflector is constant, whereas the phase of the received signal from a moving reflector fluctuates with time. Consequently, sampling with another pulsed sound wave at a later time introduces a change in the QD signal level at the point in the waveform corresponding to the depth of a moving reflector (Fig. 16-6). Each QD output is partitioned according to depth by sequentially clocked gates (Fig. 16-7). A plot of QD output from successive transmitted pulses, segmented according to depth, indicates that moving reflectors produce signals with varying magnitude (Fig. 16-8). Note that two time measurements are required to obtain the information in Fig. 16-8. First, the elapsed time following the transmitted pulse assigns depth; each transmitted pulse contributes one data point to the QD signal at every depth segment. Second, intermittent sampling of the QD signal at a particular depth is achieved by a succession of transmitted pulses. Data points are separated by a time interval equal to the PRP.

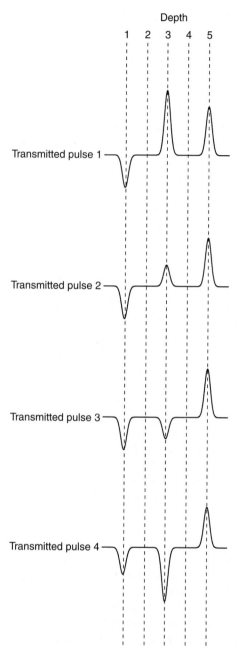

Depth
1 2 3 4 5

Transmitted pulse 1 ⸻

Transmitted pulse 2 ⸻

Transmitted pulse 3 ⸻

Transmitted pulse 4 ⸻

Fig. 16-6 Quadrature channel output from four successive pulses along the line of sight. Motion is detected by changes in the signal level at a particular time *(depth)*. The reflectors at depth segments 1 and 5 are stationary, while that at depth segment 3 is moving.

Autocorrelation is a comparison of measurements acquired from the same reflector. Processing of the echoes received from multiple depths is done concurrently. The stream of echoes along the entire scan line is examined by delaying the previous echo wavetrain obtained from the immediately preceding excitation pulse by a time equal to the PRP. This places the successive echo wavetrains on the same relative time scale, and thus reflector location is designated by the time interval following the transmitted pulse. Each echo wavetrain is divided into segments by depth.

At every location the individual echoes from consecutive samplings are multiplied together, and the product is

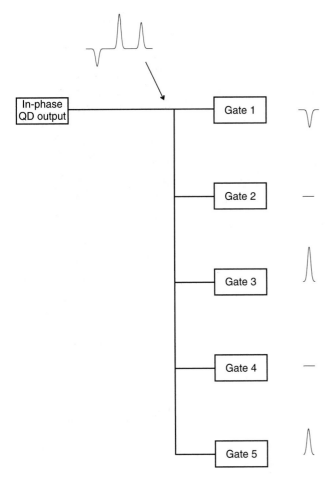

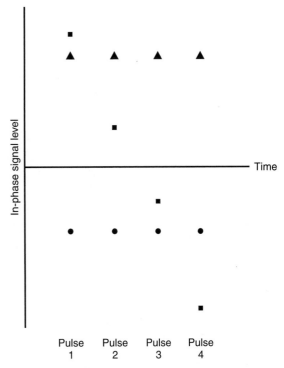

Fig. 16-8 Doppler signal generation from the quadrature detection output. Each data point for a depth segment requires one transmitted pulse. Reflectors in depth segment 1 *(triangles)*; reflectors in depth segment 3 *(squares)*; reflectors in depth segment 5 *(circles)*.

Fig. 16-7 Gating of the quadrature detection (QD) output allows the signal to be segmented according to depth. One QD channel output is shown.

added in the integrator to the values from other samplings (Fig. 16-9). Registers store the computational results while the data are accumulated for one line of sight.

Both channels of the QD circuit provide input to the autocorrelation detector. For each depth two separate registers hold the output from the autocorrelation detector. At the conclusion of sampling along the line of sight, velocity and phase are computed at each depth from the values stored in registers corresponding to that depth. The phase is equal to the arc tangent of the ratio of the output values, and the velocity is equal to the phase divided by the sampling time interval, the PRP. Variance can also be determined.

Dwell time. A minimum of three observations is required to determine the Doppler shift. Generally, each scan line is sampled 4 to 10 times, although it may be as many as 32 times. **Packet size** or ensemble length describes the number of pulses used to interrogate a single color line of sight. Large packet size (long integration time) provides the highest color definition (most accurate frequency estimates), but a long dwell time lowers the frame rate.

The dwell time for each color line using autocorrelation is now be examined. The frame rate is determined by

16-1

$$FR = \frac{1}{N \, n \, (PRP)}$$

where N is the number of scan lines per frame (lpf), and n is the packet size. For a scanning range of 8 cm (PRP of 104 μs) under the conditions of 15 fps and 64 lpf, 10 pulses are used to sample each line of sight. The dwell time is 1.04 ms. At a pulse repetition frequency (PRF) of 4 kHz or higher, autocorrelation provides rapid acquisition of the Doppler data to allow real-time imaging of the flow.

Fixed echo canceller. To lower the dynamic range of the QD input to the autocorrelation detector, strong echoes from stationary structures are often eliminated. Echoes from stationary reflectors remain unchanged in successive echo wavetrains; otherwise, varying echoes would be attributed to moving reflectors. Echoes from stationary reflectors are removed by subtracting identical echoes in consecutive pulses through the introduction of a **fixed echo canceller** (Figs. 16-10 and 16-11). The inability of mechanical transducers to generate an extremely stable beam path inhibits their use in CD imaging.

Velocity estimation. The autocorrelation detector does not depict spectral analysis of the Doppler signal from each sample volume but rather a **mean frequency estimate.** An average, not maximum, Doppler shift is determined. Although this is not ideal, a region with high mean velocity is likely to be a region with maximum velocity as well. The maximum Doppler shift could be presented, but this parameter is more sensitive to noise and spectral broadening.

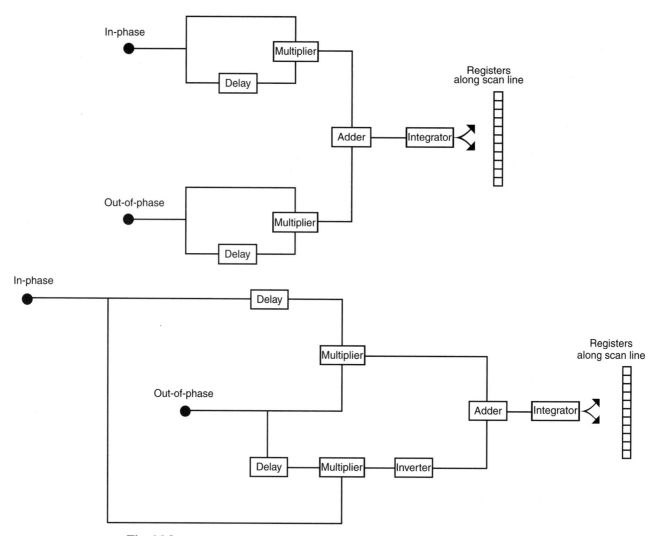

Fig. 16-9 Autocorrelation detector. The in-phase and out-of-phase quadrature detection signals from two consecutive transmitted pulses are segmented by depth and then manipulated in a series of multiplication and addition steps. An integrator sums the computational results at each depth from repeated samplings and stores them in registers.

CD imaging with autocorrelation is a PW technique that uses a relatively long pulse duration with a narrow bandwidth. Variance in the mean frequency estimate (spectral broadening) is increased when the pulse is shortened to improve axial resolution. Attenuation and diffraction of the ultrasound beam affect the velocity estimation, and the measured mean frequency of reflectors moving with the same velocity distribution is depth dependent. Attenuation selectively removes the higher frequency components of the Doppler signal.

Time Domain Correlation

Time domain correlation determines the velocity of a moving reflector by measuring the change in spatial location during a known time interval (Fig. 16-12). Successive echo wavetrains along a fixed line of sight reveal that the echo associated with a moving reflector is displaced in time (Fig. 16-13). Using the echo-ranging principle, time (Δt) is converted into distance (x) by assuming a value for the velocity of sound in the medium (c):

$$x = 1/2\ c\ (\Delta t) \qquad \text{16-2}$$

The parameter x is the distance that the reflector moves in the direction of the beam axis between transmitted pulses. Since the time between measurements is known (equal to the PRP), the velocity of the reflector (v_x) is calculated by

$$v_x = \frac{x}{PRP} \qquad \text{16-3}$$

Because sampling occurs along one direction only, Equation 16-3 yields the velocity component along the beam axis. The total reflector velocity (v) can be determined if the angle (φ) between the beam axis and the direction of motion (Doppler angle) is known:

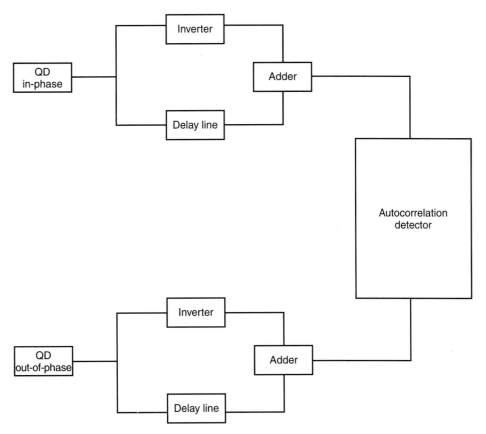

Fig. 16-10 Block diagram of the fixed echo canceller.

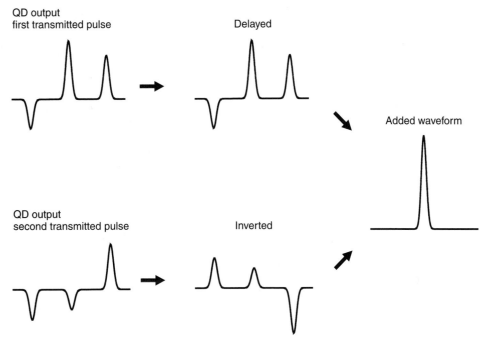

Fig. 16-11 Manipulation of echo wavetrains by the fixed echo canceller.

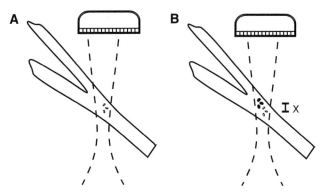

Fig. 16-12 Displacement of moving reflectors between samplings with pulsed-wave ultrasound. **A,** Location of red blood cells (RBCs) when interrogated by the initial transmitted pulse. **B,** After an elapsed time equal to the pulse repetition period, the RBCs have moved a distance *x* along the beam axis as detected by the succeeding transmitted pulse. The initial and final locations are designated by light and dark shading.

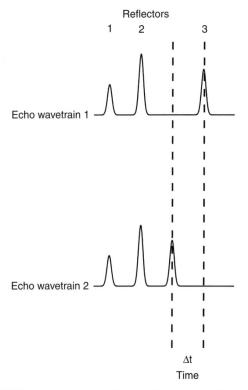

Fig. 16-13 Received echo signal level from three reflectors at different depths. Reflectors 1 and 2 are stationary. Reflector 3 moves during the time between transmitted pulses. The shift in time indicates the distance of movement.

16-4

$$v = \frac{x}{PRP \cos \varphi}$$

Echo pattern matching. The unique feature of time domain correlation is the ability to identify a particular echo signal waveform in multiple echo wavetrains consisting of many echoes and to track the individual echo signals in time. Echo pattern matching is achieved by searching for a time position with maximum correlation. The echo wavetrain is

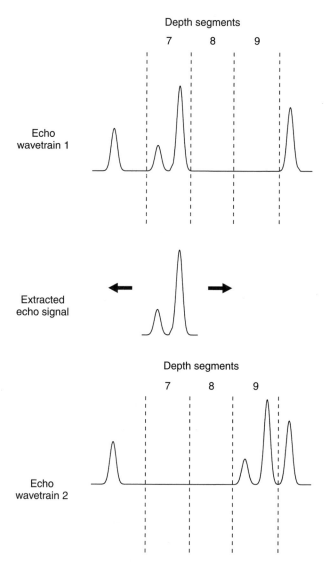

Fig. 16-14 Echo signal matching in time domain correlation. The extracted signal from segment 7 in the first echo wavetrain is compared with various segments of the second echo wavetrain. The best match occurs at segment 9.

segmented by depth, and the echo signal in each segment is extracted. A second echo wavetrain is acquired. Extracted echo signals in the first echo wavetrain are compared with echo signals at the corresponding depth and with signals at the neighboring segments in the second echo wavetrain until a match is found (Fig. 16-14). Moving reflectors are identified by a different depth assignment in the successive echo wavetrains. The time shift (Δt) between the two segments provides the measurement by which the reflector velocity can be determined.

Velocity detection limit. The time correlation function has one maximum; no ambiguity is present as occurs in PW Doppler when the phase shift exceeds one cycle (aliasing). Time shifts greater than the period of the radiofrequency signal can be measured. Consequently, the velocity limits imposed by time domain correlation are less restrictive than those with PW Doppler techniques. A velocity limit does arise, however, because the reflector must remain within the sampling volume during successive transmitted pulses.

The displacement for a reflector moving at a velocity of 1 m/s is 0.25 mm when the sampling rate is 4000 Hz. This distance is well within the spatial resolution of segmental divisions of the echo wavetrain. In PW Doppler the maximum velocity limit is 77 cm/s if the transducer is operating at a frequency of 2 MHz. A higher center frequency imposes a more severe restriction on the maximum detectable velocity.

For time domain correlation a broad-bandwidth transducer is used to shorten the pulse duration (similar to B-mode). The decreased spatial pulse length improves axial resolution of the color display. Pixels in gray scale and color are comparable in size.

Two-Dimensional Speckle Tracking

The speckle pattern produced by echoes from moving red blood cells (RBCs) is tracked in successive images (**speckle tracking**). The distance traveled in the acquisition interval between frames yields the velocity. Both axial and lateral components of the motion are determined. A 2D image of blood flow is constructed by tracking multiple regions within the FOV. The velocity for each region is color encoded and superimposed on the gray-scale image.

Tracking of the speckle pattern is accomplished by identifying a small region (called a kernel) in the first image and then searching the subsequent image for the matching region (Fig. 16-15). The search area in the second image is limited to a small region surrounding the kernel. The

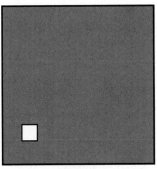

Image 1

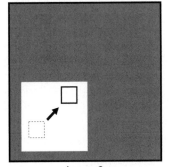

Image 2

Fig. 16-15 Speckle tracking. The reflectors producing the signal from a pixel in image 1 move from the original location *(dotted line)* to a new location *(solid line)* in image 2. The search area is denoted in white.

location of the match for the kernel indicates the distance moved by the RBCs in the time between frames.

Recent developments in computer technology have enabled speckle tracking to be performed in real time at a frame rate of 30 fps. Spatial resolution of the color-encoded velocity display is inferior to that in gray-scale images, because the pixel size is twice as large. The maximum detectable velocity is 1 to 2 m/s but, in theory, could be as high as 8 m/s.

The major advantage of speckle tracking is that an angle-independent color map of flow is produced. *Conventional color flow imaging, in which sampling is performed along one line of sight, provides mapping of only the axial component of motion.* Consequently, quantitative assessment of flow velocity is compromised, because the Doppler angle is not accurately known.

TYPES OF COLOR DOPPLER IMAGING DEVICES

CD imaging scanners are classified as **asynchronous** or **synchronous** based on how the scanner acquires the 2D gray-scale and velocity information. Asynchronous devices collect imaging and flow data at different times, whereas synchronous systems collect the two data sets simultaneously.

ASYNCHRONOUS COLOR DOPPLER IMAGING DEVICES

We can use a linear array to see how the 2D gray-scale and flow data are acquired separately and later superimposed to form the asynchronous image. The gray-scale image is obtained by generating sequential, dynamically focused beams along the length of the array. Parallel lines of sight compose the 2D gray-scale image, which allows for sampling perpendicular to the blood movement (the vessel is assumed to be parallel to the skin surface). This geometry is ideal for imaging but not for assessing flow (for which the interrogation angle would be 90 degrees). To place the beam at a more appropriate Doppler angle for measuring flow, it is steered at an angle to the array (Fig. 16-16). The beam angle is adjustable by the operator.

Separate, complete FOV sweeps for 2D gray-scale and flow imaging displace stationary tissue position and flow in time. Consequently, small groups of steered and unsteered lines of sight are alternated in a time-sharing scheme. These scan lines are interwoven in a digital scan converter to compose the final image (Fig. 16-17).

Fig. 16-18 diagrams an asynchronous autocorrelation system. Separate transmitters form either the steered or the unsteered beam. If the beam is steered, the induced signal is directed to the Doppler channel. Otherwise, the gray-scale channel is active. The image data are processed and sent to the scan converter. In the Doppler channel a quadrature detector coupled with autocorrelation quantifies forward and reverse flow signals, which are numerically encoded and placed in the scan converter. The numerical values in the scan converter are translated into gray and color levels before being displayed on the monitor.

The asynchronous autocorrelation scanner allows the transmitted beam to be optimized for both Doppler and 2D gray scale, because each component is collected independently of the other. The transducer frequency and transmit power may be adjusted for each component. Transmitted pulses can be switched between a gray-scale frequency of 5 MHz and a Doppler frequency of 3 MHz. The dual-frequency transducer entails some compromises: Sensitivity is reduced, and beam manipulation becomes more difficult as the frequency is offset from the center frequency. Although a narrow beam width is desirable for good lateral resolution in the 2D gray-scale mode, it causes spectral broadening in the Doppler mode. Transmitted power in the Doppler mode can be increased to improve detection of weak flow signals.

Because the FOV is scanned twice for each frame, the frame rate is reduced. Most of the acquisition time is

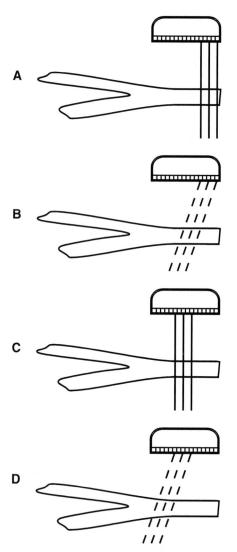

Fig. 16-17 Asynchronous linear array with time sharing. A small portion of the field of view (FOV) is sampled with gray-scale, **A**, and then color, **B**, lines of sight before the next section of the FOV is probed, **C** and **D**.

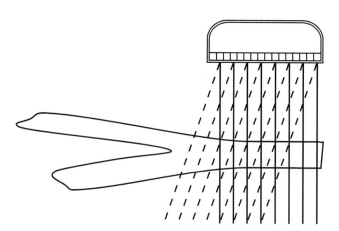

Fig. 16-16 Asynchronous linear array with gray-scale lines of sight *(solid)* and steered color lines of sight *(dotted)*.

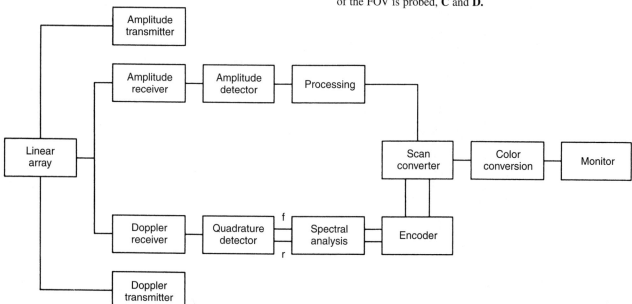

Fig. 16-18 Asynchronous autocorrelation scanner.

devoted to collecting the flow image. Only one pulse per scan line is required for the 2D gray-scale mode, although multiple pulses are necessary to compose a color line. To compensate partially for the longer acquisition time, fewer lines of sight, a smaller FOV, a higher-frequency threshold for the minimum displayed velocity, or a combination of these is used in the color mode (Figs. 16-19 and 16-20). Interpolating between lines fills in the gaps (spatial persistence). *The axial sampling interval for Doppler is*

usually greater (as much as several millimeters), which means that the Doppler and 2D gray-scale spatial resolution are not the same.

SYNCHRONOUS COLOR DOPPLER IMAGING DEVICES

In a synchronous autocorrelation scanner (Fig. 16-21), amplitude, phase, and frequency of the detected echo are

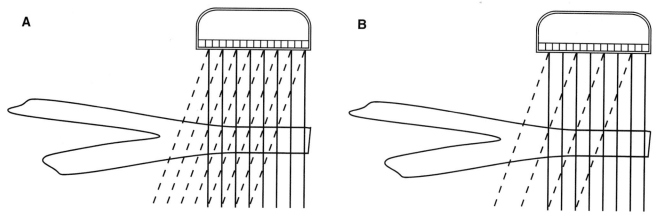

Fig. 16-19 Frame rate can be increased by reducing the color line density across the field of view. Color lines of sight are shown as dotted lines. **A,** High density. **B,** Low density.

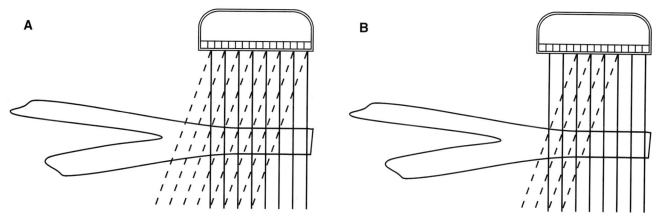

Fig. 16-20 Frame rate can be increased by reducing the width of the color field of view (FOV). Color lines of sight are shown as dotted lines. **A,** Wide FOV. **B,** Narrow FOV.

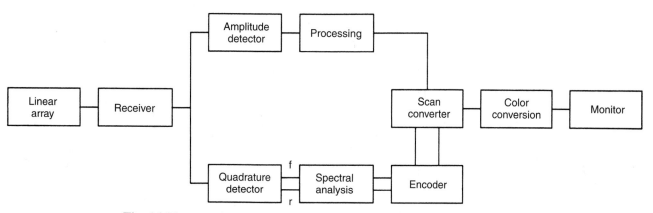

Fig. 16-21 Synchronous autocorrelation scanner.

analyzed simultaneously. After reception, the induced signal is divided into two parts and then processed separately for 2D gray-scale and flow information. Image manipulation and color encoding are similar to those described for the asynchronous scanner, the major distinctions being generation of the ultrasound beam and initial routing of the induced signals in the receiver circuit.

The synchronous scanner uses a linear array transducer to direct the transmitted beams perpendicular to the array. Electronic sweeping of the beam is avoided so that the intensity of side lobes is reduced. Each sampling site throughout the FOV, on a pixel-by-pixel basis, is evaluated for gray scale and color. Sampling interval is typically one wavelength in length (0.3 mm at 5 MHz). The FOV and spatial resolution are the same for both gray scale and Doppler.

A suitable Doppler angle is necessary for the detection of flow. If the direction of flow is perpendicular to the transducer line of sight, flow will not be visualized. A mechanical standoff wedge can be used with linear arrays to change the relative orientation of the moving reflectors so an adequate Doppler angle is achieved. The fluid-filled wedge should not attenuate the ultrasound beam nor change the focusing characteristics of the beam, but be relatively echo free. The standoff wedge lowers the PRF, because the path length is increased. Some systems can alter beam steering and permit the operator to select the insonation angle.

Because the transmitted beam is used for both the 2D gray-scale and Doppler modes, the optimum pulse length and other beam characteristics are sacrificed. High-frame rates are possible, however, because 2D gray-scale and flow information is collected concurrently.

COLOR DOPPLER PARAMETERS

Commercially available CD instruments have multiple controls that affect the color image. These operator-adjustable parameters contribute markedly to the overall complexity of CD imaging. Fortunately, many of the controls have a function similar to that described for CW and PW Doppler. The terminology used to label the controls has not become standardized, however, and each manufacturer has adopted its own set of descriptors.

Autocorrelation Scanners

Echoes from blood are weak compared with echoes from tissue. This property (in the form of signal amplitude) is evaluated using an echo-versus-color threshold to differentiate flow from moving tissue. Strong reflections that exceed the threshold value are assigned a gray level. Weak echoes from tissue are sometimes depicted in color at low gain settings. Proper gray-scale gain creates an image in which tissue is free of color. Excessive gray-scale gain can suppress color within the vessel and mask the flow.

The **velocity scale** specifies the range of velocities that are presented in the color display. The PRF is set by the velocity scale and the depth of scanning. For applications

in peripheral vascular imaging, in which a low-velocity flow is encountered, decreasing the PRF lowers the maximum detectable velocity and improves the velocity resolution. Some manufacturers alter the transducer frequency in response to a shift in velocity scale.

The center of the velocity scale is initially set at zero so the magnitude limits for forward and reverse flow are equal. The **baseline control** shifts the center of the velocity scale up or down to display a greater range of velocities in one direction. The total velocity range is unchanged. For example, if the initial velocity range was −0.5 to 0.5 m/s, an adjustment in baseline could establish a new velocity range as −0.2 to 0.8 m/s. (Higher velocities in the forward direction are displayed without aliasing.)

Color gain is the amplification applied to the Doppler component during signal processing. High color gain increases the system's sensitivity for color and expands the number of pixels encoded with color.

The **color gate** adjusts the axial length of the Doppler sampling volume. Increasing the color gate enlarges the region from which PW Doppler signals are examined. The ability to separate flow and nonflow is improved but with a sacrifice in spatial resolution. The sampling interval can extend several millimeters. The pixel size encoded with color may not be identical to the gray-scale pixel size.

Color reject sets the threshold below which weak flow signals are not included in the color display. The basis for rejection is the amplitude and not the frequency of the Doppler signal. This is a noise-reduction technique. Lowering the threshold increases the amount of color within the image. In the asynchronous autocorrelation scanner, color reject is independent of gray-scale gain and time gain compensation.

For asynchronous autocorrelation scanners, the region of interest selected by the operator controls which portion of the gray-scale image will be subjected to CD analysis. The width of the color region has a considerable impact on frame rate. The dwell time for a color line is long, because multiple pulse repetitions are required for the Doppler analysis (denoted by packet size). *In general, as the color FOV is expanded, more lines of sight are necessary, and the frame rate is reduced.* Many scanners, however, automatically adjust packet size and line density as a function of field width to optimize the frame rate for a particular application.

Color persistence is a temporal smoothing technique to reduce noise. Images are displayed at a rapid rate (e.g., 30 fps). By combining previous frames with the most recently acquired frame, the color in the displayed image is averaged. The time interval of the averaging is controlled by the number of frames added together. Color persistence may enhance regions with a low-velocity flow.

A **color map,** similar to a gray-scale map in real-time imaging, assigns flow velocities to various color shades. The "blue away, red toward" (BART) and "red away, blue toward" (RABT) formats use color saturation to code for velocity. Deep shades represent low velocities, and light shades high velocities. Maps consisting of rainbow-colored hues also encode flow information. Red progressing to yellow allows rapid flow in opposite directions to be more easily differentiated.

The **velocity tag** function emphasizes a selected range of velocities by highlighting regions of flow within this range with a contrasting color (usually green or white). The color bar adjacent to the displayed image indicates (with the same contrasting color) that portion of the velocity scale selected for tagging.

The color image is not limited to a display of mean velocity, however. Additional information (e.g., the spread of velocities within a sampled region) can also be depicted. The **variance** is a statistical measure of the velocity distribution within each sampled volume. Regions with plug flow demonstrate little spread, whereas those with laminar flow exhibit more variation. The turbulence or variance map provides a means of displaying the spatial variance.

The **capture function** displays the highest mean velocity detected at each pixel during an elongated acquisition time (1 to several seconds). Each small region within the FOV is scanned repeatedly for moving reflectors. On the first pass, if motion is detected at a particular point, the color level associated with the mean velocity is displayed on the monitor. This initial color level remains until replaced by a new value. As the data collection continues, measurements may yield a subsequent velocity of greater magnitude at a particular point. The color level associated with this velocity replaces the existing color level on the monitor. Low-velocity color levels are discarded. Thus an image is built up in which the maximum mean velocity detected at each pixel is displayed. For vessels with intermittent Doppler signals, the capture function is useful in defining whether flow extends to the wall of the vessel.

As the angle of insonation relative to the vessel segment approaches 90 degrees, low-frequency Doppler shifts are generated that may not be depicted in the image. When a steered beam collects the Doppler signal, the angle of insonation can be selected to provide a more favorable geometry between the direction of flow and the ultrasound beam.

Time Domain Correlation

Color flow imagers based on the time domain correlation principle use many of the same controls as described for autocorrelation scanners. These include transmit power, color map, velocity scale, baseline adjustment, velocity tag, color persistence (enhance), capture function (quantify), restrictive color FOV, and beam insonation angle.

A flow-angle marker establishes the direction of flow relative to the beam axis. By correcting for insonation angle, the velocity scale indicates the absolute velocity of reflectors. If multiple vessels are present within the FOV or the vessel is tortuous, the color-coded velocity may not be correct. The magnitude of the velocity scale is adjusted by altering the PRF. Operation in slow flow mode is susceptible to color flash, since sensitivity for motion is maximized.

Frame rate is adjusted by changing the width of the color FOV and by selecting the appropriate resolution versus speed setting. The latter control increases the frame rate by reducing the line density. Decreasing the depth of the color FOV typically does not alter the frame rate.

Thresholding designates the low velocity cutoff. Measured velocities below the threshold value are not displayed. Color noise, in which weak stationary reflectors are depicted with color, occurs if the threshold is set too low.

COMBINED DOPPLER MODE

Regardless of the velocity-detection method, a 2D mapping of flow within the FOV is produced. In the CD image a single parameter, usually the mean velocity, is represented by the variation in color. A more detailed presentation of the distribution of the velocity profile requires an FFT time-dependent power spectrum. The **combined Doppler mode** displays the CD image and the Doppler spectral analysis (Fig. 16-22). Since the beam must be shared between gray scale, color Doppler, and PW Doppler, the refresh rate of the color image is slowed to a new frame every 1 to 5 seconds.

To obtain information regarding the individual velocity components, range-gated PW Doppler with FFT analysis is performed for selected regions of interest. A specific sampling volume for spectral analysis is identified on the CD image. Since areas with abnormal flow pattern are rapidly identified, CD imaging reduces examination time by facilitating placement of the sampling volume for FFT analysis.

Spectral invert displays the negative velocity components in the power spectrum above the baseline. Spectral smoothing averages information along the velocity or time axes. Smoothing is a technique to reduce rapid fluctuations in the displayed spectrum. Smoothing in time is accomplished by combining the results of the most recent FFT analysis with the preceding power spectra. The smoothing effect is enhanced by increasing the number of power spectra added together. Smoothing in velocity averages the magnitudes of adjacent Doppler shifts.

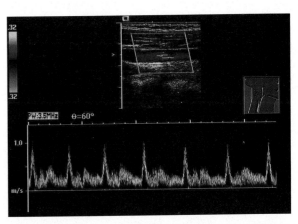

Fig. 16-22 Combined Doppler mode. The color Doppler image with the sampled region identified is shown with the Doppler spectral analysis. (See Color Plate 6.)

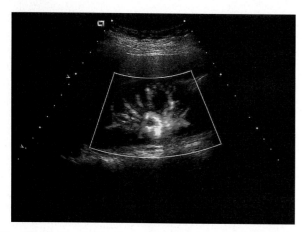

Fig. 16-23 Power Doppler image of the kidney. (See Color Plate 7.)

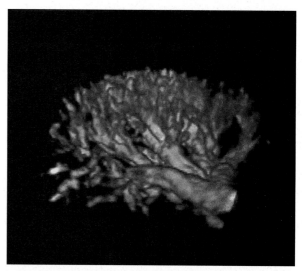

Fig. 16-24 Three-dimensional power Doppler image of the kidney. (See Color Plate 8.) (Courtesy Siemens Medical Solutions USA, Inc., Ultrasound Division, Malvern, Penn.)

POWER DOPPLER

Power Doppler imaging (also called energy mode Doppler imaging) portrays the intensity (amplitude) of the Doppler signal without an indication of the velocity (Fig. 16-23). The signal intensity depends on the number of RBCs within the sampled volume and the attenuation of the intervening tissue. Power Doppler emphasizes the quantity of blood flow. The autocorrelation detector to estimate flow velocity can also yield the total power of the Doppler signal. Consequently, on many scanners the operator can switch easily from velocity mode to power mode.

Because all phase shifts (moving reflectors) contribute to the amplitude signal, Doppler imaging is essentially nondirectional and therefore not subject to aliasing. However, the color coding does not indicate the velocity or direction of flow; pulsatility and flow reversal cannot be evaluated. This flow information must be obtained from the CD image. The total power Doppler signal is less dependent than color Doppler on the insonation angle.

Vessel wall definition is usually improved with power Doppler imaging. Compare the relative signals arising from a sampling volume near the vessel wall with one partially overlapping the vessel wall. For velocity measurements the frequency shift will be small, because both sampling volumes contain moving RBCs. The color mapping will display the pixels in similar shades. However, for the amplitude measurements, the total number of RBCs is very different, creating a much lower signal for the sampling volume that includes the vessel wall.

The major advantage of power Doppler imaging is the ability to differentiate between regions with flow and no flow. This is usually described as increased sensitivity to depict small vessels in color, which is derived from expanded dynamic range to extend the color priority to weaker signals. Increased persistence is also employed to image flow in small vessels. Tissue motion (e.g., heart) often creates flash artifacts, which limits the applicability of this imaging mode to regions where tissue motion is more subdued.

Power Doppler flow information is used in conjunction with extended FOV imaging and three-dimensional (3D) imaging. Regions of flow are color encoded and superimposed on the 2D or 3D gray-scale presentation of anatomy. The 3D display formats include multiplanar, polyhedron, and volume rendering. The vasculature of the organ or structure of interest including liver, kidney, uterine fibroid, and fetal lung is portrayed (Fig. 16-24).

The characteristics of Power Doppler imaging are summarized in Table 16-1.

■ **Table 16-1**　Characteristics of Power Doppler Imaging

Advantages	Disadvantages
Visualization of flow in small vessels	Motion artifacts
Independent of flow direction	No velocity information
Independent of velocity	No directional information
Reduced angle dependence	Low temporal resolution
No aliasing	Qualitative observations
Good lumen definition	

DOPPLER TISSUE IMAGING

In CD imaging a threshold is set that rejects strong echoes from moving reflectors with the assumption that echoes of this magnitude must originate from tissue and not flowing blood. Only weak echoes from moving reflectors are processed and displayed as color. Doppler tissue imaging reverses the selection process so that only strong echoes from moving reflectors are processed and displayed as color. In this way a color image of tissue motion is portrayed.

COLOR DOPPLER IMAGE QUALITY

CD image quality is characterized by four factors: **motion discrimination,** temporal resolution, spatial resolution, and uniformity. The term *color sensitivity* has also been applied to describe this collection of factors.

Color is associated with movement, but it does not necessarily indicate flow. Movement of the transducer, peristaltic motion, and cardiac motion all may contribute spurious color to the image and give an artifactual impression of flow. The ability to distinguish moving blood from moving tissue and at the same time depict subtle flow patterns is the ultimate goal. Low-frequency shifts from slowly moving tissue are selectively removed with a wall filter. Various filters are used depending on the application. Often the PRF is adjusted automatically to be as high as possible for the depth of interrogation. The wall filter is altered in conjunction with this change in PRF. Unfortunately, this technique is not completely effective in eliminating high-amplitude, low-frequency Doppler shifts associated with vessel wall movement. Also, this high-pass filter excludes low-velocity flow components. To better differentiate flowing blood from stationary fluid and moving soft tissue, the amplitude and the Doppler shift are examined. Weak reflections are associated with blood and other fluids. Gray-scale values are assigned to strong echoes. An alternative method called multivariate motion discrimination evaluates several parameters of the motion (not only velocity and amplitude) to ascertain whether the motion is characteristic of tissue or flowing blood.

Flow hemodynamics varies throughout the cardiac cycle. The ability to detect changing flow patterns depends on the frame rate. Temporal resolution is improved as the frame rate is increased. A high frame rate is achieved by reducing the number of color scan lines, the lateral extent of the color FOV, the dwell time, or a combination of these.

Spatial resolution characterizes a scanner's ability to depict small structures at the proper location. The axial dimension of the Doppler sampling volume is defined by the sampling time interval (color gate). The out-of-plane dimension (slice thickness) is determined by the beam size along that direction. The beam width and scan line density affect the lateral resolution. As the interrogated volume is reduced in size, weaker-amplitude signals that are less likely to be encoded in color are generated (lower signal-to-noise ratio). The precision of the Doppler shift measurement also deteriorates. Spatial filtering is a technique to diminish random color variations throughout the image. Pixels are encoded in color only if they neighbor other pixels previously encoded in color. Small vessels with weak flow must be visualized with the spatial filter off. Another type of spatial filtering (sharp/smooth processing) manipulates the presentation of the boundary between color and gray-scale pixels.

Generally, real-time imaging provides superior gray-scale spatial and temporal resolution compared with CD imaging. The CD temporal and frequency resolution of the Doppler shifts is less than that obtained by spectral analysis in which the sampling time is typically 8 to 15 ms with 60 to 125 Hz frequency resolution.

Uniformity implies that vessels with identical properties are depicted in a similar manner regardless of their respective locations within the FOV; that is, vessel size and color pattern should not be altered by a change in position.

Dynamic focusing enables pixels of constant size to be portrayed throughout the FOV. Pixel size for color Doppler and 2D gray-scale modes may not be the same, however.

COLOR DOPPLER ARTIFACTS

Specific artifacts for the various scanning modes have been considered in other chapters—real-time imaging artifacts in Chapter 12 and aliasing and spectral broadening for PW Doppler in Chapter 15. The subject of imaging artifacts with color Doppler is now considered.

Because color Doppler imaging is a portrayal of the Doppler shifts in two dimensions, artifacts identified with imaging and PW Doppler are also possible in the color presentation. These potential artifacts include shadowing, reverberation, mirror image, misregistration from grating lobes, depth ambiguity, and aliasing. In addition, artifacts such as color bleed, color flash, and color noise are unique to CD imaging.

Echo Mapping

Enhanced attenuation by overlying solid structures may cause no color to be displayed within the vessel although flow is present. In Fig. 16-25, shadowing by a calcified plaque masks flow through the vessel.

When an anechoic wedge is used with a synchronous linear array to provide a more favorable angle of insonation, multiple reflections from interfaces formed by the wedge may introduce reverberation artifacts. Steering the asynchronous linear array to improve the Doppler angle increases the number and intensity of the grating lobes, which can cause misregistration of interfaces.

Under conditions of high PRF, high gain, and low transmitter frequency, deep Doppler shifts may be depicted in a more superficial location. This depth ambiguity occurs because echoes originating beyond the set scanning depth are detected after the next pulse has been emitted. Flow can be portrayed in a region where no flow actually exists. Clinically this is not a common problem (except in cardiac scanning), because attenuation reduces the echo amplitudes

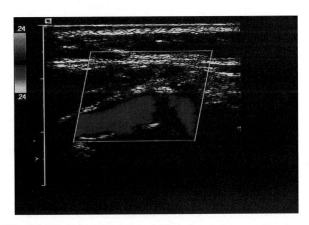

Fig. 16-25 Shadowing by a calcified plaque obscures flow in the common carotid artery. (See Color Plate 9.)

from deep-lying reflectors and allows the color reject to exclude these signals from color encoding.

Aliasing

Because moving reflectors are sampled intermittently along the color line of sight, aliasing occurs if the flow exceeds the velocity range set by the operator. A high-frequency shift above the Nyquist limit, but less than twice the Nyquist limit, is detected as a low-frequency shift with opposite phase. The reversal in phase is interpreted as flow in the opposite direction, and thus a color change is induced. Often, aliasing is readily identified as an inappropriate color progression in which a pale shade of red or blue is surrounded by a light shade of the contrasting color, or, in the case of the rainbow color map, contrasting colors representing maximum flow in opposite directions are contiguous (Fig. 16-26). At a very high velocity (i.e., greater than twice the Nyquist limit) flow is depicted incorrectly, with a low-velocity color level in the correct direction.

Aliasing is reduced by increasing the Doppler angle, decreasing the frequency of the transmitted pulse, expanding the velocity scale, or shortening the scanning depth (Fig. 16-27). The latter two techniques act to raise the PRF.

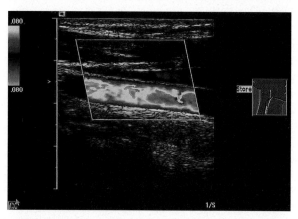

Fig. 16-26 Color Doppler aliasing. See Color Plate 10 to note the improper color progression—red to yellow to green to blue. If reverse flow were present, red and blue would be separated by a black region. (See Color Plate 10.)

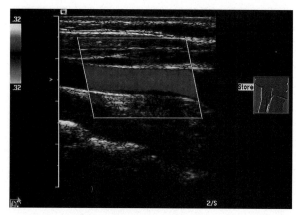

Fig. 16-27 Increasing the velocity range removes the aliasing artifact in Fig. 16-26. (See Color Plate 11.)

Incorrect Velocity Assignment in Time Domain Correlation

Time domain processing depends on the fidelity of echo pattern matching to determine the spatial shift in echo origin between transmitted pulses and ultimately the velocity of flow. The echo signature of the group of RBCs is unique, and a match should be obtained only at the new translated location and nowhere else. Unfortunately, the echo signals are weak and have high noise content, which corrupts the matching algorithm. Often, a region near the transducer is improperly matched with the echo pattern from the RBCs. When this occurs the incorrect velocity is assigned based on the perceived displacement associated with this RBC group (Fig. 16-28).

Multiple-Angle Artifact

A sector transducer interrogates a linear segment of a vessel oriented parallel to the skin surface with a variable angle of insonation (Fig. 16-29). The angle is greatest in the center of the FOV and decreases toward the periphery. Progressing across the FOV, a vessel with constant flow is depicted first by color in the reverse direction, then with no color, and finally by color in the forward direction (Fig. 16-30).

Comparatively, a linear array with a constant angle of insonation demonstrates uniform color throughout the FOV. Power Doppler imaging, because of its independence with respect to insonation angle, is not susceptible to this artifact (Fig. 16-31 and Color Plate 13).

Nonuniform angle of insonation can also occur when a tortuous vessel is imaged with a linear array transducer. An apparent velocity deviation at the bend of the vessel is attributed to a change in Doppler angle (Fig. 16-32).

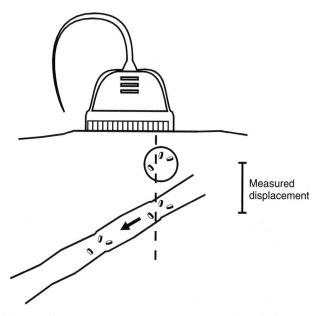

Fig. 16-28 If the echo pattern from red blood cells is incorrectly matched to a region outside the vessel near the transducer, then improper velocity is assigned based on the perceived displacement.

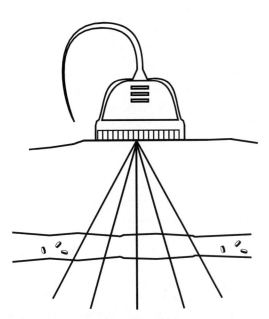

Fig. 16-29 A steered beam from a linear phased array interrogates the vessel at different insonation angles.

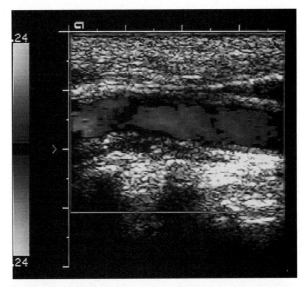

Fig. 16-32 A tortuous vessel with unidirectional flow is depicted in changing colors, which suggests a reversal of flow. (See Color Plate 14.)

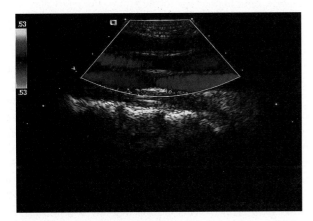

Fig. 16-30 Color Doppler image of two vessels acquired with a vector transducer. (See Color Plate 12.)

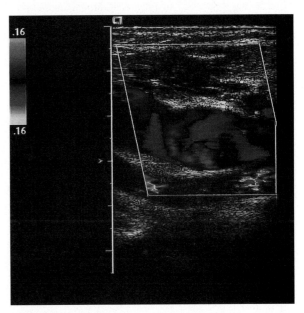

Fig. 16-33 Flow reversal. (See Color Plate 15.)

Flow reversal must be distinguished from aliasing and multiple-angle artifact. The color filter removes low-frequency Doppler signals, thereby setting a velocity threshold below which color is not assigned to the image. Flow reversal is characterized as a black region separating areas with different-color, low-velocity directions (Fig. 16-33).

Mirror Image Artifact

A mirror image of the color flow is produced when the vessel is in front of a highly reflective interface, resulting in color encoding at the wrong location. This type of artifact is also called ghosting. Spectral analyses of the real and virtual images are identical. For example, the lung acts as a strong reflector to form a mirror image of the subclavian

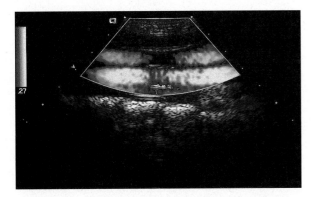

Fig. 16-31 Power Doppler image of two vessels acquired with a vector transducer. (See Color Plate 13.)

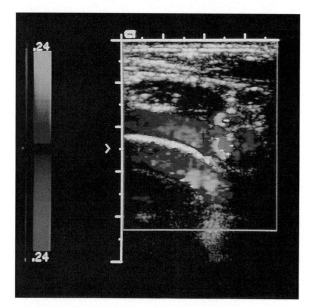

Fig. 16-34 Color Doppler mirror image artifact of the subclavian artery. (See Color Plate 16.) (Courtesy Rob Steins.)

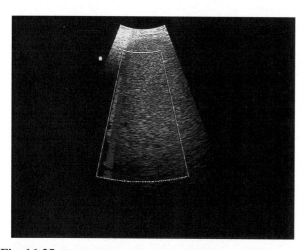

Fig. 16-35 Flash artifact. Color is improperly assigned to stationary tissue (phantom material) caused by movement of the transducer. (See Color Plate 17.)

artery (Fig. 16-34). Mirror images of the carotid and brachial arteries also can occur. Reducing the power, decreasing the color gain, changing the angle of insonation, or a combination of these eliminates this artifact.

Misregistration of Color

The flash artifact is a sudden burst of color that encompasses a wide region within the frame. The improper assignment of color is caused by movement of the transducer or tissue (Fig. 16-35). Cardiac motion, general pulsatility of the arteries, and respiratory movements are all responsible for a change in interface position, which is color encoded. The flash artifact is suppressed by increasing the color filter, decreasing the persistence, and reducing the width of the color FOV. Increasing the color filter removes a greater amount of low-velocity components associated with these

motions. On a more limited basis, tissue movements are conveyed to nonvascular structures with low echogenicity, which are color encoded. Motion discriminators are less effective when the returning echoes are weak. Flow within dilated bile ducts, cysts, or the gallbladder may be incorrectly assigned. Doppler spectral analysis is necessary to distinguish these from flow areas.

Color Bleed

Color bleed is the extension of color beyond the region of flow to the adjacent tissue. This artifact is eliminated by decreasing the transmit power and color gain.

Color Noise

Induced signal amplitude is often used to suppress color. Strong echoes are assigned a gray-scale value, but weak echoes are permitted a color assignment if other criteria are met (i.e., Doppler shift). If Doppler gain is set too high or the Doppler reject is set too low, random variations in echo measurements cause hypoechoic regions to fill with color. Fluid collections or thrombosed vessels may be color encoded by this color noise. Color noise can be differentiated from flow by spectral analysis.

Color Bruit

A bruit is a low- to high-pitched squirting sound caused by severe stenosis of the vessel (usually between 60% and 95% stenosis). The sound occurs during systole and can be auscultated with a stethoscope. The strong vibrations are radiated into the surrounding tissues, which are encoded in color. These color disturbances around the vessel are centered at the stenotic source of the bruit. The color bruit in the Doppler image provides a valuable diagnostic tool for the location of the stenotic area and for identification of the involved vessel. Decreasing the low velocity setting enhances the color disturbance caused by the bruit. Many sonographers classify the color bruit as an artifact, but Doppler imaging in this case does accurately detect tissue motion.

CLINICAL APPLICATIONS OF COLOR-FLOW IMAGING

The presence of flow, direction of flow, characteristics of flow, and existence of focal differences in velocity within the vessel are all assessed by CD imaging. Specific clinical applications are listed in Box 16-1. For cardiac applications, temporal resolution is essential. To achieve high frame rates, the sonographer needs to minimize the FOV width, scanning depth, and line density. Often, when a larger FOV is selected, line density is adjusted automatically to maintain a high frame rate. Slow flow in peripheral vessels is analyzed by a low PRF, long dwell time, and low wall filter setting. The Doppler transmit frequency influences the limit for the lowest velocity that can be detected. High frequency reduces the low-velocity limit. Under the same conditions the low-

Box 16-1 Clinical Applications of Doppler Imaging

Diagnosis of vascular stenosis
Portrayal of small vessel flow
Visualization of organ perfusion
Tumor vascularity
Detection of extravascular flow
Examination of large vascular territories
Imaging of the heart

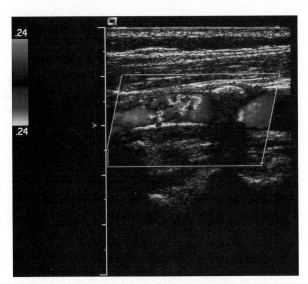

Fig. 16-36 In this color flow image the internal carotid shows turbulence distal to the stenosis. (See Color Plate 18.)

Table 16-2 Characteristics of Color Doppler Imaging

Advantages	Disadvantages
Spatial display of blood flow	Aliasing
Global overview of flow	Motion artifacts
Real-time frame rates (10 frames per second)	Limited frame rate
	Mean velocity displayed
More sensitive than B-mode to show flow in vessels	Accuracy of velocity limited by sampling time
Guides placement of pulsed wave sampling volume	Low-density scan lines or limited field of view
	Poor lumen definition
	Qualitative observations

not include the correction for Doppler angle. Short pulses optimized for gray-scale imaging are interspersed with longer pulses that provide Doppler information. The pulsing sequence and extensive computations limit the frame rate. A wide dynamic range of greater than 110 dB is necessary in the receiver circuit to accommodate both the echoes and the Doppler signals.

The color encoding is not a sensitive indicator of velocity variation. Color assignment is based on the direction of flow but can be reversed. The direction of flow in the vessel of interest should be established by the orientation of the vessel with respect to the transducer or by reference to another vessel of known origin.

The presence of gas also produces color artifacts, because the velocity of sound in air is not the same as in tissue. The highly focused beam is readily attenuated by a calcified plaque. Shadowing obscures the lumen of the artery and gives the impression of an absence of flow. Vessel tortuosity, poor scanning technique, and weak Doppler signal may also cause flow not to be visualized in an image.

SUMMARY

Color flow imaging combines gray-scale imaging with 2D mapping of flow velocity in real time. Motion is depicted throughout the FOV by color encoding the flow information. In color flow imaging the mean velocity at each sampling site is depicted by hue or intensity of color. In power Doppler imaging the signal strength of moving reflectors at each sampling site is encoded by color. Regional flow patterns within the color FOV are portrayed.

Two detection methods are used in Doppler imaging. Autocorrelation is based on frequency differences and intercompares successive echo wavetrains to compute the flow components. Time domain correlation is a measurement technique in which the distance moved by a reflector between samplings yields the velocity directly. Improved color spatial resolution and reduced susceptibility to aliasing artifacts are attractive features of time domain correlation.

The distribution of velocity components is not available from autocorrelation and time domain correlation and must be obtained by another method, such as FFT spectral analysis.

velocity limit is 15 cm/s and 6 cm/s for 3 MHz and 7.5 MHz, respectively. Deep slow flow in the abdomen requires a low frequency to penetrate tissue and a narrow FOV to counteract the effect of a long dwell time and low PRF on the frame rate.

The major advantage of CD imaging is that the pattern of flow throughout the vessel within the FOV is visualized instantaneously as the hemodynamics change during the cardiac cycle (Fig. 16-36). Vessels too small to be discerned with real-time gray-scale imaging are located with CD imaging. Improved ease of vessel identification allows for examination of large vascular territories. In addition, vascular and nonvascular structures are more readily differentiated. Determination of the presence or absence of flow in peripheral vessels is also enhanced.

COLOR DOPPLER LIMITATIONS

The rapid acceptance of CD imaging indicates that this scanning technique has unique applicability in the clinical environment. Nevertheless, CD imaging is not without limitations, many of which have been discussed previously. The characteristics of color Doppler imaging are summarized in Table 16-2.

Color coding is based on the average, rather than the peak, Doppler shift. Measurement of peak velocity from the CD image is not appropriate. Velocity estimates do

Motion discrimination, temporal resolution, spatial resolution, and uniformity all contribute to overall image quality. Numerous controls including gray-scale gain, packet size, color gate, color gain, color reject, velocity map, velocity tag, and capture function are available to manipulate the collection and processing of the CD data.

Potential artifacts associated with 2D Doppler imaging include shadowing, reverberation, mirror image, misregistration from grating lobes, depth ambiguity, and aliasing. Color bleed, color flash, and color noise describe the incorrect assignment of color to tissue.

REVIEW QUESTIONS

1. What term describes the number of pulses that interrogate a color line of sight?
2. To acquire the phase shift information rapidly, color Doppler imaging uses an _____ detector.
3. What is the purpose of the fixed echo canceller?
4. What method measures velocity of a moving reflector by detecting a time shift in the echo signals from successive echo wavetrains?
5. Name several characteristics of the asynchronous scanner.
6. What are the advantages of the synchronous scanner?
7. Which Doppler imaging method is the least susceptible to aliasing artifacts?
8. What flow parameter is typically encoded by the color scale in color Doppler imaging?
9. What flow parameter is typically encoded by the color scale in power Doppler imaging?
10. The axial length of the Doppler sampling volume is set by which control?
11. What control shifts the center of the velocity scale to display a greater range of velocities in one direction?
12. In color Doppler imaging what adjustment is made to improve the velocity estimates of the moving reflectors?
13. What adjustments are made in color Doppler imaging to increase the frame rate?
14. Name four color Doppler imaging artifacts.

BIBLIOGRAPHY

Barber WD, Eberhard JW, Karr SG: A new time domain technique for velocity measurements using Doppler ultrasound, *IEEE Trans Biomed Eng* 32:213-229, 1985.

Bohs LN et al: Real-time system for angle-independent ultrasound of blood flow in two dimensions: initial results, *Radiology* 186:259-261, 1993.

Bonnefous O, Pesque P: Time domain formulation of pulse-Doppler ultrasound and blood velocity estimation by cross correlation, *Ultrason Imaging* 8:73-85, 1986.

Boote EJ: Doppler ultrasound techniques: Concepts of blood flow detection and flow dynamics, *Radiographics* 23:1315-1327, 2003.

Foley WD, Erickson SJ: Color Doppler flow imaging, *AJR Am J Roentgenol* 156:3-13, 1991.

Forsberg F: Principles of Doppler imaging. In Goldman LW, Fowlkes JB, eds: *Categorical course in diagnostic radiology physics: CT and US cross-sectional imaging,* Oak Brook, Ill, 2000, Radiological Society of North America.

Hoeks APG et al: A novel frequency estimator for sampled Doppler signals, *IEEE Trans Biomed Eng* 31:212-220, 1984.

Kasai C et al: Real time two-dimensional blood flow imaging using an autocorrelation technique, *IEEE Trans Son Ultrason* 32:458-464, 1985.

Kremkau FW: Doppler principles, *Semin Roentgenol* 27:6-16, 1992.

Loupas T, McDicken WN: Low-order complex AR models for mean and maximum frequency estimation in the context of Doppler color flow mapping, *IEEE Trans Ultrason Ferroelectr Frequency Control* 37:590-601, 1990.

Merritt CRB: Doppler color flow imaging, *J Clin Ultrasound* 15:591-597, 1987.

Mitchell DG: Color Doppler imaging: principles, limitations, and artifacts, *Radiology* 177:1-10, 1990.

Powis RL: Color flow imaging, *Radiographics* 14:415-428, 1994.

Smith H, Zagzebski J: *Basic Doppler physics,* Madison, Wisc, 1991, Medical Physics Publishing.

Taylor KJW, Burns PN, Wells PNT: *Clinical applications of Doppler ultrasound,* New York, 1988, Raven Press.

Wells PNT: Doppler ultrasound in medical diagnosis, *Br J Radiol* 62:399-420, 1989.

Zweibel WJ: Color-encoded blood flow imaging, *Semin Ultrasound CT MR* 9:320-325, 1988.

Zweibel WJ: Color duplex imaging and Doppler spectrum analysis: principle, capabilities, and limitations, *Semin Ultrasound CT MR* 11:84-96, 1990.

M-Mode Scanning

The first motion-detection device used in diagnostic ultrasound was the **M-mode** (or motion-mode) **scanner.** It emphasized the movement of interfaces, including velocity, amplitude, and pattern of motion. Also called **time-motion (TM)** or **position-motion (PM) mode,** it was first used to interrogate the mitral valve in cardiac ultrasonography.

EFFECT OF MOTION

For nonstationary interfaces the A-mode spike moves back and forth on the display, showing the changing position of the interface. The fidelity of the motion depicted depends on the pulse repetition frequency. Because most A-mode scanners are pulsed at least 1000 times per second, the motion appears continuous. The display can be recorded on videotape for viewing. Hard copy film imaging, however, is not practical, because the moving spike is frozen in one position, and the effect of motion is lost. This limits the usefulness of one-dimensional A-mode imaging for detecting motion.

Motion of interfaces during two-dimensional (2D) static B-mode scanning poses similar problems. Blurred borders around the moving interface are produced in the image. Each line of sight registers the interface at a particular position, but the interrogation of the interface from multiple lines of sight separated in time places the interface at different locations. Static B-mode imaging is not useful for detecting motion because of the poor temporal resolution.

B-mode scanning allows the depiction of moving structures, but the sampling rate must be fast compared with the motion. Temporal resolution describes the ability to image the motion dynamics with fidelity. The interdependence of frame rate, field of view, and scan line density have been discussed previously. In spite of all its advantages, B-mode scanning does not readily allow quantitative analysis of the motion. For that application M-mode scanning excels.

DATA ACQUISITION

The spatial locations of interfaces along one line of sight are combined with the dimension of time to form a 2D recording called an M-mode trace. In this scanning technique data are collected along one line of sight only (similar to A-mode), and therefore no registration arm is required (Fig. 17-1). The

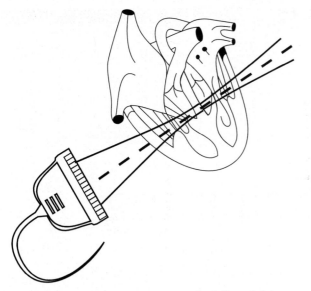

Fig. 17-1 M-mode sampling is along a single line of sight.

transducer or beam direction is moved to view another line of sight. In the spatial dimension, B-mode dots represent the depths of various interfaces encountered along the line of sight. A time sweep of the line data proceeds across the screen at a constant rate. Tick marks show the timing interval. Typical sweep rates are 25 to 100 mm/s. Other sweep rates are also possible. By rapidly repeating echo-ranging measurements, the axial position of each interface is displayed as a function of time. Stationary interfaces are recorded as straight lines on the display, whereas moving interfaces produce oscillating waveforms (Fig. 17-2).

Echo intensity varies greatly depending on the properties of the interface. The strength of the detected echo is depicted in the display by shades of gray, color brightness, or different hues of color. With gray-scale mapping the brightness of the dot increases as signal level is increased. Color mapping is useful to enhance subtle soft tissue differences. *The 2D M-mode trace contains four types of information: reflector depth, signal level of each reflector,*

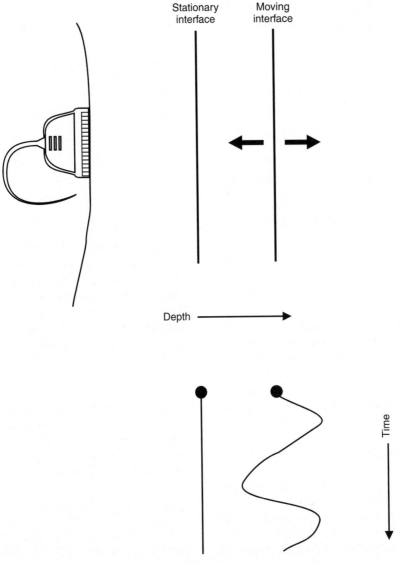

Fig. 17-2 Principle of M-mode scanning. The depth of each interface encountered along the line of sight is monitored by repeated measurements during the observation time. M-mode display of a stationary and moving interface.

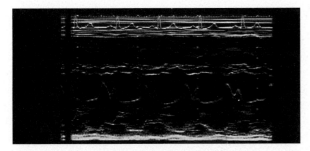

Fig. 17-3 M-mode trace of a normal mitral valve.

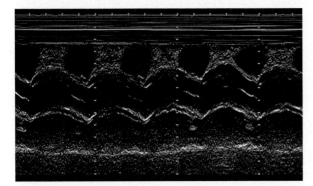

Fig. 17-4 M-mode trace of normal aortic valve.

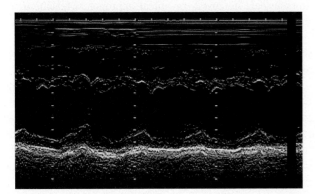

Fig. 17-5 M-mode trace showing right and left ventricular wall movement.

relative positions of the reflectors at each sampling time, and change in axial position of each reflector with time.

The M-mode traces in Figs. 17-3, 17-4, and 17-5 illustrate strong specular reflection from the ventricular wall and the low-amplitude nonspecular reflection (scatterers). The sweep rate can change the pattern of the M-mode trace, depending on the speed of the moving interface (Fig. 17-6).

M-MODE AND TWO-DIMENSIONAL IMAGING

The screen is divided into two sections to show a 2D real-time image and the M-mode trace. A line cursor is placed on the B-mode image to denote the line of sight for the M-mode acquisition (Fig. 17-7). Updates of the image are suspended (or less frequent) while the M-mode trace is collected. The 2D image facilitates sampling of the desired structures and provides correlation between the two scanning modes.

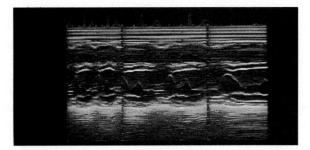

Fig. 17-6 M-mode traces of normal mitral valve at 25 mm/s, 50 mm/s, and 100 mm/s. The pattern is changed (elongated in the time direction) as the trace speed is increased.

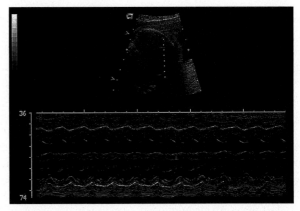

Fig. 17-7 M-mode with two-dimensional B-mode imaging. Four-chamber view of the fetal heart. The line of sight for the M-mode trace denoted on the B-mode image interrogates ventricular mechanical events.

COLOR M-MODE

Color M-mode imaging combines M-mode with 2D Doppler information encoded in color. A line cursor on the color Doppler image denotes the sampling direction with respect to flow. In this manner data along one line of sight are evaluated for both interface motion and blood flow. The flow data and M-mode trace are displayed in conjunction with the corresponding segment of the cardiac cycle given by the electrocardiogram (ECG). Color M-mode thus provides important information about timing of flow across the valve.

OPERATOR CONTROLS

In many ways the informational content of the single line of sight M-mode acquisition is similar to 2D B-mode imaging. The operator controls are also similar in function. These include gain, log compression, preprocessing, postprocessing, strip speed, freeze function, and magnification.

Gain is applied to the induced signals from along the sampling direction. This is usually independent of the image gain. Log compression changes the dynamic range and usually is applied to suppress low signals and noise. Preprocessing is an edge filtering technique to sharpen or smooth borders of moving structures.

The gray-scale map or color map is selected as a post-processing option. Signal strength is translated into brightness level or color depending on the map. Gray-scale inversion represents the highest signal levels in black tones.

The freeze function suspends M-mode data collection and displays the last few seconds of the M-mode trace for prolonged viewing. The spatial dimension of the M-mode trace can be magnified by reducing the length of the line cursor to correspond to a particular range of depths. The effect is that structures in close proximity can now be separated in the display.

RECORDING

M-mode traces in real time can be recorded on film from a persistence cathode ray tube (CRT) or with a strip chart recorder. Film development of this type is time consuming and expensive. The scroll feature allows viewing of information stored in the memory. The length of viewing depends on the sweep rate. A stored M-mode trace may be recorded on videotape, a strip chart, or CD-ROM.

One common archiving method uses the **strip chart recorder,** which provides a continuous reproduction of the trace. The M-mode trace is recorded in a line-by-line sequence as the recording paper moves past a specialized CRT. The CRT has a narrow band of phosphor deposited on the glass plate. An electron beam sweeps horizontally across the phosphor and is modulated in response to the echoes detected along the path. To prevent diffusion of the light and subsequent blurring of the trace, light from the phosphor strip is transferred to the recording paper via fiberoptic light guides (Fig. 17-8). Thousands of optic fibers are placed parallel to each other across the phosphor plate to provide continuity. The speed of the recording paper can be varied. Some paper is sensitive to ultraviolet light; other paper requires development by a thermal or film processor. The latter two methods improve the gray-level reproduction.

The freeze function captures a few seconds of the most recent M-mode trace, which then can be recorded on transparency film as a static image. The time range of the recording is limited but often is sufficient to show physiologic findings. Film provides good contrast and gray-scale reproduction.

VELOCITY MEASUREMENT

M-mode is a 2D data-presentation technique that provides a plot of distance (i.e., the depth of the interfaces relative to the face of the transducer along one line of sight) versus time. The M-mode trace is descriptive of the speed of the interface, the distance traveled by the interface, and the direction and type of motion of the interface. The velocity of the interface is obtained by the slope of the trace (Fig. 17-9). A line drawn tangent to the trace at the point of interest yields the instantaneous change in position (x) with time (t). Velocity is calculated by the ratio of these components:

$$17\text{-}1$$

$$v = \frac{x}{t}$$

M-mode scanning gives an excellent evaluation of the object's size and amplitude of motion in the axial direction.

APPLICATIONS

An M-mode trace can be acquired by using dedicated units with a circular, pencil-type, fixed-focus, single-element transducer or a multi-element transducer. For echocardiology the scan is obtained from the left parasternal, suprasternal, subcostal, or apical approach. Measurements are usually made at end diastole and end systole, as denoted by a simultaneously recorded ECG. Recommendations for performance measurements using M-mode techniques have been published.

The parameters assessed by M-mode scanning include dimensions and a cross-sectional area of the left ventricle, dimensions of the ventricular septum, left ventricular wall thickness at end systole and end diastole, and left ventricular volume. Various indices derived from these parameters (e.g., fractional shortening, fractional area change, and ejection fraction) are used as indicators of cardiac function. Measurements of the left atrium; right ventricle; and the mitral, aortic tricuspid, and pulmonic valves during systole and diastole are also performed. An M-mode trace demonstrating mitral valve prolapse is shown in Fig. 17-10. Special analysis packages are available for making necessary calculations after the appropriate scans have been collected.

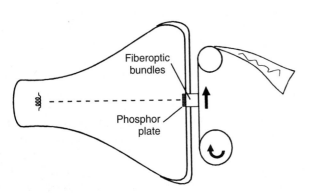

Fig. 17-8 Strip chart recorder.

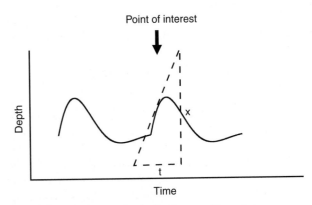

Fig. 17-9 Calculation of velocity from an M-mode trace.

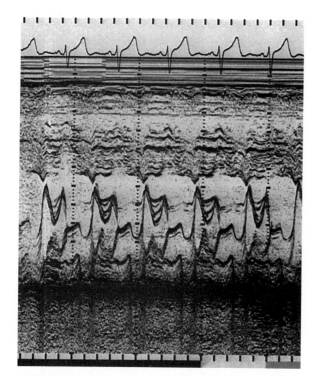

Fig. 17-10 M-mode trace showing mitral valve prolapse.

ADVANTAGES AND DISADVANTAGES

The M-mode scan is interpreted by pattern recognition, but it does not replicate the usual 2D structural anatomy as depicted in real-time imaging. Although the axial and temporal resolution is excellent, motion in the lateral direction (perpendicular to the beam axis) is not portrayed because of the limited field of view (sampling is along one line of sight only).

Another limitation of M-mode scanning is based on assumptions of geometric shapes when measurements along one dimension are extrapolated to calculate 2D areas and three-dimensional volumes. Only real-time 2D imaging techniques can portray lateral motion and depict shape.

Because of its simplicity, high axial resolution, and superior temporal resolution, M-mode scanning will continue to play an important role in echocardiology.

SUMMARY

M-mode scanning evaluates the motion of an interface. Reflector depth and position relative to other structures, signal level, and changes in position with time (velocity and amplitude of the motion) are depicted by the M-mode trace. A single line of sight is repeatedly sampled. The detected echoes from each transmitted pulse are displayed as distance from the transducer, and multiple transmitted pulses provide the temporal changes in each reflector's position. The high pulse repetition frequency allows very rapid motion to be characterized faithfully. However, motion can be evaluated only along the sampling direction. When combined with 2D real-time imaging or color Doppler imaging, the M-mode sampling direction can be specified with respect to the visualized structures.

REVIEW QUESTIONS

1. The M-mode trace is a two-dimensional (2D) plot of _____ versus time in real time.
2. The M-mode trace of a stationary interface produces a _____ on the display.
3. The M-mode trace yields all the following except
   _____.
   A. Reflector movement pattern
   B. 2D spatial relationships
   C. Reflector echo amplitude
   D. Distance between reflectors
4. Which characteristic of M-mode scanning is particularly useful for the evaluation of heart valves?
5. Color is employed in the M-mode trace to depict _____ of the reflectors encountered along the line of sight.
6. Color M-mode scanning combines _____ imaging with M-mode data collection.
7. What is the advantage of combining 2D B-mode with M-mode?
8. Name three devices that are used to record the M-mode trace.
9. The sweep rate is changed from 25 mm/s to 100 mm/s. What is the effect on the M-mode trace?

BIBLIOGRAPHY

Hagen-Ansert SL: *Textbook of diagnostic ultrasonography,* St Louis, 1995, Mosby-Year Book.
Lee RM, Riesen BE: Diagnostic cardiology: noninvasive imaging techniques. In Come PC, ed: *Diagnostic cardiology: non-invasive imaging techniques,* Philadelphia, 1985, JB Lippincott.
McDicken WN: *Diagnostic ultrasonics: principles and use of instruments,* ed 3, New York, 1991, Churchill Livingstone.
Zagzebski JA: *Essentials of ultrasound physics,* St Louis, 1996, Mosby-Year Book.

Contrast Agents

The purpose of contrast agents in ultrasound is to improve image quality by introducing a change in the acoustic properties (backscatter, attenuation, or speed of sound) of tissues in which the material resides. Generally, contrast is enhanced by the increased reflectivity of selected tissues—whether normal tissue, blood pool, or lesion—depending on the biodistribution of the agent. Attenuation effects are subtle, but they can be inferred by observing enhanced or diminished beam penetration distal to the localized material. Speed of sound shifts are not discernible in real-time images and require specialized equipment to measure the changes.

Another application of contrast agents is to improve transmission of the ultrasonic beam along the line of sight. Displacement of air from the ultrasound beam path (e.g., in the gastrointestinal tract) increases sound transmission to the underlying structures.

The initial research focused on the increased signal produced in the region where the contrast agent was local-ized. As contrast agent technology evolved, applications have expanded to include assessment of physiologic function by manipulating the acoustic power and acquisition techniques. That is, both biokinetic properties of the contrast agent and scanning parameters contribute to the diagnostic information obtainable from the ultrasound examination. The use of contrast agents is not limited to improving image quality but offers additional information content.

TYPES OF CONTRAST AGENTS

Contrast agents must demonstrate preferential tissue uptake, stability during examination, low toxicity, and safe elimination through a biologic or metabolic pathway. Types include free gas bubbles, encapsulated gas bubbles, particulates (colloidal suspensions), emulsions, and aqueous solutions.

1. Free gas bubbles may preexist in a liquid or may be produced by rapid injection of a liquid through a narrow passage. They are excellent scatterers of sound energy, with low toxicity, but are removed by the lungs. Localization in soft tissue following venous injection is not possible with them. Applications are limited to intraarterial injection for imaging parts of the cardiovascular system and to direct injection into the bile ducts.

2. Encapsulated gas bubbles are gas-filled microspheres with a thin outer chemical coating. The introduction of

a gas interface increases the echogenicity of the tissue in which the contrast resides. Backscatter depends on the size and concentration of the **microbubbles** as well as on the imaging frequency. Bubble size is typically a few microns in diameter; thus the lung capillaries can be safely crossed for systemic distribution following intravenous (IV) injection. The composition of the coating is varied to alter the distribution of gas-filled microbubbles (tissue specificity) and to prolong stability.

Air-filled albumin microspheres are used as a blood pool agent in echocardiography to increase the reflectivity of the right and left chambers of the heart. Left ventricular border definition and wall motion visualization are improved. The microspheres also improve evaluation of both flow dynamics within the ventricular cavity and valvular regurgitation. As vascular agents, the microbubbles adhere to thrombi, facilitating the diagnosis of venous disease. Infertility in women can be assessed with these agents (i.e., contrast-enhanced sonohysterosalpingography).

Galactose stabilized by free fatty acids is also used to encapsulate gas bubbles. This contrast agent has vascular applications, including visualization of small vessels in the pancreas, kidney, and liver; evaluation of tumor vascularity; and assessment of peripheral vascular disease.

3. Small particles, approximately 1 μm in diameter, of iodipamide ethyl ester accumulate in the reticuloendothelial system, particularly the Kupffer cells of the liver. Liver metastases, however, do not capture this contrast agent, since tumors lack Kupffer cells. The high mass density of iodipamide produces increased backscatter according to the concentration of these particles in the liver. Contrast between liver parenchyma and the lesion can be enhanced. Iodipamide is eliminated within 2 days.

4. Perflubron emulsion is a brominated fluorocarbon in lecithin that persists in the blood for many hours after IV injection and is slowly taken up by the liver and spleen. Patients with hepatic metastases have shown increased tumor echogenicity following administration of this agent.

5. Buffered sodium citrate and calcium disodium ethylenediaminetetraacetic acid (EDTA) exhibit higher acoustic impedance as molar concentration is increased. These materials have been proposed to create transiently enhanced tissue backscatter in highly vascularized organs like the kidney. Compared with encapsulated gas bubbles, however, aqueous solutions are poor scatterers, and a large target volume is necessary to produce an observable effect.

ABDOMINAL IMAGING

Imaging of the abdomen is often compromised by shadowing from gas in the adjacent and overlying bowel. The acoustic impedance mismatch, as well as differences in acoustic velocity between soft tissue and gas, causes a loss of ultrasound intensity and various image artifacts. The displacement of bowel gas by an orally administered gastrointestinal contrast agent creates an acoustic window for improved visualization of the stomach and duodenum. Potential gastrointestinal contrast agents must have low toxicity, mild side effects, adequate bulk, and appropriate surface tension (cohesiveness). Studies have reported that cellulose-based suspensions allow distinct bowel wall layers in the body and antrum of the stomach and in the duodenum to be visualized. Cellulose does not induce gallbladder contraction or excessive gas formation.

PROPERTIES OF MICROBUBBLES AS CONTRAST AGENTS

The properties of the ideal microbubble contrast agent are listed in Table 18-1. The size of the microbubble must be less than 6 μm to cross the pulmonary capillary bed. Air in the microbubble escapes into the surrounding fluid by diffusion. Stability of microbubbles has been improved by encapsulation and by replacement of entrapped air with a gas having a low diffusion coefficient. Encapsulation assumes different forms: Sites on a particle surface (sugar matrix) trap the gas, or a shell encompasses spherical bubbles. Microspheres of albumin, lipids, or polymers are used to entrap the gas and form the capsule. Perfluorocarbon gases are insoluble in water and exhibit a lower diffusion rate than air. Scattering efficiency increases as the sixth power of the radius. Micron-size gas bubbles are very efficient scatterers.

The characteristics of contrast agents that have been evaluated for clinical use are summarized in Table 18-2.

GAS BUBBLE DYNAMICS

The gas in the microbubble is compressible, but the surrounding liquid is relatively incompressible. When a small gas bubble (radius less than the wavelength of the sound wave) is subjected to an acoustic field, the bubble oscillates and scatters sound energy. As the bubble is reduced in size, less scattering occurs. That is, a bubble with a 1-μm radius scatters less of the incident energy than a bubble with a 3-μm radius. For each radius size a particular driving frequency produces a peak response for scattering (Table 18-3).

■ **Table 18-1** Ideal Microbubble Contrast Agent

Property	Reason
Nontoxic	Minimal side effects
Intravenous administration	Ease of use
Transpulmonary	Available for uptake by organs or perfused tissues
Tissue specific biodistribution	Uptake by organ designated for study
Stable to reach site	Available for imaging
Stable during ultrasound	Repeated ultrasound measurements
Low cost	Acceptance for clinical use

■ **Table 18-2** Characteristics of Clinical Contrast Agents

Agent	Physical Components	Size (μm)	Stability	Transpulmonary	Application
Albunex	Air, human albumin shell	3.8	<1 min	Yes	Endocardial border delineation
Echovist	Air, galactose matrix	2	<1 min	No	Right heart cavities, cardiac shunts
Levovist	Air, galactose matrix with palmitic acid	2	<5 min	Yes	Heart, liver, kidney imaging
EchoGen	Dodecafluoropentine	2-5	>5 min	Yes	Cardiac
Optison	Octafluoropropane	2-4.5	>5 min	Yes	Opacification of heart chambers, left ventricular endocardial border
SonoVue	Sulfurhexafluoride polyethylene glycol, phospholipids, palmitic acid	2.5	> 5 min	Yes	Opacification of heart chambers; left ventricular endocardial border; cerebral, carotid, and peripheral arteries; breast and liver vascularity
Definity	Liposome encapsulated perfluoropropane	1.1-3.3	<10 min	Yes	Opacification of heart chambers, left ventricular endocardial border, prostate

■ **Table 18-3** Peak Scattering for Air Bubbles

Radius (μm)	Frequency (MHz)
1	4
2	1.8
3	1
6	0.5

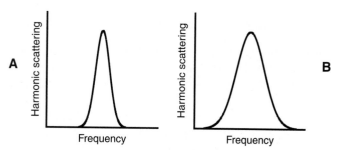

Fig. 18-1 A, Harmonic scattering from bubbles uniform in size has a well-defined peak frequency. **B,** The frequency response for harmonic scattering broadens if the bubbles vary in size.

The expansion and contraction of the bubble does not maintain synchrony with the pressure-varying applied field as power is increased. This nonlinearity leads to the generation of harmonics (2 f, 3 f) and subharmonics (0.5 f), which are emitted in all directions. Harmonic scatter production is maximized at the resonant frequency. Generally, the second harmonic scatter component from the microbubble is much higher in intensity than harmonics formed by nonlinear propagation through tissue.

Stabilized Gas Bubbles

The capsule or matrix used to stabilize the gas bubble alters the response of the bubble when exposed to ultrasonic fields. The presence of these materials resists the displacement when subjected to ultrasonic force. The stiffness shifts the resonant frequency to a higher value (approximately a factor of 2). The amplitude of the oscillations is less, reducing the second harmonic energy that is scattered. Microbubbles administered as contrast agents are not uniformly the same size but extend over a range of radii. The distribution of bubble sizes broadens the response to insonation frequencies that generate harmonics (Fig. 18-1).

INFLUENCE OF ACOUSTIC POWER

At low power levels, the microbubbles oscillate at the insonation frequency and produce scattering at that same frequency. Shell stiffness, gas density, and bubble size

influence the scattering intensity. At higher power levels the amplitude oscillations are no longer synchronized with the applied ultrasound beam, and scattering with harmonic frequencies ensues.

Further increases in acoustic power cause the microbubbles to break apart after a few oscillations. The released gas rapidly diffuses into the surrounding liquid. The destruction of microbubbles produces an intense transient echo rich in harmonics. Contrast agent destruction by the incident ultrasound beam limits the signal that can be obtained by repeated samplings. As acoustic power is increased, both tissue and microbubbles generate harmonics. The separation of harmonic signals to identify the source becomes more difficult.

IMAGING TECHNIQUES

Conventional B-mode imaging detects the presence of contrast agent by the strong scattering component. Liquid cavities that contain contrast agent are opacified. The informational content available from the use of contrast agents is much more extensive than an enhanced real-time image. Multiple imaging techniques have been developed to take advantage of the unique properties of contrast agents and to expand the clinical utility.

Intermittent Imaging

High acoustic power is applied to image and at the same time to destroy the contrast agent within the ultrasonic field. Subsequent images are obtained at the same high power level. Each image shows the contrast agent present but in the process destroys it. Following each image, perfusion replenishes the tissue with contrast agent. This technique shows the amount of contrast agent returning to the tissue in the time interval between images. In order to extend the persistence of the contrast agent, the sampling rate is reduced to one frame every one to four cardiac cycles.

High acoustic power is applied to destroy the contrast agent within the ultrasonic field. The region is then monitored in real time at low acoustic power to avoid further bubble destruction as microbubbles return. Measurements of contrast agent concentration with time characterize **reperfusion imaging** (Fig. 18-2). The slope of the reperfusion curve is indicative of blood flow.

Contrast Harmonic Imaging

Harmonic imaging minimizes echogenic contributions from tissue devoid of contrast agent by detecting reflected sound waves at twice the transmitted frequency (Fig. 18-3).

Gas bubble dynamics predict that the small microbubbles resonate and emit sound waves at the harmonic frequencies. **Contrast harmonic imaging** isolates the second harmonic frequency component in the received echo signals for imaging. By tuning the receiver to a harmonic frequency only, it is possible to enhance contrast by reducing the contributions from tissue. Nonlinear propagation through tissue gives rise to frequencies within this range, although generally at much weaker signal levels compared with those from the microbubbles.

Image contrast can be enhanced further by the post-processing technique of background subtraction. The pre-injection image is subtracted from the postinjection image to yield the net signal attributed to the presence of contrast agent. The harmonic components present in both images are eliminated from the processed image. However, the subtracted image is subject to motion artifacts caused by the time delay between data collections.

At relatively high power levels, intermittent sampling during contrast harmonic imaging must be used to preserve contrast agent. A further modification combines low-power real-time imaging to depict anatomic structures with harmonic imaging at high power. The continuous real-time image and harmonic image obtained during bubble destruction are presented simultaneously in a dual display on the monitor.

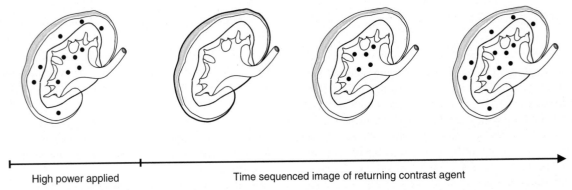

High power applied   Time sequenced image of returning contrast agent

Fig. 18-2 Reperfusion imaging. After destruction of the contrast agent within the field of view, the increase in backscatter signal with time is monitored as contrast agent returns to the region.

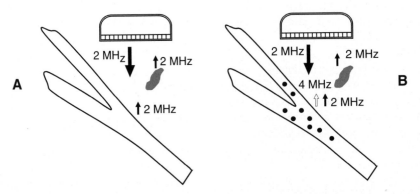

Fig. 18-3 **A,** In conventional imaging all echo-induced signals from tissue and flow are processed at the transmitted frequency. **B,** The contrast agent produces harmonic scattering at twice the transmitted frequency. The signals from tissue at the transmitted frequency are suppressed, while harmonic scattering from microbubbles increases signals from those regions containing the contrast agent.

Digital Subtraction Harmonic Imaging

An image of the structures containing the contrast agent is obtained at high power so that the contrast agent is destroyed. A background image is acquired immediately following the destruction of the microbubbles and then subtracted from the contrast-enhanced image. The resulting image depicts the echoes generated by the contrast agent only and shows the distribution of contrast agent. Because the background image is acquired within a few milliseconds of the contrast image, motion artifacts are reduced.

Color Doppler Imaging

Conventional color Doppler imaging shows a color mosaic where contrast agent was present and then destroyed by insonication. Areas in which contrast agent was absent are shown as a color void. The color image has little or no dependence on blood flow. Other descriptive names for this technique include stimulated acoustic emission and **loss of correlation** imaging.

Microbubble annihilation is not uniform throughout the ultrasonic field. (Enhancement is most pronounced within the focal zone.) Also, only one to three images can be acquired before the contrast agent is depleted.

One possible application is phagocytosis of the contrast agent by Kuppfer cells in the liver. The contrast agent is not taken up by tumors that lack Kuppfer cells. Normal liver parenchyma, which collects microbubbles, is displayed in color mosaic while the tumor, from which the contrast agent is excluded, is free of color.

Harmonic Power Doppler

The harmonic component of the echo-induced radio-frequency signals is isolated and then processed in an autocorrelation circuit to obtain the power Doppler signal. Doppler detection is sensitive to change in the echo pattern along the line of sight. Transient destruction of the bubbles within the sampling volume creates strong echoes followed by weak echoes. The changing amplitude is interpreted as a nonstationary structure and encoded in color. Color is associated with the concentration of contrast agent and not the velocity of movement. As with other destructive techniques, intermittent sampling is required.

DYNAMIC IMAGING

Intercorrelation of echo wavetrains from consecutive pulses along the scan line detects harmonic signals from microbubbles and eliminates static tissue signals. Real-time imaging is possible if low power without significant contrast agent destruction yields sufficient signal. The potential to image organ perfusion and flow in small, deep vessels and hypoperfused lesions now exists. **Pulse inversion harmonic imaging** and **power pulse inversion harmonic imaging** are two types of **dynamic imaging** that employ multiple transmit pulses to isolate the signal originating from the contrast agent.

Pulse Inversion

Pulse inversion isolates the harmonic component generated by scattering from microbubbles by combining the echo signals from consecutive pulses that are reversed in phase. This method enables broadband transmission while maintaining the ability to isolate harmonic components in the echo signals. If tissue harmonic response and tissue movement are negligible, then in the absence of contrast agent the sum of the out-of-phase signals is zero. The introduction of contrast agent under the same conditions creates a nonzero sum signal, if the microbubbles exhibit harmonic behavior. A relatively low power setting is necessary for continuous real-time imaging and has the additional advantages of interrogating microbubbles without destruction and low nonlinear contributions from tissue.

Pulse Inversion Harmonic Imaging

Pulse inversion harmonic imaging, mentioned earlier, is gray-scale imaging in which the harmonic signal is detected with pulse inversion. Signal strength is measured by the amplitude of the inverted sum signal. Microbubbles, if present in the ultrasonic field, generate harmonic scattering, which contributes to the sum signal. In the absence of microbubbles, the sum signal is zero. The real-time image depicts the distribution and concentration of the microbubbles.

Power Pulse Inversion Harmonic Imaging

A background tissue image obtained at the conventional frequency is overlayed with pulse inversion harmonic signals encoded in color. However, the ability to cancel the fundamental components with pulse inversion in the color image is inhibited by tissue motion. The relative time shifts of the echo signals caused by tissue motion retain a strong fundamental component when these inverted signals are combined. By expanding the number of pulses transmitted in a series and using complex mathematic schemes to combine the echo signals from multiple transmit pulses, the fundamental components associated with tissue motion are suppressed.

Real-time myocardial perfusion imaging is possible with power pulse inversion harmonic imaging. Since multiple images are acquired during the cardiac cycle, wall motion abnormalities can be depicted.

CLINICAL APPLICATIONS

Encapsulated microbubbles injected intravenously are used as vascular contrast agents to depict small vessels, detect small tumors in low-sensitivity areas, evaluate tumor vascularity, and distinguish tumors from pseudotumors. Potential clinical applications are summarized in Table 18-4.

Clinical examples of differential uptake of contrast agent are illustrated in Figs. 18-4 and 18-5. Lesions in the liver that do not contain microbubbles are shown as signal voids. (See Fig. 18-4.) Fig. 18-5 depicts a mass with high signal content compared with liver parenchyma during the initial

■ **Table 18-4**   Clinical Applications of Contrast Agents

Technique	Application
Improved Doppler sensitivity	Small vessels, low volume flow, deep-lying vessels, poor insonation angle
Perfusion imaging	Liver and renal lesions, myocardial perfusion
Contrast-enhanced signal	Traumatic parenchymal damage of the kidneys, spleen, liver
Directly to body cavity (bladder)	Renal reflux
Blood pool tracers	Functional indices
Therapeutic applications	Site-specific administration of drugs

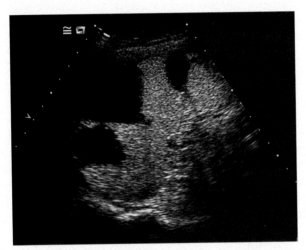

Fig. 18-4 Sonogram of the liver showing the distribution of contrast agent. Three lesions that failed to accumulate contrast agent are present. (See Color Plate 19.) (Courtesy Siemens Medical Solutions USA, Inc., Ultrasound Division, Malvern, Penn.)

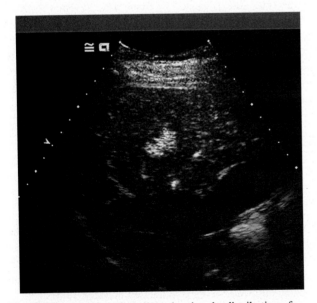

Fig. 18-5 Sonogram of the liver showing the distribution of contrast agent. A mass with enhanced signal content is observed. (See Color Plate 20.) (Courtesy Siemens Medical Solutions USA, Inc., Ultrasound Division, Malvern, Penn.)

introduction of the contrast agent. Since the enhanced signal does not extend to the boundary of the mass, hemangioma is ruled out, but neoplasm is suspected.

THERAPEUTIC APPLICATIONS

Microspheres are loaded with fibrinolytic or chemotherapeutic drugs, which are subsequently released by the application of high power ultrasound when the microspheres are present near the desired site. Therapeutic applications are in the investigational stage and have not been approved for clinical use.

ARTIFACTS

Since microbubbles scattered most of the incident energy, shadowing may obscure structures distal to the regions containing the contrast agent. If the scanner does not have sufficient dynamic range, the strong backscattered signals from contrast agents cause color blooming. Inappropriate color Doppler settings may also contribute to color blooming. Decreased color gain or power may reduce this artifact. Measured systolic peak velocity may increase by 50% during periods of high-level signal content.

SUMMARY

Contrast agents have been developed to improve Doppler and B-mode image quality by altering selected tissue echogenicity. Most ultrasound contrast agents are stabilized microbubbles that increase the backscattered signal intensity from the regions in which they reside. Specialized imaging techniques designed to amplify signals originating from contrast agents have been invented. Enhancement of Doppler signals improves imaging of tumor vascularization, ischemic areas, deep-lying small vessels, vessels with slow flow, vessels with low flow volume, and vessels with limited access (poor Doppler angle).

■■■■■   **REVIEW QUESTIONS**   ■■■■■

1. Why is the size of encapsulated gas bubbles typically a few microns in diameter?

2. Name two functions of the coating for the encapsulated gas bubbles.

3. The nonlinear expansion and contraction of the gas bubble when subjected to an ultrasonic field creates scattering with _____ frequencies.

4. Destruction of microbubbles can be instigated by the application of ultrasound with high _____.

5. Why does color Doppler imaging of the contrast agent produce a color mosaic?

6. One imaging method to extend the lifetime of contrast agent is to apply _____.

7. Name two methods of dynamic flow imaging.

BIBLIOGRAPHY

Barnhart J et al: Characteristics of Albunex: air-filled albumin microspheres for echocardiography contrast enhancement, *Invest Radiol* 25:S162-164, 1990.

Behan M et al: Perfluorooctylbromide as a contrast agent for CT and sonography: preliminary clinical results, *AJR Am J Roentgenol* 160:399-405, 1993.

Correas J et al: Ultrasound contrast agents: properties, principles of action, tolerance, and artifacts, *Eur Radiol* 11:1316-1328, 2001.

Fowlkes JB, Averkiou M: Contrast and tissue harmonic imaging. In Goldman LW, Fowlkes JB, eds: *Categorical course in diagnostic radiology physics: CT and US cross-sectional imaging,* Oak Brook, Ill, 2000, Radiological Society of North America.

Goldberg BB, Liu J, Forsberg F: Ultrasound contrast agents: a review, *Ultrasound Med Biol* 20:319-333, 1994.

Lund PJ et al: Cellulose as a gastrointestinal US contrast agent, *Radiology* 185:783-788, 1992.

Mattrey RF: Sonographic enhancement of Doppler signals and perfused tissues with perfluorooctylbromide, *Invest Radiol* 25:S158-159, 1990.

Ophir J, Parker KJ: Contrast agents in diagnostic ultrasound, *Ultrasound Med Biol* 15:319-333, 1989.

Robbin ML: Ultrasound contrast agents: a promising future, *Radiol Clin North Am* 39:399-414, 2001.

Violante MR, Parker K, Lerner R: Particulate contrast agents for improved ultrasound detection of liver metastases, *Invest Radiol* 25:S165-166, 1990.

Image-Recording Devices

The two-dimensional scan produces an image that is normally displayed on a monitor. The screen is erased and updated with the most recent information each time a new scan is acquired. If the displayed image demonstrates relevant clinical findings, a **hard copy** must be generated by an image-recording device interfaced to the scanner. The recorded image must render a faithful reproduction of the displayed image. Various image-recording devices—including multiformat cameras, laser cameras, and video printers—are available for this purpose.

The quality of the recorded image is primarily judged by the WYSIWYG—"what you see is what you get"—criterion. Repeatability, stability, ease of use, downtime, and cost are also considerations by which image-recording devices are evaluated.

The reasons for hard copy recording are threefold. First, the physician who interprets the results of the study does not necessarily scan the patient. A means to communicate observations from the operator to the diagnostician must be included as part of the examination. Second, images from follow-up examinations can be compared with those obtained from previous examinations. And, finally, documenting clinical findings for legal purposes is essential.

Long-term electronic storage and soft copy interpretation within a picture archiving and communication system (PACS) environment offer a viable alternative to hard copy recording. However, most facilities still use **transparency film.** And transparency film establishes the standard by which all other image recording and display are judged.

FILM CHARACTERISTICS

Based on previous experience with radiographic procedures, transparency film is well accepted by the medical community. The archival lifetime of film is several years, very likely longer than the clinical interest in the study. Storage space and retrieval problems are severe disadvantages, however, which have provided the impetus for electronic archiving methods.

Film is constructed by coating a polyester base with an emulsion layer, the active component. The emulsion consists of a large number of small silver halide grains suspended in a gelatin matrix. Gelatin maintains the distribution of silver halide grains and is porous to liquids used in processing.

The transparent base provides physical support for the emulsion and resists warping with age.

To form an image, the film is first exposed to light and then processed in a series of chemical solutions. It is darkened where light was incident, the degree of darkening depending on the intensity of the light.

Absorption of light photons causes electrons to be released and move through the silver halide crystal, where they are trapped at sensitivity specks in the crystal lattice. A sensitivity speck is an imperfection in the crystalline structure (e.g., sulfur at a location where bromine normally is positioned). Negatively charged electrons migrate within the crystal to combine with the positively charged silver ions and form metallic silver. Deposits of silver atoms accumulate only in the exposed grains. The number of exposed grains increases with the intensity of the light. Information transmitted as variable light intensity applied across the film is captured by the distribution of metallic silver, which is referred to as the **latent image.** The latent image is not observable, but it does act as a template for visual image formation when subjected to chemical processing. The sensitivity speck acts as a catalyst for the conversion of additional silver ions to metallic silver during development. The silver halide crystal is transformed to a visible black silver particle in the emulsion. As the silver particles increase in concentration, the film becomes darker.

The amount of darkening is quantified by the **optical density,** which is defined as the logarithm of the ratio of incident to transmitted light. The relationship between optical density and the percentage of light transmitted is shown in Table 19-1.

Film is generally characterized by a plot of optical density versus exposure or log exposure (Fig. 19-1). The resulting curve, called the **H and D curve** (named for Hurter and Driffield), describes the speed, latitude, and contrast of the film. Film speed determines the location of the curve with respect to the exposure scale and specifies the sensitivity (amount of exposure necessary to cause a particular optical density). Fast film requires less exposure for darkening. Speed is influenced by the number of sensitivity specks per grain, the concentration of grains, the size and shape of the grains, and the presence of chemical sensitizers in the emulsion. Latitude refers to the exposure range over which contrast is sufficient to be useful (e.g., optical density is between 0.25 and 2.5). The straight-line portion of the curve provides the highest contrast (change in gray level per increment of exposure). The maximum slope of the curve is the film gamma. The average slope of the curve is the average gradient.

FILM PROCESSING

An automatic processor performs the chemical operations necessary to transform the latent image into a visual pattern of shades of gray. This four-step sequence involves development, fixing, washing, and drying. A roller system transports the film to the various chemical baths and to the drying chamber. The transport rate determines the time allowed for each processing step (established by the manufacturer). For 90-second processing, the time for each step is partitioned as follows:

	Time in (seconds)
Development	22
Fixing	22
Washing	20
Drying	26

The developer solution consists of several chemical components. *The primary task of the developing agent is to supply electrons so that silver ions can be reduced to metallic silver.* Phenidone and hydroquinone, working in synergy, fulfill this requirement. Other chemical components include an accelerator (sodium carbonate) to control hydrogen ion concentration, a preservative (sodium sulfite) to inhibit oxidation of the developing agent by air, a restrainer (potassium bromide) to limit the reaction rate of the developing agent with unexposed grains, and a hardener (glutaraldehyde) to control emulsion swelling. At the conclusion of development, latent image grains have been converted to particles of metallic silver, and unexposed silver halide grains remain distributed throughout the gelatin.

The fixing solution contains acetic acid to stop the action of the developing agent and sodium thiosulfate to remove the undeveloped silver halide grains. A preservative (sodium sulfite) and hardener (aluminum chloride) are also present.

■ **Table 19-1** Relationship between Optical Density and the Amount of Transmitted Light

Optical Density	Percent Transmitted
0	100
1	10
2	1
3	0.1

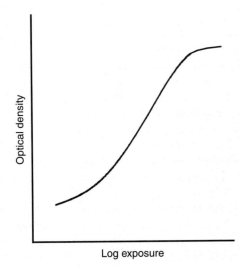

Fig. 19-1 H and D curve to characterize a film (sensitivity, latitude, and contrast).

Fresh tap water washes the film to remove the fixer. If thiosulfate is retained, a yellow-brown stain is formed as the film ages. After washing, the film is transported to a drying chamber, where hot circulating air dries the film.

Variations in film processing alter density and contrast. The composition of the processing solutions is different depending on the manufacturer. The chemical formulation must be compatible with the automatic processor and film. Developer concentration must be proper and uniform throughout the tank. A pump recirculates and agitates this solution. Contamination of the developer (a base) with the acidic fixing solution renders the developer inactive. Processing also consumes chemicals, which must be replaced. Replenishment of both developer and fixer is automatic based on the size of the film processed. Development time and temperature must be regulated within very narrow limits; otherwise, fluctuations in optical density will occur.

Automatic processors have increased efficiency (the processing time is reduced from 1 hour when done manually to 90 seconds) and provide rapid feedback of the recorded information. More important, consistent image quality is achieved by the tightly controlled processing conditions.

FILM SELECTION

A single-emulsion film, compatible with automatic processing, is recommended for hard copy cameras. Image-recording devices have different operational characteristics, and these must be considered when selecting a film to be used with a specific device. For example, the light source may be blue or green (multiformat cameras) or red or infrared (laser cameras), and thus film with the appropriate spectral sensitivity is required. The polyester base may be clear or have a blue tint as preferred by the interpreting physician. The film gamma is typically 1.9 to 2.2. A light-absorbing antihalation layer, which prevents reflection from the base into the emulsion, improves the sharpness of the image. The recommendations of the manufacturer should be followed when selecting film and film processing chemicals.

MULTIFORMAT CAMERA

One or more images are recorded on a single sheet of transparency film (typically 8- × 10-inch size) by the **multiformat camera.** The number of images per sheet is usually fixed as 1, 2, 4, 6, or 9 depending on the model. Some devices have changeable formats, in which the size of the recorded image can be varied.

Transparency film exhibits good gray-scale characteristics (wide range of optical densities that are perceived as separate shades of gray). Development of the film is accomplished by the standard automatic processors common in imaging departments.

Components

Information from the ultrasound scanner is communicated to an internal cathode ray tube (CRT) in the multiformat

camera via an analog or digital interface. The analog form uses the 525- or 1050-line video signal. This type of multiformat camera is also called a video imager.

The components of the multiformat camera include an ultrahigh-resolution monochrome CRT, optical system, photometer, and film cassette. The CRT produces a visible light image for recording. Fine crystalline phosphors in the screen provide small dot size, homogeneous dot shape, and uniform light output. Different types of phosphors (green or blue) are used. Therefore the spectral response of the film must be matched to the emitted light to ensure proper contrast.

Light Output

The brightness of individual dots associated with different portions of the image is controlled by the incoming electronic signal, which regulates the beam current striking each small region on the CRT phosphor screen. Light from the CRT is directed toward the film via a system of mirrors. A lens focuses the image in the film plane (the geometric relationship between CRT, lens, and film determines image size, and thus format), and a shutter controls the length of exposure (Fig. 19-2). The shutter is opened for a time ranging from a fraction of 1 second to several seconds. To record multiple images on a single sheet of film, the film cassette or optical system must move to a new position after

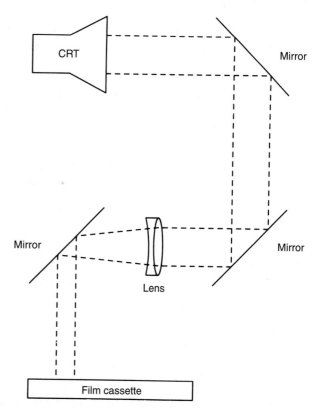

Fig. 19-2 One possible configuration of a multiformat camera. A system of mirrors directs the light from the cathode ray tube to the film. A lens focuses the image in the film plane. Multiple images are placed on a single sheet of film by moving the film cassette after each exposure.

each exposure. Double-sided film cassettes hold two sheets of film, which are individually exposed.

The light output from the CRT, given identical input signals, is not constant over time. A photometer is incorporated into the multiformat camera to maintain consistent optical density. A photocell measures the light emitted from a calibration pattern displayed on the CRT. The intensity of the light is converted to a voltage signal, which is compared with a reference level. The CRT brightness is automatically adjusted until the measured output signal matches the reference signal. The image is then displayed on the CRT; the proper brightness is based on monitoring of the calibration pattern, and exposure now takes place. This feedback circuit is designed to provide reproducible optical density. If the initial setup is in error and light or dark films are produced, this condition will be propagated until corrected by recalibrating the device.

Operator Controls

Adjustments for contrast, brightness, and exposure time can be manipulated to optimize the fidelity of the recording. The contrast control establishes the range of black and white levels of the gray scale. The brightness control changes the midpoint of the gray scale. The overall optical density is varied by shortening or lengthening the exposure time. The effect of improper brightness and contrast settings is illustrated in Fig. 19-3. Signal levels from 0 to 255 are represented as various shades of gray by a properly calibrated device. Improper settings exclude some signal levels from being reproduced on film or prohibit the full extent of possible shades of gray from blacks to whites.

A common misconception is that proper gray-scale presentation on the display monitor is invariably reproduced on the film. *The internal CRT in the multiformat camera is not controlled by the external monitor and must be adjusted independently.* This becomes a practical problem in the clinical environment. To provide assurance that what is seen on the monitor is recorded on film, quality-control tests must be performed.

The operator selects a positive or negative mode for recording. The positive mode is described as white on black, which depicts strong echoes as white and weak echoes as black. This is the preferred mode for most applications in ultrasound. The negative mode displays strong echoes as black and weak echoes as white (the inverse of the positive mode).

Problem Areas

Multiformat cameras are not without their problems. If the phosphor is deposited on a curved face of the CRT, the image in the film plane is distorted, because the depth of field is not constant. A nearly flat CRT (which is expensive) must be used. A uniform phosphor thickness is required to minimize the variation in light output across the screen.

The lens must be of high quality and flat-field corrected. An aperture restricts the incident light to a small central area of the lens. For the best image quality, a line drawn from the CRT to the center of the image on the film should pass through the center of the lens. This geometry is most easily maintained by moving the film cassette to change the image position.

Raster scanning with the video signal input interlaces two 1/60-second fields to compose one frame (similar to television). Distracting raster lines are sometimes present in the static images on film. To de-emphasize this line structure, successive video fields are shifted slightly in the vertical direction to fill in the space between raster lines. Multiple video frames (at least eight) spread the raster lines over a larger area so each horizontal line merges with neighboring lines. The camera shutter must be synchronized

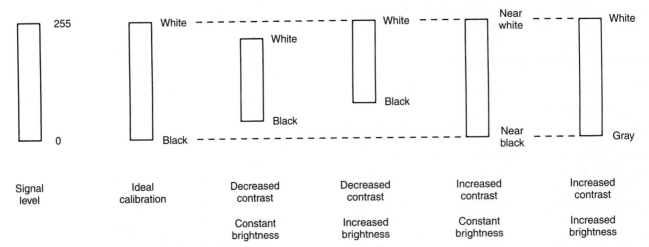

Fig. 19-3 Effect of contrast and brightness controls on the gray scale. An ideal calibration allows the complete range of pixel values (0 to 255) to be expressed as various shades of gray from black to white. A change in brightness and/or contrast settings compared with the ideal calibration causes an incomplete use of all possible shades of gray (from black to white) or compresses the gray scale over a narrower range of pixel values.

with the start of a video frame; otherwise, a partial field included in the exposure will cause the optical density throughout the image to be inconsistent.

Some multiformat cameras contain density step patterns that can be printed on film and read with an internal densitometer after film development. The measured H and D curve is compared with the H and D standard curve stored in computer memory. Adjustment of the light intensity at each gray level is then made to achieve the desired optical density. This calibration corrects for film emulsion and processor variations and can be performed daily.

Spatial resolution is limited not by the film but by the video format (or pixel size in the digital format) and phosphor size.

LASER CAMERA

The major weakness of the multiformat camera is the CRT and optical system. Light-output variation related to phosphor nonuniformity and to electronic drift produces an inaccurate gray scale. Off-axis focusing (i.e., the light path is not through the center of lens) and the curved screen cause distortion. Phosphor dot size limits spatial detail. These image quality issues have caused the multiformat camera to be replaced with the laser camera in many facilities.

System Components

A laser (light amplification by stimulated emission of radiation) replaces the CRT as the light source in the **laser camera.** The intensity and size of the laser beam are precisely controlled. Laser beam diameter is 0.1 mm or less. Two types of lasers are in common use: helium-neon and solid-state diode. The helium-neon laser emits light at a wavelength of 633 nm in the red region of the spectrum. The solid-state diode emits light with a wavelength of 820 nm (infrared).

In one manufacturer's design the digital or video signal from the scanner is loaded in an image-storage memory. Multiple images can be stored simultaneously. Film is removed from the supply magazine and placed on a drum platen. The laser beam sweeps across the film, forming one line of the image. The intensity of the incident light is modulated according to the stored values in memory. A rotating mirror in the light path directs the laser beam to 4096 points along the line. Successive lines are formed by rotating the drum until 5120 lines are generated. When the exposure is completed, the film is transported to an attached film processor for immediate processing or to a receive magazine for remote processing.

An alternate scheme that does not use the revolving platen employs a series of rollers to maintain the film in a flat configuration while linearly advancing the film for line-by-line scanning by the laser beam.

In both methods many pixels compose the image (i.e., there is a potential for excellent spatial resolution). Each pixel can be represented in 256 to 4096 different shades of gray with a high degree of reproducibility (i.e., it provides excellent contrast resolution). Also, a wide dynamic range is achieved.

Image Presentation

When multiple images are recorded on a sheet of film, the area between images is exposed. The darkened borders around each image remove the glare of the viewbox light and improve the visual perception of contrast. Conventional multiformat film has unexposed areas adjacent to the recorded image that hinder contrast discrimination.

Adjustments for contrast, brightness, window width, window level, and gray-scale mapping are available to manipulate the recorded image. Controls for contrast and brightness operate in the same manner as described for the multiformat camera. Window width and level allow for contrast enhancement by defining the range of pixel values distributed throughout the gray scale. Gray-scale maps specify the conversion of the pixel value to a particular shade of gray.

A single-emulsion film with antihalation backing is also used in a laser camera. However, red-sensitive or infrared-sensitive film is required to match the light produced by the laser. As a cautionary note, the usual safelight filter in most radiology darkrooms is not proper for use with laser camera film.

Quality Control

For purposes of quality control, several test patterns are available for imaging to evaluate uniformity, pixel registration, and gray-scale reproducibility. For example, the optical density of each step from a gray-scale bar test pattern recorded on film can be measured and then communicated to the laser camera via a keypad. The laser camera processes this information to adjust the exposure so the resulting optical density for each step is within certain tolerance limits. Many laser cameras have an internal densitometer for monitoring optical density in a reference pattern.

Advantages and Disadvantages

The laser camera provides a fast and highly reliable method of recording hard copy images on film. It can accommodate different film sizes, and the image format can be varied. In addition, multiple imaging devices can be interfaced to it, and batch processing of examinations is possible. The expense of a laser camera dedicated to ultrasound, however, may be difficult to justify. If one has been purchased for another modality (e.g., MRI, CT, or DSA), consideration should possibly be given to interfacing the ultrasound scanner to it.

GRAY-SCALE MAPPING

As discussed in Chapter 10, gray-scale maps assume different functional shapes to highlight certain informational content in the image. The linear map distributes gray levels equally throughout the range of pixel values (echo strengths). The logarithmic map enhances the contrast of weak echoes. The inverse logarithmic map emphasizes variations in high-strength echoes. Usually gray-scale maps, available as postprocessing options in the scanner, are used to enhance contrast so its effect on the image can be visualized before recording.

Many image-recording devices using transparency film incorporate selectable gray-scale maps. The hard copy camera can alter the translation of pixel values to a particular shade of gray to improve contrast. This manipulation of the recorded image is independent of the displayed image. Linear, logarithmic, inverse logarithmic, exponential, squared, and square root maps are available.

Often a hard copy camera gray-scale map is applied to compensate for differences in response between the monitor phosphor screen and the film. Matching displayed brightness levels with film optical densities is essential for the faithful reproduction of a displayed image.

TRANSPARENCY FILM WITH DRY PROCESSING

In the past few years high-quality hard copy image recording without wet chemistry has been introduced. Wet chemistry is the most likely source of variation in optical density and contrast in the recording system. Just as the laser replaced the weakest component of the multiformat camera (light source), the **dry processing** systems confront the weakest component of the wet laser (film processing with liquid chemistry).

The transfer of digital or analog video image information to film and the development of film with dry processing are accomplished within the same unit. Hard copy image recording with dry processing offers many advantages, including consistent film quality, no need for a liquid chemistry film processor, compactness, no darkroom requirement, no handling of chemicals, and no disposal of government-regulated effluents. Four methods of dry processing are currently commercially available for image recording. These printing technologies include photothermography, direct thermal silver behenate, thermography, and dye-sublimation.

Photothermography

Photothermography is a dry processing technique introduced in 1995. The film has a clear or blue base coated with a silver halide (light sensitive) and silver behenate (light insensitive) emulsion that is developed by exposure to heat. The latent image is formed in the usual manner by scanning the film with a modulated infrared laser beam. Development of the latent image is accomplished by moving the film across a heated drum (250° F for 15 seconds). Thermal energy causes the silver behenate to diffuse to the latent image centers and release silver to form visible silver grains. In those regions where latent image centers do not exist, no silver is released, and transparency is maintained.

The matrix format for a 14- × 17-inch film is 4620 × 5596 or approximately 325 dpi. The optical density range is 0.02 to 3.2 with 4096 shades of gray. Processing rate is 60 to 130 films per hour. A density pattern read with an internal densitometer provides a feedback mechanism via look-up tables to maintain proper optical density without operator intervention.

Unlike wet processing, the developer chemistry is not removed during photothermographic processing. The potential exists for the unprocessed chemicals to develop at a later time. Film subjected to high heat conditions and bright light may undergo optical density changes. Continued darkening of films is called "print-up." Dark areas may fade. Transfer of image from one film to another also occurs. Image instability and archiving difficulties have been significantly reduced since this product was initially introduced. Films should not be exposed to acids, alkalis, or solvents. Dust on the laser causes streaks on the processed film. Film emulsion particles can collect on the drum, which are transferred to succeeding films.

No difference in ultrasound diagnostic accuracy has been observed between dry-processed films with photothermography and wet-processed films.

Direct Thermal Silver Behenate

The film consists of a heat-sensitive layer composed of silver behenate crystals between a protective layer and base. Localized heating by the scanning laser causes silver release in that region. The amount of silver deposition depends on the laser beam intensity. Optical density is thus regulated by varying the laser beam intensity as it is scanned throughout the film.

Thermography

In thermography a thermal print head is scanned across the film. The heat-sensitive layer of film contains dye precursor microcapsules and developer. When heat is applied, the walls of the microcapsules become permeable and allow the developer to enter the microcapsule. The dye precursor and developer react to form a black dye. As the film is cooled, the capsules once more become impermeable, and dye formation stops (Fig. 19-4). The temperature of the print head and the time of heating regulate optical density. The starting temperature for development is 100° C. Microcapsules with different heat sensitivities are used to control the gray scale.

Since the film is not sensitive to light, daylight operation is possible. The spatial resolution is 300 dpi with 4096 shades of gray. Processing rate is 90 films per hour.

Dye-Sublimation

A sublimation process (conversion of solid to gas) is used to transfer the dye from the ribbon to transparency film (Fig. 19-5). When heated, the dye on the ribbon is converted to a gas and transferred to the film. The density of the gas

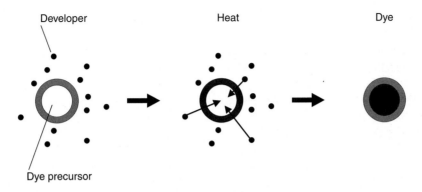

Fig. 19-4 Dry processing method of thermography. The dye precursor contained within the microcapsule is converted into dye when the developer is allowed to enter the microcapsule. The application of heat makes the microcapsule permeable to the developer. Upon cooling, the microcapsule hardens and retains the dye.

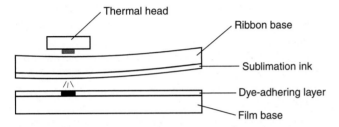

Fig. 19-5 Dye-sublimation. Localized heating by the thermal print head causes the dye to vaporize and then be deposited on the film. The print head is scanned across the width and length of the film.

and, consequently, the quantity of dye infused onto the film is increased as more heat is applied to the print head. The spatial resolution is typically 300 dpi with 256 shades of gray.

Advantages of Dry Processing

The characteristics of the various types of dry processing devices are compared in Table 19-2.

The purchase price for most dry processors is similar to that for a laser camera. Lower cost is achieved by eliminat-ing the expense of chemicals purchased for wet processing. In the current market more than 80% of the recently purchased laser systems incorporate dry processing. However, film throughput for some dry imagers is a limiting factor.

Video inputs and computer interfaces allow multiple scanners to be connected to a single image-recording unit with the capability of batch processing. The transition to computer networks is ideally suited for central processing. The total number of image-recording devices can be reduced while providing redundancy if more than one dry imager is connected to the network.

Adjustments for brightness, contrast, gray-scale map-ping, sharpness, and positive/negative mode are available.

Hard copy image recording with dry processing is particularly well suited for ultrasound departments or stand-alone clinics where wet processing of transparency film (e.g., in mammography) is not required. The lack of environ-mental constraints (no plumbing needed and small size) allows the image-recording system to be conveniently placed in the work area (next to an individual scanner or in a central location where quality control review of films takes place). Staff productivity has been reported to increase by 30% with dry processing.

■ **Table 19-2** Characteristics of Dry Processing Image-Recording Devices

Type	Method	Pixels	Resolution (dots per inch)	Shades of Gray	Film Size	Films/hr
Photothermography	Laser diode	4361 × 5223	325	4096	14 × 17	60
Photothermography	Laser diode	3520 × 4280 or 5080 × 7200	254 or 508	4096	14 × 17 10 × 14 8 × 10	130
Thermal	Dye precursor	4084 × 4984	300	4096	14 × 17	90
Direct Thermal	Silver behenate	6962 × 8408	508	4096	14 × 17 11 × 14 10 × 12 8 × 10	100
Thermal	Dye-sublimation	2548 × 4196	300	256	8.5 × 14 8 × 10	60

VIDEO PRINTER

The video printer (also called a video graphics printer) provides a black-and-white hard copy recording of an image displayed on the monitor. Three methods have been developed to form a black-and-white image on a paper receptor—impact, photo, and thermal.

Methods

In impact printing the print head strikes a ribbon, which places a black dot on the paper. The color of black is created by placing multiple dots within a small area on the paper. Impact printers are not used with ultrasound scanners, because the gray-level representation is poor.

Either light-sensitive (photo) or heat-sensitive (thermal) paper acts as the receptor medium for video printers currently in use. The paper is supplied in long rolls of several hundred feet and is cut to size within the device. The thermal method has gained popularity, because exposing heat-sensitive paper to light does not render it useless, as is the case with light-sensitive paper.

A video signal sent to the video printer is captured as one or two fields and stored in computer memory. The signal level in memory controls the exposure source (amount of light or heat applied to the paper).

In the photo method a dry silver-coated paper is pulled past the face of a CRT. A single scan line is illuminated on the CRT and updated to correspond to successive lines of the image. As the paper moves past the CRT, it is exposed line by line. The exposed paper is heat developed by passage over a mechanical heater or by the application of an electrical current to the conductive back surface. Adjustments include contrast and brightness on the CRT and development temperature.

An alternative method for transferring the image data to paper employs a thermal print head instead of a CRT. This device scans chemically treated paper line by line. The heat generated by the print head is varied to correspond to changes in signal level. The application of heat cures the paper (forms deposits of black carbon). As more heat is applied, more carbon is created at that location, and the area appears darker. The number of gray levels is typically 64 to 128. The dot density, indicative of spatial detail, is 3 to 7.7 dots per millimeter. A print is processed in approximately 10 seconds.

Operator Controls

The operator selects how much of the video signal is stored in memory for printing by selecting the field or frame mode. Spatial resolution is sacrificed in the field mode, because a reduced number of raster lines is available to compose the image. Consequently, the frame mode should be used, if possible. Black-white reversal (also called positive-negative) inverts the gray scale to display blacks as whites and vice versa.

Adjustments for contrast, brightness, and sharpness are available. The contrast control changes the video-signal amplification and alters the translation of the video signal into gray level. The brightness control sets the overall optical density. Edges in the image are enhanced by the sharpness control.

Imaging Characteristics

Video printers offer several advantages compared with multiformat cameras. These include ease of processing, convenience, speed, and low cost. The paper print has a limited optical density range (maximum optical density is 1.6), however, and less archival stability.

COLOR VIDEO PRINTER

A color image on paper is viewed by sensing the reflected light from colored dyes distributed across the paper surface. The incident white light from a conventional light source, consisting of all colors, strikes the paper, and varying amounts of its constituent colors are selectively removed by the absorbing dyes. The color of the reflected light is altered. This process is repeated at every pixel throughout the printed image and results in the visual spatial pattern of colors.

Typical primary colors of the dyes are cyan, magenta, and yellow, which absorb red, green, and blue. Black is formed when all three primary colors are present. In some devices a separate black dye is used. The absence of dye yields white. A combination of the two primary colors magenta and yellow forms the reflected color red; all colors in the incident light are absorbed except red. Similarly, green and blue are produced by different combinations of two primary colors (cyan/yellow and cyan/magenta).

The color video printer provides a color hard copy recording of the image displayed on the monitor. One or more images are printed on a paper sheet. Heat-activated dyes are transferred to the paper without the processor chemicals required for film. This device is used extensively for recording color Doppler images.

A video signal sent to the color video printer is captured as one or two fields and stored in computer memory. One 512×512 color image requires 0.75 megabytes of computer memory. The video input can assume different formats to code for the color information (e.g., composite video, Y/C [luminescence and chrominance], and red-green-blue analog). The colors yellow, magenta, and cyan are printed on the paper. A separate Mylar ribbon coated with dye is necessary for each color. The paper is printed three times— once for each color—which accounts for the increased printing time compared with black-and-white video printers.

The chemically treated paper with a smooth surface is attached to a platen, which rolls around and is scanned line by line with a miniature thermal print head. A sublimation process (conversion of solid to gas) is used to transfer the dye from the ribbon to the paper. The dye on the ribbon is in solid form. When heated, the dye is converted to a gas. The density of the gas and, consequently, the quantity of dye infused into the paper is increased as more heat is applied to the print head. The amount of heating at a particular location is controlled by the information stored in memory. During each rotation of the platen, a different-colored dye ribbon is placed next to the thermal print head for transfer to the paper.

Color gradations are controlled by superimposing varying amounts of each dye on the paper. The number of color levels ranges up to several million. Each primary color is coded in 8 bits (24 total bits per pixel). A color selection table translates the video signal into various color levels. The number of lines printed is typically greater than 500; thus the video signal and not the device limits the spatial resolution. Three hundred dots per inch are printed. The printing time is usually less than 90 seconds.

The operator selects the number of images printed on a sheet (full or split mode) and how much of the video signal is stored in memory (field or frame mode). Spatial resolution is sacrificed in the field mode, because a reduced number of video lines is available for image formation. Adjustments for contrast, brightness, color intensity, and tint can be manipulated to optimize the fidelity of the image recording. The contrast control changes the video signal amplification and alters the translation of the video signal into color level. The brightness control, in essence, determines the amount of dye used to print the image. The purity or shading of the color is established by the color control. The tint control adjusts the mixing of the three basic colors.

MAGNETIC TAPE RECORDER
Standard Video Home System

Recording a series of images for subsequent playback in real time is often accomplished with magnetic tape recorders. The **videocassette recorder (VCR)** has dominated the **video home system (VHS)** market. A 1/2-inch tape is enclosed in a cassette for ease of loading and unloading. The polyester tape is coated with a magnetic substance. Tiny regions called dipoles in this coating are aligned when subjected to an external magnetic field, and they maintain their induced orientation until a new magnetic force redirects them. During recording, the tape is mechanically driven past the writing head at a constant velocity. The writing head converts the input video signal to a rapidly changing magnetic field that extends beyond the head to the region of the tape. This fluctuating magnetic field varies the alignment of dipoles along the tape. During playback, the magnetic field associated with the aligned dipoles induces an electrical signal in the writing head as the tape moves past. The induced video signal, consisting of 525 lines, is sent to the television monitor for display. VHS, however, can preserve the spatial detail of only 240 lines; thus image quality is degraded.

Two writing heads mounted 180 degrees apart on a rapidly revolving drum each write a video field as an individual track with every revolution of the drum. In the VHS format a track width is 29 μm, with a gap between adjacent tracks to reduce interference or cross-talk. One or more linear sound tracks are included on the tape for audio capability.

The tracking control adjusts for small variations in tape speed caused by tape stretch or inconsistent tape transport. To reduce noise, only one head is active during playback. In the record mode, both heads are sent the video signal, but only the head in contact with the tape writes the track to tape.

The amount of tape in the cassette can be increased to extend recording time (30 to 180 minutes). The physical size of the cassette is unchanged, but the diameter of the center hubs is made smaller to accommodate more tape. Longer recording times are also possible by reducing the tape speed. The fidelity of the recording is compromised, however, by slower tape speed.

Super Home Video System

The latest generation of video format, introduced in 1987, is **super VHS.** A high-density oxide tape in the standard cassette shell is used. The cassette is notched to identify the type of tape (standard or super). Super VHS videocassette recorders operate with a higher-frequency bandwidth, which allows 425 lines of horizontal resolution compared with 240 lines in standard VHS. Image quality is superior with super VHS, because the information contained in the video signal is preserved.

Limited compatibility exists between super VHS and conventional units. A recording in the super VHS format cannot be played on a conventional VCR. Tapes in the standard format can be interchanged between super VHS and standard VHS equipment.

The low cost makes videotape recording very attractive. Voice commentary can be added to the audio track. Unfortunately, tape wear from contact with the writing head limits tape life to a few hundred plays. Also, the recommended shelf life of 2 years prohibits long-term archiving. The freeze-frame option stops movement of the tape, and a single track is repeatedly read for the video signal. This allows selected images consisting of one video field to be annotated and transferred to a multiformat camera or video printer for hardcopy recording. Measurements can be performed on the stop-framed image.

Cleaning Writing Heads

Dirt and magnetic particles from the tape collect on the writing head and must be removed periodically. The overuse of head cleaners, however, promotes headwear since cleaning is accomplished by scraping the head surface. Consequently, cleaning should be performed only when the playback picture becomes noisy.

The indirect method uses a special head-cleaning cassette that is loaded into the tape recorder. The cleaning material replaces the tape and is driven across the head surface. In the direct method a nonwoven, low-abrasive, lint-free cleaning pad is moved across the head in one direction only. Back-and-forth and up-and-down motions can damage the writing head. A Freon-based cleaning solution leaves no residue. Alcohol should be avoided, because any remaining moisture will cause the tape to seize.

CD-ROM

Computer technology incorporated into ultrasound instrumentation alters its design and function. Increasingly, the digital format dominates how data are represented and processed. *Electronic storage of images and cine (video) clips on CD-ROM provides a low-cost option to communicate the results of the examination to another facility.* This is also a means to make a record of the examination available to the patient. Software installed on the CD-ROM with the images allows the user to select and view images on the computer monitor. Hard copy recording would be limited to the printers that are interfaced to the computer.

Even though the CD-ROM can store thousands of static images, this is not a long-term solution to the archival problem. Higher capacity is required with almost immediate access to the images. This is a problem for PACS, which is considered in the next chapter.

SUMMARY

The traditional image-storage medium is transparency film. Its cost, image quality, and long-term stability are the standards against which those features of alternative media are compared. Paper is less expensive, has slightly inferior spatial and contrast resolution, and is less stable with time. The laser camera (because of its excellent image quality) and the video printer (because of its low cost) experience widespread use. The dry-processed transparency film offers an alternative to the laser camera for high-quality image recording and is rapidly becoming the method of choice in imaging departments. Color video printers seem particularly well suited for recording color Doppler images. VCRs or CD-ROMs offer a means of recording dynamic studies for subsequent playback in real time. Magnetic tape cannot function as a permanent storage medium, and consequently appropriate frames from the video recording must be selected for hard copy recording, if other means to store video clips are not available.

Quality assurance of the entire ultrasound system, including the recording devices, must be monitored periodically to ensure that the recorded image matches that of the monitor.

REVIEW QUESTIONS

1. What is the major disadvantage of transparency film as an image storage medium?
2. The latent image is retained in which component of transparency film?
3. What is the major weakness of the multiformat camera?
4. Why is adjustment of brightness/contrast controls on the display monitor inappropriate during scanning?
5. Which image-recording devices allow playback of a real-time study?
6. Which image-recording devices offer a low-cost option to provide patients with images of their examinations?
7. Color video printers use a thermal _____ process to form the image.
8. The advantage of the super VHS format compared with the standard VHS format is that _____ is improved.
9. When image data transfer is accomplished with a video signal, the video signal provides an ultimate limit for _____ regardless of the image-recording device.

BIBLIOGRAPHY

Gray JE et al: Multiformat video and laser cameras: history, design considerations, acceptance testing, and quality control. Report of AAPM Diagnostic X-ray Imaging Committee Task Group no 1, *Med Phys* 20:427-438, 1993.

Lu ZF, Nickoloff EL, Terilli T: Monthly monitoring program on DryView laser imager: one year experience on five Imation units, *Med Phys* 26:1817-1821, 1999.

Russ JC: *The image processing handbook,* ed 4, Boca Raton, Fla, 2002, CRC Press.

Starkweather GK: Digital color printing, *Physics Today* 45:60-65, 1992.

Thompson TT: Laser applications in radiology, *Radiographics* 5:627-629, 1985.

Trefler M: Inside the multiformat camera, *Radiographics* 4:785-786, 1984.

Picture Archiving and Communication System

A picture archiving and communication system (PACS) is a computer system that allows digitized images from various imaging modalities to be stored electronically for later retrieval, display, manipulation, interpretation, and distribution to remote locations. In addition, text and patient demographic data must also be stored in such a manner as to allow the appropriate information to be associated with the corresponding images. A PACS must be fully integrated with the digital acquisition devices as well as workstations, printers, image-recording devices, and medical information systems (Fig. 20-1).

In the **network** scheme, redundancy of certain hardware devices can be reduced. Hard copy image-recording devices are not required at each scanner; rather, a single laser camera can provide image recording for multiple imaging modalities. Image-processing workstations can also be centralized. Images from multiple scanners can be routed to a single workstation. At the same time, workstations and review stations may be located as needed throughout the institution.

Clinical implementation of PACSs has proceeded at a rapid rate during the past few years. To acquire, replace, maintain, and repair PACSs, a major financial commitment and a dedicated, highly trained staff are necessary. Continued expansion will depend on demonstrated performance (reduced costs, increased throughput, and improved patient care).

DIGITAL IMAGING AND COMMUNICATION IN MEDICINE

Standards for PACS technology have been developed by the American College of Radiology and the National Electrical Manufacturers Association. The collection of standards is called **Digital Imaging and Communication in Medicine (DICOM).** DICOM established standardized file formats for patient data and images as well as criteria for the transfer, storage, and display of this information.

DATA MANAGEMENT

Extremely large quantities of image and nonimage data are present on the PACS. These data must be managed so

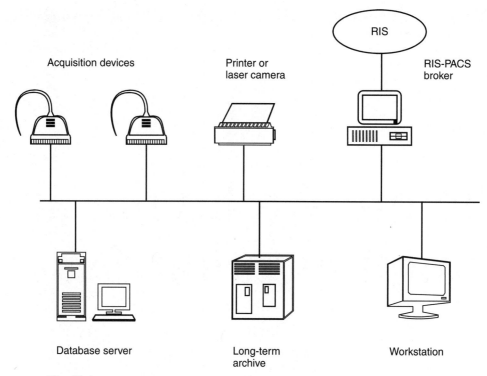

Fig. 20-1 Components of a picture archiving and communication system network.

that the proper images with the associated attributes, as well as patient demographics, go to the correct location at the proper time within the network. The network provides the framework for data communication among the various components of a PACS. The aspects of data management are summarized below:

- Control data transfer through the network
- Access patient demographics and reports
- Generate modality work lists
- Provide a dynamic list showing studies for interpretation
- Archive image data
- Serve as a medical information system interface

MEDICAL INFORMATION SYSTEMS

A medical information system such as the **radiology information system (RIS)** or the **hospital information system (HIS)** is a computer system that acts as a dynamic database for patient information. Patient demographics, examination schedules, billing status, and interpreted reports are stored, updated, and distributed as needed. A PACS relies on the RIS as the primary source of patient information. The single pathway of data entry via the RIS when the patient initially registers avoids patient data duplication and data inconsistencies. One time entry improves workflow, since demographics are not entered for each subsequent visit or at each imaging modality, but only when changes occur.

The standard communication language for medical information is called HL7. A robust communication link must be established between the PACS and the RIS. Often

an interface is accomplished through a **broker,** where the exchanged data are translated from HL7 to DICOM and vice versa. However, data transfer is not completely error free. A fully integrated PACS and RIS is now offered by some vendors.

TOPOLOGY

The acquisition, display, archiving, hard copy, and computer components of a PACS must be interconnected in the form of a local area network (LAN). The term **topology** is used to describe the configuration in which these components are linked together in a network. Each device on the network constitutes a node with a unique address (identification number for each device).

A bus topology employs a common communication path shared by every device in the network; that is, all devices are, in essence, connected to the same cable. Transmission is not continuous (information would become garbled) but is in the form of packets. Each packet contains the source and destination addresses in addition to the data for transfer. The components in the network monitor the communication medium for packets addressed to them and copy only these packets from the network.

In star topology, all devices are connected directly to a central computer through which all data must pass. In ring topology all components are linked together in a ring, and each is restricted to communicating with the neighbor on each side only. Each position on the ring contains a repeater, which allows the information to be relayed to other components around the ring. Other topologies are also possible.

Each configuration has advantages and disadvantages, although no single topology has yet emerged as the one of choice.

A **server** is one or more computers that provide a service (data locator, storage, or printing) to other computers within the network. The database server maintains a directory of the locations of all images, image attributes, and patient data. Some PACSs have a second database server to provide redundancy in the event of device failure or system maintenance.

DATA TRANSMISSION

Transmitting large quantities of data in a timely fashion within the clinical setting is a major consideration in PACS. The speed of transfer of information is characterized by the number of bits transmitted per second. Twisted-pair cable, coaxial cable, and optical fiber cable are commonly used as communication media. The first two pass electrical signals, whereas the third allows one-way transmission with a light-emitting diode at one end and a photodiode receiver at the other. Two cables are necessary for two-way communication. The maximum speed at which information is transmitted varies over a wide range—1 to 10 megabits per second (Mbps) for twisted-pair cable, 10 to 50 Mbps for coaxial cable, 100 to 1000 Mbps for optical fiber. The process of coordinating information transfers in the network reduces transmission rates below these idealized values.

The transfer time for image data depends on the bandwidth (rate of transmission) of the network. Technology with very fast data transfer rates is desirable to provide instant access to images. The transfer times required to send one ultrasound image to another location by different communication technologies are compared in Table 20-1.

SCANNER INTERFACE

Ultrasound scan data are communicated to the network digital interface, which transfers the image and demographics directly to the network from the scanner. Most ultrasound scanners can be purchased with DICOM output for this direct communication link to a PACS. Another method digitizes the analog video signal with a video frame grabber.

DATA STORAGE REQUIREMENTS

A PACS must be capable of storing enormous quantities of data for long periods while allowing the user rapid access to the stored information. As an example of the storage capacity required, one ultrasound study consisting of 20 images in the $512 \times 512 \times 8$-bit format would use 5 megabytes (MB) of storage. The demographic data are not included in this calculation and would require additional storage allocation. For an average-sized radiology department, all imaging modalities could easily generate 10,000 or more MB per day.

■ Example 20-1

Calculate the storage requirements in MB for a study consisting of 80 images in a 512×512 matrix with 256 gray levels.

One byte is required to represent a pixel with 256 gray levels. Each image has 262,144 pixels or 262,144 bytes (0.25 MB). A total of 20 MB is required to store 80 images of 0.25 MB each.

ARCHIVAL SYSTEMS

The **archival system** is responsible for the electronic storage of image data and the associated patient information. An impediment to the adoption of PACS has been the high cost of archival storage. However, the cost of digital storage media continues to decrease while capacity continues to increase. This combination has made PACS more cost effective.

Electronic storage compared with film is less labor intensive and less subject to filing error and lost images. Retrieval of images and reports is faster and can be linked to a database so that related records become readily available.

Storage Devices

The primary devices used for data storage are magnetic disk, optical disk, magnetic tape, DVDs, and **redundant array of independent disks (RAID)**. A comparison of archival technologies is shown in Table 20-2.

A magnetic disk provides relatively fast access but is expensive and has limited capacity (10 to 200 gigabytes [GB]). In the past, cost considerations limited the magnetic disk to scanner and workstation local storage and to

---

■ **Table 20-1** Bandwidth and Transfer Time for Various Communication Technologies

Technology	Bandwidth (Mbps)	Transfer Time (sec)*
Modem	0.056	132
T-1	1.54	4.8
Ethernet	10	0.74
Fast Ethernet	100	0.074
Asynchronous transfer mode	155	0.048
Gigabit Ethernet	1000	0.007

Mbps, Megabits per second; *sec*, seconds.
*One ultrasound image of 0.88 megabytes.

■ **Table 20-2** Archival Technologies for Picture Archiving and Communication System

Device	Access Time	Capacity	Relative Cost per GB
Magnetic disk	1-50 ms	10-200 GB	1
Optical disk	min	10+ GB	0.4
Tape	min	10-100 GB	0.2
DVD	sec	10-100 GB	0.8
RAID	<300 ms	10s TB	8

GB, Gigabyte; *ms*, milliseconds; *min*, minutes; *sec*, seconds; *RAID*, redundant array of independent disks; *TB*, terabytes.

short-term archive storage. However, capacity and the performance-to-cost ratio are increasing rapidly.

Magneto-optical disks are configured as multiple platters (100 or more) within a jukebox to expand storage capacity (terabytes [TB]) and serve as long-term permanent storage. A mechanical media-movement device selects the appropriate disk for read/write. Erasable optical disks are slower but have lower costs compared with magnetic disks.

The high cost and lack of uniform standards has inhibited the incorporation of DVDs into PACSs as storage media. As this technology matures with its very high storage capacity, increased applications in PACSs are anticipated.

Tape is also removable storage medium that is arranged in a jukebox. The major advantages of tape are low cost and high capacity (TB when configured in a jukebox). However, access time for retrieval is long (several seconds to minutes). Tape has been used primarily for disaster backup and long-term permanent storage.

System Design

A combination of storage devices is used to meet the diversified storage and retrieval requirements. A computer with the imaging device provides rapid access of the recently acquired studies via magnetic disk. After initial review, the digitally formatted data are transferred to a fixed magnetic disk drive for short-term storage. Because the magnetic disk drive has limited capacity, the information must be transferred once more to a slower but much higher-capacity device (e.g., optical disk or magnetic tape) for permanent storage.

Magnetic disks offer high capacity with rapid access when configured as a RAID. Data are stored at multiple locations within the array of disks. This technique provides redundancy and lessens the potential for data loss. RAID is now a viable option for long-term archive storage.

DATA COMPRESSION

To reduce the storage requirements of a digital image, a technique called **compression** is applied to reformat the image into fewer bytes. Typically, an ultrasound image is stored in a matrix format, wherein each byte holds one value that is associated with a particular pixel in the image. For other imaging modalities there is a 1:1 or 2:1 relationship between bytes and pixels depending on the dynamic range

or number of gray levels. For example, an image consisting of 1024 pixels and 256 gray levels requires 1024 bytes; images with more pixels use more bytes. If decreasing the number of pixels or the bit depth reduces storage requirements, spatial resolution or contrast is sacrificed. An alternative method is to code the pixel values in a new format.

Often, many redundant pixel values occur in an image. Instead of repeating these values over and over in the matrix format, an instruction coding for the number of repetitive pixels and the pixel value can be substituted. Various coding methods are available. The DICOM standard supports run-length encoding and Joint Photographic Experts Group (JPEG) compression protocols. If the original image data can be regenerated from the reformatted data with no loss of information, the compression is reversible or lossless (e.g., run-length encoding). If a loss of information occurs, then the original image data cannot be regenerated from the reformatted data, and the compression is lossy.

A typical lossless compression ratio is 3:1, which means that the storage requirements have been reduced by a factor of 3. A greater gain in compression (with some loss in image quality) is possible if perfect reproduction of the original image is not necessary. An irreversible compression ratio of 7:1 to 20:1 is obtainable without significant image degradation. *Compression techniques are critically important for reducing PACS design requirements for data storage and transmission rates.*

Dynamic Clips

A color Doppler image with a 640×480 matrix encoded in 24 bits is 0.88 MB in size. An ultrasound examination is not limited to a single image but rather is a series of freeze-frame images and cine clips. The storage requirements for various combinations of image formats with and without compression are shown in Table 20-3.

Remote viewing of dynamic clips is of particular interest. Uncompressed video would require extensive transmission time and thus is impractical. Lossy compression enables remote viewing of dynamic clips. Each frame is compressed independently during acquisition or by command of the system user. The compressed data are transmitted to the remote site, where they are reformatted for viewing. Lossy compression with a ratio of 26:1 is comparable to information loss when real-time imaging is recorded with super VHS videotape.

■ **Table 20-3** Storage Requirements in Megabytes

Image Type	Uncompressed	Lossless Compression 3:1	JPEG Lossy Compression 20:1
Static image	0.88	0.29	0.044
1-sec video	26.4	8.8	1.32
50 static images	44	14.7	2.2
30-sec video, 20 static images	810	270	40.5
20-min video	31,680	10,560	1584

WORKSTATIONS

Image review and manipulation take place at workstations located throughout the network. A **workstation** is an interactive minicomputer with specialized graphics capabilities. The random access memory (RAM) capacity is 1 to 2 GB. A high-resolution cathode ray tube (CRT) or liquid crystal display (LCD) is required for image display. These workstations each have access to any study stored in the PACS network. Previous studies are available for review and comparison with the current image data.

Displayed image quality, system speed, and image processing options are the primary considerations in workstation design. The spatial resolution, contrast resolution, distortion, noise, and viewing conditions imposed by the workstation should be such that the information content of the image data is not degraded significantly when displayed. System speed determines the time required to retrieve, display, and manipulate image data. Image processing can enhance the presentation of the image data to facilitate interpretation.

Monitors

Performance of monitors is a combination of several factors:
- Spatial resolution (number of pixels)
- Distortion
- Contrast resolution
- Aspect ratio
- Maximum luminance
- Dynamic range
- Uniformity
- Persistence
- Refresh rate

The question of appropriate matrix size has been a topic of debate. The 1K monitor has 1000 pixels along one dimension, while the 2K monitor has twice this number. The time required to refresh the image depends on the number of pixels and the speed of the video card (increased component costs). Also, the maximum luminance and contrast resolution are lower for high-resolution monitors. High light output extends the dynamic range and is generally desirable, but ultimately the monitor must be judged with respect to all performance capabilities. Maximum luminance for different monitors is shown in Table 20-4.

In a multimodality workstation the matrix size and gray-level requirements are established by radiography. A large-format, 21-inch, progressive raster-scanned CRT is used as the high-resolution display device. This unit displays an image matrix of 2560 × 2048 with 128 gray levels, corresponding to 200 dots per inch. This matrix size is also available with LCDs. Other 1K high-resolution monitors are limited to a matrix size of 1280 × 1024. Either type is acceptable for the display of ultrasound images, which typically consist of 512 × 512 pixels and each pixel coded in 8 bits.

Compared with transparency film, monitors have inferior spatial and contrast resolution. The luminance of the screen is much lower than that obtained from the viewbox. Visual acuity and perception of luminance differences (contrast) depend on the luminance level. Veiling glare (scattering of light from regions of high luminance to regions of low luminance) also degrades perceived contrast. The image-processing technique of gray-scale mapping (window and level) compensates for the inherent weakness of monitor contrast resolution. Light output from the phosphor decreases as the phosphor ages. Long, persistent phosphors cause blurring when rapid updates of the screen occur.

Viewing Conditions

The low luminance of monitors compared with film view-boxes necessitates adherence to proper ambient viewing conditions. Glare (reflection from bright objects) and illumination from room lighting cause loss of contrast in the displayed image. The reading room design should include indirect incandescent lighting at low luminance levels (<50 lux and preferably <10 lux), no windows, and walls with low reflection.

Image Display

The time for image retrieval is determined mainly by the speed of the storage device. To achieve a retrieval time of 1 to 2 seconds, workstations are usually equipped with a high-capacity magnetic disk drive. Studies on the system storage device are transferred via the network to the magnetic disk at the workstation.

After a study is selected, the image data are loaded from the magnetic disk into a frame buffer and then modified by means of look-up tables before placement in the video buffer. Video RAM can accommodate 2560 × 2048 pixels with a bit depth of 8. Rapid readout of the video buffer enables the screen to be refreshed at a rate of 75 times per second. The frame buffer holds more image data than the video buffer, but the video buffer configuration allows rapid updating of the screen when other image data are viewed.

The selection, positioning, and sequencing of images displayed on the CRT are specified by the operator. Tile mode places the images side by side on the screen. Stack mode allows sequential viewing of images, one at a time. Dynamic studies can be displayed in cine mode, which is the sequential projection of temporally contiguous images. The type of study and the preferences of the interpreting physician usually dictate the viewing format. An automatic viewing scheme for a study consisting of a predetermined

■ **Table 20-4** Maximum Luminance of Display Devices

Display Device	Luminance (nits)
Viewbox	1500
CRT	800
LCD	400-500
Color LCD	200

CRT, Cathode ray tube; *LCD*, liquid crystal display.

number of images and views can be defined. The workstation must have the capability of manipulating the displayed image. These image-processing techniques include window and level, gray-scale mapping, zoom, panning, smoothing, and edge enhancement. Volumetric display, contour extraction, and spatial measurements are available on most workstations. Interactive mode requires time-efficient image processing, and thus the system must meet the demand for high computational ability.

Operator instructions are communicated to the computer via a graphical user interface. Selectable tasks are each indicated by an icon or pictorial representation of the operation displayed on the screen. A mouse is used to move a cursor to the appropriate icon, which is then selected by depressing a mouse button.

WORKFLOW

Patient information is entered once via RIS and not repeated by the sonographer at the time of the examination. Modality work lists show the schedule of patient examinations for each imaging device. Completed and pending examinations are easily tracked. At the conclusion of the examination, images are sent electronically to the PACS, and the technologist does not need to leave the scan room to develop or retrieve films. Procedure time is reduced, although continuous patient contact is maintained. Since the patient is not left unattended, patient satisfaction is improved. Also, technical staff can now devote the majority of time to the patient care tasks that they are uniquely qualified to do.

Unread studies are listed for interpretation and can be directed to a particular workstation or physician. Lost films, which go unread, are virtually eliminated with PACS. Faster response time is also possible.

Statistics related to workflow are becoming increasingly important for financial management in health care and are easily tracked with PACS. Total number and average time of examinations by procedure, by sonographer, and by interpreting physician are all readily available.

MINI-PICTURE ARCHIVING AND COMMUNICATION SYSTEM IN ULTRASONOGRAPHY

The incorporation of all imaging modalities into a PACS network is expensive and a technically complex endeavor. Ultrasound scan data are in digital format and easily adapted to a mini-PACS environment consisting of ultrasound scanners only as acquisition devices. In Fig. 20-2, four scanners are interfaced to the network. A laser camera, workstation, and disk storage device are also included in the network. The sonographer selects the images that comprise the patient study and sends these images to the PACS. Image review and processing for any study archived on the network are performed at the workstation.

Recently, equipment manufacturers have introduced digital management systems for ultrasound. Image data including video clips, patient demographics, and instrument settings are recorded electronically and distributed throughout the network. The ability to interface scanners from different manufacturers is now possible through DICOM. However, these image management systems are expensive and currently undergoing technical developments. The major advantage of these dedicated systems is the ability to view video clips immediately after acquisition.

REMOTE ACCESS

One application of PACS technology is the electronic transfer of images from one location to another. The computer at the remote site receives and decodes the transmitted information. The image data are placed in computer memory and displayed. If the image data had been compressed, the recovery algorithm must be applied before display. Various software packages are available to enhance the interpretation process. These include the ability to transmit text and images and image-manipulation techniques.

The time to transmit an image depends on the acquisition matrix, the extent of compression, and the method of transmission. Potential transmission methods include telephone lines, coaxial cables, fiberoptic cables, microwave dishes, satellites, and T-1 (multiple) telephone lines. For telephone lines the transmission rate is called the baud rate, which corresponds to the number of bits per second. If a system has a maximum rate of 56,000 baud (which is relatively slow compared with other methods), approximately 1 minute will be required to transfer a $512 \times 512 \times 8$-bit image matrix. In practice, the actual transmission time is longer than anticipated, because the maximum transmission rate is not attained. A decrease in transmission time can be achieved by sending a compressed image that is converted to matrix format at the receiving station.

◼ **Example 20-2**

Calculate the transmission time (T) for a $512 \times 512 \times 8$-bit ultrasound image sent at a rate of 56,000 bits per second.

$$T = \frac{\text{Total bits}}{\text{Transmission rate}}$$

The total number of bits is 2,097,152.

$$T = \frac{2,097,152 \text{ bits}}{56,000 \text{ bps}}$$

$$T = 37 \text{ sec}$$

◼ **Example 20-3**

Calculate the transmission time (T) for a $512 \times 512 \times 8$-bit ultrasound image that has undergone a 3:1 compression. The transmission rate is 56,000 bits per second. The total number of bits is 699,051.

$$T = \frac{\text{Total bits}}{\text{Transmission rate}}$$

$$T = \frac{699,051 \text{ bits}}{56,000 \text{ bps}}$$

$$T = 12.5 \text{ sec}$$

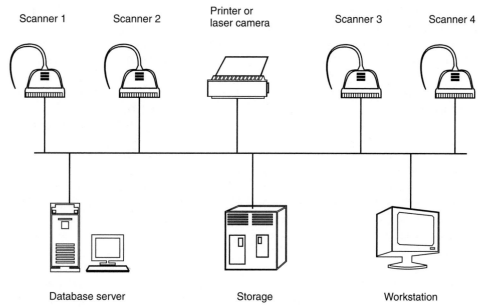

Fig. 20-2 Configuration of a mini–picture archiving and communication system network.

The digital subscriber line (DSL) telephone system designed for digital data communication can achieve a transmission rate of 1.5 Mbps. A 512-matrix image can thus be transferred in less than 2 seconds. Analog television cable modem has a transfer rate of 2 Mbps. Remember, an ultrasound examination consists of multiple static images and dynamic clips. As shown in Table 20-3, the volume of data expands dramatically as the number of images increases.

Web Server

Remote access is often provided by a Web server with image display software installed. This allows distribution of images and data via the established network (Internet) without the costly extension of a PACS to remote locations. Security, speed, and displayed image quality are important concerns regarding Internet access. Encryption is essential to protect patient privacy. The distribution of large data sets is avoided by designating the most important images that demonstrate clinical findings for remote access. Since most Internet access is via personal computers (PCs), images are normally viewed with the monitor installed with the PC. The monitor may need to be upgraded to improve displayed image quality. However, the same performance criteria applied to the workstation is not necessary. In general, review stations have lower performance standards than workstations used for interpretation.

SECURITY

Referring physicians and other health care professionals need ready access to images and reports from interpreted studies. At the same time, unauthorized access to patient data must be prohibited. Also, software and data must be protected from modification or loss by users or hackers.

A **firewall** is a router or computer connection between two networks that controls the flow of information from one network to the other. One security technique is packet filtering. All packets are examined at the firewall with respect to source, destination, and purpose to determine if this is an approved application established by the PACS administrator. If the packet meets the appropriate criteria, then the firewall forwards it to the destination. If the packet does not meet the appropriate criteria, then the packet is discarded. A PACS network connected to the Internet may have anyone with Internet access attempt to retrieve patient data from the PACS. Obviously, the release of this information must be very selective. Only approved users with proper identification and authorization should be able to access a PACS.

Other security techniques include encryption, authentication, and integrity. Encryption encodes the transmitted information at the source, which must be converted to the original form by the recipient. Authentication is a means to verify that the sender/recipient are who they are stated to be. Integrity describes the condition in which the transmitted information is received unaltered. Tests of the received information should yield certain results to confirm that the received data are the same as those sent.

RELIABILITY

Software and data must be protected from sabotage and accidental loss. Redundancy both in system critical function and file storage is necessary. System critical function is hardware/software, without which PACS ceases to function clinically. Duplication of all patient information should reside in long-term archival storage. Often, redundant storage for disaster recovery is located off site. If a disk drive fails, then whatever patient information and software contained on that disk should be available elsewhere so that the PACS continues without interruption. If connection to the RIS fails, then other means to enter patient demographics on a temporary basis must be provided. A well-designed system with reliable components minimizes downtime.

QUALITY CONTROL

In a PACS the primary means of image interpretation is by soft copy display on a CRT or LCD monitor. These devices can deviate from established operating parameters and require routine quality control checks to analyze monitor performance. In particular, luminance changes over time, and periodic recalibration is necessary. Decreased maximum luminance with time ultimately causes many monitor failures.

Monitor quality control procedures should include cleaning the screen, maximum and minimum luminance measurements, luminance uniformity, and image quality assessment with video test patterns. Sample tests to check monitor performance are shown below:

1. Maximum luminance level must be greater than 50 foot-Lambert (fL) or 170 candela per meter squared (cd/m^2) and should be at least 70 fL or 240 cd/m^2. The conversion factor between foot-Lambert and candela/meter squared is 1 fL equals 3.426 cd/m^2. An alternate unit for 1 cd/m^2 is the nit. A white box corresponding to 10% of the full image area is used for this measurement. A calibrated photometer is required.
2. Minimum luminance level (black) should be less than 0.3 fL or 1 cd/m^2.
3. Luminance levels for 20%, 40%, 60%, 80% of maximum output or some other combination of intermediate gray levels.
4. Ambient light level must be less than 50 lux and should be less than 10 lux.
5. Luminance uniformity at five locations (10% box moved to different points) should be within 20%, and 10% to 15% is desirable.
6. All-white image to check for glass and screen defects including bad pixels.
7. All-black image to check for bad pixels.
8. Video test pattern to evaluate image quality.

ADVANTAGES AND DISADVANTAGES

A major disadvantage of the current film archiving methods is that the hard copy cannot be readily viewed by several observers in various locations simultaneously. Accountability of the film file becomes problematical. In the PACS scheme simultaneous requests for the same study or same patient file can be accommodated with short retrieval times. The problem of lost films is also eliminated.

The electronic archiving of images is expected to decrease film costs. Communication between the imaging service and referring physicians can be improved by the electronic distribution of images and reports.

Advantages of a PACS include the following:
- Decreased film costs
- No lost films
- Current list of studies for interpretation
- Prompt access to images from multiple modalities
- Multiple clinicians can view the same images simultaneously
- Compact storage of patient data
- Image processing
- Computer-aided detection
- Electronic transfer to remote locations
- Reduced file room personnel

The primary disadvantages of a PACS are high cost, changing technology, complexity, and the digital conversion of all imaging modalities. The demand for instant access has also impeded the acceptance of PACS. Imaging specialists are often hesitant to replace transparency film, the image-recording standard for the past 100 years.

Disadvantages of a PACS in summary are as follows:
- Capital costs of equipment
- Recurring equipment costs
- Labor cost for technical personnel
- Conversion to digital format
- Lossy image compression
- Monitor viewing of images (light levels, dynamic range)
- Interfacing equipment from different manufacturers
- Changing technology
- Security
- Reliability

Conversion to filmless imaging represents a completely new approach to clinical workflow. A PACS requires extensive planning before implementation.

SUMMARY

Computer acquisition and digital manipulation of images has assumed a dominant role in ultrasound imaging. The digital format and DICOM standards enable ultrasound scanners to be readily interfaced to PACS. PACS has the potential to increase efficiency, improve patient care, and reduce long-term costs. The electronic distribution of images and reports decreases response time and creates a high level of satisfaction among referring physicians.

Computer performance versus cost is doubling every 2 years. The rapid development of computer capabilities will enhance the attractiveness of PACS networks. They must be modular and upgradeable, however, to adapt to these technologic changes.

▰▰▰ REVIEW QUESTIONS ▰▰▰

1. What is the importance of Digital Imaging and Communication in Medicine (DICOM) standards?
2. Why is data compression important for cost reduction in a picture archiving and communication system (PACS)?
3. Name two classifications of data compression with respect to the ability to change the compressed data back to the original image.

4. What are the primary advantages of a PACS?
5. Why is redundancy of data and software a necessary requirement with PACS?
6. Which types of storage devices are used for long-term permanent archive?
7. Calculate the transmission time for a $512 \times 512 \times 8$-bit ultrasound image that is transmitted at a rate of 1 million bits per second.
8. The term that describes the number of bits per second transmitted via the analog telephone line is the _____.
9. State the proper viewing conditions for a workstation.
10. What digital processing technique is used to enhance contrast resolution on the monitor?
11. What characteristics of the monitor are important for image interpretation?

BIBLIOGRAPHY

Arenson RL et al: The digital imaging workstation, *Radiology* 176:303-315, 1990.

Groth DS et al: Cathode ray tube quality control and acceptance testing program: initial results for clinical PACS displays, *Radiographics* 21:719-732, 2001.

Samei E et al: General guidelines for purchasing and acceptance testing of PACS equipment, *Radiographics* 24:313-334, 2004.

Seibert JA, Filipow, LJ, Andriole KP: *Practical digital imaging and PACS. American Association of Physicists in Medicine, 1999 Summer School Proceedings,* Madison, Wisc, 1999, Medical Physics Publishing.

CHAPTER 21

Intensity and Power

KEY TERMS

Acoustic output levels
  (equipment)
Intensity
Intensity descriptors
Mechanical index
Output display standard (ODS)
Peak negative pressure

Pulse average
Spatial average
Spatial peak
Temporal average
Temporal peak
Thermal index

The need to quantify intensity and power is twofold. Increasingly, clinical applications such as tissue harmonic imaging (THI) and contrast agent imaging are predicated on acoustic output level. Nonlinear propagation in tissue, destruction of microbubbles, and harmonic response of microbubbles are regulated by varying power. To assess biologic effects, we must know the dose of ultrasound. Dose in this instance has a meaning similar to that of radiation absorbed dose (rad). Therefore dose is the quantity of energy absorbed per unit mass of absorbing medium (e.g., tissue). Closely related to energy absorption throughout the medium is the point-by-point variation of intensity in the medium.

SPECIFICATION OF INTENSITY

Intensity is the rate of energy flow through a unit area. Unfortunately, state-of-the-art measurement techniques await a good method whereby the intensity (or some other parameter, such as pressure, from which intensity is calculated) could be ascertained at a particular point within tissue (classified as an in situ measurement). Typically the ultrasound device is characterized by using free-field experimental conditions in which the parameter of interest is determined in water without reflectors or other disturbances to the ultrasonic field. Free-field measurements do not assess the attenuation by tissue, focusing by anatomic structures, production of standing waves, or effect of reflecting boundaries. Nevertheless, free-field testing does provide measurable physical entities that characterize the ultrasound beam and allow comparisons between devices.

Because of the pulsing and scanning techniques employed, diagnostic ultrasound equipment produces complex and time-varying acoustic fields in space. Quantification of these patterns is impractical and difficult to correlate with the bioeffect potential of the ultrasound beam. Thus characterization of the ultrasonic field is accomplished by a few select parameters, usually related to energy, such as acoustic power, intensity, or peak negative pressure. Some researchers, however, have argued that other parameters (e.g., particle displacement, particle velocity, or particle acceleration) are more indicative of potential damage. The spatial and temporal dependence of the intensity complicates this descriptive process. Several shorthand methods have been developed to describe intensity.

Temporal Dependence

As the transducer emits pulses, it causes large fluctuations of intensity in the region through which the pulses move. Each pulse consists of multiple cycles that produce intensity variations within the pulse itself—the maximum intensity, designated **temporal peak (TP)**; the intensity averaged over the duration of a single pulse, designated **pulse average (PA)**; and the intensity averaged over the longer interval of the pulse repetition period, designated **temporal average (TA).** For a given pulse sequence, TP has the highest value, followed by PA, and finally by TA (Fig. 21-1).

The TA intensity is related to the PA intensity by the duty factor (DF):

$$TA = DF \times PA \qquad \text{21-1}$$

or by the pulse duration (PD) and pulse repetition frequency (PRF):

$$TA = PD \times PRF \times PA \qquad \text{21-2}$$

For example, if the pulse duration is 1 μs and the pulse-repetition period is 1 ms, the duty factor is 0.001. The PA intensity is 1000 times greater than the TA intensity. A determination of the TP intensity from the PA intensity requires knowledge of the pulse shape. The ratio TP/PA is typically in the range of 2 to 10.

The relationship between intensity peak and intensity averaging is an important concept. The following analogy may help illustrate it: Suppose a row of sand castles has been built along the seashore, as in Fig. 21-2. Each castle corresponds to a single pulse. The height of the tallest point of a castle represents the temporal peak. If a castle is flattened so the sand is spread evenly over its base, the level of the sand will be lower than the original peak. This corresponds to the pulse average. If the sand is distributed over the area between castles, it will be even lower than the original height of the peak. This represents the temporal average.

Spatial Dependence

The additional factor of space must now be considered in the shorthand description of intensity. Once more, the peak or average value with respect to the variable (in this case space) is used. The TP intensity, PA intensity, or TA intensity is mapped as a function of position. The variation in intensity

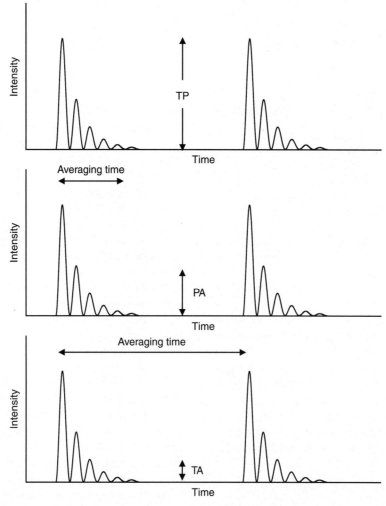

Fig. 21-1 Specification of intensity with respect to time. **A,** Temporal peak *(TP).* **B,** Pulse average *(PA).* **C,** Temporal average *(TA).*

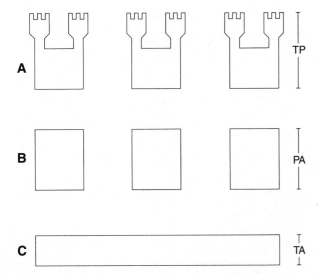

Fig. 21-2 Temporal averaging. **A,** The highest points on the sand castles *(turrets)* correspond to the temporal peak *(TP)*. **B,** Sand making up the turrets has been flattened and distributed across the base of each castle. This corresponds to the pulse average *(PA)*. **C,** The sand has been flattened to cover the area between the castles. This corresponds to the temporal average *(TA)*.

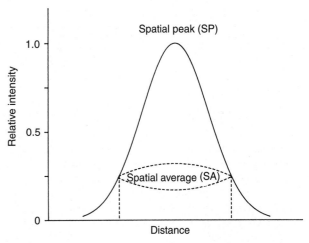

Fig. 21-4 Relationship of spatial peak *(SP)* and spatial average *(SA)* intensities. The curve represents the intensity profile across the width of the beam. The SA intensity is found by averaging the intensity over the beam width. In this case the boundary is defined at 0.25 SP.

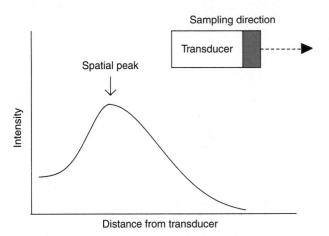

Fig. 21-3 Axial intensity profile. The intensity is maximal at a particular distance from the face of the transducer. This point is called the spatial peak intensity.

along the axis of propagation is illustrated in Fig. 21-3. The maximum intensity of all measured values within the sound field is designated as the **spatial peak (SP)**. Thus three combinations are possible depending on which temporal intensity is mapped:

I(SPTP)—Spatial peak, temporal peak intensity
I(SPPA)—Spatial peak, pulse average intensity
I(SPTA)—Spatial peak, temporal average intensity

The designation of spatial peak is not clearly defined. In some applications it refers to the maximum intensity in a plane perpendicular to the beam axis at a particular distance from the transducer. More commonly, however, it denotes the maximum intensity throughout the ultrasonic field, which usually occurs along the beam axis. The focusing of

the transducer is the most important determinant of spatial peak.

Spatial averaging over the cross-sectional area of the beam for each temporal intensity is also specified. A cutoff point of 0.25 times the SP intensity has been established to limit the area over which the intensity is averaged. Fig. 21-4 shows the intensity profile through the cross section of the beam and the location at which the **spatial average (SA)** is obtained. Again, three combinations are possible:

I(SATP)—Spatial average, temporal peak intensity
I(SAPA)—Spatial average, pulse average intensity
I(SATA)—Spatial average, temporal average intensity

For nonfocused transducers, the SP is usually greater than the SA by a factor of 2 to 6. The SP intensity is often converted to an SA by multiplying the peak value by one third. In the case of focused transducers, the degree of focusing influences this factor greatly. The ratio of SP to SA ranges from 5 to 50.

Alternative Intensity Descriptors

Other **intensity descriptors** have been used to specify the ultrasonic field. The instantaneous peak intensity (i_p) is the maximum intensity with respect to space and time and is the same as I(SPTP). The term maximum intensity (I_m), when used as a shorthand descriptor, refers to the time-averaged intensity over the largest half-cycle in the pulse at the spatial peak. For a perfect sine wave, I_m equals I(SPPA), although generally for pulsed ultrasound, the temporal-peak intensity is greater than the maximum intensity, which is greater than the PA intensity. Cycle-averaged intensity (I_a) is an alternative term for I(SPPA). The symbol I_T denotes the I(SATA) at the transducer, which has been spatially averaged over the area of the radiating surface (acoustic power divided by area of the transducer equals I_T). The intensity (I) of continuous-wave (CW) devices usually refers to a temporal-averaged intensity.

■ **Table 21-1** Intensity Descriptors

Parameter	Symbol
Instantaneous peak intensity (maximum intensity with respect to space and time)	I(SPTP) or i_p
Maximum intensity (at SP, time-averaged intensity over largest half-cycle)	I_m
Pulse-averaged intensity at spatial peak (averaged over the duration of the pulse)	I(SPPA) or I_a
Spatial peak, temporal average intensity	I(SPTA)
Spatial average, temporal peak intensity	I(SATP)
Spatial average, pulse average intensity	I(SAPA)
Time-averaged intensity at the transducer averaged over the area of the radiating surface	I_T
Spatial average, temporal average intensity	I(SATA)
Intensity of continuous wave (time-averaged intensity)	I
Instantaneous intensity	i

SP, Spatial peak.

A summary of various intensity descriptors is presented in Table 21-1.

Instantaneous Intensity

All the intensity parameters just discussed have been derived by averaging the instantaneous intensity (i) with respect to space, time, or both. The instantaneous intensity is determined from the measured acoustic pressure (p) using the equation

$$i = \frac{p^2}{\rho c} \tag{21-3}$$

where c is the speed of sound, and ρ is the density of the medium.

Table 21-2 shows the conversion between instantaneous intensity (in watts per square centimeter [W/cm²]) and pressure (in megapascals [MPa] and standard atmospheres [atm]). Frequently, pulsed-wave (PW) ultrasound is characterized by a **peak negative pressure** (expressed in MPa). The peak negative pressure is also called the peak rarefactional pressure (Fig. 21-5).

Clinical Usage

For continuous waveforms, time averaging is usually employed with an intensity specification of I(SATA) or I(SPTA). PA descriptors are not applicable for CW ultrasound.

These definitions of intensity descriptors must be modified slightly for real-time scanners. In autoscanning, consideration of the dwell time (i.e., time the ultrasound beam is directed toward a particular region) and the spatial sampling method must also be included in the averaging process.

■ **Table 21-2** Relationship between Intensity and Pressure

Intensity (W/cm²)	Pressure (MPa)	(atm)
0.001	0.004	0.04
0.01	0.0126	0.126
0.1	0.04	0.4
1	0.126	1.26
10	0.4	4
100	1.26	12.6

W/cm², Watts per centimeter squared; *MPa*, megapascal; *atm*, standard atmosphere.

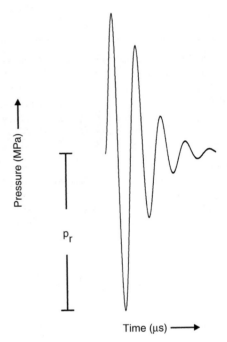

Fig. 21-5 Pressure variation as a function of time at a point in the ultrasonic field. The peak rarefactional pressure is designated p_r.

The most frequently quoted intensity is the I(SATA), which is approximated by the ratio of ultrasonic power to beam cross-sectional area (scan cross-sectional area for autoscanning systems). In practice, the temporal average of the power is determined by placing a plane absorber or plane reflector in the beam and measuring the resultant force. The power and, subsequently, the I(SATA) are computed from the radiation force. (See Chapter 24 for more information on the radiation force technique.)

Approximate values of the intensity descriptors for an illustrative set of conditions are listed in Table 21-3. The acoustic power is assumed to be 1 milliwatt (mW), and the beam cross-sectional area 1 cm². All the intensity descriptors are derived from I(SATA) using the SP/SA and TP/TA ratios defined previously. The duty factor is taken as 0.001. The ranking of intensity descriptors demonstrates that I(SPTP) has the highest value and I(SATA) the lowest. Although these parameters describe the same ultrasonic field, their values differ by a factor of 100,000 or more. The

■ **Table 21-3** Calculated Intensity Parameter Values*

Descriptor	Nonfocused	Focused
SATA[†]	1 mW/cm^2	1 mW/cm^2
SAPA	1 W/cm^2	1 W/cm^2
SATP	2 to 10 W/cm^2	2 to 10 W/cm^2
SPTA	2 to 6 mW/cm^2	5 to 50 mW/cm^2
SPPA	2 to 6 W/cm^2	5 to 50 W/cm^2
SPTP	4 to 60 W/cm^2	10 to 500 W/cm^2

Modified from O'Brien WD Jr: *Semin Ultrasound CT MR* 5:105-120, 1984.
PA/TA, 1000; TP/PA, 2 to 10; SP/SA for nonfocused transducers, 2 to 6;
SP/SA for focused transducers, 5 to 50.
SATA, Spatial average, temporal average intensity; *mW*, milliwatt; *cm^2*,
centimeter squared; *SAPA*, spatial average, pulse average intensity; *W*,
watt; *SATP*, spatial average, temporal peak intensity; *SPTA*, spatial peak,
temporal average intensity; *SPPA*, spatial peak, pulse average intensity;
SPTP, spatial peak, temporal peak intensity.
*Ultrasonic power of 1 mW and beam cross-sectional area of 1 cm^2.
[†]Evaluated at the radiating surface.

PA intensity can vary considerably depending on the ring-down characteristics of the transducer. The relative ranking of I(SPPA) and I(SATP) for a specific transducer is dictated by the pulse length and the degree of focusing.

OUTPUT DISPLAY STANDARD

The "standard for real-time display of thermal and mechanical acoustic output indices on diagnostic ultrasound equipment" was adopted by the American Institute of Ultrasound in Medicine (AIUM) and the National Eclectic Medical Association (NEMA) in 1992 with minor revisions in 1996 and 1998. This benchmark, which has become known as the **output display standard (ODS),** developed a formalism to calculate in real time the effect of operator-selected parameters on acoustic output. Two acoustic output parameters, the **thermal index (TI)** and the **mechanical index (MI),** were devised. The thermal index, in essence, gives the maximum temperature rise in tissue caused by energy absorption, and the mechanical index describes the maximum negative peak pressure in tissue.

OUTPUT LEVELS FROM DIAGNOSTIC EQUIPMENT

The intensity and power levels from commercial diagnostic instruments are now examined. The output characteristics from diagnostic devices vary considerably depending on their designed application. Units are classified according to the major categories—linear arrays, phased arrays, mechanical sector scanners, CW obstetric Doppler systems, CW peripheral vascular Doppler systems, CW fetal heart monitors, pulsed obstetric Doppler systems, pulsed peripheral vascular Doppler systems, and pulsed cardiac Doppler systems. In addition, among units of the same type, the intensity and power levels differ over a wide range of values.

Although many real-time pulse-echo imaging systems operate with an I(SPPA) in the range of 0.4 to 933 W/cm^2, most operate at less than 250 W/cm^2. Because the pulse duration is on the order of microseconds, with PRFs of approximately 1000 per second, the high intensity levels within a pulse are reached only a small fraction of the scan time. This produces an I(SPTA) in the 1 to 50 mW/cm^2 range. Acoustic power output is typically less than 50 mW.

PW Doppler units have the highest I(SPTA) values, because the temporal pulse length is relatively long compared with those generated in real-time scanners. Also, sensitivity (by increasing the power) must be improved to detect the weak scattering from RBCs. The I(SPTA) is usually less than 2 W/cm^2.

The acoustic power output, I(SPPA), and peak negative pressure of M-mode units are comparable to those found in B-mode scanners. The I(SPTA) for M-mode equipment, however, is generally higher.

The time-averaged intensity for CW peripheral vascular Doppler units is much higher than that obtained from CW obstetric Doppler units. The SATA intensities are typically 400 mW/cm^2 and 15 mW/cm^2, respectively. The pulsed Doppler units used in cardiology have SATA intensities of 3 to 32 mW/cm^2.

The various intensities produced by diagnostic devices are summarized in Tables 21-4 and 21-5. The data represent a collection of the output levels reported by several investigators. The American Institute of Ultrasound in Medicine (AIUM), the National Council on Radiation Protection and Measurements (NCRP), and the Bureau of Radiological Health have compiled similar tables. More

■ **Table 21-4** Survey of Acoustic Output Parameters in Diagnostic Ultrasound Equipment

Type	Power (mW)	I(SPTA) (mW/cm^2)	Peak Negative Pressure (MPa)
B-mode	0.3-360	0.3-991	0.45-5.5
M-mode	0.5-350	2.4-440	0.45-5.5
Pulsed wave Doppler	8.7-500	110-9500	0.2-6.3
Color Doppler	15-440	21-2050	0.46-4.2

From Henderson J et al: *Ultrasound Med Biol* 21:699-705, 1995; and
Duck FA, Martin K: *Phys Med Biol* 36:1423-1432, 1991.
I(SPTA), Spatial peak, temporal average intensity; *mW/cm^2,* milliwatt per centimeter squared; *MPa,* megapascal.

■ **Table 21-5** Survey of Acoustic Output Parameters for Intracavity Probes

Type	I(SPTA) (mW/cm^2)	Peak Negative Pressure (MPa)
M mode	2-210	0.66-3.5
B-mode	0.8-284	0.66-3.5
Pulsed wave Doppler	97-1440	0.97-3.5
Color Doppler	4-465	1.1-3

From Henderson J et al: *Ultrasound Med Biol* 21:699-705, 1995.
I(SPTA), Spatial peak, temporal average intensity; *mW/cm^2,* milliwatts per centimeter squared; *MPa,* megapascal.

recent surveys of the **acoustic output levels** of diagnostic ultrasound equipment have demonstrated the trend toward higher output intensity.

Unfortunately, measurements of acoustic output are not normally performed in the clinical environment due to limited resources and time-consuming measurement procedures. Independent verification of the manufacturer's stated values is not readily available. Since 1991, surveys of acoustic output have been conducted primarily in the United Kingdom.

Food and Drug Administration Requirements

In the United States manufacturers and importers of diagnostic ultrasound equipment are required to submit to the Food and Drug Administration (FDA) a report on the safety and testing of their products before the products are introduced on the market. This submission is called 510(k) notification, since section 510(k) of the Food, Drug, and Cosmetic Act established the requirement. The FDA has, in essence, set limits on the acoustic output intensity levels by stating that the intensity of diagnostic ultrasound equipment should be no greater than that measured for commercially available equipment manufactured before 1976. Intensity measurements for each transducer are made under the worst-case condition of highest power setting.

The initial FDA guidelines for acoustic output intensity levels measured in water are listed in Table 21-6. In 1985 the FDA revised the guidelines to include calculations of focal intensity in situ–based propagation through a homogeneous medium with an attenuation rate of 0.3 dB/cm/MHz. Maximum values of I(SPTA) and I(SPPA) in tissue were established (Table 21-7). Following the creation of the ODS, the FDA in 1997 increased the maximum output levels for cardiac, obstetric, and general purpose applications to be the same as the highest values previously measured for peripheral vascular systems. The ODS of mechanical index replaced I(SPPA) in the regulatory guidelines. *With the exception of ophthalmology, all systems have the I(SPTA) limit in tissue of 720 mW/cm² (Table 21-8), if the mechanical index is maintained to less than 1.9.* However, manufacturers can opt to follow I(SPPA) from 1985 or the

■ **Table 21-6** Food and Drug Administration Guidelines for Acoustic Output Intensities of Diagnostic Ultrasound Equipment (1976)*

Clinical Application	I(SPTA) (mW/cm²)	I(SPPA) (W/cm²)
Adult		
Peripheral vessel	1500	350
Cardiac	730	350
Abdominal, small organ, cephalic	180	350
Ophthalmic	68	110
Pediatric and fetal	180	350

I(SPTA), Spatial peak, temporal average intensity; *mW/cm²,* milliwatts per centimeter squared; *I(SPPA),* spatial peak, pulse average intensity; *W/cm²,* watts per centimeter squared.
*All measurements in water.

■ **Table 21-7** Food and Drug Administration Guidelines for Acoustic Output Intensities of Diagnostic Ultrasound Equipment (1985)

Application	I(SPTA) in Tissue (mW/cm²)	I(SPPA) in Tissue (mW/cm²)
Fetal imaging, neonatal, pediatric, and other general purpose	94	190
Cardiac	430	190
Peripheral vascular	720	190
Ophthalmic	17	28

I(SPTA), Spatial peak, temporal average intensity; *mW/cm²,* milliwatts per centimeter squared; *I(SPPA),* spatial peak, pulse average intensity.

■ **Table 21-8** Food and Drug Administration Guidelines for Acoustic Output Intensities of Diagnostic Ultrasound Equipment (1997)

Application	I(SPTA) in Tissue (mW/cm²)	MI
Fetal imaging, neonatal, pediatric, and other general purpose	720	1.9
Cardiac	720	1.9
Peripheral vascular	720	1.9
Ophthalmic	50	0.23

I(SPTA), Spatial peak, temporal average intensity; *mW/cm²,* milliwatts per centimeter squared; *MI,* mechanical index.

mechanical index limit. The two acoustic output parameters in the FDA guidelines, I(SPTA) and MI, address the primary concerns: rate of energy transfer to tissue and peak pressure (maximum intensity).

Acoustic Power Limits

The FDA's current guideline for acoustic intensity limit is not based on a risk-versus-benefit analysis of potential biologic effects but rather on the highest known output value an ultrasound device could produce in 1976. Measurements of intensity were SPTA intensity with a maximum of 720 mW/cm².

The continued restriction to the 1976 limit is controversial. Higher power output levels for diagnostic ultrasound units could increase penetration for B-mode, enhance nonlinear propagation for harmonic imaging, improve the performance of color Doppler imaging, allow greater use of contrast agents, and generally increase the signal-to-noise ratio. Research opportunities for new scanning techniques are not pursued because of this power limit.

The perception by clinicians is that the current output limit is completely safe. Manufacturers are reluctant to increase power limits since the potential improvements are not well defined, the expense to redesign transducers is high (transducers fail at the higher heating levels produced at higher power outputs), and additional training must be provided.

Industry Standards

Manufacturers have an obligation to characterize their units with respect to standards established by scientific and industry organizations. The results of these measurements should be communicated to potential buyers. Center frequency, bandwidth, peak negative pressure, I(SPTA), maximum power, and spatial profile of beam intensity should be specified. Examples of manufacturer's specifications for three transducers operating in B-mode and color Doppler mode are shown in Tables 21-9, 21-10, and 21-11.

Unfortunately, the acoustic output levels required to obtain a certain level of performance for particular applications are not established. Performance criteria including image quality are not well defined. Acoustic output level will depend on receiving and signal processing components. For B-mode scanners, the maximum I(SPTA) values in water range from less than 1 to 990 mW/cm². The benefits of a thousandfold increase in intensity should be characterized so that sonographers can make informed decisions regarding clinical use of ultrasound scanners.

American Institute of Ultrasound in Medicine Statement

The following AIUM statement, titled "Manufacturers Are Encouraged to Publish Acoustic Parameters," was approved in June 2003:

The AIUM Board of Governors believes that it is in the interest of the ultrasound community at large that a sufficient set of Acoustic Parameters of Ultrasound Systems be well documented and openly available. This information is necessary for the prudent and informed clinical use of ultrasound. The Board strongly endorses all efforts to require manufacturers to provide this information.*

SUMMARY

Characterization of the ultrasound beam is essential if the relationship between induced effects and the ultrasonic dose is to be described in a consistent and predictable manner. The most important beam parameters are intensity and pressure. Intensity exhibits wide spatial and temporal variation. Shorthand descriptors have been developed that designate a peak or average value with respect to both space and time. Although various combinations are possible, the most commonly used are SPTP, SPTA, and SATA. Pressure also fluctuates over a wide range, but ultrasound beams are usually denoted by a single pressure descriptor (called the peak negative pressure).

The Output Display Standard was developed to provide the operator with acoustic output information in real time.

*From American Institute of Ultrasound in Medicine: Manufacturers Are Encouraged to Publish Acoustic Parameters, http://www.aium.org/provider/statements/statements.asp, retrieved September 9, 2004.

Table 21-9 Manufacturer's Specification for a Linear Array

Parameter	B-mode	Color Doppler
Frequency (MHz)	6.9	7.2
Pulse duration (µs)	0.47	1.3
PRF (Hz)	2750	5610
Power (mW)	27	25
Peak pressure in tissue (MPa)	1.7	2.3
Pulsed average intensity (W/cm₂)	123	288
MI	0.63	0.85
TIB	0.9	0.87
TIC	0.98	1.8

MHz, Megaherz; PRF, pulse repetition frequency; Hz, hertz; mW, milliwatts; MPa, megapascal; W/cm², watts per centimeter squared; MI, mechanical index; TIB, thermal index (bone); TIC, thermal index (cranial bone).

Table 21-10 Manufacturer's Specification for a Curvilinear Array

Parameter	B-mode	Color Doppler
Frequency (MHz)	5.2	5
Pulse duration (µs)	0.48	1
PRF (Hz)	1440	2640
Power (mW)	53	32
Peak pressure in tissue (MPa)	2.4	2.1
Pulsed average intensity (W/cm²)	223	196
MI	1	0.92
TIB	1.5	0.91
TIC	1.3	1

MHz, Megaherz; PRF, pulse repetition frequency; Hz, hertz; mW, milliwatts; MPa, megapascal; W/cm², watts per centimeter squared; MI, mechanical index; TIB, thermal index (bone); TIC, thermal index (cranial bone).

Table 21-11 Manufacturer's Specification for a Linear Phased Array

Parameter	B-mode	Color Doppler
Frequency (MHz)	3.3	2.7
Pulse duration (µs)	0.61	0.94
PRF (Hz)	8750	664
Power (mW)	136	127
Peak pressure in tissue (MPa)	2.2	2
Pulsed average intensity (W/cm²)	251	210
MI	1.2	1.2
TIB	2.9	2.1
TIC	3.2	2.8

MHz, Megaherz; PRF, pulse repetition frequency; Hz, hertz; mW, milliwatts; MPa, megapascal; W/cm², watts per centimeter squared; MI, mechanical index; TIB, thermal index (bone); TIC, thermal index (cranial bone).

The mechanical index indicates the likelihood of cavitation based on peak negative pressure, and the thermal index predicts the maximum temperature rise in tissue caused by absorption of ultrasound energy.

The intensity and power from commercial diagnostic equipment vary over a wide range of values depending on application and model. For all applications except ophthalmic, the FDA has set a maximum limit of 720 mW/cm^2, if the mechanical index is maintained at less than 1.9.

REVIEW QUESTIONS

1. For a pulsed, focused ultrasound beam from a B-mode scanner, measurements of intensity were carried out in water. Rank the following intensity descriptors from highest to lowest: SPTP, SATP, SATA, SPTA.
2. What are the units for peak negative pressure?
3. What factors affect the temporal average of ultrasound intensity?
4. The instantaneous intensity is directly proportional to the _____ of the acoustic pressure.
5. The 1997 Food and Drug Administration guidelines specify limits for the _____ intensity and the output display standard of _____.
6. The location of the spatial peak intensity is influenced by the _____ characteristics of the transducer.
7. Free-field intensity measurements are made in _____ without the interference of other reflectors in the ultrasonic field.

BIBLIOGRAPHY

American Institute of Ultrasound in Medicine: Safety standard for diagnostic ultrasound equipment: appendix B—survey of exposure levels from current diagnostic ultrasound systems, *J Ultrasound Med* 2:S1-S50, 1983.

Duck FA: Output data from European studies, *Ultrasound Med Biol* 15(suppl 1):61-64, 1989.

Duck FA, Martin K: Trends in diagnostic ultrasound exposure, *Phys Med Biol* 36:1423-1432, 1991.

Federal Food and Drug Administration: *510(k) Guide for preparing reports on radiation safety of diagnostic ultrasound equipment,* Rockville, Md, 1993, Center for Devices and Radiological Health.

Henderson J et al: A survey of the acoustic outputs of diagnostic ultrasound equipment in current clinical use, *Ultrasound Med Biol* 21:699-705, 1995.

NCRP Report 140: *Exposure criteria for medical diagnostic ultrasound: II. Criteria based on all known mechanism,* Bethesda, Md, 2002, National Council on Radiation Protection and Measurements.

NCRP Report 74: *Biological effects of ultrasound: mechanisms and clinical implications,* Bethesda, Md, 1983, National Council on Radiation Protection and Measurements.

O'Brien WD Jr: Safety of ultrasound with selective emphasis for obstetrics, *Semin Ultrasound CT MR* 5:105-120, 1984.

Steward HF, Stratmeyer ME: An overview of ultrasound: theory, measurement, medical applications, and biological effects, *HHS Pub (FDA)* 82-8190, 1982.

Zagzebski JA: Acoustic output of ultrasound equipment: summary of data reported to the AIUM, *Ultrasound Med Biol* 15(suppl 1):55-59, 1989.

Biologic Effects

The medical applications of ultrasound have experienced considerable growth during the past 30 years. The development and subsequent incorporation of new technology into reasonably priced, commercially available devices have made ultrasound readily accessible. The increased acceptance of this modality, however, can be attributed in large part to one especially attractive feature—ultrasound does not use ionizing radiation. Obstetrics seems particularly well suited for ultrasonic techniques, which include amniocentesis, fetal heart monitoring, estimation of fetal age, determination of fetal position, diagnosis of multiple pregnancy, and placental localization. Indeed, ultrasound has completely replaced x-ray pelvimetry as a means of evaluating the maternal pelvis and fetal head before childbirth. Fetal exposure to ionizing radiation, which has the potential for latent biologic injury at diagnostic x-ray levels according to current radiation protection philosophy, is completely eliminated in ultrasound.

Besides its applicability in obstetrics, ultrasound can be used in cardiology (for the detection of pericardial effusion, valvular dysfunction, or wall-motion abnormalities), in vascular studies, in ophthalmology (for the detection of vitreous hemorrhage, retinal detachment, or intraocular foreign bodies), and in gastroenterology (especially for the assessment of an abdominal mass).

AREAS OF RESEARCH

No acute harmful effects have been reported after diagnostic ultrasound examinations. Nevertheless, when large populations are exposed to any diagnostic modality, it is appropriate to investigate any potential long-term effects, which may not be evident on an individual case-by-case basis. Any risk (i.e., potential harmful effect) versus benefit (i.e., diagnostic information derived) analysis requires an assessment of the risk factors. Quantification of risk is not currently available and, most likely, will never be precisely known. Ethical considerations preclude experimentation on human subjects, although such studies would provide the necessary data. Instead, the potential harmful effects to the exposed human population must be inferred from other avenues of investigation. Several of these can contribute to an overall comprehensive picture:

- Development of measurement techniques to quantify the ultrasonic dose received by a patient or test system

- Identification of mechanisms by which ultrasound interacts with matter
- In vitro studies of biologically significant molecules and various cell types
- Animal studies with intensity levels comparable to those used in diagnostic ultrasound
- Epidemiologic studies of human populations that will undergo or have undergone diagnostic ultrasound examination

Predictive Models

Because of the observed bioeffects, most research has been conducted at higher intensity levels and with longer exposure times than those used clinically. *The validity of results from these studies is limited when extrapolated to predict potential effects from medical exposures.* The problem posed is not unique to ultrasound. If we wanted to know the hazard (or benefit) of the thermal effects resulting from taking a warm bath, the effect to 100° C could readily be measured using relatively few subjects. However, we would encounter some difficulty in constructing a model that permitted the extrapolation of resulting data to temperatures slightly above 37° C. To perform the study at 40° C, for example, would require an epidemiologic comparison of possibly a million subjects in which the control and test populations were matched perfectly. For the study of any effect, as the probability of that effect approaches zero, the number of individuals necessary to quantitate this probability approaches infinity. In most situations we attempt to avoid large risks and accept risks that may be nonzero but that are too small to measure accurately.

Threshold versus Nonthreshold Effects

Intensity levels below a certain value may be incapable of inducing an effect if a **threshold** exists. Effects reported for high intensity levels will not be present at levels lower than the threshold. If the biologic response has no threshold, however, any exposure to the physical agent carries some risk; the question then becomes whether incidence rate per unit dose at low intensity is the same as that at high intensities for which the effects are observed. In addition, the dependency of the response on other factors such as frequency, pulse sequence, pulse width, and exposure time must be considered.

Early Research

Unfortunately, much of the early work published in the scientific literature is seriously flawed. Many experiments have lacked proper controls; furthermore, the conditions of irradiation have not been specified, particularly with respect to defining the ultrasound field intensity. The term irradiation describes the process wherein ultrasonic energy is transmitted as a wave; it does not mean that the sound wave is ionizing. The early animal experiments were important for demonstrating acute functional or gross structural

alterations at very high intensity levels (e.g., the production of lesions in the brain or the interruption of nervous conduction in the spinal cord). Recently, more research has been directed toward elucidating potential effects at intensity levels produced by diagnostic devices.

INTERACTIONS OF ULTRASOUND WITH MATTER

Three mechanisms by which ultrasound interacts with matter have been identified: acoustic radiation force, thermal, and cavitation. These are microscopic effects as compared with the macroscopic interactions of ultrasound in tissue (see Chapter 1). Other phenomena—microstreaming and altered chemical reaction rates—have been linked with experimental end points, but these are initiated by one of the aforementioned mechanisms of action.

Mechanical Interactions

The first mechanism by which damage can be induced, **radiation force,** is sometimes called direct and generally includes all but thermal and cavitational effects. The ultrasound wave propagates through the medium by interactions between neighboring particles. The particles undergo considerable changes in velocity and acceleration. A discrete object with a density different from that of the surrounding medium experiences a force in the ultrasound field, because acoustic pressure is applied over its surface. This causes translational or rotational motion of the object. The translational motion may transport biologic particles (e.g., cells) to highly localized regions within the ultrasound field. The rotational motion may give rise to acoustic streaming (i.e., circulatory flow of the fluid), and spinning of intracellular particles may be induced. At high intensities, high-velocity gradients are formed near solid boundaries. The resulting microstreaming (i.e., rapid movement of fluid in a localized area) can fragment the macromolecules in these regions.

Thermal Interactions

The second mechanism by which damage can be induced is **thermal.** With the ultrasound beam propagation through the medium, its intensity decreases as the sonic energy is absorbed and converted to heat. The increased temperature has the potential to cause irreversible tissue damage. The rate of temperature rise depends on the temporal average intensity, the absorption coefficient of the medium, the cross-sectional area of the beam, the duration of exposure, and the heat-transport processes (thermal conductivity and blood flow). Within the frequency range of 1 to 10 MHz, the absorption coefficient increases with frequency.

Thermal effects dominate the low-megahertz frequencies and tend to mask other (nonthermal) effects. To observe cavitation and other nonthermal effects, it is necessary to minimize the thermal component by cooling the medium or by some other means (e.g., lowering the pulse repetition frequencies [PRFs]).

Cavitation Interactions

The third mechanism by which damage can be induced is **cavitation.** As the ultrasound wave propagates through the medium, regions of compression and rarefaction are created. Thus localized regions are subjected to increases and decreases in pressure in an alternating fashion, and these cause gas bubbles to form and grow and to exhibit dynamic behavior. This phenomenon is known as cavitation, and it can be either stable or transient.

Stable cavitation. In **stable cavitation,** microbubbles already present in the medium expand and contract during each cycle in response to the applied pressure oscillations. The bubbles may also grow as dissolved gas leaves the solution during the negative-pressure phase, a process called rectified diffusion. Each bubble oscillates about the expanding radius for many cycles without collapsing completely. At a characteristic frequency (which is a function of the size of the bubble) the vibration amplitude of neighboring liquid particles is maximized. This condition is called volume resonance.

The action of the gas bubble in the liquid is analogous to a child's swinging on a swing. An external force (push) applied to the child at the proper point in the oscillatory path increases the height of the swing. If the force is repeated over and over at the proper frequency, the motion of the swing will be amplified. If the child is pushed opposite the direction of movement, the height of the swing will decrease. The interplay between the rate of pushing and the physical characteristic of the swing (e.g., length of rope between the pivot point and the seat) is essential for maximum effect. Similarly, in cavitation, the interaction between the size of the gas bubble (i.e., the swing) and the frequency becomes critically important.

A free air bubble in water undergoes resonance at 1 MHz when its radius is 3.5 μm. At higher frequencies, the size of the bubble required for resonance decreases. Bubbles somewhat smaller than resonance size tend to grow, whereas those significantly larger than resonance size do not sustain stable cavitation. Oscillations of a gas bubble may produce high shearing forces in the nearby surrounding areas. Stable cavitation may also give rise to microstreaming. The radial oscillatory motion of the bubble is not always spherically symmetrical. An adjoining solid boundary may distort the motion of the bubble and cause eddies near the air-liquid interface. High-velocity gradients are created in the localized region of the oscillatory boundary layer. Biomolecules or membranes subjected to such gradients can fragment or rupture.

Stable cavitation has been reported in mammalian tissue at the continuous-wave (CW) spatial peak intensity of 80 mW/cm[2].[1] O'Brien[2] has theorized that a CW spatial peak intensity as low as 0.1 mW/cm[2] is sufficient to cause stable cavitation. The pulse sequence may have considerable importance and appears to be a resonant effect acting over several cycles.

Transient cavitation. Transient cavitation is a more violent form of microbubble dynamics in which short-lived bubbles undergo large size changes over a few acoustic cycles before completely collapsing.

During the rarefaction phase, bubbles may be formed by dissolved gases leaving the solution or bubbles of submicron dimensions may already exist in the medium. High viscosity and surface tension inhibit bubble growth. A rarefaction phase of long duration enhances bubble growth.

During the compression phase, changing pressure causes the bubbles to collapse and produce highly localized (within 1 μm[3]) shock waves. In addition, very high temperatures (up to 10,000° K) and pressures (10^8 pascals or higher) are created within the bubbles, resulting in the decomposition of water to free radicals. These pressures and temperature changes may also drive chemical reactions.

The release of enzymes when shock waves rupture lysosomal membranes may also enhance DNA and protein synthesis.

The general consensus is that transient cavitation is a threshold effect. The intensity levels necessary for cavitation to develop in tissue are a matter of debate. The pressure threshold for transient cavitation in water is 0.3 MPa at 1 MHz if gas bodies of optimal size are present (0.5 μm radius).[3] At higher frequencies, increased pressure or intensity is required.[4] The threshold for transient cavitation in tissue without preexisting gas nuclei is most likely 1500 W/cm[2] I(SPTP) (instantaneous peak intensity [maximum intensity with respect to space and time]) or greater.[5] Theoretic analysis suggests that the I(SPTP) threshold for transient cavitation in tissue is in the range of 1 to 10 W/cm[2] for microsecond-pulsed ultrasound if gas bubbles of optimal size are present.[6]

Apfel and Holland[3] have predicted that a negative peak pressure of 0.3 MPa at 1 MHz is sufficient to cause cavitation in blood under the conditions of short pulse length (5 μs) and low duty cycle (0.1%). *The threshold of the peak negative pressure increases with frequency, exhibiting an $f^{0.5}$ dependence* (Fig. 22-1). As the peak negative pressure is increased above the threshold value at a certain frequency, bubbles of different size can also undergo transient cavitation, which generally extends bubble activity to more sites. Transient cavitation has been demonstrated in mammalian systems at pressure levels generated by diagnostic imaging equipment.

Cavitation-Induced Effects

Organisms that contain small stable gas bodies are more likely to incur damage by cavitation when exposed to ultrasound. Cavitation has been demonstrated to be responsible for the death and abnormal development of *Drosophila* (fruit fly) larvae exposed to ultrasound. The contribution of thermal effects is eliminated by using very low temporal average intensities to prevent heating. The larvae contain air-filled tubes, which function as a respiratory apparatus. These naturally occurring gas bodies may serve as sites for cavitation. Peak intensity rather than temporal averaged intensity is the most important physical predictor of the effects induced by cavitation.

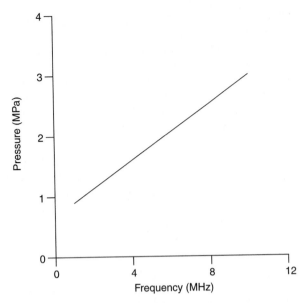

Fig. 22-1 Threshold for cavitation in situ. Negative peak pressures for biologic effects show a dependence on the square root of frequency.

Attributing biologic effects to cavitation in animals is more difficult, because gaseous nuclei have not been identified, and the associated heating in cavitation experiments interferes with the interpretation of data. Some evidence for the existence of gas bubbles in mammalian tissues has been presented in the literature. Raising the hydrostatic pressure increased the intensity threshold for hind limb paralysis in neonatal mice.[7] Ter Haar and Daniels[1] observed stable bubbles in the hind limb of a guinea pig following exposure to a commercial ultrasound-therapy device operating at 0.75 MHz and 0.68 W/cm² I(SATA) (spatial average, temporal average intensity). In separate studies, cavitation damage has been responsible for lung hemorrhage in dogs and mice exposed to a shock wave lithotripter.[8,9]

Lung hemorrhage in mice, rats, pigs, rabbits, and monkeys exposed to microsecond-pulsed ultrasound demonstrated a threshold for damage.[10-13] From multiple studies, the pressure threshold to cause hemorrhage was generally between 1 and 2 MPa for the frequency range 0.5 to 5 MHz. Beam diameter and temporal-averaged intensity did not influence the pressure threshold. These findings are consistent with the cavitation phenomenon. The response showed a pressure divided by the square root frequency dependence, which also supports the hypothesis of cavitation-induced damage in vivo.

The pressure threshold for hemorrhage in murine intestine is similar to that observed for lung hemorrhage.[14] The fetal intestine, which presumably contains no bubbles, showed no damage under the same exposure conditions that produced damage in 100 percent of the dams.[15] Hemorrhage near fetal bone in mice has a pressure threshold of 2.5 MPa at 1 MHz.[16]

Little damage has been observed in fetal lung exposed to a peak pressure of 20 MPa.[9] Mouse kidney showed essentially no damage at peak pressures almost 10 times greater than the threshold for lung hemorrhage.[17] The presence of appropriate-sized bubbles in the lung predisposes this organ to damage.

EFFECTS ON BIOMOLECULES

The observed biologic effect on mammalian systems exposed to ultrasound is most likely the end product of a long chain of events involving physical, chemical, and physiologic processes. The initial step is absorption of energy, generally considered to take place at the macromolecular level. Numerous studies on biomolecules in solution have identified the types of damage and elucidated the mechanisms by which damage is induced.

The in vitro experimental conditions have been extremely diverse. In many studies the physical aspects of ultrasound exposure and, consequently, the intensity field to which the biomolecules were exposed have not been well defined. The presence of reflecting boundaries distorts the ultrasonic field. Dissolved gas in solution, which cannot be controlled adequately, enhances cavitation.

Inactivation of enzymes in vitro has been demonstrated at very high intensities (e.g., 10^4 W/cm²).[18] Cavitation appears necessary to produce damage in protein molecules. Certainly, most of the work has been directed toward DNA and its component parts (i.e., bases, nucleotides, and nucleosides). Base damage similar to that induced by ionizing radiation via free radical formation has been identified. The bases appear to react with free radicals produced by cavitation. Degradation of DNA in solution is most often associated with intensities above 25 to 72 W/cm² as a result of cavitation.[19-22] One study, however, reported partial degradation of DNA in solution for intensities as low as 200 mW/cm².[23] Extrapolation to the in vivo case is difficult, because the viscosity of cytoplasm necessitates higher intensity levels to produce comparable velocity gradients.[24] Also, DNA is not in a free state within the living organism but is part of an intricate structure that may protect it. Finally, the presence of gaseous bodies in solution may enhance damage.

In general, the damage to biomolecules in solution is associated with the cavitation type of mechanism.

EFFECTS ON CELLS

Cells are typically irradiated in an aqueous solution or monolayer state attached to the surface of a culture dish. An extremely diverse variety of cell types—including human red blood cells, human lymphocytes, human platelets, cells in culture, protozoa, ameba, and bacteria—has been investigated. The criticisms outlined in the previous section regarding biomolecules pertain to experiments involving cells.

Cell lysis is caused by cavitation at high intensity levels.[25] Cell killing has also been attributed to microstreaming near cavitating bubbles and to free radical production. In addition, altered morphology of cultured mammalian cells has been observed.[26,27] Both positive and negative neoplastic transformation of cultured cells has been reported, although the studies with positive findings were criticized for low plating efficiency and a lack of certain types of transformed loci.[27,28]

Survival and growth rate for some cell types are reduced following exposure to ultrasound. Cell-surface function as assessed by the transport of ions across membranes, by electrophoretic and phagocytic activity, and by attachment to surfaces is altered by shear forces generated from stable cavitation. Cell-cycle sensitivity has been reported, but researchers are not in agreement regarding the most sensitive phase of the cell cycle.

Few effects have been observed under conditions in which cavitation does not occur. The presence of gas nuclei is critical for damage to occur. In an experiment not involving cultured cells, chick embryos *in ovo* were insonated with pulsed-wave (PW) ultrasound.[29] The exposure parameters were 1.1 MHz, PRF of 2000 per second, temporal pulse length of 75 μs, and exposure time of 10 minutes. No effect on cell proliferation and migration of chick motoneurons was observed.

EFFECTS ON MAMMALS

Focal lesions are observed in the brain following ultrasound exposure when the product of the I(SPTA) (spatial peak, temporal average intensity) and the square root of the time for a single pulse exceeds a threshold of 200 $Ws^{0.5}/cm^2$.[30] This relationship holds for a large range of exposures (100 μs to 10 minutes). The threshold for irreversible structural change is higher for other organs (e.g., liver, kidneys, and testes). When the spinal cords of neonatal mice were irradiated, hind limb paralysis was induced at a threshold approximately 25% of that for brain lesions.[31]

Accelerated tissue regeneration has been demonstrated in some cases when the injured tissue was subjected to periodic exposure to ultrasound.[32]

The combined application of ultrasound and ionizing radiation to solid tumors has produced a synergistic effect, reducing tumor volume and extending survival time.[33] Ultrasound heats the tumor site to approximately 43° C at the same time that ionizing radiation is delivered to the site. This treatment (called hyperthermia) has evolved into a highly specialized modality in radiation oncology.

Little evidence of biologic effect exists for an I(SPTA) of less than 100 mW/cm^2, regardless of the duration of exposure.

GENETIC EFFECTS

Mutations

In studies with yeast, bacteria, and fruit flies exposed to diagnostic levels of ultrasound, no evidence of increased mutations has been observed. Negative findings have also been reported for intensity levels greater than those used in clinical practice. Early work with *Drosophila,* presumably at high intensities, has shown that there is an induction of dominant lethal mutations. However, these mutations have been attributed to heat, which is mutagenic in *Drosophila.*[34]

Free radicals have been shown to cause DNA damage that may be expressed as a mutation. Hydroxyl radicals and hydrogen atoms are formed in aqueous solutions by transient cavitation. Free radical generation in aqueous solutions exposed to ultrasound pulses at diagnostic levels has also been reported.[35] If DNA is located near the site of free radical formation, mutations are possible.

The potential for DNA damage in cells exposed to ultrasound is unclear. Repair synthesis, an indirect indicator of DNA damage, has been shown to be both present and absent following insonation of intact cells.[27,36] Thymine base damage in the DNA of cells has also been reported.[37]

Kaufman[26] observed mutations in cultured mammalian cells in suspension exposed to 1 MHz CW ultrasound at a spatial peak intensity of 35 W/cm^2. The mutation rate was very low but increased with exposure times ranging from 60 to 180 seconds. Another study involving hamster cells and human lymphoblasts found that CW ultrasound at 35 W/cm^2 increased the mutation rate by a factor of approximately 2.[38] Experiments with human-hamster hybrid cells containing human chromosome 11 following insonation with CW and PW ultrasound failed to demonstrate mutagenic effects.[39] The assay method used in the latter study is generally very sensitive to mutation caused by most agents.

Single-strand DNA breaks have been observed in Chinese hamster ovary cells exposed to an I(SPTA) of 8 W/cm^2.[40] Cell killing was extensive, however, and the breaks were in nonviable cells. Mutations cannot be propagated by nonviable cells.

Aberrations

During the early 1970s, MacIntosh and Davey[41,42] reported an increase in the frequency of chromatid and chromosomal aberrations of human lymphocytes irradiated in vitro with a fetal heart monitor. These authors observed a threshold of 8.2 mW/cm^2 for a 1-hour exposure at 2.25 MHz. Their reports generated controversy as well as concern, because this intensity level is in the diagnostic range, and patients would definitely be at risk. Numerous investigations by other researchers have failed to support MacIntosh and Davey's observation of increased chromosomal aberrations at peak intensities of 300 W/cm^2. Indeed, MacIntosh et al.[43] subsequently repeated the experiments and found no evidence of chromosomal aberrations.

Several investigators have tested for chromosomal aberrations in lymphocytes isolated from neonates exposed in utero.[44-46] No significant differences in either type or number were found between the exposed and control groups.

Nonclassical chromosomal aberrations have been reported for Vicia faba root tips exposed to ultrasound (8 W/cm^2 for 1 minute at 2 MHz).[47] The chromosomal damage was in the form of bridged prophases and metaphases and agglomerated mitotics, which would not have been detected in the standard chromosomal aberration–scoring technique. The significance of this type of damage is unknown.

Lyon and Simpson[48] exposed the gonads of mice to approximately 1 W/cm^2 of either CW or PW ultrasound (pulse width 30 μs, duty factor 0.02) at 1.5 MHz. They tested for translocations in spermatocytes and dominant lethal mutations and found none. Only a small number of animals were examined, however. Mutation rates would have to have been high to be detected.

Sister Chromatid Exchange

During mitosis, every chromosome must be replicated so each daughter cell receives identical genetic material. The chromosomes consist of two identical chromatids, which are joined together during the prophase and metaphase. Chromatids on the same chromosome can exchange DNA, generally at the same relative position. The process is called sister chromatid exchange (SCE). Although SCEs have been linked to mutagenic agents (e.g., ultraviolet radiation, x-rays, and certain drugs), their biologic importance has not been established. Controversy regarding the potential of ultrasound at diagnostic levels to cause SCEs has evolved over the past several years.

An increased frequency of SCEs in human lymphocytes following exposure to a diagnostic ultrasound device has been observed by Liebeskind et al.[49] A different cell type (HeLa cells) from this same laboratory showed no difference in SCE frequency.[27] Additional studies by other researchers have also found an increased frequency in SCEs following exposure to ultrasound.[50,51] The majority of studies, however, including those that attempted to replicate Liebeskind's work and those using much higher intensity levels, have demonstrated no effect on the frequency of SCEs.[52-57] Because some researchers who reported positive results failed to include positive controls, the validity of their results remains in question. Nevertheless, the magnitude of the SCE effect is probably small, and the variability reported in the literature can be attributed to undefined experimental conditions in vitro.

Assays of DNA Damage

Other in vitro experiments have examined the effect on genetic material of exposure to ultrasound, with positive findings. As noted in the previous section, purified DNA is degraded by ultrasound. Transformation of cells, altered DNA synthesis, and formation of glycols have also been reported. Unwinding of the DNA following exposure to diagnostic levels of ultrasound is suggested by the observation of increased immunoreactivity to antinucleoside antibodies in cultured cells. This is classified as an immune effect, because the assay method involves an immune technique—not because a response of the immune system was evoked. Although they are not proof of a genetic effect, these results are suggestive of one.

Mutagenic Potential

The conflicting results obtained from mutagenicity studies of mammalian cells in culture remain unresolved. If ultrasound is a mutagen, its mutagenic action is relatively weak compared with that of x-rays. Furthermore, intensity levels sufficient to produce cavitation are required. The site of cavitation must be close to the DNA so the free radicals produced can migrate to the DNA.

TERATOGENIC EFFECTS

The sensitivity of embryonic and fetal tissues to chemical and physical agents (e.g., ionizing radiation) is well documented. The extensive use of ultrasound in obstetrics combined with an anticipated increased sensitivity of tissues to ultrasound has led to the question whether diagnostic ultrasonic techniques can affect the developing embryo or fetus. The subject may be addressed from two approaches—one involving experiments with prenatal ultrasound exposure of animals, usually mammals, and the other involving epidemiological studies of human populations. These avenues are discussed in the following sections.

Experimental Observations

Much experimental work has been published regarding the possible effects following prenatal ultrasound exposure. Because of the diverse experimental conditions, these studies are difficult to consolidate in a consistent pattern. Single and multiple exposures to PW and CW ultrasound at different intensity levels have been used at various stages of gestation. Fetal deaths in rats and mice have been induced following such exposures. This effect is associated with a rise in temperature of the amniotic fluid. The initial rate of the temperature rise and the absolute evaluation in temperature are dependent on the intensity of the ultrasonic beam.

Some researchers have reported on congenital malformations and fetal mortality rates.[58] The type of malformation produced is a function of the developmental stage during which exposure occurred and is similar to that obtained with ionizing radiation and thermal insult. Most of these studies, however, were conducted using intensities above diagnostic levels. In addition, there were many reports of negative findings, even at high intensities.[58]

In vivo exposure to CW ultrasound at intensities of less than 1 W/cm² during the preimplantation period does not appear to affect development in rodents. When early rat embryos were exposed in vitro to CW ultrasound at 0.65 W/cm² for 1 hour, retardation in development and abnormal morphologic characteristics were observed.[59] These were attributed to a thermal mechanism, because embryos subjected to the same temperature increase without ultrasound exposure demonstrated similar results. Another study reported embryolethality and weight reduction in rats exposed to pulsed ultrasound during the preimplantation period.[60] Peak intensity has been estimated to be 1 W/cm², but the dosimetry aspects are questionable. Researchers from other laboratories have been unable to replicate this finding for intensities as high as 10 W/cm².[61]

Warwick et al.[62] found no significant differences in fetal weight, litter size, resorption rate, or number of abnormalities among groups of mice irradiated for 5 minutes on different gestational days with an I(SPTP) as high as 490 W/cm². Shoji et al.,[63,64] however, reported some very controversial findings: Pregnant mice irradiated for 5 hours on the ninth day of gestation with CW ultrasound from a commercial fetal Doppler device, intensity level 40 mW/cm², had statistically significant increases in fetal mortality and congenital abnormalities. These observations have been attributed to the stress associated with physical restraint of the animals for 5 hours or to possible temperature elevation during the long exposure time. The results have not been confirmed by an independent research group.

Diagnostic Intensity Levels

Two studies have linked PW ultrasound exposure at diagnostic intensity levels with congenital abnormalities via a nonthermal mechanism. Takabayashi et al.[65] reported that pulsed ultrasound with an I(SATP) (spatial average, temporal peak intensity) threshold of 60 W/cm² produced malformations in mice. A repeat of this study by another laboratory, however, yielded completely negative results, and additional experiments with microsecond PW ultrasound exposure to mouse fetuses under hyperbaric conditions showed no malformations for an I(SAPA) of 100 W/cm².[66] Taylor and Dyson[67] observed congenital abnormalities following ultrasound exposure to chick embryos. The experimental conditions were 20 μs temporal pulse length, 5000 pulses per second, 1 MHz, intensity of 25 W/cm², and exposure time of 5 minutes. PW ultrasound provided a low TA intensity so the effects of heating were eliminated. At intensity levels of less than 10 W/cm², no congenital abnormalities occurred. A long temporal pulse length and high PRF are not characteristic of real-time instrumentation. Less controversial is the finding that high-pressure shock waves from lithotripsers (≥10 MPa) will induce malformations in chick embryos.[68]

Thermal Damage

Thermal-induced damage is a threshold phenomenon; that is, no biologic effects are observed unless the temperature elevation exceeds a particular value for a minimum time duration. The threshold for thermal bioeffects, including fetal abnormalities, is shown in Fig. 22-2. A temperature increase of 2.5° C must be present for 2 hours to cause fetal abnormalities. At higher temperatures, the time necessary to induce damage is shortened dramatically (e.g., at 43° C it is 1 minute).

Nonthermal Damage

Certainly exposure durations of 1 hour at TA intensities capable of increasing the temperature 3° C to 4° C can induce fetal abnormalities in small mammals. Whether nonthermal mechanisms also contribute to fetal abnormalities is less certain. In an extensive research effort, fetal weight reduction in mice was linked to a dose parameter (intensity squared times the exposure time) for intensities greater than

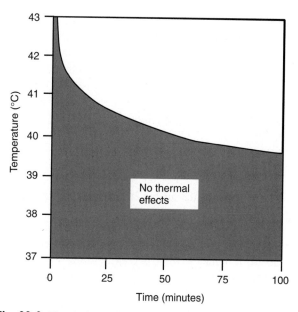

Fig. 22-2 Threshold for thermal biologic effects. No adverse effects are observed for time-temperature combinations in the shaded region.

diagnostic levels.[56] With this model, the fetal weight reduction predicted at diagnostic intensity levels was considered to be insignificant. Fetal weight reduction in rats has not been detected at spatial-averaged intensities below 30 W/cm².

Subtle changes in some reflex responses for rodents after in utero exposure have been reported by a number of researchers. The effects were noted at or near diagnostic intensity levels. Such observations imply that in utero ultrasound exposure affects prenatal growth and development.

Beam Size

Most in vivo studies on mice and rats have been done using transducers from the clinical setting. Relatively speaking, these transducers produce large-sized beams for the animal subject. The rodent fetus is usually completely enveloped by the beam, whereas only part of the human fetus would be included within the ultrasonic field. The fraction of tissue exposed, which is much less for humans, may influence the amount of damage induced.

EPIDEMIOLOGIC STUDIES

Although experimentation on animals has provided some insight into and reassurance regarding the potential effects from ultrasound exposure at diagnostic levels, the application of these data to human populations is limited. *The ultimate assessment of biologic effects induced in human populations exposed to ultrasound lies with **epidemiologic studies***. Observational investigations of human populations attempt to answer the question whether individuals exposed to a particular agent have a higher risk of developing impaired health than nonexposed individuals do.

The major complication in epidemiologic studies is the influence of other risk factors. The agent of interest is most likely not the sole determinant of an adverse effect;

furthermore, the risk of a potential effect is not the same for all members of the population. Modification of the incidence of an adverse effect by other factors is called confounding.

If the additional risk to an exposed population is small, large sample sizes will be required to distinguish the agent-induced effects from disorders that occur spontaneously. Sample size limits the minimum level of excess risk detectable in a particular study.

Detection of Adverse Effects

The ability to identify an adverse effect in a population exposed to a particular agent (e.g., drug, x-ray, or ultrasound) depends on the visibility of the effect and its probability in the exposed as well as unexposed population. The absence of a thumb at birth is readily observable; a small decrease in visual acuity at 10 years of age is not.

For a new or very rare event (one whose occurrence in the unexposed population is highly unlikely), the risk can be quantified by surveying the exposed population for the number of times that the event has occurred. All events are attributable to the agent, because the incidence rate in the unexposed population is zero or very nearly zero.

Consider, for example, the rare event of red eyes in humans. Assume that a 0.1% incidence rate of red eyes at birth is induced in a population exposed in utero to a particular agent. A survey of 100,000 neonates exposed to this agent would yield 100 cases of red eyes (or very nearly 100, based on the probability distribution of sampling 100,000 individuals with an incidence rate of 0.1% for the effect). If different researchers examined a different group of 1000 neonates exposed to the agent, however, at least one case of red eyes in a particular group might or might not be present. By random chance, different studies addressing the same question can obtain contradictory results. Absence of positive findings in an exposed population does not mean that a potential effect does not occur, but it does establish an upper limit for the incidence rate of the effect. Obviously, surveys of increasingly larger populations with no positive findings reduce the upper boundary of the risk estimate.

Very likely, the adverse effect attributed to a particular agent is an event that occurs naturally in the unexposed population. The exposed population is expected to have a higher incidence rate than the unexposed population. The ability to identify the adverse effect depends on the relative increase in incidence rate and the number of individuals observed. Epidemiologic studies are designed to assess by statistical methods the occurrence of adverse effects in populations exposed to a particular agent.

Factors that may influence the relative incidence rates of a given outcome following in utero exposure include pregnancy complications, gestational age at the time of irradiation, maternal age, ethnic origin, diet, and geographic location. The selection of a control group with the same characteristics is essential. Ideally, the only difference between the exposed and unexposed groups would be the agent of interest. In practice, this is very difficult to achieve and is the major criticism of many epidemiologic studies.

If the relative risk is small, a large sample size is required to distinguish the agent-induced effects from disorders that occur spontaneously in the population. Sample size limits the minimum level of relative risk detectable in a particular study.

The possibility of a long latent period (i.e., the delay between exposure and observable effect) must be considered. To assess risk factors accurately, it is necessary to examine these populations over a period of many years. Collecting data for a large population over a long time is an extremely expensive undertaking and subject to many difficulties.

Experimental Designs

Two commonly used experimental designs for assessing the association between exposure to an agent and its long-term effect are case-control (retrospective) and cohort (prospective) studies.

Case-control studies identify individuals with a particular health problem (cases) and research the histories of these individuals, particularly past exposure to the agent of interest. Past exposure to the agent is also examined for a reference group (control), which is free of the health problem. Ideally, the control group has similar attributes (e.g., socioeconomic status, age, ethnic origin, sex) as the case group. An excess of exposure to the agent by the case group compared with the control group indicates an association. Relative risk is estimated by the ratio of the fraction of subjects in each group exposed to the agent. For example, a relative risk of five is assigned following a case-control study in which 50% of the case group and 10% of the control group were exposed to a particular agent.

Cohort studies identify a population that is initially free of the potential adverse effect. During the investigation, observations regarding exposure to the agent, other potential etiologic factors, and changes in health status are made. The occurrence of an adverse outcome between the exposed and unexposed portions of the population is compared. Many health end points can be assessed within the study, and the absolute incidence rates can be determined. The major advantage of the prospective study is that the selection of individuals in the cohort is inherently unbiased, because their disease status is not yet known, although bias in the diagnosis of health effect is possible.

Study design usually involves the inclusion or withholding of the supposed cause to one group. The addition or removal of the agent is generally believed, but not yet proven, beneficial to the members of that group. If clear benefit to one group is demonstrated, then ethical considerations dictate that the study is terminated and all members are provided the same access to health care. This inhibits risk estimates but is a recognized limitation when humans are subjects of investigation.

Confounding factors that modify the relative incidence rates between the two groups may be present. In some studies, attempts are made to eliminate the influence of these factors by matching the control and exposed groups initially with respect to several attributes (e.g., age, sex, race, and marital status). For large groups, however, this technique of matching is not feasible.

A different form of the cohort experimental design is the historical prospective study, which investigates events that have occurred during an earlier time. A cohort exposed to an agent in the past is identified, and the health experience of this population over the ensuing years is examined. Rather than identifying subjects at the present time for future follow-up (spanning possibly many years), the investigators study consequences from past exposure to the agent in the population. The need for lengthy follow-up and the associated high costs of a prospective study are eliminated.

In a retrospective study the observations have been recorded in the past for some unrelated purpose, and the investigators reexamine this collected information to test a particular hypothesis regarding exposure to the agent and its potential adverse effect. The data in many cases are incomplete, because the original design of the information-gathering process did not specify the agent for special consideration. The possibility of biased recall of exposure to the agent exists. The selection of an appropriate control group is problematic. Case-control studies compared with cohort studies have certain advantages, however—including lower cost, smaller sample size, and shorter time interval to conduct the study (faster availability of results). For studying rare health effects, the case-control design is the method of choice.

Rarely does a single study become the definitive work regarding identification of an adverse effect and the level of risk from exposure to a particular agent. The overall assessment must be based on multiple studies conducted under diverse conditions involving different populations. Epidemiologic studies are often flawed either in experimental design or by incompleteness of the data. To establish an agent as potentially harmful, a pattern must develop whereby the results from different studies associate the same biologic effect(s) with prior exposure to the agent, produce a dose-dependent rate of occurrence, and demonstrate a similar time sequence with respect to onset of the adverse effect.

Clinical Surveys

Surveys of clinical ultrasound users incorporating more than 400,000 patient examinations have shown no obvious increase in any anomalies that occur naturally, though rarely, in the general population.[69,70] These surveys, however, rely on the judgment of respondents who differ in scientific training and ability to perceive changes in patient status. The results nevertheless indicate that clinicians believe ultrasound to be safe for their patients.

Limitations of Exposure-In-Utero Studies

The most important issue that epidemiologic studies must address is whether ultrasound exposure in utero at diagnostic intensity levels produces adverse effects. The current estimate is that 3 million children born each year in the United States were examined in utero with ultrasound. Because large numbers of fetuses are exposed to ultrasound, the ability to demonstrate that the risk of adverse effects is extremely small becomes critically important.

Before reviewing reports of epidemiologic studies of ultrasound exposure in utero, we must consider the limitations of these studies. Many retrospective clinical investigations contain methodological flaws—including small sample size, lack of controls, and limited information regarding characteristics of the population. The prevalence of in utero exposures creates difficulties in identifying a well-matched control group. The exposed group should be characterized by the following:

- Reason for the examination
- Gestational age at the time of the examination
- Number of examinations
- Exposure parameters

If an individual is not assigned to the exposed group at random, a biased selection process may lead to an invalid finding. A patient with a clinical problem is more likely to be assigned to the exposed group, because the diagnostic information obtained from the ultrasound examination is desirable for the management of that patient; patients with no clinical problems are preferentially assigned to the unexposed group. The suspected clinical problem may often result in an observed biologic effect (e.g., low birth weight). Therefore an analysis of this end point would show a difference between the exposed and unexposed groups, but a question would still remain as to whether ultrasound exposure or the selection process was the cause of the adverse outcome.

For populations exposed in utero, the information gained from the ultrasound examination could be used clinically to alter patient health and distort the findings of the study. For example, fetuses with structural abnormalities could be identified, and the pregnancy therapeutically terminated, thus selectively eliminating these fetuses from the analysis of biologic end points evaluated at birth.

Experience with teratogenic agents (e.g., ionizing radiation) has shown that the induction of structural abnormalities is dependent on gestational age at the time of exposure. Negative findings from a study in which the exposure occurred at a gestational age of 32 weeks would not allow the conclusion to be made that exposure at any time during pregnancy was without effect. If harm were caused by ultrasound, the probability and severity of the adverse effect would be expected to increase with the dose as monitored by the number of examinations and exposure parameters. Unfortunately, the exposure parameters are not well defined in most studies, and consequently, quantitative risk estimates have not been possible if a positive finding was obtained.

Results of Exposure-In-Utero Studies

Low birth weight, fetal chromosome abnormalities, structural fetal anomalies, altered neurologic development, cancer, and hearing disorders have been investigated as possible adverse effects from fetal exposure to ultrasound. A summary of the findings from various studies is presented in Table 22-1.

Several studies, including three randomized clinical trials, have found no association between low birth weight and in utero exposure.[71-74] Moore et al.,[75] however, did report a positive correlation between low birth weight and insonation in utero. In their first study, 2135 births during the late 1960s and early 1970s in Denver were investigated. The reason for the examination, the physical size of the mother, and whether the mother smoked were not delineated, which could have introduced bias. An analysis of the Denver data by Stark et al.[76] contradicted Moore's conclusion by arguing that the complications affecting birth weight were not comparable in the exposed and control groups.

In a subsequent study, Moore[77] acknowledged that the association of ultrasound with low birth weight was probably a result of confounding maternal and fetal factors. Women with problems during pregnancy are more likely to have an ultrasound examination, and complications are more likely to affect birth weight. In other words, intrauterine growth retardation would have been more prevalent in the group exposed to ultrasound even if the ultrasound exposure had not occurred. Thus designing a study to adjust for all potential confounding factors by matching exposed and unexposed infants is difficult.

In a randomized clinical trial, women with a single pregnancy were selected to receive multiple ultrasound examinations from 18 to 38 weeks' gestational age.[78] Higher intrauterine growth restriction expressed as birth weight less than the tenth percentile was observed. The difference in mean birth weight between the ultrasound group and controls was not significant.

The final conclusion regarding low birth weight and in utero exposure to ultrasound is based primarily on the four

■ **Table 22-1** Epidemiologic Studies of Ultrasound Exposure In Utero

Study	Number of Subjects Exposed	Findings
Bernstine (1969)	720	Rate of congenital anomalies less than in reference population
Hellman (1970)	1114	Fetal abnormalities no more common than in the general population
Serr (1971)	150	Suggested damage to chromosomes of fetal cells but not statistically significant
Abdulla (1971)	35	No increase in chromosome abnormalities in fetal lymphocytes
Falus (1972)	171	Height and weight within normal range for age 6 mo to 3 yr; no development disorders
Ikeuchi (1973)	98	No chromosome damage
Scheidt (1978)	297 amniocentesis and ultrasound; 661 amniocentesis only (949 controls)	More abnormal grasp reflexes and abnormal tonic neck reflexes in amniocentesis with ultrasound group; no difference between the group with both ultrasound and amniocentesis and amniocentesis alone; 121 other outcomes negative, including low birth weight
Lyons (1979)	2428	No increased incidence of congenital malformations, chromosome abnormalities, neoplasms, speech disorders, hearing disorders, or development problems
Lyons (1980)	500	Increase in low birth weight infants
Wladimiroff (1980)	341 (364 controls)	Negative findings for low birth weight infants
Moore (1982)	2135	Association between ultrasound and low birth weight
Stark (1984)	425 (381 controls)	Higher incidence of dyslexia but not statistically significant; no association between ultrasound and low birth weight
Bakketeig (1984)	510 (499 controls)	Negative findings for low birth weight, physical status, mortality
Kinner Wilson (1984)	1731 cancer patients (1731 matched controls)	No difference in two populations with respect to exposure in utero
Cartwright (1984)	555 cancer patients (1110 controls)	No association between exposure in utero and childhood cancer
Moore (1988)	1594 (944 controls)	Association between exposure in utero and low birth weight infants
Lyons (1988)	149 sibling pairs	Exposure in utero did not affect growth in childhood up to age 6 yr
Salvesen (1992-1993)	2161	No decrease in school performance; no increase in dyslexia, sensory deficits, or impaired neurologic development; increase in non–right handedness
Ewigmann (1993)	7812 (7718 controls)	No significant differences in rates of preterm delivery or birth weight
Newnham (1993)	2834	Higher intrauterine growth restriction
Campbell (1993)	72	Association between exposure in utero and delayed speech in children
Salvesen (1999)	4715	No association between ultrasound in utero and non–right handedness
Naumburg (2000)	752	Ultrasound in utero does not influence the risk of childhood leukemia

studies in which the subjects were randomly selected for exposure. No difference in birth weight was observed between the exposed and control groups. The finding of reduced birth weight in two retrospective studies has had little clinical importance. However, the low percentile of birth weight for gestational age cannot be discounted and requires further study.

Several other studies have found no association between ultrasound exposure in utero and fetal structural anomalies.[79-84] In 1969 Bernstine[79] compared the incidence of congenital anomalies in an ultrasound-exposed population with a U.S. Navy statistic for incidence of congenital anomalies. Presumably, this control incidence rate was derived from a reference population that was similar to the patient population identified by Bernstine. The study concluded that examining pregnant women by Doppler ultrasound did not place the fetus at increased risk for structural anomalies. Hellman et al.[81] examined 1114 neonates for anatomic abnormalities following in utero ultrasound exposure. The gestational age at the time of examination varied from 10 weeks to 40+ weeks, and some patients had multiple examinations. Both CW and PW regimens were used. The frequency of fetal abnormalities in this population was compared with the frequency in a large survey of 63,000 births. The number of abnormalities did not exceed that expected from the general population. In both studies mentioned previously, however, the lack of a well-matched control population casts doubt on the validity of the conclusions.

A study involving small groups of infants whose mothers had received either amniocentesis and ultrasound or amniocentesis alone showed no association between ultrasound exposure and abnormalities.[84] Lyons et al.[83] reported that the offspring of 10,000 women exposed to ultrasound during pregnancy showed no increased incidence of speech or hearing disorders, neoplasia, or congenital anomalies. This study is difficult to evaluate, because many data underlying the conclusions were not included in the report.

In a randomized clinical trial, the Routine Antenatal Diagnostic Imaging with Ultrasound (RADIUS) study tested the hypothesis that routine screening at 15 to 22 weeks and again at 31 to 35 weeks reduces perinatal morbidity and mortality.[85] The results did not improve outcome compared with selective ultrasound examination when clinically indicated. This conclusion is in marked contrast with the findings from other randomized clinical trials.[86,87] Only low-risk pregnant women were included in the RADIUS study. A decrease in perinatal mortality in other clinical trials may be attributed to a relatively high rate of induced abortion of malformed fetuses compared with the RADIUS study.[87]

No association between in utero ultrasound exposure and fetal chromosome abnormalities,[44-46] cancer,[88-90] and hearing disorders[76,84] has been demonstrated. The studies examining childhood cancer appear to be well designed and involve large numbers of subjects. Two independent studies had contradictory findings regarding the association of delayed speech in children with ultrasonography in utero.[91,92] The

RADIUS clinical trial reported no increase in congenital abnormalities.

Because migration of neurons within the developing brain takes place at a gestational age of 14 to 22 weeks, ultrasound delivered to the fetus during this period may affect neurologic development. Scheidt et al.[84] reported abnormal grasp and tonic neck reflexes in infants exposed to ultrasound in utero. These results may be attributable to random chance, because 123 different end points were examined. Stark et al.[76] identified dyslexia as a possible learning disorder of children exposed in utero. All three hospitals in this study had higher incidence rates of dyslexia in the exposed population, although the increases were not statistically significant. Salvesen and co-workers found no association between ultrasound in utero and impaired neurologic development.[93-96]

Assessment of Results

Results of the epidemiologic studies have been generally negative, which indicates that damage, if any, is subtle, delayed, or infrequent. The number of subjects in a study reporting negative results places an upper limit on the incidence rate of an adverse effect, but it does not exclude the induction of the effect by ultrasound. The association of ultrasound exposure with a particular outcome does not absolutely establish ultrasound as the causative agent. The association may be the result of shared underlying factors. The overall assessment is that no firm epidemiologic evidence exists to conclude that a causal relationship exists between diagnostic ultrasound and adverse effects.

Since ultrasonography is a rapidly developing technical field with new capabilities, past epidemiologic studies have only recently investigated biologic effects at the intensity levels associated with current medical practice. Well-designed epidemiologic surveys involving large numbers of subjects are still needed. The information derived from such studies is essential for assessing risk. The very nature of epidemiologic surveys, which precludes the ability to control all factors, necessitates that numerous studies be undertaken, rather than a single study be relied on. It is hoped that this approach will reveal a consistent pattern of cause and effect.

AIUM EVALUATION OF BIOEFFECTS DATA

The Bioeffects Committee of the American Institute of Ultrasound in Medicine (AIUM) was established to examine the current knowledge concerning bioeffects and to assess the risk of clinical diagnostic ultrasound. This Committee regularly publishes critiques of research reports and issues statements regarding the safety of diagnostic ultrasound. Its conclusions are acknowledged to be safety guidelines throughout the ultrasound community.

Statement on Mammalian In Vivo Biologic Effects

In August 1976 the Bioeffects Committee reviewed all the data pertaining to biologic effects attributable to ultrasound irradiation of mammalian tissue. Its evaluation of the scientific literature was summarized in a statement that was subsequently revised in October 1992. The statement is as follows:

Information from experiments utilizing laboratory mammals has contributed significantly to our understanding of ultrasonically induced biological effects and the mechanisms that are most likely responsible. The following statement summarizes observations relative to specific ultrasound parameters and indices. The history and rationale for this statement are provided in *Bioeffects and Safety of Diagnostic Ultrasound* (AIUM, 1993).

In the low megahertz frequency range there have been no independently confirmed adverse biologic effects in mammalian tissues exposed in vivo under experimental ultrasound conditions, as follows.

   a. When a thermal mechanism is involved, these conditions are unfocused–beam intensities* below 100 mW/cm^2, focused[†]–beam intensities below 1 W/cm^2, or thermal index values less than 2. Furthermore, such effects have not been reported for higher values of thermal index when they are less than 6 – (log t/0.6) where t is exposure time ranging from 1 to 250 minutes, including off-time for pulsed exposure.

   b. When a nonthermal mechanism is involved[‡] in tissues that contain well-defined gas bodies, these conditions are in situ peak rarefactional pressures below approximately 0.3 MPa or mechanical index values less than approximately 0.3. Furthermore, for other tissues, no such effects have been reported.[§]

The low-megahertz frequency range is considered to be 0.5 to 10 MHz. CW and PW ultrasound, as well as focused and unfocused beams, are included. The intensity is designated SPTA, as measured under free-field conditions.

With the availability of later information, the Committee statement has been modified to incorporate specifications that are more suitable for the clinical environment. In the most recent reassessment, very low PRFs (<100 Hz) have been excluded, and the intensity of focused beams has been evaluated explicitly. A diagnostic unit with high PRFs may produce an I(SPTA) above 100 mW/cm^2, the previous statement level for both focused and unfocused beams. Generally, bioeffects data have been obtained under the conditions of high-power, broad-beam, and CW irradiation. A focused beam is less damaging than an unfocused beam of equal I(SPTA). Most bioeffects are attributable to the thermal mechanism, and the temperature rise is a critical function of beam width. A small beam (<4 mm in diameter) transfers heat more rapidly from the irradiated volume than a large beam does, and the corresponding increase in temperature is only 1/10 to 1/100 that for a wide beam. The I(SPTA) estimate of 1 W/cm^2 for a focused beam is conser-

vative, since this level is 10 times the level for an unfocused beam.

Thermal damage is dependent on the temperature elevation and the duration of exposure, which is addressed by the mathematic relationship between TI and exposure time. The threshold for nonthermal damage is considered a peak pressure of 0.3 MPa or a mechanical index of 0.3.

Since 1992 several researchers have examined the effects of PW ultrasound with short temporal pulse lengths at diagnostic intensity levels using the acoustic output indices to correlate ultrasound exposure with potential biologic effects.

The AIUM Bioeffects Committee also developed the "Statement of In Vitro Biological Effects" (November 2003) and the "Statement on Safety in Training and Research" (March 1997).

AIUM Statement of In Vitro Biologic Effects

It is often difficult to evaluate reports of ultrasonically induced in vitro biologic effects with respect to their clinical significance. The predominant physical and biologic interactions and mechanisms involved in an in vitro effect may not pertain to the in vivo situation. Nevertheless, an in vitro effect must be regarded as a real biologic effect.

Results from in vitro experiments suggest new end points and serve as a basis for design of in vivo experiments. In vitro studies provide the capability to control experimental variables and thus offer a means to explore and evaluate specific mechanisms. Although they may have limited applicability to in vivo biologic effects, such studies can disclose fundamental intercellular or intracellular interactions. While it is valid for authors to place their results in context and to suggest further relevant investigations, reports that do more than this should be viewed with caution.*

AIUM Statement on Safety in Training and Research

Diagnostic ultrasound has been in use since the late 1950s. There are no confirmed adverse biologic effects on patients resulting from this usage. Although no hazard that would preclude the prudent and conservative use of diagnostic ultrasound in education and research has been identified, experience from normal diagnostic practice may or may not be relevant to extended exposure times and altered exposure conditions. It is therefore considered appropriate to make the following recommendation:

In those special situations in which examinations are to be carried out for purposes other than direct medical benefit to the individual being examined, the subject should be informed of the anticipated exposure conditions, and of how these compare with conditions for normal diagnostic practice.[†]

---

*Free-field spatial peak, temporal average (SPTA) for CW and pulsed exposures.
[†]Quarter-power (−6 dB) beam width smaller than four wavelengths or 4 mm, whichever is less at the exposure frequency.
[‡]For diagnostically relevant ultrasound exposures.
[§]From American Institute of Ultrasound in Medicine: Mammalian In Vivo Ultrasonic Biological Effects, http://www.aium.org/provider/statements/statements.asp, retrieved September 8, 2004.

---

*From American Institute of Ultrasound in Medicine: In Vitro Biological Effects, http://www.aium.org/provider/statements/statements.asp, retrieved September 8, 2004.
[†]From American Institute of Ultrasound in Medicine: Safety in Training and Research, http://www.aium.org/provider/statements/statements.asp, retrieved September 8, 2004.

SCIENTIFIC REVIEWS

Several scientific organizations including the National Council on Radiation Protection and Measurements (NCRP), AIUM, World Federation for Ultrasound in Medicine and Biology, and European Committee for Ultrasound Radiation Safety have published reports summarizing the biologic effects of medical ultrasound. In addition to these, the reader is referred to several review articles in the literature.[97-104]

SUMMARY

Three mechanisms for the interaction of ultrasound with matter have been identified: radiation force, thermal, and cavitation. These physical processes may give rise to the secondary actions of microstreaming and altered chemical reaction rates.

Early studies using high intensity levels and long exposure times reported numerous biologic effects—including protein denaturation, changes in membrane permeability, membrane rupture, chromosomal breakage, nerve block, cataracts, brain lesions, and fetal developmental anomalies. Much of this work lacks the necessary dosimetric details.

During in vitro studies, the particular molecule of interest is usually dissolved in aqueous media and then exposed to ultrasound. This experimental setup does not mimic the physical environment of the biomolecule in nature and thus creates the possibility of introducing microbubbles into the system, which may enhance cavitation. These types of studies are useful for identifying biomolecules sensitive to ultrasound, the type of damage induced, and the mechanisms of interaction; but their applicability to the assessment of risk is limited.

Although animal studies provide a good indication of potential damage and can aid in the establishment of reasonable levels of safety, they possess certain limitations when extrapolated to humans. Species sensitivity variation has been demonstrated, and there is no assurance that humans will respond in the same manner as certain species of animals. The amount of attenuation and the relative target size are also factors that must be considered. Nevertheless, dose-effect observations in animals are critically important to determining the mechanisms of interaction and assessing the risk in humans.

At current diagnostic intensity levels and scan times, no biologic effects of ultrasound have been observed in humans. The AIUM has reviewed available data and established intensity guidelines. A safe level of 100 mW/cm² I(SPTA) is often mentioned in the literature. The adoption of 1 W/cm² I(SPTA) as a safe level for focused beams by the AIUM has also become widely accepted. Thermal and mechanical acoustic output indices offer a clinically relevant approach to controlling ultrasonic exposure of patients and providing assurance of safety.

REVIEW QUESTIONS

1. Name the three mechanisms of interaction of ultrasound with matter.
2. Why should reports of experimental studies include irradiation conditions and specifications of beam parameters?
3. Why are epidemiologic studies important for risk assessment?
4. Why is it essential to identify harmful effects and corresponding risk factors from fetal exposure?
5. According to the AIUM's evaluation of scientific data in 1992, no biologic effects have been observed in mammalian systems below an intensity level of _____ for unfocused beams and _____ for focused beams. How is this intensity specified?
6. Damage induced by the thermal mechanism shows a threshold, which is dependent on temperature elevation and _____ .

REFERENCES

1. Ter Haar GR, Daniels S: Evidence for ultrasonically induced cavitation in vivo, *Phys Med Biol* 26:1145-1149, 1981.
2. O'Brien WD Jr: Biological effects of ultrasound. In Fullerton GD, Zagzebski JA, eds: *Medical physics of CT and ultrasound: tissue imaging and characterization,* New York, 1980, American Institute of Physics.
3. Apfel RE, Holland CK: Gauging the likelihood of cavitation from short pulse, low-duty cycle diagnostic ultrasound, *Ultrasound Med Biol* 17:179-185, 1991.
4. Flynn HG: Physics of acoustic cavitation in liquids. In Mason WP, ed: *Physical acoustics,* New York, 1964, Academic Press.
5. Gross DR, Miller DL, Williams AR: A search for ultrasonic cavitation within the canine cardiovascular system, *Ultrasound Med Biol* 11:85-97, 1985.
6. Carstensen EL, Flynn HG: The potential for transient cavitation with microsecond pulses of ultrasound, *Ultrasound Med Biol* 8:L720-L724, 1982.
7. Frizzel LA et al: Involvement of ultrasonically induced cavitation in the production of hind limb paralysis of the mouse neonate, *J Acoust Soc Am* 74:1062-1065, 1983.
8. Delius M et al: Biological effects of shock waves: lung hemorrhage by shock waves in dogs: pressure dependence, *Ultrasound Med Biol* 13:61-67, 1987.
9. Hartman C et al: Lung damage from exposure to the fields of an electrohydraulic lithotripter, *Ultrasound Med Biol* 16:675-679, 1990.
10. Child SZ et al: Lung damage from exposure to pulsed ultrasound, *Ultrasound Med Biol* 16:817-825, 1990.
11. Holland CK et al: Direct evidence of cavitation in vivo from diagnostic ultrasound, *Ultrasound Med Biol* 22:917-925, 1996.
12. Zachary JF, O'Brien WD Jr: Lung lesions induced by continuous- and pulsed-wave (diagnostic) in mice, rabbits, and pigs, *Vet Pathol* 32:43-54, 1995.
13. Tarantal AF, Canfield DR: Ultrasound induced lung hemorrhage in the monkey, *Ultrasound Med Biol* 20:65-72, 1994.
14. Dalecki D et al: Intestinal hemorrhage from exposure to pulsed ultrasound, *Ultrasound Med Biol* 21:1067-1072, 1995.

15. Dalecki D et al: A test for cavitation as a mechanism for intestinal hemorrhage in mice exposed to piezoelectric lithotripter, *Ultrasound Med Biol* 22:493-496, 1996.

16. Dalecki D et al: Hemorrhage in murine fetuses exposed to pulsed ultrasound, *Ultrasound Med Biol* 25:1139-1144, 1999.

17. Carstensen EL et al: Test for kidney hemorrhage following exposure to intense, pulsed ultrasound, *Ultrasound Med Biol* 16:681-685, 1990.

18. Coakley WT, Dunn F: Interaction of megahertz ultrasound and biological polymers. In Reid JM, Sikov MR, eds: *Interaction of ultrasound and biological tissues, HEW Publication (FDA) 73-8008:43,* Washington, DC, 1972, Government Printing Office.

19. Coakley WT, Dunn F: Degradation of DNA in high intensity focused ultrasonic fields at 1 MHz, *J Acoust Soc Am* 50:1539-1545, 1971.

20. Hawley SA, Macleod RM, Dunn F: Degradation of DNA by intense, noncavitating ultrasound, *J Acoust Soc Am* 35:1285-1287, 1963.

21. Hill CR: Ultrasonic exposure thresholds for changes in cells and tissues, *J Acoust Soc Am* 52:667-672, 1972.

22. Peacocke AR, Pritchard NJ: Some biophysical aspects of ultrasound, *Prog Biophys Mol Biol* 18:187-208, 1968.

23. Galperin-Lemaitre H, Kirsch-Volders M, Levi S: Fragmentation of purified mammalian DNA molecules by ultrasound below human therapeutic doses, *Humangenetik* 29:61-66, 1975.

24. Thacker J: Ultrasound and mammalian DNA, *Lancet* 2:770, 1975.

25. Fu YK et al: Ultrasound lethality to synchronous and asynchronous Chinese hamster V-79 cells, *Ultrasound Med Biol* 6:39-46, 1980.

26. Kaufman GE: Mutagenicity of ultrasound in cultured mammalian cells, *Ultrasound Med Biol* 11:497-501, 1985.

27. Liebeskind D et al: Diagnostic ultrasound: effects on the DNA and growth patterns of animal cells, *Radiology* 131:177-184, 1979.

28. Harrison GH, Balcer-Kubiczek EK: Pulsed ultrasound and neoplastic transformation in vitro, *Ultrasound Med Biol* 17:627-632, 1991.

29. Yip YP et al: Ultrasound effects on cell proliferation and migration of chick motoneurons, *Ultrasound Med Biol* 17:55-63, 1991.

30. Fry FJ et al: Threshold ultrasonic dosages for structural changes in mammalian brain, *J Acoust Soc Am* 48:1413-1417, 1970.

31. Dunn F, Fry FJ: Ultrasonic threshold dosage for the mammalian central nervous system, *IEEE Trans Biomed Eng* 18:253-256, 1971.

32. Dyson M et al: The simulation of tissue regeneration by means of ultrasound, *Clin Sci (Colch)* 35:273-285, 1968.

33. Kremkau FW: Cancer therapy with ultrasound: a historical review, *J Clin Ultrasound* 7:287-300, 1979.

34. Martin AO: Can ultrasound cause genetic damage? *J Clin Ultrasound* 12:11-19, 1984.

35. Carmichael AJ et al: Free radical production in aqueous solutions exposed to simulated ultrasonic diagnostic conditions, *IEEE Trans Ultrason Ferroelectr Freq Control* 33:148-155, 1986.

36. Wegner RD, Obe G, Meyenburg M: Has diagnostic ultrasound mutagenic effects? *Hum Genet* 56:95-98, 1980.

37. Dooley DA, Sacks PG, Miller MW: Production of thymine base damage in ultrasound-exposed EMT6 mouse mammary sarcoma cells, *Radiat Res* 97:71-86, 1984.

38. Doida Y et al: Confirmation of an ultrasound-induced mutation in two in vitro mammalian cell lines, *Ultrasound Med Biol* 16:699-705, 1990.

39. Ritenour ER et al: Absence of mutagenic effects of continuous and pulsed ultrasound in cultured AL human-hamster hybrid cells, *Ultrasound Med Biol* 17:921-930, 1991.

40. Miller DL, Thomas RM, Frazier ME: Single strand breaks in CHO cell DNA induced by ultrasonic cavitation in vitro, *Ultrasound Med Biol* 17:401-406, 1991.

41. MacIntosh IJC, Davey DA: Chromosome aberrations induced by an ultrasonic fetal pulse detector, *Br Med J* 4:92-93, 1970.

42. MacIntosh IJC, Davey DA: Relationship between intensity of ultrasound and induction of chromosome aberrations, *Br J Radiol* 45:320-327, 1972.

43. MacIntosh IJC, Brown RC, Coakley WT: Ultrasound and in vitro chromosome aberrations, *Br J Radiol* 48:230-232, 1975.

44. Abdulla U et al: Effects of diagnostic ultrasound on maternal and fetal chromosomes, *Lancet* 2:829-831, 1971.

45. Ikeuchi T et al: Ultrasound and embryonic chromosomes, *Br Med J* 1:112, 1973.

46. Serr DM et al: Studies on the effect of ultrasonic waves on the fetus. In Huntington PJ et al, eds: *Proceedings of the second European congress on perinatal medicine,* London, 1971, The Congress.

47. Cataldo FL et al: A description of ultrasonically induced chromosomal anomalies in Vicia faba, *Radiat Biol* 13:211-213, 1973.

48. Lyon MF, Simpson GM: An investigation into the possible genetic hazards of ultrasound, *Br J Radiol* 47:712-722, 1974.

49. Liebeskind D et al: Sister chromatid exchanges in human lymphocytes after exposure to diagnostic ultrasound, *Science* 205:1273-1275, 1979.

50. Barnett SB et al: Increased sister chromatid exchanges in Chinese hamster ovary cells exposed to high intensity pulsed ultrasound, *Ultrasound Med Biol* 14:397-403, 1988.

51. Stella M et al: Induction of sister chromatid exchanges in human lymphocytes exposed to in vitro and in vivo therapeutic ultrasound, *Mutat Res* 138:75-85, 1984.

52. Ciaravino V et al: Lack of effect of high-intensity pulsed ultrasound on sister chromatid exchange and in vitro Chinese hamster ovary cell viability, *Ultrasound Med Biol* 11:491-495, 1985.

53. Miller MW et al: Lack of induced increase in sister chromatid exchanges in human lymphocytes exposed to in vivo therapeutic ultrasound, *Ultrasound Med Biol* 17:81-83, 1991.

54. Miller MW et al: Sister chromatid exchanges in Chinese hamster ovary cells exposed to high intensity pulsed ultrasound: inability to confirm previous positive results, *Ultrasound Med Biol* 15:255-262, 1989.

55. Morris SM et al: Effect of ultrasound on human leucocytes: sister chromatid exchange analysis, *Ultrasound Med Biol* 4:253-258, 1978.

56. O'Brien WD Jr: Safety of ultrasound with selective emphasis for obstetrics, *Semin Ultrasound CT MR* 5:105-120, 1984.

57. Wegner RD, Meyenburg M: The effects of diagnostic ultrasonography on the frequencies of sister chromatid exchanges in Chinese hamster cells and human lymphocytes, *J Ultrasound Med* 1:355-358, 1982.

58. Sikov MR: Effects of ultrasound on development, Part 2, Studies in mammalian species: an overview, *J Ultrasound Med* 5:651-661, 1986.

59. Akamatsu N: Ultrasound irradiation effects on preimplantation embryos, *Acta Obstet Gynaecol Jpn* 33:969-978, 1981.

60. Pizzarello DJ et al: Effect of pulsed low power ultrasound on growing tissues. I. Developing mammalian and insect tissue, *Exp Cell Biol* 46:179-191, 1978.

61. Child SZ, Carstensen EL, Davis H: A test for the effects of low-temporal-average intensity, pulsed ultrasound on the rat fetus, *Exp Cell Biol* 52:207-210, 1984.

62. Warwick R et al: Hazards of diagnostic ultrasonography: a study with mice, *IEEE Trans Sonics Ultrasound* 5417:158-164, 1970.

63. Shoji R et al: An experimental study on the effects of low-intensity ultrasound on developing mouse embryos, *Hokkaido Igaku Zasshi* 18:51-56, 1971.

64. Shoji R et al: Experimental studies on the effect of ultrasound on mouse embryos (abstract), *Teratology* 6:119, 1972.

65. Takabayashi YA et al: Effects of pulse-wave ultrasonic irradiation on mouse embryo, *Cho-Onpa Igaku* 8:286-288, 1981.

66. Child SZ et al: Pulsed ultrasound and the hyperbarically exposed mouse fetus, *Ultrasound Med Biol* 17:367-371, 1991.

67. Taylor KJW, Dyson M: Toxicity studies on the interaction of ultrasound on embryonic and adult tissues. In deVliger M, White DN, McCready VR, eds: *Ultrasonics in medicine: proceedings of the Second World Congress on Ultrasound in Medicine (Amsterdam), Excerpta Medica,* New York, 1974, American Elsevier, pp 353-359.

68. Hartman C et al: Effects of lithotripter fields on development of chick embryos, *Ultrasound Med Biol* 16:581-585, 1990.

69. Environmental Health Directorate: *Safety code 23: Guidelines for the safe use of ultrasound. I. Medical and paramedical applications, Report 8-EHD-59, Environmental Health Directorate of Canada, Health Protection Branch,* Ottawa, 1981.

70. Ziskin MC: Survey of patient exposure to diagnostic ultrasound. In Reid JM, Sikov MR, eds: *Interaction of ultrasound and biological tissues,* HEW Pub (FDA) 73:203-205, 1972.

71. Bennett MJ et al: Predictive value of ultrasound measurement in early pregnancy: a randomized controlled trial, *Br J Obstet Gynecol* 89:338-341, 1982.

72. Falus M et al: Follow-up studies on infants examined by ultrasound during the fetal age, *Orv Hetil* 13:2119-2121, 1972.

73. Lyons EA et al: In utero exposure to diagnostic ultrasound: a six-year follow-up, *Radiology* 166:687-690, 1988.

74. Wladimiroff JW, Laar J: Ultrasonic measurement of fetal body size: a randomized controlled trial, *Acta Obstet Gynecol Scand* 59:177-179, 1980.

75. Moore R Jr, Barrick M, Hamilton P: Effects of sonic radiation on growth and development (abstract), *Am J Epidemiol* 116:571, 1982.

76. Stark CR et al: Short- and long-term risks after exposure to diagnostic ultrasound in utero, *Obstet Gynecol* 63:194-200, 1984.

77. Moore RM, Diamond EL, Cavalieri RL: The relationship of birth weight and intrauterine diagnostic ultrasound exposure, *Obstet Gynecol* 71:513-517, 1988.

78. Newnham JP et al: Effects of frequent ultrasound during pregnancy: a randomized controlled trial, *Lancet* 342:887-891, 1993.

79. Bernstine RL: Safety studies with ultrasonic Doppler technic: a clinical follow-up of patients and tissue culture study, *Obstet Gynecol* 34:707-709, 1969.

80. Bakketeig LS et al: Randomised controlled trial of ultrasonographic screening on pregnancy, *Lancet* 2:207-211, 1984.

81. Hellman LM et al: Safety of diagnostic ultrasound in obstetrics, *Lancet* 1:1133-1134, 1970.

82. Lyons EA, Coggrave-Toms M: *Long-term follow-up study of children exposed to ultrasound in utero. Proceedings of the twenty-fourth annual meeting of the American Institute of Ultrasound Medicine,* Montreal, August 1979.

83. Lyons EA, Coggrave M, Brown RE: *Follow-up study in children exposed to ultrasound in utero: analysis of height and weight in the first six years of life, Proceedings of the twenty-fifth annual meeting of the American Institute of Ultrasound in Medicine,* New Orleans, September 1980.

84. Scheidt PC, Stanley F, Bryla DA: One-year follow-up of infants exposed to ultrasound in utero, *Am J Obstet Gynecol* 131:743-748, 1978.

85. Ewigman BG et al: Effect of prenatal ultrasound screening on perinatal outcome. RADIUS Study Group, *N Engl J Med* 329:821-827, 1993.

86. Thacker SB: Quality of controlled trials: the case of imaging in obstetrics: a review, *Br J Obstet Gynecol* 92:437-444, 1985.

87. Saari-Kemppainen A et al: Ultrasound screening and perinatal mortality: controlled trial of systematic one-state screening in pregnancy, *Lancet* 336:387-391, 1990.

88. Cartwright RA et al: Ultrasound examinations in pregnancy and childhood cancer, *Lancet* 2:999-1000, 1984.

89. Kinner Wilson LM, Waterhouse JAH: Obstetric ultrasound and childhood malignancies, *Lancet* 2:997-999, 1984.

90. Naumurg E et al: Prenatal ultrasound examinations and risk of childhood leukemia: case-control study, *BMJ* 320:282-283, 2000.

91. Campbell JD, Elford RW, Brant RF: Case-control study of prenatal ultrasonography exposure in children with delayed speech, *CMAJ* 149:1435-1440, 1993.

92. Salvesen KA et al: Routine ultrasonography in utero and speech development, *Ultrasound Obstet Gynecol* 4:101-103, 1994.

93. Salvesen KA et al: Routine ultrasonography *in utero* and school performance at age 8-9 years, *Lancet* 339:85-89, 1992.

94. Salvesen KA et al: Routine ultrasonography *in utero* and subsequent handedness and neurological development, *BMJ* 307:159-164, 1993.

95. Salvesen KA, Eik-Nes SH: Ultrasound during pregnancy and birthweight, childhood malignancies and neurological development, *Ultrasound Med Biol* 25:1025-1031, 1999.

96. Salvesen KA, Eik-Nes SH: Ultrasound during pregnancy and subsequent childhood non-right handedness: a meta-analysis, *Ultrasound Obstet Gynecol* 6:293-246, 1999.

97. AIUM: *Bioeffects and safety of diagnostic ultrasound,* Laurel, Md, 1993, American Institute of Ultrasound in Medicine.

98. Barnett SB et al: The sensitivity of biological tissue to ultrasound, *Ultrasound Med Biol* 23:805-812, 1997.

99. Barnett SB et al: International recommendations and guidelines for the safe use of diagnostic ultrasound in medicine, *Ultrasound Med Biol* 26:355-366, 2000.

100. EFSUMB (European Federation of Societies for Ultrasound in Medicine and Biology): Tutorial paper: diagnostic ultrasound: genetic aspects, *Eur J Ultrasound* 1:91-92, 1994.

101. NCRP: *Biological effects of ultrasound: mechanisms and clinical implications, NCRP Report 74,* Bethesda, Md, 1983, National Council on Radiation Protection and Measurements.

102. NCRP: *Exposure criteria for medical diagnostic ultrasound: II. Criteria based on all known mechanisms, NCRP Report 140,* Bethesda, Md, 2002, National Council on Radiation Protection and Measurements.

103. WFUMB: Barnett SB, Kossoff G, eds: World Federation for Ultrasound in Medicine and Biology Symposium on safety and standardisation in medical ultrasound; issues and recommendations regarding thermal mechanisms for biological effects of ultrasound, *Ultrasound Med Biol* 18(9):731-810, 1992.

104. WFUMB. Barnett SB (ed): World Federation for Ultrasound in Medicine and Biology Symposium on safety of ultrasound in medicine conclusions and recommendations on thermal and non-thermal mechanisms for biological effects of ultrasound, *Ultrasound Med Biol* 24:1-55, 1998.

Clinical Safety

We now discuss several important concepts that have a bearing on the practice of diagnostic ultrasound: risks versus benefits, thermal considerations (including minimum threshold), acoustic output indices, nonlinear propagation, clinical efficacy in obstetrics, recommendations of professional societies, education and training, and potential exposure limits.

RISKS VERSUS BENEFITS

Although harmful effects of ultrasound have not been demonstrated after exposure at diagnostic levels, the data are not sufficient to permit unquestioned acceptance of its safety. The potential for harm does exist. Interactions of ultrasound with biologic tissue are not fully understood, and until the risks are accurately defined, the prudent course of action must be to apply objective criteria in the selection of patients for an ultrasound examination and to minimize exposure. Exposure in this sense consists of the intensity (or peak pressure) and the exposure time.

A diagnostic ultrasound examination should be conducted only when medically indicated. *Medically indicated* implies that some benefit can be expected from the information obtained. Furthermore, an intensity consistent with the objectives of the examination should be used. A low intensity that reduces the ultrasound exposure but does not provide the desired diagnostic information exposes the patient unnecessarily. Although the exposure is low, no benefit is gained. The same principles apply to an examination so limited in time as to compromise the validity of the study.

The selection process for new instruments should include consideration of the intensity specifications of the various units.

If future work succeeds in quantifying risk factors for small animals exposed to diagnostic levels of ultrasound, the risk factors may not be readily extrapolated to human beings. The human in vivo situation likely provides some reduction in risk compared with that observed for small animals. The attenuation of an ultrasound beam by overlying tissues lowers the dose delivered to deeper structures. Also, since only part of an organ intercepts the beam, only a fraction of it is at risk. During scanning, a particular volume of tissue is irradiated for only a portion of the examination time. In addition, focusing, reflections from body interfaces, and the formation of standing waves are all conditions that can increase the risk by creating locally intense ultrasound fields.

Damage induced by chronic exposure to ultrasound may be cumulative. The ability to repair the damage and thus reduce the overall effect must be investigated. Findings from such studies could have implications in the clinical setting with regard to the frequency of examination and the total number of procedures performed.

The identification of adverse effects attributable to diagnostic ultrasound would not necessarily preclude its medical application. A certain amount of risk is justified if morbidity and mortality can be reduced by the information gained thereby. An important example of this risk-versus-benefit concept in the healing arts is the use of ionizing radiation. Radiation doses are delivered to various organs during nuclear medicine, computed tomography, and radiographic procedures. If the dose-risk relationship is assumed to be linear, with no absolute dose threshold, a small increase in the cancer incidence rate can be expected for persons who have undergone such examinations. These high-technology specialty areas, however, provide such extensive diagnostic information that the small accompanying risk is overshadowed by the high standard of medical care. For example, if a study produces a mortality risk of one per million and a yield of 1% (in terms of saving life), the risk of not performing the procedure is 10,000 times greater than the risk of performing it.

When the risk factors become available, physicians must evaluate the risks associated with a particular procedure compared with the diagnostic information to be gained. Consideration must be given to the various types of examinations (e.g., ultrasound versus x-ray) that can provide the desired diagnostic information. The procedure with the lowest risk and necessary diagnostic information content should be performed.

AIUM Statement on Clinical Safety

The American Institute of Ultrasound in Medicine (AIUM) has performed a risks-versus-benefits analysis and formulated the following statement regarding clinical safety that was approved in March 1997:

Diagnostic ultrasound has been in use since the late 1950s. Given its known benefits and recognized efficacy for medical diagnosis, including use during human pregnancy, the AIUM therein addresses the clinical safety of such use:

There are no confirmed biological effects on patients or instrument operators caused by exposures from present diagnostic ultrasound instruments. Although the possibility exists that such biological effects may be identified in the future, current data indicate that the benefits to patients of the prudent use of diagnostic ultrasound outweigh the risks, if any, that may be present.*

---

*From American Institute of Ultrasound in Medicine: AIUM Official Statements: Clinical Safety, http://www.aium.org/provider/statements/statements.asp, retrieved September 8, 2004.

THERMAL CONSIDERATIONS

For life processes to be maintained, the body temperature must stay within a narrow range. Although a variation of 1° C is tolerable (and indeed common), thermal-mediated fetal abnormalities can result from an elevation of 2.5° C for 2 hours. Avoiding a local rise in temperature above 1° C will ensure that no biologic effects are induced.

Acoustic energy is converted to heat as the ultrasound beam passes through tissue. The heat production rate (q) in a small volume is determined by the absorption coefficient of the tissue (α) and the local time-averaged intensity of the ultrasound beam (I_{TA}):

23-1

$$q = 0.002 \, \alpha \, I_{TA}$$

Heat production rate, absorption coefficient, and intensity are expressed in joules per cubic centimeter per second (J/cm³/s), nepers per centimeter (Np/cm), and milliwatts per square centimeter (mW/cm²), respectively. The rate of absorption for most tissues increases linearly with frequency. Variations in the heat production rate occur because of different tissue types and nonuniformity of the ultrasound field.

For example, the initial temperature rise caused by an ultrasound beam (3.5 MHz, 1000 mW/cm² temporal-averaged intensity) incident on soft tissue is compared with one incident on bone. The heat capacity of a substance is the amount of energy required to raise the temperature 1° C. Dividing the heat production rate by the heat capacity yields the initial temperature rise. Table 23-1 lists the parameters necessary for this calculation. The initial temperature rise is approximately 50 times higher in bone.

The initial rate of temperature rise cannot be maintained. Heat removal by conduction and perfusion quickly slows it. Focused beams create small, localized regions of heating. The removal of heat from small volumes is very rapid. Continuous insonation ultimately produces a steady state condition in which the maximum temperature does not change (Fig. 23-1). Results of experiments quantifying the

■ **Table 23-1** Initial Temperature Rise in Soft Tissue and Bone*

Parameter	Soft Tissue	Bone
Absorption coefficient (Np/cm/MHz)	0.05	1.5
Absorption coefficient at 3.5 MHz (Np/cm)	0.175	5.25
q (J/cm³/s)	0.35	10.5
Heat capacity (J/cm³/° C)	3.8	2.5
Initial temperature rise (° C/s)	0.09	4.2

Np/cm/MHz, Neper per centimeter per megahertz; *q (J/cm³/s),* heat production rate (joule per cubic centimeter per second).
*Time-averaged intensity is 1000 milliwatts/cm². Transducer frequency is 3.5 MHz.

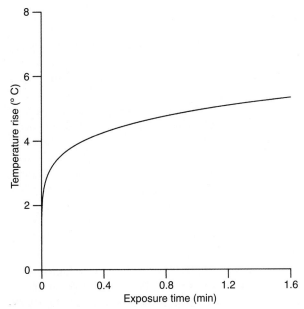

Fig. 23-1 Heating of rat skull bone with a focused ultrasound beam. The temperature rise depends primarily on intensity and the cross-sectional area of the beam. The rapid initial rate of temperature rise is not sustained. After the ultrasound beam has been applied for some time, a steady state condition of maximum temperature rise is approached.

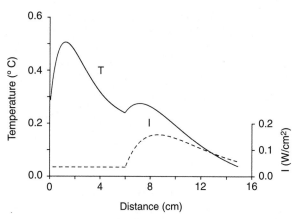

Fig. 23-2 Temperature and intensity profiles along the axis of a focused beam. Exposure conditions include frequency 3 MHz, transducer diameter 2 cm, radius of curvature 10 cm, absorption coefficient 0.15 Np/cm, power 0.1 W. (Adapted from American Institute of Ultrasound in Medicine: *J Ultrasound Med* 7:S1-S38, 1988.)

heating of rat skull bone exposed to a focused ultrasound beam form the basis for thermal models involving the insonation of bone.

By converting acoustic energy into heat, an absorbing object in the ultrasound beam becomes a heat source. Some fraction of the available acoustic energy (e.g., 0.2) is transformed into heat. As the total energy absorbed encompasses a larger and larger volume, the efficiency of the beam in heating tissue becomes diminished. The total energy per unit time (the power) incident on an object is found by summing the intensity over the entire region where heat generation is taking place. More simply, in situ power ($W_{in\ situ}$) (in mW) is determined by

23-2

$$W_{in\ situ} = I_{in\ situ}\ A$$

where A is the effective cross-sectional area (in cm²) of the ultrasound beam. Power then becomes a very important parameter that describes the heating of an object within the ultrasound beam.

TEMPERATURE PROFILES

Temperature profiles along the axis of a focused beam through a homogeneous medium can be generated for a given set of conditions: transducer diameter, frequency, intensity, absorption coefficient of tissue, and degree of perfusion (Fig. 23-2). From the temperature profiles for a wide range of parameters, a conservative estimate of the acoustic power output (W) (in mW) necessary to maintain

the maximum temperature rise to less than 1° C at any point along the ultrasonic path is given as

23-3

$$W = \frac{(230\ \text{W-MHz/cm})\ d}{f}$$

where d is the diameter of the transducer in centimeters, and f is the frequency (in MHz). Equation 23-3 is applicable for diameters of 1 to 2 cm and frequencies between 2 and 10 MHz. As the total energy absorbed encompasses a larger area, the effectiveness of heating tissue becomes less; therefore an increased diameter of the transducer raises the acoustic power limit (W is proportional to d). The energy of the sound beam is more readily converted to heat as the frequency is increased, which reduces the acoustic power limit (W is inversely proportional to f). The 1° C value of the I(SATA) (spatial average, temporal average intensity) at the transducer is calculated by dividing the acoustic power limit by the transducer area.

AIUM MODEL TO LIMIT FETAL TEMPERATURE RISE

For examinations of fetal soft tissues, the AIUM has estimated the in situ I(SATA) required to raise the temperature 1° C within the focal zone (Table 23-2). The model employed for these calculations assumes that the diameter of the focal zone is constant for several centimeters and that the absorption coefficient in the region before the focal zone is relatively low compared to the absorption coefficient within the focal zone. The latter condition is important for ensuring that heating in the intervening tissues does not contribute to the temperature rise within the focal zone. As shown in Table 23-2, the in situ I(SATA) decreases as the frequency and diameter of the focal zone increase; that is, the heating of tissue is more effective when high-frequency ultrasound is applied over a large area. The heat energy in a

◼ **Table 23-2** Predicted In Situ Intensity in mW/cm² (Averaged over the Focal Area) for Which the Temperature Rise is 1° C or Less

Focal Diameter (mm)	Frequency (MHz)			
	2	4	6	8
1	—	3500	2450	1900
2	—	1100	770	605
3	1070	570	405	320
4	680	365	260	205
5	480	260	185	145
6	365	200	140	115
7	290	160	115	91
8	240	130	94	76

Adapted from American Institute of Ultrasound in Medicine: *J Ultrasound Med* 7:S1-S38, 1988.

small volume of tissue traversed by the ultrasound beam is readily transferred to the surrounding region, which is at a lower temperature. When the irradiated volume is increased, removal of heat energy becomes less rapid, and the local temperature rises.

The model, as presented by the AIUM, does not consider the thermal effect if fetal bone is present in the ultrasound beam. If fetal bone has a high absorption coefficient and exposure times are several seconds in duration, the local temperature rise may be greater than 1° C.

Currently the in situ I(SATA) cannot be measured. By correcting for attenuation along the path from the transducer to the focal zone, however, the in situ I(SATA) at the depth of interest can be estimated. This calculation depends on the thicknesses and attenuation coefficients of the intervening tissues. For example, consider a transducer operating at a frequency of 3 MHz with a focal diameter of 5 mm. Carson has determined that attenuation by the overlying maternal tissues is a function of gestational age. A minimum value of 1.4 dB is obtained for the attenuation at 3 MHz. From Table 23-2, it can be seen that the 1° C in situ I(SATA) is 370 mW/cm², which when corrected for attenuation corresponds to an intensity in water of 510 mW/cm². If the measured free-field I(SATA) is not greater than 510 mW/cm², the temperature rise in vivo should not exceed 1° C.

ACOUSTIC OUTPUT INDICES

Diagnostic ultrasound has well-established medical applications with known benefits and recognized efficacy. No acute harmful effects have been reported after its use. Two potential interactions through which it may induce biologic effects, however, are mechanical and **thermal mechanisms.** Thermally produced teratologic effects have been demonstrated in various laboratory animals, including nonhuman primates. Mechanical mechanisms are considered to include cavitation. In vitro experiments and animal studies suggest that cavitation may occur at peak pressures and frequencies used in some diagnostic equipment.

Prudent Use

The statement on clinical safety by the AIUM recommends prudent use of ultrasound in the clinical environment. The term "prudent use" was not defined initially. In a subsequent statement in May 1999, nonmedical use of ultrasound for psychosocial and entertainment purposes is discouraged. Viewing the fetus without medical indication is inappropriate.

In our opinion, objective criteria should be applied in the selection of patients for an ultrasound examination. Furthermore, knowledgeable users should conduct the examination at minimum intensity levels and exposure times to obtain the desired diagnostic information. The principle of ALARA (as low as reasonably achievable) is applied in other areas, particularly x-ray imaging, to evaluate whether the conditions of use are prudent. If the sonographer is to practice ALARA, then an indication of exposure levels must be provided at the time of examination. Exposure of the patient may be minimized by adjusting acquisition parameters while maintaining the desired information content. Safety guidelines based on scientific knowledge concerning the interactions of ultrasound with tissue must be established to delineate prudent use.

Output Display Standard

In response to this need, the AIUM and the National Electrical Manufacturers Association (NEMA) adopted in 1992 the voluntary standard for display of acoustical output information (**Output Display Standard [ODS]).** Two acoustic output parameters, called the **thermal index (TI)** and the **mechanical index (MI),** are defined as indicators of the potential for biologic effects. The thermal index, in essence, gives the maximum temperature rise in tissue that can be predicted as a result of the diagnostic examination, and the MI describes the likelihood of cavitation. Three thermal indices corresponding to soft tissue (TIS), bone (TIB), and cranial bone (TIC) have been developed depending on whether bone is encountered along the path, and if it is, whether bone is located near the transducer or in the interior of the body. TIS applies when the ultrasound beam passes through soft tissue only and bone is not present (examinations of the abdomen and fetus during the first trimester). If bone is encountered near the transducer, then TIC is used (examinations of pediatric and adult head). TIB applies if the ultrasound beam, after passing through soft tissue, impinges on bone near the focal zone (examinations of the fetus during the second and third trimesters).

Determining acoustic intensity distributions along various tissue paths for diverse equipment and operating modes in use today is an overwhelming task. Thermal and mechanical indices are generated from simplified models using conservative worst-case situations. The indices provide upper limits for the assessment of risk. The agreement among manufacturers to standardize acoustic output information allows sonographers to apply the same safety principles to all diagnostic ultrasound equipment regardless of manufacturer.

Derating Acoustic Output

Acoustic output is generally denoted by the power at the radiating source or by an intensity descriptor that characterizes the ultrasonic field. Peak pressure is also used as an output parameter. Intensity (or pressure) is measured at multiple points throughout the ultrasound field in a water medium. To quantify the tissue exposure to ultrasound, the free-field intensity or pressure must be converted to an in situ value.

When soft tissue replaces water along the ultrasonic pathway, a decrease in the intensity is expected, because soft tissue has a much higher rate of attenuation. The fractional reduction in intensity caused by attenuation is denoted by the **derating factor:**

23-4
$$\text{Derating factor} = 10^{(-0.1\,afz)}$$

where a is the attenuation coefficient in dB/cm/MHz, f is the transducer frequency, and z is the distance along the beam axis between the source and the point of interest (Fig. 23-3). In Table 23-3 the derating factor is shown as a function of frequency and distance. The attenuation coefficient is assigned a value of 0.3 dB/cm/MHz in conjunction with the homogeneous soft tissue model, which is applied in later calculations of acoustic output indices. The derated intensity ($I_{\text{SPTA.3}}$) represents the intensity in soft tissue and is calculated by

23-5
$$I_{\text{SPTA.3}} = I_{\text{SPTA}}\,10^{(-0.1\,afz)}$$

where I_{SPTA} is the spatial peak time-averaged intensity measured in water.

Power and peak pressure also decrease as the ultrasound beam penetrates tissue. A similar calculation can be performed to determine the derated power or peak pressure. The derating factor for power is identical to that specified for intensity in Equation 23-4. The derating factor for pressure is found by taking the square root of the intensity derating factor.

Tissue Models

A homogeneous tissue model is assumed for soft tissue. Tissue in this model has low fat content and does not contain calcifications or large gas-filled spaces. Thermal conduction is the same as in water. The attenuation coefficient is uniform and equal to a value of 0.3 dB/cm/MHz. The probability of scatter is low, which allows the absorption rate to be represented by the attenuation coefficient. If bone is present, 60% of the incident energy is assumed to be absorbed within the volume of a thin disk.

Temperature elevation depends on power, transducer aperture, tissue types, beam dimensions, and scanning mode. Scanned mode or autoscanning refers to the steering of successive ultrasound pulses through the field of view. In

■ **Table 23-3** Intensity Derating Factor

Distance (cm)	Frequency (MHz)			
	1	3	5	7.5
1	0.9332	0.8128	0.708	0.5957
2	0.871	0.6607	0.5012	0.3548
3	0.8128	0.537	0.3548	0.2113
4	0.7586	0.4365	0.2512	0.1259
5	0.708	0.3548	0.1778	0.075
6	0.6607	0.2884	0.1259	0.0447
7	0.6166	0.2344	0.0891	0.0266
8	0.5754	0.1906	0.0631	0.0158

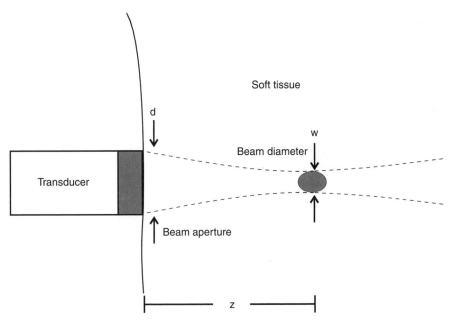

Fig. 23-3 Focused transducer operating in the nonscanned mode. Note the parameters of beam aperture diameter *(d)*, beam diameter *(w)*, and distance *(z)* from the transducer to the location of interest *(shaded region)*.

the nonscanned mode, emission of ultrasound pulses occurs along a single line of sight, which does not change until the transducer is moved to a new position.

Six thermal models have been developed to mimic possible clinical situations (Table 23-4). Figs. 23-4 to 23-8 diagram these models. The homogeneous soft tissue model is used in determining the MI.

Thermal Index

The thermal index is defined as the ratio of the in situ acoustic power ($W_{.3}$) to the acoustic power required to raise tissue temperature by 1° C (W_{deg}). The in situ acoustic power is calculated from the measured power in water corrected for attenuation by the derating factor. The subscript 0.3 indicates the attenuation rate is assumed to be 0.3 dB/cm/MHz.

■ **Table 23-4**   Thermal Models

Number	Composition	Mode	Specification
1	Soft tissue	Nonscanned	Large aperture
2	Soft tissue	Nonscanned	Small aperture
3	Soft tissue	Scanned	Evaluated at surface
4	Soft tissue and bone	Scanned	Soft tissue at surface
5	Soft tissue and bone	Nonscanned	Bone at focus
6	Soft tissue and bone	Nonscanned or scanned	Bone at surface

23-6

$$TI = \frac{W_{.3}}{W_{deg}}$$

A conservative estimate of the acoustic power in milliwatts necessary to produce a 1° C temperature elevation in soft tissue is given by

23-7

$$W_{deg} = \frac{210 \text{ mW-MHz}}{f}$$

where f is the frequency in MHz. This relationship was derived from experimentally measured absorbed power levels from multiple transducers. The absorbed power per unit path length necessary to cause a 1° C temperature rise was surprisingly consistent. An absorption coefficient of 0.1 Np/cm/MHz and an average perfusion rate designated by a perfusion length of 1 cm when applied to the measured data for absorbed power per unit path length yields Equation 23-7. The reference power (W_{deg}) in this equation is used in the estimation of thermal indices for situations depicted by Models 1 through 4 (see later).

The power necessary to cause a 1° C temperature elevation in bone is considerably less, since acoustic energy absorption by bone is higher than by soft tissue. The equation for the reference power becomes

23-8

$$W_{deg} = (40 \text{ mW/cm}) Kw$$

where K is a beam shape factor that describes the radial nonuniformity of the intensity distribution, and w is the beam diameter (in centimeters) at the depth of interest. The beam shape factor is set as 1 (uniform beam) or 1.1 (all

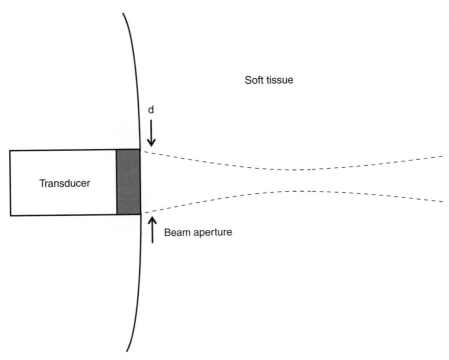

Fig. 23-4 Thermal model for evaluating the temperature elevation in soft tissue. Transducer operating in the nonscanned mode with the entrance beam area greater than 1 cm² (Model 1) or less than 1 cm² (Model 2).

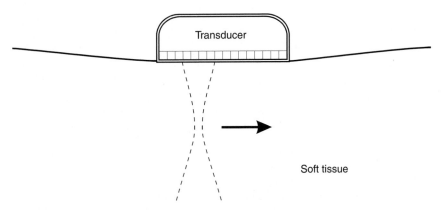

Fig. 23-5 Thermal Model 3 for evaluating the temperature elevation in soft tissue at the surface. Transducer operating in the scanned mode.

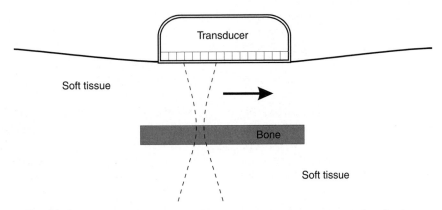

Fig. 23-6 Thermal Model 4 for evaluating the maximum temperature elevation in soft tissue at the surface. Transducer operating in the scanned mode with bone located in the focal zone.

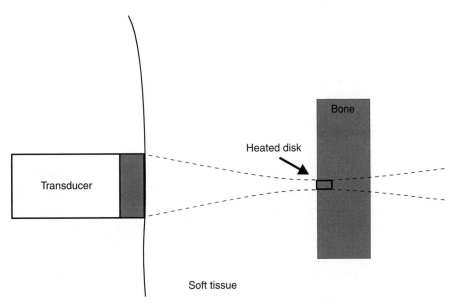

Fig. 23-7 Thermal Model 5 for evaluating the temperature elevation in bone. Transducer operating in the nonscanned mode with bone located in the focal zone.

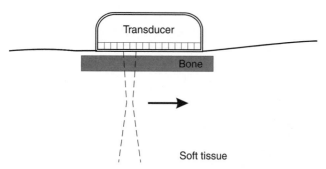

Fig. 23-8 Thermal Model 6 for evaluating the temperature elevation in bone. Transducer operating in the scanned mode with bone located near the surface.

other cases). For narrow nonscanning beams, the beam diameter is considered to be no smaller than 0.1 cm. For autoscan systems, beam diameter is replaced by aperture diameter, since the beam sweeps across the entrance surface. The reference power in Equation 23-8 is used in estimating the thermal index for situations depicted by Models 5 and 6 (see later).

Model 1 (Soft Tissue, Nonscanned, Large Aperture). The entrance area is more than 1 cm². At some distance from the transducer, the beam may be focused. If the beam area is less than 1 cm², power controls the temperature rise. For broader beams, intensity controls the temperature rise. The derated intensity over a designated area ($I_{SPTA.3} \times 1$ cm²) and derated power ($W_{.3}$) are calculated for each point along the beam axis. For each pair of calculated values, the minimum of these two functions (designated the power parameter) determines the amount of heating at that location. The maximum power parameter for all points along the propagation axis causes the maximum temperature increase and is used in Equation 23-6 to estimate the thermal index (TIS):

23-9

$$TIS = \frac{f\{[W_{.3}(z), I_{SPTA.3}(z) \times 1 \text{ cm}^2]_{min}\}_{max}}{210 \text{ mW-MHz}}$$

The verbal explanation of this equation is difficult to express in clear and unencumbered language. A TIS calculation using profiles of the derated power and intensity functions is illustrated in Table 23-5. The derated power and derated intensity multiplied by 1 cm² are calculated for several points along the propagation axis. For each pair of calculated values, the minimum is assigned as the power parameter for that distance. The maximum of all power parameters along the z-axis (in this example, 45 mW) is substituted for the factor within the brackets in Equation 23-9. Assuming a transducer frequency of 5 MHz, thermal index is calculated to be

$$TIS = \frac{(5 \text{ MHz}) (45 \text{ mW})}{210 \text{ mW-MHz}} = 1.1$$

Model 2 (Soft Tissue, Nonscanned, Small Aperture). For a small aperture in which the entrance area is less than 1 cm², the in situ power is maximal at the surface and equal to the source acoustic power, W_o. The thermal index (TIS) is estimated as

■ **Table 23-5** Calculation of Thermal Index (TIS) (Model 1)*

z (cm)	$W_{.3}$ (mW)	$I_{SPTA.3} \times 1$ cm² (mW)	Power Parameter (mW)
1	70.8	40	40
2	50.1	45	45†
3	35.5	40	35.5
4	25.1	60	25.1
5	17.8	150	17.8
6	12.6	125	12.6
7	8.9	60	8.9
8	6.3	6	6

z, Distance along beam axis; *cm,* centimeter; *mW,* milliwatts; $I_{SPTA.3}$, intensity in soft tissue.
*Focused transducer (weak focus); transducer frequency is 5 MHz; acoustic source power equals 100 mW.
†Maximum power parameter is 45 mW.

23-10

$$TIS = \frac{f W_o}{210 \text{ mW-MHz}}$$

Model 3 (Soft Tissue at Surface, Scanned) and Model 4 (Soft Tissue with Bone at Focus, Scanned). Maximum temperature rise occurs at the surface for scanned modes such as real-time B-mode and color Doppler. Even if bone is present at the focus, this model predicts that the temperature increase is generally highest at the surface. The in situ power is set equal to the source acoustic power; however, if the active transmitting area is large (more than 1 cm²), a modification is applied to the measurement of source power. Power for the central portion of the radiating surface is determined over a scan width of 1 cm. In this measurement format, power is designated W_{o1}. The thermal index (TIS for Model 3 or TIB for Model 4) is calculated in an identical manner:

23-11

$$TIS \text{ (or TIB)} = \frac{f W_{o1}}{210 \text{ mW-MHz}}$$

Model 5 (Soft Tissue, Nonscanned, Bone at Focus). Bone is assumed to be located in the focal region, where the product of the derated intensity and power is maximal (worst-case situation). The diameter of the beam in the focal region is defined by the ratio of the derated power to the derated intensity:

23-12

$$w = \sqrt{\frac{4 W_{.3}}{\pi I_{SPTA.3}}}$$

Substituting this expression for w and with 1.1 as the beam shape factor in Equation 23-8,

23-13

$$W_{deg} = (50 \text{ mW/cm}) \sqrt{\frac{W_{.3}}{I_{SPTA.3}}}$$

The in situ power at the focal region is the derated power, $W_{.3}$. Thus

23-14

$$TIB = \frac{\sqrt{W_{.3} I_{SPTA.3}}}{50 \text{ mW/cm}}$$

In the case of small-diameter beams, a minimum value of $(0.227 \text{ mW}^{-1}) \times W_{.3}$ is assigned to TIB.

At the highest I(SPTA) (spatial peak, temporal average intensity) allowed by the Food and Drug Administration (FDA) of 720 W/cm², the TIB is estimated as 12 multiplied by the beam diameter. For a 0.3-cm diameter beam, the TIB is 3.6.

Model 6 (Bone at Surface, Scanned or Nonscanned). The transducer is placed in contact with the head of an adult or infant. The sound beam crosses a thin layer of skin before striking bone. Because little attenuation occurs, the derating factor is essentially unity. The area of bone exposed is the same as the active area of the transducer (both scanned and nonscanned modes). Summing the time-averaged intensity over the active area yields the acoustic power at the source, W_o. The in situ power is considered equal to the transmitted power. The thermal index formula for this model is

23-15

$$TIC = \frac{W_o}{(40 \text{ mW/cm}) \, d}$$

where d is the aperture diameter (in centimeters). For example, if acoustic power is 12 mW and the beam diameter is 0.3 cm, then TIC is 1.

The algorithm for TIC is the simplest and most firmly based on experimental data. Measurements have characterized temperature rise at the outer surface of the rat skull during exposure to ultrasound. The model includes consideration of thermal conductivity and perfusion.

Limitations of Thermal Index

Along a poorly attenuating path such as when fluid is present, the derated peak rarefactional power is lower than the in situ value, and an underestimate of the TI occurs. For those situations in which a long sound path is encountered before reaching the point of interest (obese patients, large muscular patients, and deep-lying structures), the TI may overestimate the temperature rise for that region. In the circumstance of nonlinear propagation, TI may underestimate temperature rise in tissue at high power levels.

For poorly perfused tissue in contact with the transducer, the temperature rise may be higher than that predicted by the TI. TIS is calculated at the transducer surface and overestimates the temperature rise in tissue at the focus. The dwell time from scanning is often less than the time required to reach steady state, and in that circumstance, TI overestimates the temperature rise in tissue.

AIUM Statement Regarding Heat

The AIUM has summarized the clinically relevant findings regarding temperature elevation from exposure to ultrasound. The AIUM statement "Conclusions Regarding Heat" was approved in March 1997:

1. Excessive temperature increase can result in toxic effects in mammalian systems. The biological effects observed depend on many factors, such as the exposure duration, the type of tissue exposed, its cellular proliferation rate, and its potential for regeneration. Age and stage of development are important factors when considering fetal and neonatal safety. Temperature increases of several degrees Celsius above the normal core range can occur naturally; there have been no significant biological effects observed resulting from such temperature increases except when they were sustained for extended time periods.

   a. For exposure durations up to 50 hours, there have been no significant, adverse biological effects observed due to temperature increases less than or equal to 2° C above normal.

   b. For temperature increases greater than 2° C above normal, there have been no significant, adverse biological effects observed due to temperature increases less than or equal to $6 - [(\log_{10} t)/0.6]$ where t is the exposure duration ranging from 1 to 250 minutes. For example, for temperature increases of 4° C and 6° C, the corresponding limits for the exposure duration t are 16 minutes and 1 minute, respectively.

   c. In general, adult tissues are more tolerant of temperature increases than fetal and neonatal tissues. Therefore, higher temperatures and/or longer exposure durations would be required for thermal damage.

2. The temperature increase during exposure of tissues to diagnostic ultrasound fields is dependent upon (a) output characteristics of the acoustic source such as frequency, source dimensions, scan rate, power, pulse repetition frequency (PRF), pulse duration, transducer self heating, exposure time and wave shape and (b) tissue properties such as attenuation, absorption, speed of sound, acoustic impedance, perfusion, thermal conductivity, thermal diffusivity, anatomical structure and nonlinearity parameter.

3. For similar exposure conditions, the expected temperature increase in bone is significantly greater than in soft tissues. For this reason, conditions where an acoustic beam impinges on ossifying fetal bone deserve special attention due to its close proximity to other developing tissues.

4. Calculations of the maximum temperature increase resulting from ultrasound exposure in vivo should not be assumed to be exact because of the uncertainties and approximations associated with the thermal, acoustic and structural characteristics of the tissues involved. However, experimental evidence shows that calculations are capable of predicting measured values within a factor of two. Thus, it appears reasonable to use calculations to obtain safety guidelines for clinical exposures where temperature measurements are not feasible. To provide a display of real-time estimates of tissue temperature increases as part of a diagnostic system, simplifying approximations are used to yield values called Thermal Indices.* Under most clinically relevant conditions, the soft-tissue thermal index, TIS, and the bone thermal index, TIB, either overestimate or closely approximate the best available estimate of the maximum temperature increase (ΔT_{max}). For example, if TIS = 2, then ΔT_{max} is 2° C.

5. The current FDA regulatory limit for $I_{SPTA.3}$ is 720 mW/cm². For this, and lesser intensities, the best available estimate of the

---

*The Thermal Indices are the nondimensional ratios of the estimated temperature increases to 1° C for specific tissue models (see the *Standard for Real-Time Display of Thermal and Mechanical Acoustic Output Indices on Diagnostic Ultrasound Equipment,* AIUM/NEMA, 1992).

maximum temperature increase in the conceptus can exceed 2° C.
6. The soft-tissue thermal index, TIS, and the bone thermal index, TIB, are useful for estimating the temperature increase in vivo. For this purpose, these thermal indices are superior to any single ultrasonic field quantity such as the derated spatial-peak, temporal-average intensity, $I_{SPTA.3}$. That is, TIS and TIB track changes in the maximum temperature increases, ΔT_{max}, thus allowing for implementation of the ALARA principle, whereas $I_{SPTA.3}$ does not. For example,
   a. At a constant value of $I_{SPTA.3}$, TIS increases with increasing frequency and with increasing source diameter.
   b. At a constant value of $I_{SPTA.3}$, TIB increases with increasing focal beam diameter.*

WFUMB EVALUATION OF THERMAL DATA

At the second symposium on safety and standardization in medical ultrasound conducted by the World Federation of Ultrasound in Medicine and Biology (WFUMB) in 1992, the safety of the technique was evaluated with respect to thermal considerations.

B-mode imaging. Known diagnostic ultrasound equipment as used today for simple B-mode imaging operates at acoustic outputs that are not capable of producing harmful temperature rises. Its use in medicine is therefore not contraindicated on thermal grounds. This includes endoscopic, transvaginal, and transcutaneous applications.

Doppler. It has been demonstrated in experiments with unperfused tissue that some Doppler diagnostic equipment has the potential to produce biologically significant temperature rises, specifically at bone/soft tissue interfaces. The effects of elevated temperatures may be minimized by keeping the time for which the beam passes through any one point in tissue as short as possible. Where output power can be controlled, the lowest available power level consistent with obtaining the desired diagnostic information should be used.

Although the data on humans are sparse, it is clear from animal studies that exposures resulting in temperatures less than 38.5° C can be used without reservation on thermal grounds. This includes obstetric applications.

Transducer heating. A substantial source of heating may be the transducer itself. Tissue heating from this source is localized to the volume in contact with the transducer.[†]

MECHANICAL INDEX

The pulsed ultrasound wave, consisting of multiple cycles, causes large fluctuations in pressure as it moves through the medium. *Cavitation is more likely to occur at high pressures and low frequencies.* Scientific research has indicated that cavitation-induced effects may be possible at peak pressures and frequencies within the operational range of diagnostic equipment. Specifically, lung and intestinal hemorrhages in mice have been reported at diagnostic output levels. The cavitation threshold under optimal conditions with pulsed ultrasound is predicted by the ratio of the peak negative pressure in situ to the square root of the frequency.

Measurement of peak rarefactional pressure is performed in water for the transducer under well-defined operating conditions. The location of measurement is specified at the point along the beam axis where the derated pulse intensity integral is a maximum. The pulse intensity integral is the total energy per unit area carried by the wave during the time duration of the pulse. The measured values of the pulse intensity integral as a function of depth along the beam axis are corrected for attenuation using the homogeneous tissue model. At the maximum derated pulse intensity integral, the peak rarefactional pressure is measured and then corrected for attenuation for the tissue path. The derated peak rarefactional pressure is used to calculate the MI:

23-16

$$p_{r.3} = p_r e^{-azf}$$

where a is the attenuation coefficient and has a value of 0.035 Np/cm/MHz, f is the transducer frequency, and z is the distance along the beam axis between the source and the point of interest.

For a specific transmit pattern, the MI is defined as

23-17

$$MI = \frac{C\,p_{r.3}}{\sqrt{f}}$$

where $p_{r.3}$ is the derated peak rarefactional pressure in megapascals (MPa), and f is the frequency in MHz. A constant C is equal to $(1\ MHz)^{0.5}/(1\ MPa)$; thus the MI is expressed as a dimensionless quantity. For water, cavitation cannot be produced if the MI is less than 0.7 over the frequency range 1 to 10 MHz.

The FDA replaced the maximum I(SPPA) (pulse-averaged intensity at spatial peak, averaged over the duration of the pulse) limit of 190 W/cm² with an MI value of 1.9. Manufacturers, at their option, were permitted to meet either of these criteria for the introduction of new equipment. An MI of 1.9 corresponds to a peak negative pressure of 3.3 MPa at a frequency of 3 MHz. The pulse-averaged intensity at an MI of 1.9 is 360 W/cm², which is an effective increase in acoustic power level permitted by the FDA guidelines.

Limitations of Mechanical Index

The position in tissue at which the MI is calculated may shift as output power is changed. ODS indicates the numerical value of the index, but the specific site is not communicated to the operator. The spatial distribution of pressure amplitudes is unknown. Along a poorly attenuating path such as when fluid is present, the derated peak rarefactional pressure is lower than the in situ value, and an underestimate of the MI occurs. For those situations in which a long sound path is encountered before reaching the point of interest

---

*From American Institute of Ultrasound in Medicine: AIUM Official Statements: Conclusion Regarding Heat, http://www.aium.org/provider/statements/statements.asp, retrieved September 8, 2004.
[†]From WFUMB Symposium on Safety and Standardization in Medical Ultrasound: *Ultrasound Med Biol* 18(9)(Special Issue):731-810, 1992.

(e.g., obese patients, large muscular patients, deep-lying structures), the MI may overestimate the pressure for that region. In the circumstance of nonlinear propagation, MI may underestimate pressures in tissue at high power levels.

DISPLAY OF OUTPUT INDICES

The following display guidelines apply to all thermal and mechanical indices. Ultrasound equipment, which has the potential to produce an index value above 1, must be able to display that index. If the index value falls below 0.4, it is unnecessary to display it. The display increments are no greater than 0.2 for index values less than 1 and no greater than 1 for index values greater than 1.

TIS and TIB may be displayed simultaneously or independently. If the equipment is intended for adult cephalic applications exclusively, only the display of TIC is necessary. When operated in B-mode, scanners are not capable of producing a temperature rise above 1° C, and thus the MI will be displayed during this mode of operation. Display of MI and TI should be possible, although not necessarily simultaneously, for a transducer that operates in a mode other than real-time B-mode. For multimode ultrasound equipment, the MI is displayed during real-time B-mode imaging and the thermal index during pulsed-wave Doppler, M-mode, and Doppler imaging—provided that the display criteria mentioned earlier are met.

OUTPUT INDICES AS RISK INDICATORS

The determination of thermal index is a conservative estimate based on a worst-case scenario. Although the calculated temperature elevation is subject to many uncertainties, it provides an upper limit of the actual temperature rise from typical clinical examinations. Insonation of long duration is necessary for achieving the steady state temperature rise predicted by the thermal index.

Cavitation is generally believed to be a threshold phenomenon. The presence of gas cavities escalates the potential for cavitation. The presence of gaseous spaces in the aerated lung, undissolved gas in the gastrointestinal tract, and gaseous contrast agents are the principal areas of concern. Lung hemorrhage has been observed for peak negative pressure ranging from 0.6 to 2.2 MPa in the frequency range of 1 to 4 MHz (MI values vary from 0.6 to 1.4). The cavitation threshold for the fetal lung is much higher, because this tissue does not contain undissolved gas.

By tracking peak rarefactional pressure and frequency, the MI provides an estimate of the potential for mechanical biologic effects. Even if cavitation does occur at isolated sites, however, the affected area is extremely small, and a small number of cells may be killed. The only situation in which the loss of a few cells would be of concern is when the subject is a fetus.

The acoustic output indices serve as risk indicators. If the index value is below the threshold level for bioeffects (considered to be 0.5), then a further decrease in acoustic output would not improve safety and may compromise the quality of the diagnostic examination. At an index value less than 0.5, the possibility of adverse effect associated with tissue heating and cavitation is low. If the index value is greater than 0.5, the physician must evaluate the risks associated with a particular ultrasound procedure against the diagnostic information to be gained. TIBs for commercially available systems range from 0.1 to 10 for fetal scanning. At the highest TIBs, scanning for more than a few seconds may cause harm.

An additional protective measure is to limit the exposure time when the thermal index exceeds 1. Experiments on the effects of temperature elevation on fetal development have shown no abnormalities if the time and temperature elevation were less than 10 minutes and 3° C. The maximum safe exposure time in minutes is

$$t = 10 \times 0.25^{(TI-3)}$$

23-18

However, if the patient is febrile, the exposure time limit is reduced by incrementing the term −3 in the exponent by +1 for each degree centigrade the body temperature exceeds 37° C. For example, if the patient's body temperature is 38° C, the maximum safe exposure time is reduced to 2.5 minutes for a TI of 3.

NONLINEAR PROPAGATION

The calculation of ODS indices requires estimates of the in situ values for pressure, intensity, and power. The acoustic field parameter is measured in water, then a derating factor is applied to obtain the value in tissue. For low-power waveforms, this method works reasonably well. However, if measurements are performed under high-power conditions, the derated pressure (or intensity) underestimates the actual pressure (or intensity) in tissue.

Effect on Mechanical Index

As power levels are increased, nonlinear propagation distorts the wave shape and creates harmonic frequencies. The relationship between the source intensity and pressure at the focal point is no longer linear (Fig. 23-9). The presence of harmonics accelerates the attenuation loss. (The high-frequency components are removed more rapidly.) Because attenuation along the propagation path to the focal zone is less in water, water compared with tissue deviates from linearity at a lower source intensity, although saturation occurs at similar source intensity. Saturation describes the phenomena in which the pressure (or other parameter) in the ultrasonic field becomes independent of the source power. The consequence of this nonlinear behavior is that the negative pressure derated from water underestimates the value in tissue by a factor of 2 or more.

A numerical example illustrates this problem. Suppose the nonlinear propagation intensity is measured as 400 W/cm² at the focal distance of 8 cm in water. At an operating frequency of 3 MHz, the derating factor is 0.19, assuming 0.3 dB/cm/MHz. The derated intensity would be

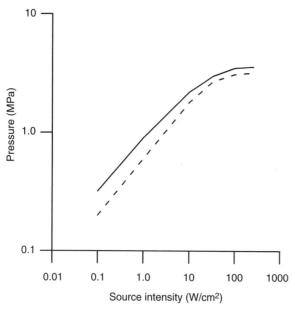

Fig. 23-9 Acoustic pressure in the focal zone for water *(solid line)* and soft tissue *(dotted line)* as a function of source intensity. At high power levels, the response becomes nonlinear. The proportionality between water and soft tissue is not maintained at high power levels.

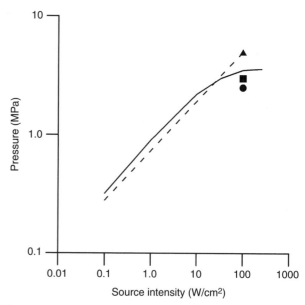

Fig. 23-10 Estimation of the acoustic pressure in soft tissue based on water measurements *(solid line)*. *Circle,* derated from water at high intensity. *Triangle,* derated from water at low intensity and extrapolated to high intensity *(dotted line)*. *Square,* actual tissue value.

76 W/cm^2 versus the true tissue value for nonlinear propagation of approximately 150 W/cm^2.

A modified measurement protocol for nonlinear propagation has been proposed:

1. Measure the acoustic parameter in water at a low-power level.
2. Apply the derating factor to the measured value in water.
3. Perform a linear extrapolation to the machine setting for power.

This algorithm, which overestimates the actual tissue value, is illustrated in Fig. 23-10.

Effect on Thermal Index

The generation of harmonics increases the rate of local absorption and thus the heat production per unit volume. As power is raised further, local absorption becomes greater until at very high power levels the saturation effect causes the intensity at the point of interest to be nearly constant. The heating at the point of interest is now independent of source power.

This phenomenon occurs first along the central beam axis (highest relative spatial intensity levels) and then spreads to off-axis sites as power is increased. Before saturation is reached on the axis, the heating pattern is narrower than the beam width, heat diffusion is higher, and the rise in steady state temperature is less than expected based on the axial heating rate. When saturation is approached, the heating pattern becomes broader, heat diffusion is reduced, and the rise in steady state temperature is more than expected based on the axial heating rate alone.

As the small amplitude absorption coefficient for the medium is reduced, nonlinear propagation enhancement of the heating rate becomes greater. In water with a small low-amplitude absorption coefficient, this effect is pronounced. The absorption rate is low until the shock wave is formed, at which point the absorption increases markedly. The shock wave near the focal point is efficiently converted into heat, and immense local heating takes place. Homogeneous soft tissue also demonstrates enhanced local heating before saturation, but the magnitude is significantly less than that observed in water. Nonlinear propagation has little change on the heating patterns in fat, since fat has a high absorption coefficient.

Fortunately, the effect of nonlinear propagation on the steady state temperature rise in soft tissue is small. The highest temperatures occur in the near field, but the predicted increase is less than 20% (insignificant compared with the other uncertainties in the calculation of TI). The centrally peaked heating pattern is modulated by heat diffusion to the surrounding area. In the application of TI to the homogeneous tissue model, the temperature rise depends on the total energy converted into heat. Even though the axial heating rate is greater during nonlinear propagation, the heat transfer across the entire beam at the focal distance compared with linear propagation is less. Therefore the effect of nonlinear propagation can be ignored, if intensity is specified by the source intensity and not by the measured nonlinear propagation intensity in water.

AIUM Statement on Tissue Models

The AIUM has examined tissue models and their ability to accurately predict acoustic exposure in tissue. The AIUM statement "Conclusions Regarding Tissue Models and Equipment Survey" was approved in October 1997:

1. Tissue models are necessary to estimate attenuation and acoustic exposure levels in situ from measurements of acoustic output made in water. Presently available models are limited in their ability to represent clinical conditions because of varying tissue paths during diagnostic ultrasound exposures and uncertainties in acoustical properties of soft tissues. No single tissue model is adequate for predicting in vivo exposures in all situations from measurements made in water, and continued improvement and verification of these models is necessary for making exposure assessments for specific applications.

2. A homogeneous tissue model with an attenuation coefficient of 0.3 dB/cm/MHz throughout the beam path is commonly used when estimating exposure levels. The model is conservative in that it overestimates the in situ acoustic exposure when the path between the transducer and the site of interest is composed entirely of soft tissue. When the path contains significant amounts of fluid, as in many first- and second-trimester pregnancies scanned transabdominally, this model may underestimate the in situ acoustical exposure. The amount of underestimation depends on each specific situation.

3. "Fixed-path" tissue models, in which soft tissue thickness is held constant, sometimes are used to estimate in situ acoustical exposures when the beam path is greater than 3 cm and consists largely of fluid. When this model is used to estimate maximum exposure to the fetus during transabdominal scans, a value of 1 dB/MHz may be used during all trimesters.

4. Existing tissue models that are based on linear propagation may underestimate acoustical exposures when significant saturation due to nonlinear distortion of beams in water is present during the output measurement.

5. The maximum acoustical output levels of diagnostic ultrasound devices extend over a broad range of values.

   a. Historically, maximum MI values of 1.9 are known to occur for commercially available equipment. Maximum MI values are similar for real-time B-mode, M-mode, pulsed Doppler, and color flow imaging.

   b. Computed estimates of upper limits to temperature elevations during transabdominal scans were obtained in a survey of 1988 and 1990 pulsed Doppler equipment.* The vast majority of models yielded upper limits less than 1° C and 4° C for exposures of first-trimester fetal tissue and second-trimester fetal bone, respectively, for dwell times sufficient to achieve steady state conditions. The largest values obtained were approximately 1.5° C for first-trimester fetal tissue and 7° C for second-trimester fetal bone.

6. Manufacturers of diagnostic ultrasound equipment should provide acoustical output data to allow calculations of thermal and mechanical indices and maximum temperature elevations and are encouraged to implement the *Standard for Real-Time Display of Thermal and Mechanical Acoustic Output Indices on Diagnostic Ultrasound Equipment* (AIUM/NEMA, 1992). Independent investigators are encouraged to make measurements to verify output specifications and to ensure consistency of equipment operation.†

---

*Estimated maximum temperature elevations given here are for a "fixed-path" tissue model and are for devices having I$_{SPTA}$ values greater than 500 mW/cm². The temperature elevations for fetal bone and tissue were computed based on calculation procedures given in Sections 4.3.2.1 to 4.3.2.6 in *Bioeffects and Safety of Diagnostic Ultrasound* (AIUM, 1993).

†From American Institute of Ultrasound in Medicine: AIUM Official Statements: Conclusion Regarding Tissue Models and Equipment Survey, http://www.aium.org/provider/statements/statements.asp, retrieved September 8, 2004.

CLINICAL EFFICACY IN OBSTETRICS

Because ultrasound yields excellent anatomic visualization and is generally considered to be without harmful effects, it has become widely used in the practice of obstetrics. In the United States 3 million children who were examined in utero with ultrasound are born each year. Although ultrasound is assumed to contribute to the improved management and outcome of a pregnancy, its clinical efficacy has not been demonstrated in randomized research studies. This does not mean that no benefit is gained, merely that for low-risk populations, routine screening with ultrasound has not reduced perinatal mortality and morbidity beyond that achieved by selective examination based on clinical judgment. Nevertheless, routine screening with ultrasound for every pregnant patient is conducted in some European countries.

As a guide for practitioners, the National Institutes of Health (NIH) reviewed the available scientific information and concluded that ultrasound has clinical benefit for certain applications, which are listed in the box. Although ultrasonography in these circumstances is not mandatory, it is appropriate when the information gained will influence prenatal care.

Reasons for Employing Diagnostic Ultrasound Imaging in Pregnancy

Estimation of gestational age
Evaluation of fetal growth
Determination of placental location
Detection of fetal death
Location of pregnancy
Determination of fetal presentation
Determination of fetal number
Detection of anomalies
Adjunct to placement of cervical cerclage
Suspected hydatidiform mole
Adjunct to intrauterine transfusion
Determination of source of vaginal bleeding
Biophysical evaluation for fetal well-being after 28 weeks' gestational age
Adjunct to amniocentesis
Evaluation of pelvic mass
Suspected polyhydramnios or oligohydramnios
Suspected abruptio placenta
Evaluation of fetal condition in late registrants for prenatal care

Currently the routine screening of every pregnancy is not recommended by the NIH. Ultrasonography during pregnancy should be performed for a specific medical indication and should be discouraged for the sole purpose of viewing the fetus by the mother or determining its sex (these are potential secondary benefits of a medically indicated examination). Additionally, feedback—in the form of viewing the monitor screen with explanation of the images—may improve maternal perception of the fetus and maternal-infant bonding. The maternal attitude can influence fetal outcome by causing prenatal behavioral changes (e.g., cessation of smoking). Educational and commercial demonstrations of ultrasound imaging during pregnancy without medical benefit are inappropriate.

The recent trend has been to use Doppler ultrasound in the first few weeks of pregnancy. There is no published guideline by professional societies regarding ultrasound examination of the uncomplicated pregnancy during the first trimester.

OPHTHALMIC CONSIDERATIONS

The cornea, lens, and vitreous body of the eye do not have a direct blood supply, and heat removal by perfusion is slow. The lens is a collagenous structure that readily absorbs ultrasound energy. Thus the lens is susceptible to high levels of heating. Therapeutic levels of ultrasound have been demonstrated to induce cataracts. Clinical studies with diagnostic exposure levels have yet to be conducted to determine bioeffects. The FDA recognizes the potential for damage to the eye by establishing lower output limits for ophthalmic applications. The I(SPTA) is 50 mW/cm², and the MI is 0.23 instead of 720 mW/cm² and 1.9 for all other applications.

NCRP RECOMMENDATIONS

The National Council on Radiation Protection and Measurements (NCRP) was created by Congress in 1964 to promulgate information and recommendations in the public interest concerning protection against radiation. In 2002 it published a comprehensive work detailing the biologic effects of ultrasound. Contained within this document were specific recommendations regarding clinical practice, diagnostic equipment, and responsibility of users, which are reproduced here in slightly edited form.

Safety Criteria

1. Safety evaluations must consider the characteristics of the tissue being exposed. Thresholds for nonthermal biologic effects are lowest in (a) tissues that naturally contain gas bodies, for example, postnatal (including adult) lung and intestine, and (b) all tissues in the presence of introduced gas bodies, such as gaseous ultrasound contrast agents.
2. A risk-benefit decision is especially important if the anticipated acoustic pressure amplitude at the surface of aerated lung tissue exceeds 1 MPa.
3. A risk-benefit decision may be important if MI exceeds 0.5. The acoustic pressure at the site of interest may be either underestimated or overestimated by MI, and it is necessary to consider the nature of the clinical situation in order to make an informed judgment.
4. A risk-benefit decision is especially important if the anticipated temperature rise of an embryo or fetus exceeds 3° C for a duration of 10 minutes.
5. The duration expected to be important in risk management depends strongly on expected temperature.

The duration should be decreased by one half for each 0.5° C by which the rise is above 3° C and, if the temperature rise exceeds 1° C, may be doubled for each 0.5° C by which the rise is less than 3° C. (No adverse thermal effects have been observed in which the temperature rise was ≤1° C from exposures of duration up to >1000 minutes.)
6. A risk-benefit decision may be important if TIB, TIC, or TIS exceeds one. The temperature rise at the site of interest may be either underestimated or overestimated by a TI, and it is necessary to consider the nature of the clinical situation in order to make an informed judgment.

Equipment Features; Output and Product Information

1. Ultrasound systems should be designed to improve image quality and diagnostic information in general by using only those acoustic-wave amplitudes that are needed for the application.
2. Diagnostic systems should be designed where possible to keep exposures to the patient close to those required for a given examination.
3. Information on output levels should be provided to the user for guidance in risk-assessment considerations. This includes labeling on screen or in documentation accompanying the systems that include the information currently required for 510(k) applications and for compliance with International Electrotechnical Commission.
4. While output information is apparently reported responsibly by manufacturers, spot checks of system outputs should be performed by independent laboratories.
5. The data in the Acoustic Output Tables prepared by manufacturers in obtaining approval for marketing in the United States and the updates of those tables published in the users' reference manuals are in the public domain and contain valuable information relevant to safety. They should be stored in archives by a professional organization and made conveniently available to the medical community.
6. Presently available methods have proven valuable for estimating the temperature rise produced by diagnostic ultrasound, though they can and should be improved. Development and testing of theoretical and experimental methods for temperature-rise predictions should be continued.
7. The output display process, with its on-screen display of TIs and MIs, is the best source of safety information available to users of medical diagnostic ultrasound equipment. However, there should be continuous efforts to encourage users to utilize this information, and also efforts to develop methods to make the information more accurate and more complete.
8. Diagnostic ultrasound equipment should be provided with the capability for on-screen display of MI if it can exceed 0.5.

9. Manufacturers of gas-body–based ultrasound contrast agents should inform purchasers (e.g., in product package inserts and other methods) that acoustic cavitation would occur during interaction of diagnostic ultrasound with the agents.

Responsibilities of Users

1. ODS indices provide crude measures of the risk of adverse effects arising from an ultrasound examination and provide better indications of the change in risk as controls are adjusted. The final benefit/risk assessment should be performed by a user who is knowledgeable in ultrasound dosimetry and biologic effects and who takes into account the index values and the particular details of the patient being examined. Users should be helped and encouraged by development of educational materials designed specifically for evaluating benefits and risks of diagnostic ultrasound procedures. Laboratory guidelines for making these decisions and training in these decisions should be documented as part of the accreditation process.
2. For each application, a default setting for the diagnostic ultrasound system employed should be set, or reviewed, and documented by the user. The MI and all TIs should be assigned values based on the best available information on bioeffects and, also, on knowledge of the lowest values at which the system employed will yield the required diagnostic information. For example, operation when MI is less than 0.5 and all TIs are less than 1 poses negligible risk under most conditions. For some situations, the desired diagnostic information can be obtained with settings of the indices in these ranges, while for others, higher outputs should be used when justified by consideration of risk and benefit to the patient. The user may find it helpful to employ a feature of the equipment that provides a reminder signal when a user-selected value of a relevant index is exceeded.*

WFUMB RECOMMENDATIONS

Thermal effects

A diagnostic exposure that produces a maximum temperature rise of no more than 1.5° C above normal physiological levels (37° C) may be used clinically without reservation on thermal grounds.

A diagnostic exposure that elevates embryonic and fetal in situ temperature above 41° C (4° C above normal temperature) for 5 minutes or more should be considered potentially hazardous.

Nonthermal effects

Lung capillary bleeding: Currently available animal data indicate that it is prudent to reduce ultrasound exposure of human postnatal lung to the minimum necessary to obtain the required diagnostic information.

Contrast agents: Gas bodies introduced by a contrast agent increase the probability of cavitation. A physician should take this into account when considering the benefit/risk ratio of an examination.

B-mode imaging: When tissue/gas interfaces or contrast agents are not present, the use of B-mode imaging need not be withheld because of concern for ultrasound safety. This statement also applies to endoscopic, transvaginal, and transcutaneous applications. When tissue/gas interfaces or contrast agents are present, ultrasound exposure levels and duration should be reduced to the minimum necessary to obtain the required diagnostic information.

Doppler: When tissue/gas interfaces or contrast agents are not present, and where there is no risk of significant temperature elevation, the use of diagnostic Doppler equipment need not be withheld because of concern for ultrasound safety. When any of the above conditions might be present, ultrasound exposure levels and duration should be reduced to the minimum necessary to obtain the required diagnostic information.*

EDUCATION AND TRAINING

In a perceptive editorial in the *Journal of Ultrasound in Medicine,* Ziskin advocates educating physicians and sonographers as the major safeguard for patients. Well-designed instrumentation to limit exposure of the patient is an alternative measure. However, equipment safeguards can be bypassed by the operator. Knowledgeable users conduct the examination at the minimum intensity levels necessary to obtain the desired diagnostic information. In addition, the examination time is usually reduced. More important, misdiagnoses because of lack of education, inexperience, and poor examination technique are more likely to cause harm than is the potential damage from ultrasound itself.

The diagnostic efficacy of ultrasound is strongly operator dependent. Unfortunately, only about half of obstetric and gynecologic sonographers are certified. The training and education requirements for physicians are not standardized. The ability of physicians to perform and interpret ultrasound examinations varies considerably. Minimum standards of education and training for clinical users of ultrasound (both physician and sonographer) must be established by regulatory agencies or by medical specialty societies.

POTENTIAL EXPOSURE LIMITS

Acoustic output can be limited by law, or the user can be given more latitude to optimize the exposure parameters based on the desired diagnostic information and the risk to the patient. If the user has the responsibility for risk assessment, then the equipment manufacturer must provide safety indices, and the user must have knowledge of biologic effects. Standards of practice must be developed in which reasonable responses to safety issues are delineated.

When clinical studies are published, they must include a statement of the exposure conditions. These data will assist in the overall evaluation of risk. Lack of such information has in the past inhibited the development of a comprehensive theory of biologic effects. It is to be hoped that the

---

*Modified from National Council on Radiation Protection and Measurements: *Exposure Criteria for Medical Diagnostic Ultrasound; II. Criteria Based on All Known Mechanisms,* NCRP Report No. 140, Bethesda, Md, December 2002, NCRP.

*From WFUMB Symposium on Safety and Standardization in Medical Ultrasound: *Ultrasound Med Biol* 18(9)(Special Issue):731-810, 1992.

necessary parameters will become standardized; but in the meantime frequency, the I(SPTA) in water at maximum power, the attenuator setting, and the number of examinations and time duration of each examination should all be specified.

Developing equipment specifications may, in the future, limit intensity, PRF, and pulse duration for various types of scanners. Diagnostic units operating below the transient cavitation threshold will ensure that this type of cavitation does not occur. Such a restriction would be one possible consideration for an intensity limit on some types of diagnostic equipment, particularly obstetric units.

In the future it is also possible, though not probable, that permissible exposure levels for various ultrasound procedures will be established by regulatory agencies. The diagnostic yield for these procedures is generally considered to be quite high, and the risk extremely low. If there were adverse effects, they would likely have become apparent as a result of the many millions of examinations that have already been performed. Ill-conceived or inappropriately applied regulations, however, can easily interfere with the development of new procedures and instrumentation in this rapidly expanding field and must be avoided. Nevertheless, recommended intensity levels and exposure times for various examinations would be helpful for the physician in clinical practice, creating a performance standardization and reducing the overall risk of ultrasound on the population.

SUMMARY

Ultrasound is not a form of ionizing radiation. This attractive feature has resulted in its extensive use for the evaluation of pregnancy, fetal age, and fetal condition. Ultrasound also has demonstrated applications in abdominal and cardiac diagnostic studies. However, harmful effects are possible any time the human body is probed using energy that is ultimately deposited in the body, and ultrasound is no exception.

At current diagnostic intensity levels and scan times, no biologic effects of ultrasound have been observed in humans. Thermal and mechanical acoustic output indices offer a uniform approach to controlling ultrasonic exposure of patients and providing assurance of safety.

Nevertheless, sufficient data do not exist to state categorically that ultrasound is absolutely safe. The continued use of diagnostic ultrasound examinations in obstetrics and other areas is justified, because the potential risk appears to be minimal, and the benefit high. This does not imply that ultrasound should be employed indiscriminately. The selection of patients should be a result of well-defined conscious processes, and steps should be taken to minimize exposure during the examination.

REVIEW QUESTIONS

1. The thermal index indicates the maximum _____ in tissue for the current scan parameters.

2. The mechanical index (MI) gives the likelihood of _____.

3. The MI is inversely proportional to the _____.

4. What factors are used to calculate the derating factor?

5. Damage induced by the thermal mechanism shows a _____, which means that exposure kept below certain combinations of temperature rise and time is unlikely to cause harm.

6. What is the recommendation by the National Institutes of Health regarding the routine screening of every pregnancy?

7. Measurements in water at high-power levels are not recommended to estimate intensity (or pressure) in tissue for nonlinear propagation. Why?

8. Suppose a patient asks you if a diagnostic ultrasound examination is "safe." What is your reply?

BIBLIOGRAPHY

Abbott JG: Rationale and derivation of MI and TI—a review, *Ultrasound Med Biol* 25:431-441, 1999.

American Institute of Ultrasound in Medicine: Bioeffects considerations for the safety of diagnostic ultrasound, *J Ultrasound Med* 7:S1-S38, 1988.

American Institute of Ultrasound in Medicine and National Electrical Manufacturers Association: *Standard for real-time display of thermal and mechanical indices on diagnostic ultrasound equipment*, Rockville, Md, 1992, AIUM-NEMA.

Barnett SB et al: International recommendations and guidelines for the safe use of diagnostic ultrasound in medicine, *Ultrasound Med Biol* 26:355-366, 2000.

Carson PL: Medical ultrasound fields and exposure measurements. In *Proceedings of the 22nd Annual Meeting of the National Council on Radiation Protection and Measurements*, Bethesda, Md, 1988, NCRP Publications.

Carstensen EL et al: Ultrasonic heating of the skull, *J Acoust Soc Am* 87:1310-1317, 1990.

Child SZ et al: Lung damage from exposure to pulsed ultrasound, *Ultrasound Med Biol* 16:817-825, 1990.

Duck FA: Nonlinear acoustics in diagnostic ultrasound, *Ultrasound Med Biol* 28:1-18, 2002.

Hedrick WR, Hykes DL: An overview of thermal and mechanical acoustic output indices, *J Diagn Med Sonogr* 9:228-235, 1993.

Miller DL: Update on safety of diagnostic ultrasonography, *J Clin Ultrasound* 19:531-540, 1991.

National Council on Radiation Protection and Measurements: *Exposure criteria for medical diagnostic ultrasound. I. Criteria based on thermal mechanisms*, NCRP Report 113, Bethesda, Md, 1992, NCRP.

National Council on Radiation Protection and Measurements: *Exposure criteria for medical diagnostic ultrasound: II. Criteria based on all known mechanisms*, NCRP Report 140, Bethesda, Md, 2002, NCRP.

National Institutes of Health: *Diagnostic ultrasound in pregnancy: report of a consensus development conference*, DHHS, NIH Publication 84-667, Bethesda, Md, 1984, NIH.

Nyborg WL: Safety of medical diagnostic ultrasound, *Semin Ultrasound, CT, MRI* 23:377-386, 2002.

Ziskin MC: The prudent use of diagnostic ultrasound, *J Ultrasound Med* 6:415-416, 1987.

Ziskin MC: Update on the safety of ultrasound in obstetrics, *Semin Roentgenol* 25:294-298, 1990.

CHAPTER 24

Performance Testing

KEY TERMS

Axial resolution
Belt phantom
Dead zone
Distortion
Feedback microbalance
Flow phantom
Focal zone
Horizontal distance
Hydrophone
Lateral resolution

Maximum depth of
   visualization
Sensitivity
String phantom
Test object
Tissue-mimicking (TM)
   material
Uniformity
Vertical distance

Earlier chapters in this text have discussed some of the important parameters (axial resolution, lateral resolution, frequency, bandwidth, power, intensity, and sensitivity) that affect the overall performance of an ultrasound system. The purpose of this chapter is to discuss the ways in which these parameters and others can be measured to ensure proper functioning of equipment. Different tissue-mimicking (TM) phantoms are described. Acceptance testing is the initial evaluation of equipment after installation to determine whether it is operating properly and whether it meets specifications. Performance testing by independent laboratories provides confirmation that the manufacturer's specifications are factual. Specialized test procedures are discussed but may be limited in application because of the cost, unavailability of phantoms, time constraints, or complexity of the testing protocol. Most clinical facilities are limited to testing with a single TM phantom.

Phantoms can be used for practice scanning to establish proper operation of time gain compensation (TGC) controls, gain settings, display settings, and output controls. They are also useful in the training of student sonographers.

PHANTOMS

A wide variety of test objects and phantoms have been developed to monitor the performance characteristics of ultrasound scanners. A test object must be differentiated from a TM phantom. A **test object** usually consists of material in which the velocity of ultrasound is the same as in tissue (1540 m/s), but other properties with respect to ultrasound propagation vary from those of tissue. The American Institute of Ultrasound in Medicine (AIUM) test object uses a uniform liquid medium with poor scattering characteristics. Some test objects do not mimic tissue at all but are designed to test performance under nonclinical conditions. One such test object is a rectangular block of acrylic with a wedge-shaped cavity that can be filled with water. The incorporation of TM material into ultrasound phantoms has essentially eliminated the need for test objects.

TM material has similar properties of tissue with respect to velocity, scattering, and attenuation throughout the diagnostic frequency range (2 to 15 MHz). The velocity in TM material is typically within 1% of the average velocity in soft tissue (1540 m/s). The attenuation rate is specified as either 0.5 dB cm^{-1} MHz^{-1} or 0.7 dB cm^{-1} MHz^{-1}. A linear response of attenuation with frequency (mathematically stated as f^1) is recommended by AIUM. Backscatter by TM material is similar to that produced by liver parenchyma. With the development of tissue harmonic imaging propagation, nonlinearity has become an important consideration, but phantoms are not generally specified with respect to the nonlinearity parameter.

The TM phantom is composed of water-based gelatin impregnated with graphite or powered milk or polysaccharide particles and glass beads. The small-diameter particles ($\approx$1 μm) vary the attenuation rate, and the glass beads govern the backscatter levels. Small, strong reflectors (e.g., nylon rods 0.1 mm in diameter) are placed within the TM matrix in well-defined geometric patterns. This small size is necessary to avoid reverberation artifacts at frequencies above 5 MHz. For example, two sets of nylon rods (one along the vertical direction and the other along the horizontal direction) are spaced 1, 2, or 3 cm apart. These rods are used to evaluate the distance accuracy. Hypoechoic and hyperechoic cylindrical or spherical objects can also be distributed throughout the TM material. The amount of scattering from an object can be controlled by varying the concentration of scattering material (often glass beads). Reducing the concentration of scattering material by a factor of 2 results in a −3 dB backscatter level. Increasing the concentration of scattering material by a factor of 2 has the opposite effect (backscatter level increases by 3 dB). A TM phantom is ideal for testing scanners under conditions that simulate the clinical environment.

Special-purpose TM phantoms have been designed for specific applications (e.g., contrast resolution, slice thickness, beam shape determination, accommodation of endoscopic probes, and mimicking of breast tissue). Contrast-resolution phantoms assess object size resolvability for varying levels of contrast. Some phantoms have limited scan depth (a few centimeters) to test small-parts transducers only. One configuration for endosonography transducers enables the probe to be inserted into a cavity surrounded by TM material. The most commonly used phantoms have multiple applications and are designed for general purpose testing.

To preserve its acoustic properties, the phantom should be maintained at a temperature between 32° F and 150° F in a dark place, preferably in an airtight container to inhibit dehydration. Improved design of water-based gel phantoms now incorporates a polymer material covering the acoustic window to act as a vapor barrier. Proper storage will prolong the useful life of the water-base gel phantom, in some cases to 4 to 8 years. Loss of water content is monitored by periodically weighing the phantom. Manufacturers have programs to replace or regenerate the phantom when water content becomes too low.

Urethane rubber-based phantoms have also been developed to mimic the attenuation and scattering of tissue. However, the velocity in this material is about 1460 m/s. These are more stable and have a longer life than the water-based gel phantoms, but care must be taken when performing distance measurements using rubber-based phantoms. Generally, the object placement in the axial direction within the phantom is closer than the stated value so that an echo-ranging distance measurement using the calibrated velocity of 1540 m/s yields the stated separation of objects. Inaccurate focusing of the ultrasound beam caused by timing-delay errors limits the assessment of axial resolution, lateral resolution, and cyst fill-in.

General-Purpose Phantoms

Two commonly used general-purpose TM phantoms are manufactured by CIRS Inc., Norfolk, Virginia (Model 40) and Gammex-RMI, Middleton, Wisconsin (Model 403 series). Figs. 24-1 and 24-2 illustrate the structures contained within these phantoms. A comparison of the 403 series phantoms indicates that the Model 403GS contains additional gray-scale targets, which are not included in the Model 403. The specifications for these phantoms are listed in Tables 24-1 and 24-2. The Model 40 phantom is divided vertically in half so that one side has an attenuation rate of 0.5 dB cm^{-1} MHz^{-1} and the other side has an attenuation rate of 0.7 dB cm^{-1} MHz^{-1}. The Model 403 is uniform in its attenuation, either 0.5 dB cm^{-1} MHz^{-1} or 0.7 dB cm^{-1} MHz^{-1} selectable at purchase. Since penetration at high frequency has improved dramatically in the past few years, the higher value of 0.7 dB cm^{-1} MHz^{-1} is preferred by these authors for penetration measurements. Extended-field-of-view sonograms of these phantoms are presented in Figs. 24-3 and 24-4.

The phantom properties of velocity, scattering, and attenuation should mimic soft tissue throughout the diagnostic frequency range (2 to 15 MHz). The characteristics of the general-purpose phantoms including urethane-rubber material are listed in Table 24-3. If the attenuation frequency dependence is greater than f^1, then the attenuation would be greater in the phantom than in tissue at high frequency, and penetration depth measurement would be in error. The nonlinear attenuation response at high frequencies is a major disadvantage of the urethane material. However, for routine quality control (QC) testing where consistency is the primary consideration, the stability, ruggedness, ease of transport, and no requirement for a vapor barrier are positive factors. All the materials conform to the recommendation that changes in velocity due to temperature change be less than 3 m s^{-1} °C^{-1}. The effect of temperature on backscatter is negligible. Nevertheless, testing with phantoms should be conducted at or near room temperature.

Phantom Cost

Typically a good TM phantom represents a small addition to the cost of an ultrasound system (1% to 2%). Some phantoms are refillable with a water-alcohol mixture to extend

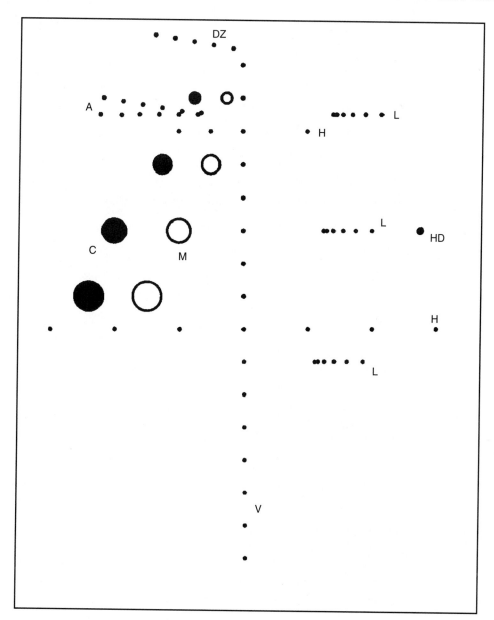

Fig. 24-1 Diagram of the Model 40 tissue-mimicking phantom. Vertical rod group *(V)*, horizontal rod groups *(H)*, dead zone rod group *(DZ)*, axial resolution rod group *(A)*, lateral resolution rod groups *(L)*, simulated cysts *(C)*, simulated solid mass *(M)*, and high density *(HD)* attenuator are indicated.

life. The total cost for a phantom seldom exceeds a very small fraction of the revenue generated by the ultrasound system over the useful life of the scanner. Also, a single phantom can be used to evaluate multiple ultrasound units, which tends to reduce its cost even further.

PERFORMANCE PARAMETERS

Numerous methods using phantoms have been developed to evaluate different aspects of scanner performance. *General-purpose TM phantoms commonly test for dead zone, axial resolution, lateral resolution, penetration, image uniformity, distance accuracy, focal zone, and cyst characteristics (size,*

shape, and fill-in). Other specialty phantoms are designed to assess contrast resolution, slice thickness, and beam width. Fidelity of the display and image recording are also evaluated with TM phantoms in conjunction with gray-scale test patterns. Power, intensity mapping, bandwidth, and echo-response patterns require expensive electronic test equipment and are usually the purview of the manufacturer and independent research laboratories.

TM phantoms are well suited for assessing the focusing of transducers at various depths in systems that have variable focal zones or dynamic focusing. These phantoms are more indicative of clinical performance, because the scattering may change the focal characteristics of a

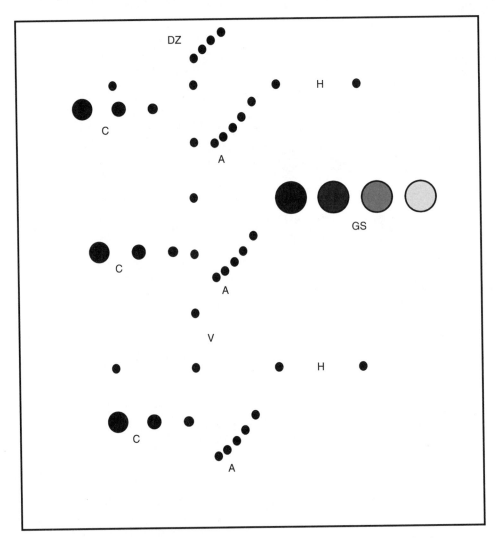

Fig. 24-2 Diagram of the Model 403GS tissue-mimicking phantom. Vertical rod group *(V)*, horizontal rod groups *(H)*, dead zone rod group *(DZ)*, axial resolution rod groups *(A)*, simulated cysts *(C)*, and gray-scale targets *(GS)* are indicated.

transducer from those specified by the manufacturer. The performance parameters evaluated with general purpose phantoms are described.

Dead Zone

The **dead zone** is the distance from the front face of the transducer to the first identifiable echo. No useful scan data are collected in this region. The dead zone is the result of transducer ringing and reverberations from the transducer–phantom (or patient) interface. Impedance matching between the transducer and the pulser/receiver is essential for prevention of electrical ringing (i.e., when part of the excitation pulse is reflected to the pulser). The transducer dead zone occurs because the system cannot send and receive at the same time. Thus performance is instrument dependent. As frequency is increased, the depth of the dead zone decreases provided that all other factors remain constant. The acoustic output also influences the depth of the dead zone.

Axial Resolution

Axial resolution describes the ability of an ultrasound system to resolve two closely spaced objects along the axis of the beam. It also determines the smallest resolvable object along the beam axis. The axial resolution is influenced by pulse length. A shorter pulse length improves the resolution.

Lateral Resolution

Lateral resolution is the ability to distinguish two objects adjacent to each other in the direction perpendicular to the beam axis within the scan plane. Decreasing the beam width improves the lateral resolution. A single object smaller than the ultrasound beam produces scattered echoes when intercepted by the beam; thus the object appears to be the same size as the width of the beam. A small beam width with high scan-line density enables small objects to become distinguishable.

■ **Table 24-1** Specifications of the CIRS Model 40 TM Phantom

Objects	Description	Specification
Near field group	Number of rods	5
	Depth range	1-5 mm
	Vertical spacing	1 mm
Vertical group	Number of rods	15
	Depth range	1-16 cm
	Vertical spacing	10 mm
Horizontal groups	Number of groups	2
	Depth of each group	3 cm and 9 cm
	Number of rods	4 and 7
	Horizontal spacing	10 mm and 20 mm
Axial resolution group	Depth	2.5 cm
	Number of rods	12
	Axial separation between rods	5, 4, 3, 2, 1, 0.5 mm
Lateral resolution group	Number of groups	3
	Depth of each group	2.5 cm, 6 cm, 10 cm
	Number of rods	6
	Horizontal spacing	5, 4, 3, 2, 1 mm
Simulated cysts	Number of cysts	4
	Attenuation coefficient	0.07 dB/cm/MHz
	Diameter	2 mm, 4 mm, 6 mm, 8 mm
	Depth	2 cm, 4 cm, 6 cm, 8 cm
High contrast masses	Number of masses	4
	Attenuation coefficient	1.23 dB/cm/MHz
	Diameter	2 mm, 4 mm, 6 mm, 8 mm
	Depth	2 cm, 4 cm, 6 cm, 8 cm
High density target	Material	Acrylic
	Diameter	1/16-in
	Depth	6 cm

■ **Table 24-2** Specifications of the Gammex-RMI Model 403GS TM Phantom

Objects	Description	Specification
Dead zone group	Number of rods	4
	Depth range	1-10 mm
	Vertical spacing	3 mm
Vertical group	Number of rods	9
	Depth range	1-16 cm
	Vertical spacing	10 mm and 20 mm
Horizontal groups	Number of groups	2
	Depth of each group	2 cm and 12 cm
	Number of rods	4
	Horizontal spacing	30 mm
Axial resolution groups	Number of groups	3
	Depth	3 cm, 8 cm, 14 cm
	Number of rods per group	5
	Axial separation between rods	2, 1, 0.5, 0.25 mm
Simulated cysts	Number of cyst groups	3
	Attenuation coefficient	0.05 dB/cm/MHz
	Diameter	2 mm, 4 mm, 6 mm
	Depth	3 cm, 8 cm, 12 cm
Gray-scale targets	Diameter	10 mm
	Depth	6 cm
	Backscatter	12 dB, 6 dB, –6 dB, anechoic

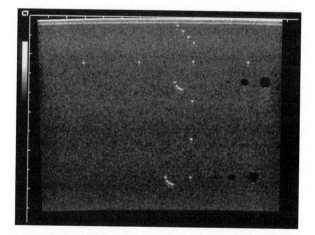

Fig. 24-4 Extended-field-of-view sonogram of the Model 403 tissue-mimicking phantom. The width of the field of view was 12 cm, and the scan depth was 10 cm. The center frequency was 6 MHz.

Distance Measurement

To facilitate the measurement of distance, area, and volume, most ultrasound systems are equipped with distance indicators, cursors, or both. Timing marks are usually superimposed on the image, which must be properly calibrated to provide accurate values. The distance measurements should be performed both near and far from the face of the

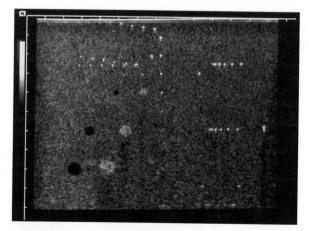

Fig. 24-3 Extended-field-of-view sonogram of the Model 40 tissue-mimicking phantom. The width of the field of view was 12 cm, and the scan depth was 10 cm. The center frequency was 6 MHz.

■ **Table 24-3** Acoustic Properties of Phantoms

Parameter	CIRS Model 40	Gammex-RMI Model 403GS	Urethane
Velocity (m/s)	1540	1540	1460
Velocity (m/s) versus f	±3	±3	±3
Velocity (m s^{-1} °C^{-1}) versus temperature	2	1.5	−2.5
Attenuation (dB cm^{-1} mHz^{-1})	0.5 and 0.7	0.5 or 0.7	0.5 or 0.7
Attenuation (dB cm^{-1} mHz^{-1}) versus f	f$^{1.3}$	f$^{1.1}$	f$^{1.8}$
Attenuation (dB cm^{-1} mHz^{-1}) versus temperature	Constant	−0.02	−0.02
Backscatter versus temperature	Constant	Constant	Constant

transducer. The total distance defined by the cursors should also be varied to check linearity.

Vertical distance is measured along the axis of the beam. The location of an acoustic interface with respect to the face of the transducer can be determined if the velocity of ultrasound in the medium and the time of flight of the ultrasonic pulse are known. In practice, the velocity of ultrasound in the phantom or patient is assumed to be constant (1540 m/s). The elapsed time between the transmitted pulse and the returning echo is measured, which permits the calculation of the distance to the interface.

Horizontal distance is measured perpendicular to the axis of the beam. The scanning mechanism determines placement of each line of sight, which in turn governs the horizontal mapping of the detected signals.

Focal Zone

The maximum intensity and narrowest beam width occur at the focal point of the transducer. The **focal zone** is the region surrounding the focal point in which the intensity is within 3 dB of maximum. This is also the region of the best lateral resolution.

Sensitivity

Sensitivity refers to the ability of the scanning system to detect weak echoes from small scatterers located at specified depths in an attenuating medium. The weak signal is detected in the presence of noise, which is indicative of the system signal-to-noise ratio (SNR). Factors that influence the strength of the detected signal include power level, gain, TGC, degree of focusing, attenuation by the medium, distance to the reflector, composition of the interface, and geometry of the reflector. The SNR is maximal within the focal zone and decreases on each side. Typically, sensitivity is related to maximum penetration of the ultrasound beam under specified conditions.

Uniformity

Ideally, a scan of a uniform object should produce an image with a consistent speckle pattern and uniform brightness throughout the field of view. This is not achieved in practice because of imprecise attenuation compensation and altered beam intensity by focusing. Nevertheless, the brightness

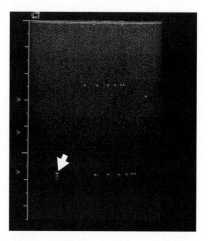

Fig. 24-5 Comet tail *(arrow)* artifact from the high-density target in the Model 40 phantom.

level at a specific depth should appear unvarying. Image nonuniformities mask subtle variations in tissue texture and increase the risk of false-negatives.

Simulated Cysts and Masses

Cysts are fluid-filled structures that are hypoechoic and usually weakly attenuating. They also have slower velocities than the surrounding tissue. The acoustic image has a distinctive pattern that should represent the size, shape, and consistency of the cyst. A nonuniform echo pattern across the cyst is referred to as cyst fill-in. Changes in output and TGC can affect cyst fill-in. Because the reflector surface is curved, fill-in is expected to occur more readily outside the focal zone, where the beam width is greater. Multiple reflections may alter cyst shape and fill-in. When a cyst is scanned with few lines of sight, a smooth border is misrepresented as an irregular border.

Solid structures consisting of strong reflectors are incorporated in some phantoms for checking size, shape, and shadowing.

High-Density Target

Small-diameter, high-density acrylic target in the Model 40 phantom mimics calcified stones and can produce shadowing and comet tail artifact (Fig. 24-5).

PERFORMANCE TESTS

A well-designed TM phantom allows the use of clinically appropriate scanner settings during testing. Dynamic range, gray-scale map, power level, gain, and TGC should be recorded for each combination of transducer and performance test. Depth of scanning and focal zone settings are adjusted as needed. In this section each parameter will be discussed individually—including its description, the reasons for testing it, the scanning and measurement procedures, and its performance limits. Although these parameters are all treated as separate scan procedures, multiple parameters can be evaluated from one image for real-time imaging systems.

Dead Zone

Description. The dead zone corresponds to the region of material adjoining the transducer in which no useful information is collected, in part because of the pulse length (transducer ringing) and reverberations from the transducer–test object (or patient) interface. The dead zone is visualized by scanning the region near the TM phantom surface. The tissue scatter from parenchyma (particle scattering) is not present in the dead zone. Beyond the dead zone, the tissue texture pattern, similar to liver parenchyma, is observed.

Reasons for Testing. A shift in the depth of the transducer dead zone reflects changes in the transducer or pulsing system, or both. Specifically, an elongated pulse caused by a cracked crystal, a loose backing or facing material, a broken lens, or a longer excitation pulse deepens the dead zone. Artifacts in the dead zone may be indicative of input power fluctuations.

Scanning Procedure. Coupling gel is used to place the transducer in contact with the scanning surface of the TM phantom. Extra gel may be required when a mechanical sector transducer is tested. The instrument settings (e.g., gain, TGC, power) are adjusted to the established baseline values (commonly a normal liver or breast technique). A scan of the rods in the dead zone target group near the top of the phantom is then performed. For the Model 403GS phantom, the rods are spaced 3 mm apart vertically and horizontally. For the Model 40 phantom, the rods are spaced 1 mm apart vertically and horizontally.

Measurement Procedure. The depth of the rod that can be visualized closest to the surface or the depth at which "normal tissue texture" begins to be seen indicates the axial extent of the dead zone (Fig. 24-6). Electronic calipers or other distance indicators (marker dots) are used to quantify the depth of the dead zone.

Performance Limits. In recent years improvements in transducer design have reduced the extent of the dead zone compared with past performance (Fig. 24-7). Note that the modern transducer used in Fig. 24-6 was operated at lower frequency and had a smaller dead zone than could be achieved by the older transducer that acquired the image in Fig. 24-7. Guidelines for dead-zone depth with respect to frequency are listed in Table 24-4. If the depth of the dead zone exceeds the guideline value, an attempt should be

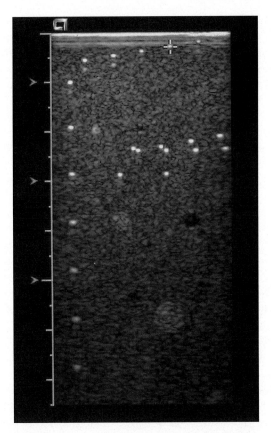

Fig. 24-6 Dead zone measurement with a Model 40 phantom. The distance from the face of the transducer to the beginning of the tissue-texture pattern is 2 mm *(cursor)*. Linear array transducer operating at 5 MHz.

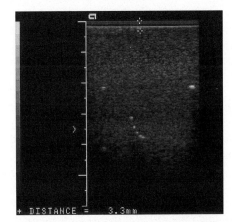

Fig. 24-7 Dead zone measurement with a Model 403 phantom for a transducer manufactured in 1993. The distance from the face of the transducer to the beginning of the tissue-texture pattern is 3.3 mm *(cursors)*. Linear array transducer operating at 7 MHz.

■ **Table 24-4** Performance Criteria for Dead Zone Measurements

Frequency (MHz)	Depth of Dead Zone (mm)
<3	<7 mm
3-7	<5 mm
≥7	<3 mm

made to correct the problem. Unfortunately, some units have dead zones in excess of 7 mm, which cannot be corrected. This poses difficulties when scanning shallow structures, as with neonatal patients. Special bolus material (similar to that used in radiation therapy) with appropriate coupling gel may enable the operator to position the structure of interest outside the dead zone. A water-filled balloon with appropriate coupling is also useful for this purpose. Careful consideration must be given to distance measurements in this case.

Vertical Distance Measurement

Description. Scanning equally spaced vertical rods provides a check of the vertical distance indicators. The separation between rods corresponds to a well-defined distance of 1 or 2 cm. If the distance indicators and the rod image separations do not correspond, either the instrument calibration is incorrect or the velocity of sound in the phantom is not equal to the value assumed for distance measurements in the equipment (1540 m/s).

Reasons for Testing. A major application of ultrasound scanning involves the measurement of length, area, or volume. Most ultrasound units employ depth markers to delineate distance on the monitor or hard copy image. The proper diagnosis depends on the accurate representation of geometric relationships. Accuracy is checked by comparing distance indicators (markers or cursors) with the known separation between rods in the phantom. Improper velocity calibration causes the scanner to fail this test.

Scanning Procedure. The transducer is positioned over the vertical set of rods in the TM phantom, and scan data are acquired. Timing or depth markers are placed vertically near the imaged rods. Electronic calipers, if available, should be used to measure the separation between rods in the image. Pressing down on the phantom with the transducer while acquiring the image may displace the rods and cause an error in the distance measurement. Scanning should be performed by applying as little pressure as possible to the acoustic window membrane. Water in a trough can also be used as a coupling medium.

Measurement Procedure. Assessment of vertical distance accuracy involves comparing the known distance between rods with the distance indicated by the timing markers, electronic calipers, or both. The image is analyzed by determining the distance between rods located near the face of the transducer, the distance between rods located far from the face of the transducer, and the distance between rods located at the extremes of the scanning depth (Fig. 24-8). The latter measurement is most likely to identify vertical depth miscalibration, because errors are compounded with longer distances. Some sector scanners have distance markers on the outside edges of the sector image with no other indicators available. Hand-held calipers must be used for distance measurements within the image on the monitor. They are also required for distance measurements on the hard copy image.

Performance Limits. The vertical distance indicators should be accurate to within 2% of the actual distance or

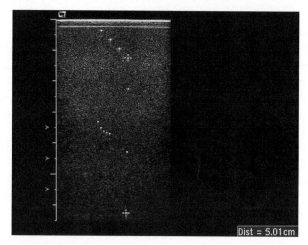

Fig. 24-8 Check of vertical distance accuracy. Measurement when the separation includes several rods in a Model 403 phantom over the scanning range. For a known distance of 50 mm, the measured separation is 50 mm. Linear array transducer operating at 6 MHz.

2 mm, whichever is less restrictive. Any discrepancy greater than this value is the result of either machine error or the fact that the velocity of ultrasound in the phantom is not equal to that in soft tissue. A second phantom is helpful in determining the source of the problem. If the distance measurements are erroneous for both phantoms, the ultrasound unit is likely at fault. If the distance measurements for only one phantom are erroneous, the phantom is probably at fault. A second ultrasound unit can be tested if only one phantom is available. If both units demonstrate similar behavior, the phantom is most likely at fault.

Some ultrasound units incorporate an electronic grid that can be superimposed on the image display. The grid pattern represents a fixed spatial relationship. The separations between rods should correspond within 2 or 3 mm to the grid lines. If they do not, the velocity of sound in the phantom is different from the assumed value of 1540 m/s.

Horizontal Distance Measurement

Description. Horizontal distance is measured perpendicularly to the beam axis within the scan plane.

Reasons for Testing. The ultrasound image is a composite of many lines of sight, each scan line representing the depth information gathered along the axis of the beam. The two-dimensional image, however, also provides spatial relationships perpendicular to the beam axis. Often information regarding the size of an object in the horizontal direction is desirable. This spatial representation depends on the number of lines of sight, output intensity, resolution of the scan converter (pixel size), resolution of the display, and beam width (lateral resolution). Changes in beam formation by a defective transducer (broken crystal, housing integrity, or scan mechanism) usually cause the scanner to fail this test. Mechanical sector and annular array transducers are particularly susceptible to loss of horizontal distance accuracy caused by motor wear.

Scanning Procedure. A scan of the horizontal rods is performed. Depth markers are placed horizontally near the imaged rods. Electronic calipers, if available, should be used to measure the separation between rods in the image.

Measurement Procedure. The distance markers are compared with the rod echo positions in a manner similar to the vertical measurement procedure discussed in the previous section (Fig. 24-9).

Performance Limits. The horizontal distance indicators should also be accurate to within 3% or 3 mm, whichever is less restrictive.

Lateral Resolution

Description. The lateral resolution, which depends on beam width, is evaluated by scanning closely spaced rods oriented horizontally. The lateral resolution is expressed as the smallest distance between any two resolvable rods at a particular depth.

Reasons for Testing. The lateral resolution of ultrasound systems depends on the beam width, the number of scan lines (lines of sight) in the image, the resolution of the scan converter and display, and the reflection and scattering properties of the medium. The beam width is transducer dependent and is affected by the distance from the transducer, the geometric shape of the piezoelectric material, and the degree of focusing. As the focusing is made weaker (provided that other factors remain constant), the beam width in the focal zone becomes larger. Circular transducer elements produce beams that are cylindrical, whereas rectangular elements (e.g., those used in linear and linear phased arrays) produce elliptical cross-sectional beams. In the latter case, beam width is not constant for the in-plane and out-of-plane directions. High-frequency transducers have an extended near field and a less divergent far field. Lateral resolution is altered by loss of transducer elements or problems with the beam former.

Scanning Procedure. A scan of the lateral resolution group or groups is obtained. In the Model 40 phantom a

lateral resolution group is located at depths of 2.5 cm, 6 cm, and 10 cm. This placement allows assessment of the lateral resolution for different focal zones and transmission frequencies. For transducers with fixed focus, lateral resolution can be determined within or very near the focal zone by selecting the appropriate group. If variable transmit focusing is available, then the focal zone can be selected to correspond with a particular lateral resolution group (Figs. 24-10 and 24-11). Switching to a higher-frequency transducer generally improves the lateral resolution.

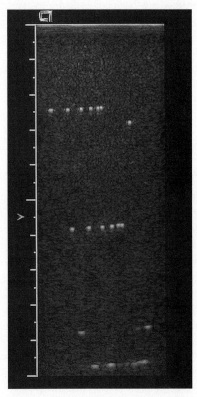

Fig. 24-10 Effect of placement of a single transmit focal zone on lateral resolution for a linear phased array transducer. The lateral resolution within the single focal zone at a depth of 6 cm is 2 mm. The lateral resolution deteriorates markedly when the focal zone is displaced from the region of interest. At a depth of 10 cm, the lateral resolution rod group is blurred. The center frequency is 4 MHz.

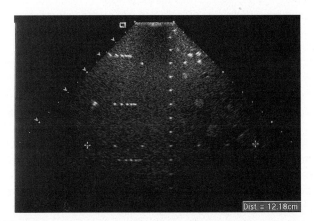

Fig. 24-9 Check of horizontal distance accuracy. Measurement when the separation includes horizontal rods in a Model 40 phantom at a scan depth of 9 cm. For a known distance of 120 mm, the measured separation is 122 mm. Linear phased array transducer operating at 4 MHz.

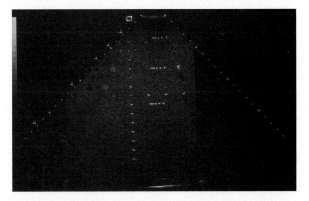

Fig. 24-11 Effect of multiple transmit focal zones on lateral resolution for a linear phased array transducer. The lateral resolution is improved throughout the field of view by applying multiple transmit focal zones. The center frequency is 4 MHz.

For those phantoms that do not contain lateral resolution rod groups, lateral resolution can be assessed by scanning the vertical rod group. The horizontal extent of the image of the rod varies with beam width.

Measurement Procedure. The rods in a rod group are spaced 5, 4, 3, 2, and 1 mm apart. Lateral resolution is determined by the smallest distance between any two separable rods. A linear transducer acquired the image in Fig. 24-10. The lateral resolution is 1 mm at a depth of 5 cm. In the alternative method the width of the rods at different depths encompassing the focal zone are measured.

Performance Limits. The lateral resolution should be within manufacturer specifications. Typical values range from 0.5 to 5 mm for the B-mode scanners, depending on the degree of focusing, frequency, and the depth of measurement. Guidelines for lateral resolution measurements are listed in Table 24-5. Lateral resolution should not vary from week to week by more than 1 mm when the TM phantom is used.

Focal Zone

Description. The beam pattern (i.e., the beam width at various depths) is obtained by scanning equally spaced vertical rods. An object produces a signal on the display the entire time it is intercepted by the beam. The rod appears as a line on the display rather than a dot. The length of the line is equivalent to the width of the beam at the depth of the rod. The beam pattern generated by scanning a set of rods at various depths permits measurements to be made of the beam width as a function of distance from the transducer (Fig. 24-12). This method also provides a means of visualizing the focal zone or zones of the transducer. The beam width is the major factor limiting the lateral resolution of an ultrasonic image.

Reasons for Testing. Ultrasound can be focused either electronically or internally with lenses or curved crystals to reduce the beam width and improve lateral resolution at a certain depth. The manufacturer specifies the location of the focal zone of the transducer. When scanning a patient, it is important that the focal zone coincide with the depth of interest. Therefore the specified location of the focal zone must be verified. Any variation in output (caused by broken lenses or crystals or by loose facing or backing material) will distort the focal zone. Because lateral resolution depends on beam width, any changes in the focal zone should be detected when they occur. Variable and dynamically focused transducers must be checked so the focal zone sweeps throughout the indicated range. The location of the

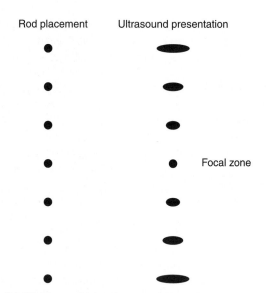

Fig. 24-12 The vertical rod group within a TM phantom when scanned yields an image of the rods with variable width. The minimum width of the imaged rod indicates the focal zone.

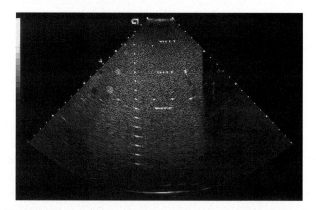

Fig. 24-13 Sonogram of the vertical rod group within the TM phantom using a single focal zone. The vertical rods within the focal zone are depicted with a narrower width than the rods located above or below this region. Linear phased array operating at 4 MHz.

focal zone can be changed by the properties of the reflective medium, which is outside the control of the sonographer.

Scanning Procedure. A scan of the vertical rods in the phantom is performed.

Measurement Procedure. Any small object creates an echo the entire time it is intercepted by the beam. A line rather than a dot is produced on the display. The length of the line is indicative of the width of the beam, but it also varies with output and gain settings. The shape of the images of the rods determines the depth of the focal zone. Rods inside the focal zone form a shorter line than the rods above or below the focal zone (Fig. 24-13). For a variable focused transducer, scans with several different focal zone settings should be performed. Fig. 24-14 is a scan obtained with a transducer in which five focal zones were selected. Units that employ dynamic receive focusing may not show a variable width of the rods on the display, but a change in intensity can be observed when the transmit focus of these transducers is adjusted.

■ **Table 24-5** Performance Criteria for Lateral Resolution Measurements

Depth (cm)	Frequency (MHz)	Lateral Resolution (mm)
>10	<3.5	<4
<10	3.5-5	<3
<10	≥5	<1.5

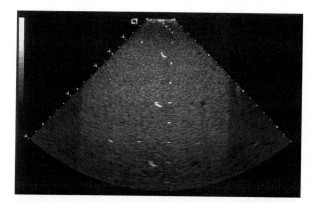

Fig. 24-14 Sonogram of the vertical rod group within a TM phantom using multiple focal zones. This narrows the beam width throughout the region of the focal zones. Note the lateral extent of the vertical rods throughout the entire scan range. Linear phased array operating at 4 MHz.

Performance Limits. The location of the focal zone should agree with the manufacturer's specifications and should not change with time. Typically, the depth of the focal zone is indicated by labeling for mechanical-sector, fixed-focused transducers. Units employing dynamic receive focusing produce very narrow beam widths over a broad range of depths.

Axial Resolution

Description. The axial resolution depends on pulse length, which in turn depends on the frequency bandwidth. If the integrity of the transducer is altered (cracked crystal, loose facing material, or loose backing material), a change in the pulse length, and hence a degradation in resolution, will result. Loss of transducer integrity may produce additional side lobes, which create image artifacts and influence the resolution.

Axial resolution is evaluated by scanning closely spaced rods oriented vertically. To prevent shadowing from the rods above, they are situated at a 15-degree angle or offset in the horizontal direction. The smallest distance between any two rods in the group that can be differentiated yields the axial resolution. The pulse length (and therefore the axial resolution) also depends on gain, power, and transducer frequency. These parameters should be recorded when axial resolution measurements are made.

A problem with a single set of resolution rods is that the axial resolution is measured at only one depth, which presents difficulties in evaluating focused transducers. The highest sensitivity of a focused transducer is in the focal zone. The position of the rods in the phantom may not correspond to the focal zone, and thus the decreased sensitivity may alter the axial resolution (strong shadowing within the focal zone deteriorates the axial resolution). When the phantom is used primarily for consistency checks, the single-resolution depth is satisfactory.

Reasons for Testing. Image quality is very dependent on the axial resolution. Damaged transducers (e.g., broken crystals, loose facing or backing material, broken electrical

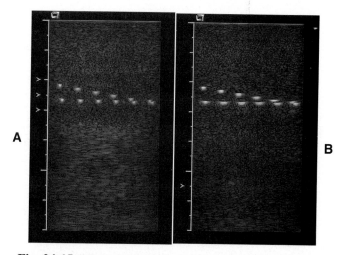

Fig. 24-15 Effect of placement of transmit focal zone on axial resolution for a linear phased array transducer using the Model 40 phantom. The center frequency is 4 MHz. **A,** Transmit focal zone at a depth of 2 to 3 cm corresponding to the location of the axial resolution rod group. **B,** Transmit focal zone at a depth of 6.5 cm. Axial resolution group is located outside the focal zone.

connections) degrade the axial resolution, because these conditions elongate the pulse length. The pulser characteristics may change, which also influences the pulse length.

Scanning Procedure. Most TM phantoms allow testing of axial resolution at several depths (e.g., the Model 403GS phantom contains the axial resolution rod groups at three depths: 3, 8, and 14 cm). The Model 40 has a single axial resolution group at a depth of 2.5 cm. The rods are offset horizontally from one another to prevent shadowing from overlying rods. Axial resolution is influenced by the beam intensity and consequently varies, depending on whether the point of measurement lies within the focal zone.

Measurement Procedure. The axial resolution is determined by measuring the smallest distance between any two rods that can be visualized as separate entities (i.e., a gap between rods). The spacing of the rods for the Model 403GS phantom is 2, 1, 0.5, and 0.25 mm and for the Model 40 phantom is 5, 4, 3, 2, 1, and 0.5 mm. Fig. 24-15 shows a scan obtained with a linear array transducer that has a resolution of 1 mm. The assessment of axial resolution should be repeated if a focused transducer has variable focal zone settings. Fig. 24-16 illustrates the axial resolution at various depths for a transducer with multiple transmit focal zones and with dynamic receive focusing. For this transducer, the axial resolution is uniform at all measured depths. Switching to a high-frequency transducer improves axial resolution (Fig. 24-17).

Performance Limits. The axial resolution should be within the manufacturer's specifications. Typical values range from 0.5 to 2 mm. The consistency from week to week should not vary by more than 1 mm for the same instrument settings.

Sensitivity

Description. The sensitivity can be checked by measuring the depth of the tissue texture pattern. Reduced

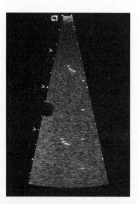

Fig. 24-16 Axial resolution for a linear phased array transducer with multiple focal zones using the Model 403 phantom. The center frequency is 4 MHz. Write zoom was applied to narrow the width of the field of view to emphasize the resolution rod groups. Good axial resolution is maintained throughout the scan range of 11 cm.

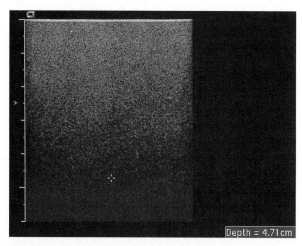

Fig. 24-18 Sensitivity testing using the Model 40 phantom. The fading of parenchyma scatterers indicates the maximum depth of penetration of 4.7 cm at a frequency of 8 MHz.

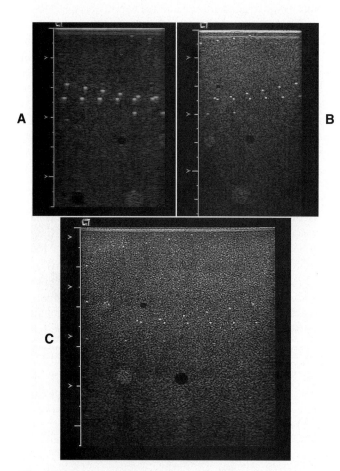

Fig. 24-17 Axial resolution measured by a Model 40 phantom is improved by increasing the frequency. **A,** The axial resolution is 1 mm for a frequency of 4 MHz. **B,** The axial resolution is 0.5 mm for a frequency of 6 MHz. **C,** The axial resolution is less than 0.5 mm for a frequency of 14 MHz.

sensitivity decreases the depth at which this pattern can be seen. A general-purpose TM phantom relatively free of embedded objects throughout the field of view is highly desirable for this test. For example, the Model 403 phantom without the gray-scale objects offers this advantage compared with the Model 403GS phantom.

Reasons for Testing. The inability to detect weak echoes restricts the tissue volume that is probed. In addition, the internal detail of organs produced by weak echoes from nonspecular reflections is degraded with a loss in sensitivity. Variations of output intensity or receiver gain and loss of transducer integrity can cause the scanner to fail this test.

Scanning Procedure. The transducer is coupled to the scanning surface of the TM phantom. Instrument settings are adjusted to a "normal" body part technique for the transducer (e.g., liver or breast), and a scan of a relatively uniform section of the phantom (free of objects such as cysts and masses) is performed. Gain and output power set at maximum with reject off is useful in testing sensitivity. This enables any changes in penetration to be more easily detected.

Measurement Procedure. The loss of the scattered echoes within the TM phantom indicates the depth of penetration. The maximum depth at which parenchyma scatterers are visualized for a well-defined scanning technique is measured. Fig. 24-18 illustrates sensitivity testing using the TM phantom. A major criticism of this test is that the determination of the **maximum depth of visualization** is subjective. The judgment of penetration becomes easier by scanning a phantom containing multiple, randomly distributed, small diameter (1 to 5 mm), hypoechoic, spherically shaped objects (Fig. 24-19). The latter technique is dependent on the beam width and thus the focusing characteristics of the transducer. This method tends to underestimate the maximum depth of penetration compared with that measured by signal loss from parenchymal scatterers.

Performance Limits. The maximum depth of visualization of parenchyma echoes is affected by transducer

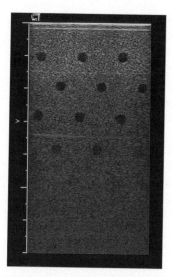

Fig. 24-19 Maximum depth of penetration is 4.5 cm at a frequency of 5 MHz using a CIRS Model 44 tissue-mimicking phantom with low scatter, spherical objects.

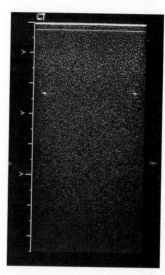

Fig. 24-20 Uniformity testing using the Model 403 phantom. At each depth the brightness is relatively constant across the field of view. Linear array transducer operating at 6 MHz.

frequency and power. Because consistency is important, any variation in sensitivity should be noted. The depth of penetration for a particular transducer should not shift by more than 1 cm for identical settings.

Uniformity

Description. Uniformity refers to the ability of the ultrasound system to display echoes of equal magnitude with the same brightness on the monitor. The test for uniformity consists of examining all regions throughout the tissue texture pattern for areas that are not displayed with equal intensity. Because TGC modifies the amplitude of the received signal, the brightness levels must be compared at the same depth. This is an excellent means of checking long-term reproducibility.

Reasons for Testing. Testing for uniformity ensures that all lines of sight of a scanner contribute equally to the image. Nonuniformity may be caused by hardware malfunctions such as bad transducer elements or poor electrical connections. Failures in image-processing hardware and software can change the uniformity of the signals from equal reflectors at the same depth.

Scanning Procedure. The scanning procedure is the same as the procedure described for sensitivity. However, images should be obtained with single and multiple focal zones.

Measurement Procedure. The tissue texture pattern of the TM phantom should be uniform in intensity at a particular depth of penetration (Fig. 24-20). Curvilinear and sector transducers do not produce a uniform pattern where the transducer is in poor contact with the phantom (Fig. 24-21). To evaluate the entire length of the radiating surface, the transducer must be rotated back and forth to establish good contact with the phantom.

Occasionally, defective scan lines are readily apparent from the clinical images (Fig. 24-22). More often, the loss

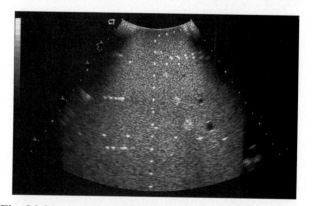

Fig. 24-21 Curvilinear transducer coupled to a tissue-mimicking phantom. Nonuniformity occurs at the periphery of the field of view because of poor contact of the phantom with the scan head.

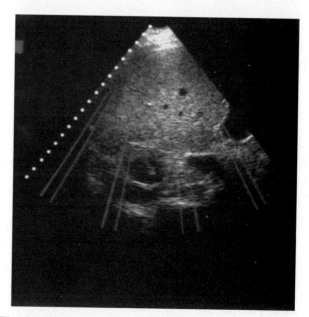

Fig. 24-22 Defective scan lines are present in this sonogram of the abdomen.

of information along scan lines is more subtle and difficult to recognize as the cause of poor image quality. An alternative test method can easily identify defective scan lines. The edge of the coin is coupled to the transducer with acoustic gel and then moved across the transducer face. Regions with decreased signal amplitude correspond to improper sampling along those lines of sight (Fig. 24-23). The lack of signal along these scan lines is very likely caused by a loss of electrical connection with the transducer elements.

Performance Limits. This is a qualitative measurement, which is difficult to assess with any numerical limits. Fig. 24-24 is a scan obtained with a linear phased array that demonstrates poor uniformity. This transducer required replacement.

Cyst Size, Shape, and Fill-in

Description. Often, cylinders, cones, or spheres of varying size are incorporated within the tissue matrix. These structures are weak reflectors compared with the background gel and usually appear anechoic. The simulated cysts

are evaluated for size, fill-in caused by overcompensation or undercompensation of gain or TGC, accuracy of shape, and enhancement distal to the simulated cyst.

Reasons for Testing. The scanner should be able to differentiate between cystic and solid structures. Contrast resolution characterizes a scanner's ability to distinguish structures with similar reflection and attenuation properties. For the purpose of evaluating contrast resolution, some TM phantoms have multiple sets of simulated cysts in the form of solid cylinders with different diameters placed at varying depths. The ultrasound system should reproduce the size and shape of the simulated cyst without fill-in. Enhancement behind the solid cylinders can be characterized using different TGC and output settings. The size of the observed simulated cyst also provides an indicator of spatial resolution.

Scanning Procedure. An image of the simulated cysts is obtained by scanning the TM phantom. Some ultrasound units are limited in their depth of penetration and may not be able to image deep-lying structures. Often, bright spots occur at the top and bottom of the anechoic objects (Fig. 24-25). These are normal specular reflections from the simulated cyst/tissue interface.

Measurement Procedure. The size of each displayed simulated cyst is measured in both vertical and horizontal directions by means of electronic calipers, distance indicators, or both. The shape of each simulated cyst and the brightness throughout the structure are noted (Figs. 24-26 and 24-27). Enhancement behind the structures is also examined.

Performance Limits. The measured size of each simulated cyst should be within 1 mm of the actual size. The geometric shape of the solid cylinders should be circular, but often linear array transducers and systems with limited numbers of pixels or lines of sight tend to square the edges of the simulated cysts. This may not be correctable. The cysts should be of uniform brightness with normal scan settings. The effects of TGC and output on fill-in and

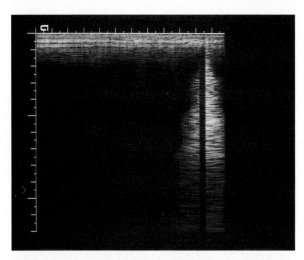

Fig. 24-23 Defective scan lines present in a linear array transducer. The image was acquired as a coin, oriented edge on, was moved across the radiating surface.

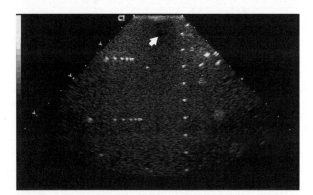

Fig. 24-24 Example of poor uniformity for a linear phased array transducer. Note the nonuniform presentation near the transducer in the central field of view *(arrow)*. Moving the transducer to other areas of the phantom yielded the same result (eliminated the phantom as the cause of the poor uniformity).

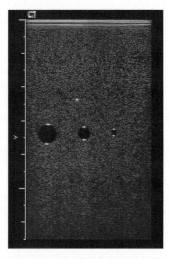

Fig. 24-25 The sonogram of simulated cysts often shows bright areas at the boundary caused by specular reflections from the cyst/tissue interface.

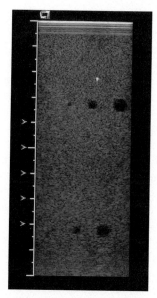

Fig. 24-26 Evaluation of cyst size, shape, and fill-in using a tissue-mimicking phantom. Three simulated cysts at a depth of 3 cm and two simulated cysts at a depth of 8 cm are seen. Fill-in is observed for the simulated cysts located at the deeper depth (displaced from the mechanical focal depth).

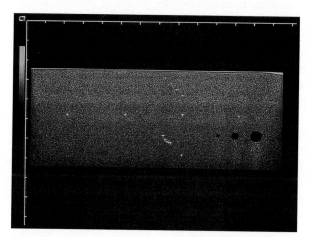

Fig. 24-27 Extended-field-of-view sonogram of the Model 403 phantom. All three simulated cysts at a depth of 3 cm are resolved. Enhancement distal to the simulated cysts is present.

enhancement behind the simulated cysts should be compared with the baseline results. Refraction defocusing artifact may be observed at the edge of the simulated cyst.

Solid Mass Size, Shape, and Shadowing

Description. Some TM phantoms (e.g., Model 40) have cylindrical structures that mimic solid tumors. These are normally more attenuating and produce more internal echoes than soft tissue does. The velocity of ultrasound is also usually faster in these structures than in normal tissues. Refraction defocusing artifact may be seen at the edges of the simulated mass.

Reasons for Testing. The scanner should be able to differentiate between solid masses and normal tissue structures. The correct size and shape of the mass should be

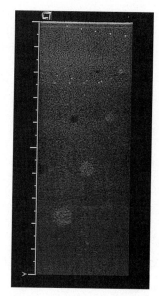

Fig. 24-28 Evaluation of mass size and shape plus shadowing behind the mass using the Model 40 phantom. Four high-contrast masses with respective diameters of 2 mm, 4 mm, 6 mm, and 8 mm are seen.

reproduced. Shadowing behind the simulated solid mass can be characterized.

Scanning Procedure. An image of the simulated solid masses is obtained by scanning from the top of the TM phantom.

Measurement Procedure. The size of each observed simulated mass should be measured in both the vertical and horizontal directions using electronic calipers or distance markers. The shape of the structures should be round with uniform brightness (Fig. 24-28). The shadowing beyond the simulated masses should be noted.

Performance Limits. The measured size of each simulated mass should be within 1 mm of the actual size. The simulated mass should appear round with uniform brightness.

EVALUATION OF CLINICAL IMAGE QUALITY

An impression of degraded image quality is difficult to assess by viewing clinical sonograms only. Testing with TM phantoms often identifies improper scanner operation. A general complaint of poor image quality from one real-time unit was rectified by a scan of the phantom, which demonstrated that a curvilinear array transducer was defective (Fig. 24-29). The one-to-one correspondence between scanned subject and the image was corrupted. Whereas anatomic structures in sonograms were blurred and indistinct, the multiple replications of a single rod set in the image of the TM phantom was immediately apparent.

HARD COPY IMAGE RECORDING

The end product of an ultrasonic scan is typically a high-quality photographic reproduction of the display—a hard

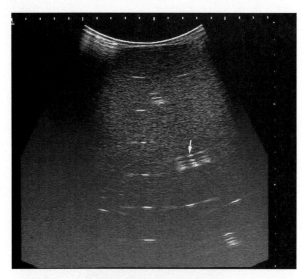

Fig. 24-29 Sonogram of a tissue-mimicking phantom with a defective curvilinear array transducer. The axial resolution rod set at a depth of 8 cm is recorded at three different locations in the image *(arrow)*.

copy visual representation of the interactions of ultrasound with tissue. The multiformat camera and laser camera both use transparency film as the recording medium. Transparency film exhibits a wide range of optical densities that are perceived as separate shades of gray. The image recorded on film must be a faithful reproduction of the image viewed on the display monitor. Gray levels must extend from black to white with multiple intermediate shades. Hard copy image quality depends on the matched response between display monitor and image-recording device as well as on proper film processing.

Photographic recording has a major impact on the quality of the final image. The fidelity of any recording with respect to resolution, distortion, and contrast is checked by comparing the display with the final hard copy image.

The photographic system should duplicate the structural detail of the displayed image. The display monitor and processed film must have the potential to exhibit a full range of shades from black to white. Also, gray-level variations on the display monitor must be reproduced on the film. Distortion should be minimal. A potential problem is a lesion observed on the video monitor that is not present on the hard copy image. This makes the diagnosis difficult to document. Often measurements are obtained by the physician from the film rather than from the displayed image. Hard copy images derived from testing also provide documentation of properly functioning equipment.

Proper adjustment of the display monitor does not ensure similar gray-scale presentation by the processed film. The image-recording device is not controlled by manipulation of the display monitor. The translation of input signals to optical density by the hard copy camera must be regulated independently via the controls of contrast, brightness, exposure time, and/or gray-scale map.

Manufacturers have incorporated various test patterns in ultrasound scanners to aid in the setup and QC of display

monitors and hard copy cameras. These test patterns usually include a gray-scale image in a set of 16 or more bars of varying brightness levels and a grid of equally spaced parallel horizontal and vertical lines. The gray scale represents the entire dynamic range of potential signal levels. The grid allows an assessment of spatial distortion.

SMPTE Test Pattern

The Society of Motion Picture and Television Engineers (SMPTE) has developed a test pattern for use in the setup, acceptance testing, and QC of display monitors and hard copy cameras. It can be generated as an analog video signal or provided in digital form.

Fig. 24-30 shows the SMPTE test pattern. Note that the background is a uniform gray at 50% video level. Low- and high-contrast bar patterns are placed at the center and at each corner. The size of the bars varies, but the smallest bar is limited by the pixel size of the digital system (i.e., the width of the smallest bar is one pixel). The low-contrast bars are modulated in contrast from 1% to 5%. The high-contrast bars have maximum contrast of 100%. A crosshatch border defines the limit of the picture area to be displayed or recorded on film. Boxes with varying brightness levels are arranged in stepwise fashion throughout the central portion of the test pattern. The entire dynamic range of potential signal levels is represented in 11 steps from 0% to 100% with 10% increments. An incremental patch with 5% contrast is inset in each box. For example, a 95% patch is positioned within the 100% box.

Unfortunately, ultrasound-equipment manufacturers have not universally adopted the standardized SMPTE video test pattern. The ready accessibility of the test pattern as a display option in each scanner would improve setup and QC monitoring. In addition, more uniform image recording by equipment from different manufacturers would then be possible.

Gray-Scale Adjustment

Setup of the display monitor is accomplished by exhibiting the gray-scale test pattern and adjusting the brightness and contrast controls. *Each bar in the test pattern should be distinguished as a separate shade of gray.* The gray levels must range from black to white, with midscale bars depicted in gray tones. If tearing or blurring of letters in the text occurs, the brightness adjustment is too high. Once brightness and contrast controls have been adjusted to achieve the proper gray-scale presentation, the knobs can be taped in place (or at least labeled) to inhibit modifying the settings. A full sheet of gray-scale test pattern images is recorded in the format and size normally used clinically (i.e., a 6:1 format requires the pattern to be printed six times). The maximum optical density for film viewed on a conventional light box that allows differences in transmitted light to be discerned as separate gray levels is 2.5. However, dark borders between images prevents glare and improves contrast resolution. For laser cameras, maximum density is

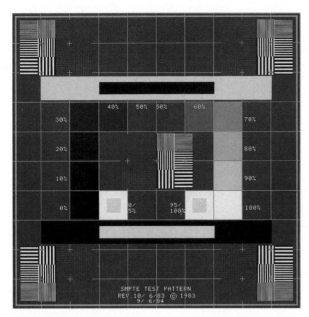

Fig. 24-30 The Society of Motion Picture and Television Engineers test pattern.

usually set at 2.5 to 3.2, and for multiformat cameras at 1.7 to 2.1. The white area must have an optical density less than 0.1 above base-plus-fog. All bars in the test pattern should be distinguishable (Fig. 24-31). A gray-scale test pattern recorded with an improperly adjusted multiformat camera is shown in Fig. 24-32.

Recording an image of the test pattern does not test all components of the ultrasound system (e.g., the transducer and processing electronics). A scan of the TM phantom can also serve as a photographic check and will indicate whether the entire system is functioning properly.

Distortion

Size, shape, and relative positions of structures in the image should be accurately presented. **Distortion** is a parameter of image quality that describes the lack of adherence to original geometric relationships. Two common methods of testing for distortion include recording the electronic grid pattern and scanning a TM phantom. In addition, critically evaluating routine clinical images can identify distortion caused by the hard copy recording device.

The first method evaluates the display and the image-recording device independent of the transducer and spatial mapping of the detected echoes. The grid pattern should appear symmetrical, with straight, equally spaced, parallel lines in both dimensions. The boxes formed by the inter-section of horizontal and vertical parallel lines should be uniform in size throughout the recorded image (Figs. 24-33 and 24-34).

The second method is a total system approach that evaluates the entire imaging chain for proper operation, including distortion in the final recorded image. A distance-calibration scale for each direction is frequently included on the monitor screen and reproduced on the hard copy, although many sector scanners contain only a vertical calib-

Fig. 24-31 Gray-scale test pattern with a properly adjusted multiformat camera. All 16 bars are resolved.

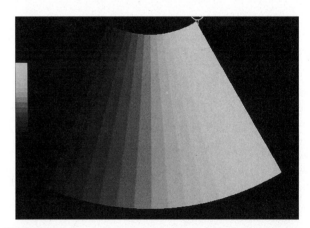

Fig. 24-32 Gray-scale test pattern with an improperly adjusted multiformat camera. The bars in the low-optical density range are not resolved.

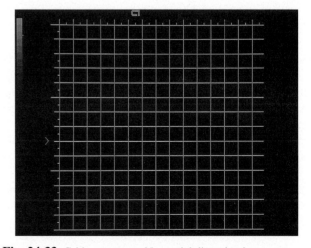

Fig. 24-33 Grid test pattern. No spatial distortion is present.

ration scale. The assumption that this single calibration scale will be appropriate for any orientation within the image is valid only if the hard copy device is properly adjusted.

When handheld calipers are used to measure distance, the measurement between any two points on the recorded image of the TM phantom should correspond to that obtained from

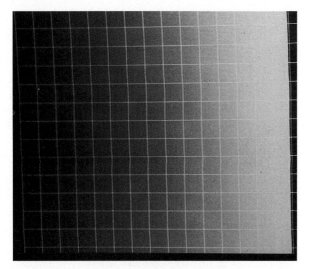

Fig. 24-34 Grid test pattern. Spatial distortion introduced by the hard copy camera.

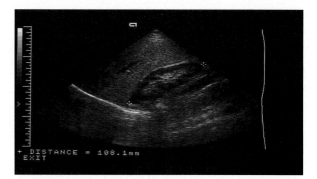

Fig. 24-36 Sonogram of a kidney recorded with an improperly adjusted laser camera. Whereas internal calipers measure the craniocaudal dimension as 108 mm, the calibration scale indicates incorrectly that the distance (between cursors) is 145 mm.

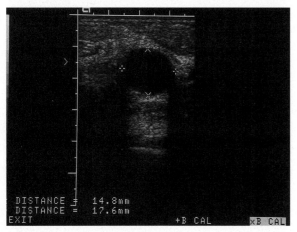

Fig. 24-35 Sonogram of a breast containing a cyst. Cursors mark the dimensions of the cyst. A properly adjusted multiformat camera recorded the hard copy image.

the display. Also, the scanner's internal calipers should yield distance values that agree with those measured from the film by the handheld calipers. Since the TM phantom has reflecting structures (rods) at known locations, every measured value obtained from the display and hard copy image should agree with the actual separation between rods in the scanned phantom.

Fig. 24-35 shows a sonogram of a breast containing a cyst. The sonogram was recorded with a properly operating hard copy camera. Distance measurements in the horizontal and vertical directions obtained by the internal calipers agree with measurements by handheld calipers. Furthermore, the graduated distance scales in both directions are equal; that is, the separation between any two points in the hard copy image should be the same whether the horizontal or vertical calibration scale is used.

Hard copy recording of the image, including the demographic information displayed on the monitor, requires data transfer to the image-recording device. To prevent geometric distortion, the aspect ratio of the monitor screen

(ratio of width to height) must be maintained on the recording medium. The hard copy image is often minified to accommodate various film formats (e.g., 15:1 on 14- × 17-inch film or 6:1 on 8- × 10-inch film). The aspect ratio of the recorded image is the same regardless of film format. The typical aspect ratio for ultrasound scanners is 4:3. A change in this ratio is accompanied by unequal magnification (or minification) in the horizontal and vertical directions.

Unequal magnification causes distortion. Circular shapes on the display monitor are elongated in the direction of higher magnification and appear elliptical on the hard copy. For example, a fetal head that is round on the display monitor would be recorded as an oval. In addition, a distance measurement along any diagonal path through the hard copy image would yield an incorrect result. Fig. 24-36 illustrates the effect of unequal magnification in the recording of a sonogram of the kidney. The size and shape of the kidney are distorted by being protracted in the horizontal direction. The calibration scale indicates that the distance between cursors is 145 mm instead of 108 mm as measured by the internal calipers. If distortion is introduced by the image-recording device, the internal calipers are unaffected by this malfunction and, consequently, the measured value for distance as designated by the cursors is correct.

The most likely circumstance for an improperly adjusted image-recording device is an incorrect initial setup (1) during installation of the scanner or (2) during replacement of the hard copy recording device (e.g., superseding the multiformat camera by interfacing the scanner to a laser camera). To ensure that the image-recording device is functioning properly, acceptance testing following these events is essential. The test methods described previously are appropriate for evaluating distortion.

Optical Density

Optical density measurements of different gray-scale bars can be obtained as listed in Table 24-6. The low-scale bar should have an optical density less than 0.1 above base-plus-fog. The maximum optical density depends on the type of recording device. The suggested levels are 2.1 for multi-

■ **Table 24-6** Suggested Optical Density Levels for Hard Copy Recording Devices Using a Gray-Scale Test Pattern

| | Optical Density | |
Gray-Scale Level	Multiformat Camera	Laser Camera
0	1.7-2.1	2.5-3.2
10	1.2-1.5	1.9
90	0.45	0.45
100	<0.1 above base + fog	<0.1 above base + fog

format cameras and 2.5 to 3.2 for laser cameras. The optical density difference between midscale bars denotes the contrast index for the processed film.

TESTING WITH SPECIALIZED PHANTOMS

Lateral Resolution Full Width at Half Maximum

One of the best methods of testing the lateral resolution is to scan a single rod target at a specific depth and measure the full width at half maximum (FWHM) of the profile in the lateral direction. These measurements are facilitated if profile plotting and analysis software is available on the ultrasound unit. The pulse-echo response profiles should be determined at several depths—at least at the focal point distance, at half the focal point distance, and at twice the focal distance—which specify the area within the focal zone. The profiles can be generated in TM attenuating media or nonattenuating media. The FWHM of these profiles at the various depths provides a measure of the beam width or lateral resolution.

Beam shape phantoms that provide an image of the actual beam shape as a function of distance from the transducer have been developed. The rods are located within a low scattering medium to reduce interference from backscattering. These phantoms are especially useful for comparing one transducer with another.

Axial Resolution Full Width at Half Maximum

The best method to quantify the axial resolution is to scan a single filament rod within a low scattering medium and measure the FWHM of the profile in the axial direction. The rods can be scanned at various output and TGC settings to determine the effects of various controls on the axial resolution. This provides a measure of total system performance with respect to the axial resolution.

Slice Thickness Phantom

Most multielement transducers (except annular arrays) are focused in the elevation direction by placing a lens in front of the crystal elements. This mechanical focusing fixes the focal length to one specific depth. The focal length is appropriate for the type of transducer and the operational frequency. For example, a small parts transducer operating

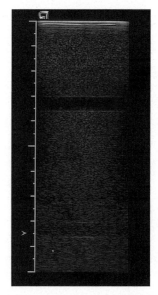

Fig. 24-37 Variation in slice thickness demonstrated by a TM phantom with cylindrical-shaped cysts containing a low concentration of scatterers. The elevation direction is into the page. The simulated cyst shown with fill-in is located within the single transmit focal zone. Displacement of the cyst from the fixed mechanical focal zone increases the sampling volume in the slice thickness direction and causes fill-in.

at 5 MHz has a minimum thickness at a depth from 1.5 cm to 3.5 cm, while the minimum slice thickness for a general purpose transducer operating at the same frequency occurs at a deeper depth of 3 cm to 6 cm.

Mechanical focusing is evaluated qualitatively by scanning anechoic cylindrical objects in a general purpose TM phantom with the scan plane oriented parallel to the length of the cylinders. The scan head is rotated 90 degrees from the typical orientation. Cyst fill-in is present where the slice thickness extends beyond the boundary of the cylindrical object (Fig. 24-37). For narrow slice thickness, cyst fill-in is less pronounced and corresponds to the depth of mechanical focus. Assessment is limited by the placement depths of the anechoic objects in the phantom.

Quantitative assessment over a continuous range of scan depths is achieved by using an inclined plane phantom. The phantom is composed of two sections forming a flat interface oriented at 45 degrees (Fig. 24-38). Both materials are uniform in their attenuation. One material containing backscattering particles forms an inclined plane; the other material containing no backscattering particles is in contact with the surface of the inclined plane. The transducer is positioned so that the scanning plane at a constant depth intercepts the inclined plane with the 45-degree angle (Fig. 24-39). For example, the row of crystal elements in a linear array cuts across the slope of the inclined plane.

The scattering plane interrogated by the beam appears as a horizontal band in the image. The axial height of the band is equal to the slice thickness. Thin slice thickness is depicted as a narrow band. The band increases in height with increased slice thickness. To view the scattering plane at different depths, the transducer is moved along the length of

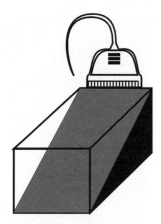

Fig. 24-38 Slice thickness phantom.

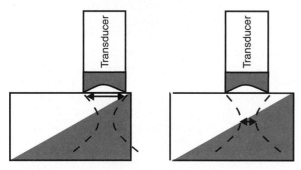

Fig. 24-39 The ultrasound beam interrogates the 45-degree interface in the slice thickness phantom. Translation of the transducer allows sampling the beam width at different depths. As beam width (slice thickness) becomes narrower, less of the 45-degree interface is included within the cross-sectional area of the beam.

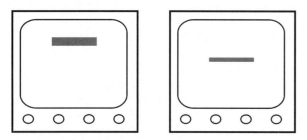

Fig. 24-40 Images obtained with the two different transducer positions shown in Fig. 24-39. The axial length of the interface in the image indicates beam width. The thinnest slice thickness is within the fixed mechanical focal zone.

the inclined plane. As slice thickness becomes narrower near the mechanical focal point, the horizontal band is reduced in size (Fig. 24-40).

Contrast Detail Phantoms

Special phantoms with "cysts" and "masses" (solids) embedded in TM material permit testing of the contrast and detail of the imaging system under simulated clinical conditions. A contrast-and-detail phantom with multiple conical targets having varying contrast (echoes vary by 20 dB) tests the system's ability to reproduce contrast and

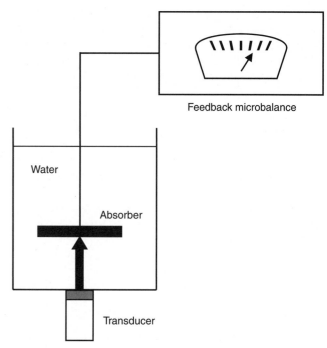

Fig. 24-41 A feedback microbalance system for measuring the ultrasonic force on an absorber.

detail in quantitative terms. This evaluation is very helpful in comparing transducers on the same system and in comparing different systems for total performance.

Limitations

TM phantoms provide an easy means for performance evaluation of the test parameters for which the phantom was designed. Power, intensity, bandwidth, and beam profiles cannot be evaluated with TM phantoms. These parameters must be measured under well-defined conditions with sophisticated test equipment.

ELECTRONIC TEST EQUIPMENT

The TM phantoms can be used on a routine basis to provide testing of ultrasonic systems. This section of the chapter deals with the more expensive and more complex test procedures, many of which must be done by the manufacturer before units are shipped to customers. Indeed, the customers should request documentation of the unit's performance, as indicated by the manufacturer's testing.

Feedback Microbalance

Power and intensity are discussed in Chapters 21 through 23 relative to biologic effects. The power is determined using a **feedback microbalance** system (Fig. 24-41). An absorber (rubber disk) placed in the ultrasonic field experiences a force arising from the pressure wave that strikes its surface. The radiation force on the absorber is measured by the microbalance. Because the response time of the balance is long compared with the period of the pressure wave, the reading represents the average force exerted on the disk. The radiation force (F_r) on a perfect absorber (with normal incidence) is related to the ultrasonic power (W) by the following equation:

24-1

$$F_r = \frac{W}{c}$$

where c is the velocity of ultrasound in the material surrounding the absorber. A power of 1 mW corresponds to 68 µg.

Power Meters

Portable power meters have been developed, making the task of determining power easier and permitting (at least relative) calibration of output and gain settings. These controls can be marked in decibels to indicate the amount of power used for a particular scan. Various combinations of TGC and gain controls may then be used to permit the best possible diagnostic image with the least patient exposure.

Hydrophone

Intensity is derived from measurements of acoustic pressure by means of a **hydrophone** placed in the ultrasonic field. The physical dimensions of the hydrophone are typically 0.5 to 1 mm in diameter; thus to minimize spatial averaging, the measurements are performed over a very small area. The spatial variation in intensity is mapped by moving the hydrophone to different locations in the field.

The ultrasound wave incident on the hydrophone induces a voltage that is directly proportional to the acoustic pressure. Because the pressure is not constant but fluctuates as the pulse passes a point in space, a time-varying waveform of the voltage is obtained (Fig. 24-42, A). The maximum peak in the waveform corresponds to the temporal peak. This process is repeated so waveforms are collected throughout the ultrasonic field. The point that gives the highest temporal peak denotes I(SPTP).

Recall the relationship between instantaneous intensity (i) and the acoustic pressure (p) is expressed as

24-2

$$i = \frac{p^2}{\rho c}$$

where c is the acoustic velocity and ρ is the density of the medium. An analog-to-digital converter transforms the voltage signal from the pressure fluctuations into digital format for signal processing. The instantaneous intensity is calculated directly from the induced voltage by squaring this value and multiplying by a constant. To determine other intensity descriptors such as the pulse-averaged intensity, the induced voltage waveform is squared and then integrated over time (Fig. 24-42, B and C). The resulting value is divided by the time duration of the pulse to yield the pulse-averaged intensity at the point of measurement. The maximum pulse-averaged intensity obtained from all points throughout the ultrasonic field is the I(SPPA). Spatial averaging is applied by combining the results from multiple points in the region of interest.

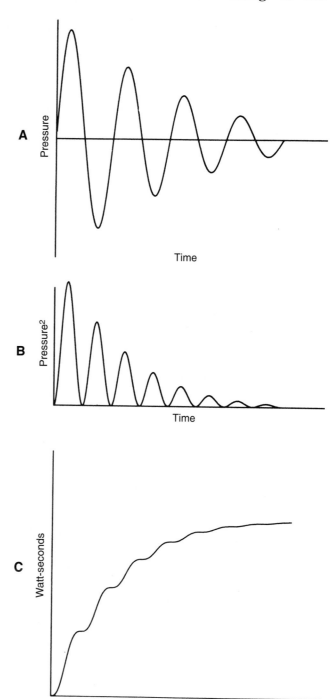

Fig. 24-42 Data for calculation of various intensity parameters. **A,** Time-varying voltage waveform detected by a hydrophone. **B,** Squared time–varying voltage waveform. **C,** Integration of the squared time–varying voltage waveform in **B** over time.

Bandwidth Measurements

A frequency-calibrated hydrophone enables the transmitted frequency profile to be obtained when the output of the hydrophone is connected to a spectrum analyzer. The frequency profile provides the center frequency (f_c)—at which the amplitude frequency spectrum is maximal—and the transmitted bandwidth. The transmitted bandwidth is the difference between frequency values ($f_2 - f_1$), where the

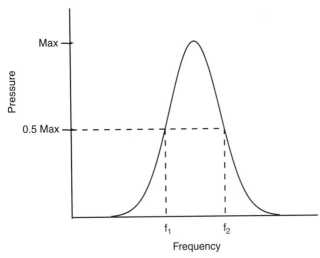

Fig. 24-43 Acoustic pressure as a function of frequency. The transmitted bandwidth is given by the frequency range at one-half maximum amplitude ($f_2 - f_1$).

acoustic pressure magnitude is –3 dB below the maximum value (Fig. 24-43). A broadband transducer (low Q) has a large frequency spread, whereas a narrow-band transducer (high Q) has a small frequency spread. More precisely, a transducer is considered to be narrow band if its fractional bandwidth is less than 15%. In general, broadband transducers are superior for medical diagnostic ultrasound imaging.

The frequency spectrum, center frequency, and frequency bandwidth may be measured by testing the transducer separately from the rest of the ultrasound system. The transducer is normally connected to a broadband pulser (e.g., a pulse-burst generator), which is used to excite it. The voltage applied to the transducer from the pulser can be made to oscillate at any desired frequency. A long pulse drives the transducer at the applied frequency.

The pulser is sequentially stepped at different frequencies throughout the bandwidth. Each ultrasound wave generated by the transducer with the pulser driven at a constant frequency is transmitted through water to a flat planar reflector. The echo from this reflector is detected by the transducer or by a hydrophone for continuous wave operation and sent to a spectrum analyzer, where a plot of signal strength versus frequency is made (Fig. 24-44). The signal strength increases as the match between driving voltage and the natural frequency of the transducer improves. The center frequency produces a signal with the greatest amplitude. Normally the excitation voltage waveform is continuous, because a short pulse causes the transducer to resonate at a frequency specified by the thickness of the crystal. The resonant frequency should be the same as the center frequency.

The bandwidth is determined from the amplitude-versus-frequency spectrum, by taking the differences in frequency at the points corresponding to half the maximum amplitude. The frequency spectrum depends on the transducer damping (Q value and backing material), the pulser, the transducer

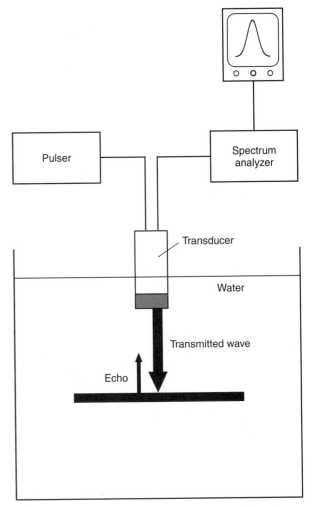

Fig. 24-44 System for determining a frequency spectrum. The pulser excites the transducer, which sends an ultrasound wave toward a planar reflector. The wave is reflected, and the received echo signal is input into the spectrum analyzer, where the amplitude for each frequency is determined.

electrical and acoustic impedances, and the total system matching. This method evaluates only the transducer-related variables and not how well the transducer is matched with the rest of the ultrasound system. Testing the transducer frequency spectrum for a complete ultrasound system is more difficult and less accurate than evaluating the transducer by itself. Test devices are currently being developed to improve these system measurements.

Echo Amplitude Profiles

The combined transmit and receive characteristics of the transducer (i.e., the response to pulse echoes) is examined by moving a small target across the beam at various depths. The usual reflector is a sphere with a diameter of 3 to 10 wavelengths. A large reflecting target may also be used. The target generates reflected ultrasound waves, which are detected and processed by the ultrasonic unit rather than by the spectrum analyzer alone. The echo-detection pattern at various depths is delineated for that particular unit

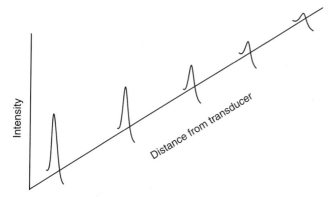

Fig. 24-45 Echo amplitude patterns of a transducer. The received echo signals are measured as a small target moves across the beam at various distances from a high-frequency, short-focused transducer.

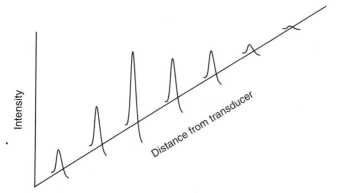

Fig. 24-46 Echo amplitude patterns of a transducer. The received echo signals are measured as a small target moves across the beam at various distances from a medium-frequency, medium-focused transducer.

(Figs. 24-45 and 24-46). These axial and transverse echo-amplitude profiles identify the focal zone and the extent of the ultrasonic field. The beam width and response with depth are illustrated. This information is obtained from the received echoes rather than from the induced voltage in a hydrophone from transmitted sound waves. The measured FWHM beam width within the focal zone should be less than the theoretical beam width (product of the wavelength and f-number):

24-3

$$FWHM = \frac{1.54\ F(mm)}{f(MHz)\ D(mm)}$$

where F is the length in millimeters, f is the frequency is MHz, and D is aperture size in millimeters.

Pressure-amplitude or echo-amplitude profiles are consolidated to denote the limits of the ultrasonic field. The point on each side of the profile peak corresponding to a 6 dB reduction is identified, and then the points along each side of the transducer axis are connected to form a boundary of the ultrasonic field (Fig. 24-47). This is the common illustrative format to designate sound wave patterns produced by a transducer.

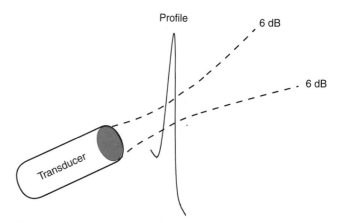

Fig. 24-47 Extent of an ultrasonic field obtained from the analysis of pressure or echo amplitude profiles. The boundary *(dotted lines)* corresponds to a 6 dB reduction in intensity.

Test Generators

Test generators can be used to evaluate the dynamic range, TGC stability, gray-scale, linearity, depth marker accuracy, SNR, photographic controls, and signal processing. These generators are connected at selected points throughout the unit to simulate scan conditions. In essence, well-known signals are introduced to ascertain the response of one or more system components. For example, when connected to the transducer, the generator furnishes an excitation pulse. Test signals can be sent to the scan converter or the display directly. Test generators normally produce exponentially decaying pulse bursts that can be triggered externally to the ultrasound system or internally with the ultrasound system transmitter. The test generators may be set for different frequencies, pulse rates, and decay rates. Information provided by the test generators is a valuable part of the manufacturer's testing.

ACCEPTANCE TESTING

It is often of value for the customer, either directly or through a medical physicist, to verify the performance of the unit at installation, independent of the manufacturer. To provide a basis for comparison at a later date, baseline performance must be clearly established when the equipment is initially installed.

DOPPLER ULTRASOUND PHANTOMS

Performance testing of stand-alone Doppler, duplex Doppler, and two-dimensional color-flow Doppler units has become increasingly important because of the dramatic increase in the clinical utility of these instruments. Duplex Doppler and color-flow imaging systems combine real-time capabilities with Doppler. The TM phantoms described previously are used to test the imaging component of these devices. The attenuation coefficient should be 0.5 dB cm^{-1} MHz^{-1} or 0.7 dB cm^{-1} MHz^{-1}. The velocity of ultrasound in the material should be 1540 m/s. To appropriately test the

TM phantom

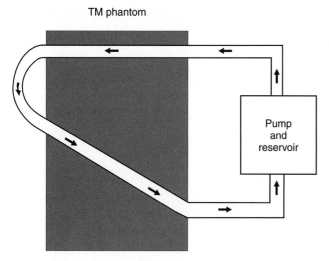

Fig. 24-48 A tissue-mimicking Doppler phantom with simulated vessels and a variable-speed control pump.

sensitivity of the imaging component, the velocity and attenuation values must be similar to those of normal tissue.

Additionally, the Doppler operation of the unit must be tested. Three types of phantoms—flow, string, and belt—have been developed to evaluate velocity or flow measurements obtained with Doppler instruments.

Flow Phantoms

Flow phantoms contain simulated vessels (i.e., latex rubber tubing) through which a blood-mimicking fluid is propelled (Fig. 24-48). In this fluid (normally a degassed water and glycerol mixture) are polystyrene microspheres to simulate the backscattering properties of red blood cells (RBCs). The attenuation coefficient is 0.1 dB cm^{-1} MHz^{-1}. The velocity of sound in the fluid is 1546 cm/s.

Special care is taken to prevent "clotting," which causes increased scattering. The blood-mimicking fluid is pumped through a closed-loop system by a variable-speed pump. Desirable characteristics of the pump include an accurate flow rate with maximum peak velocity of 1 m/s and the ability to produce steady flow, reverse flow, and physiologic pulsatile waveforms. Gear, peristaltic, and piston pumps have been used. Gear pumps provide pulsed waveforms but also cause damage to suspended particles and produce cavitation within the fluid. Peristaltic and piston pumps cannot generate steady flow and have only limited ability to produce pulsatile waveforms. All these pumps require flow monitoring with feedback to the pump to maintain the selected flow characteristics. A computer-controlled positive-displacement pump has achieved accurate flow rates between 0.1 and 40 ml per second without feedback circuitry. Care must be taken to avoid the production of cavitation air bubbles, particularly by centripetal pumps that many commercial companies use.

Variable speeds of continuous flow of the simulated blood provide a means of checking the accuracy of the Doppler shift. One problem with simulated tissue- and blood-mimicking phantoms, although "clinically" realistic, is that a single true calibration of peak flow velocity is not known. The velocity of simulated RBCs varies across the vessel, with maximum rates at the center of the vessels (i.e., the vessel walls tend to slow the "RBCs" just as in a true vessel). Flow phantoms are calibrated with respect to volume flow rate, not peak velocity. Peak velocity is based on calculations using a volume flow rate in which the velocity profile (e.g., laminar) is assumed. The actual velocity profile depends on the compliance and resistance of the tubing.

The maximum depth of a detectable Doppler signal is evaluated by placing the simulated vessel diagonally across the phantom from the bottom corner on one side to the top corner on the other. This enables the Doppler sensitivity to be evaluated for different frequency probes. At maximum acoustic power, the Doppler signal from blood-mimicking fluid is obtained near the transducer. The velocity of the moving fluid is set to be in the middle range of the instrument. The Doppler sample volume is adjusted until the maximum depth at which the signal can be detected is identified. Since the phantom attenuation is known (in dB/cm/MHz), sensitivity can be expressed in decibels by multiplying the attenuation rate times the depth times the transducer frequency.

By placing vessels at different angles through the TM material, it is possible to determine the accuracy of the Doppler angle indicator. The incorporation of various-sized vessels at different angles allows the accuracy of the sample volume cursor (position and size) to be evaluated. The phantom can also test the directional capability of the Doppler unit. Flow toward or away from the transducer is determined by reversing the pump or by routing the vessel with different orientations throughout the phantom. If the pump can be pulsed, various flow patterns are possible.

String Phantoms

String phantoms allow for accurate assessment of the flow velocity under nonclinical conditions. A loop of surgical thread (strong scatterer) or monofilament fish line (weak scatterer) is mounted on pulleys and driven at a known rate through a low-acoustic attenuating medium (degassed water or a 9% ethylene glycol–water mixture). The latter has an acoustic velocity of 1540 m/s, which allows a direct readout of velocity from the Doppler shift. Recall from Chapter 14 that the Doppler shift depends on the velocity of sound in the medium. The string can be moved at a constant speed ranging from 0.05 to 150 cm/s. A sequence of variable string speeds will produce pulsatile waveforms.

String phantoms can be used for evaluating flow angle indicators, Doppler sample volumes, wall filters, and sensitivity. When the angle of the string with respect to the fluid surface is varied, sampling is possible at different angles. The small physical size of the string, coupled with mechanical translation of the transducer, permits measurement of the Doppler sample volume in three dimensions. Removal of low-velocity components can be qualitatively checked when the wall filter setting is changed. Sensitivity is evaluated by placing additional attenuating material along the ultrasonic path.

In some designs the string is passed through air near the drive pulley. Air bubbles attach to the string and cause spectral broadening of the detected signal.

Belt Phantoms

The **belt phantom** contains a 2-cm thick layer of scattering material mounted on a belt that is moved at a constant but adjustable speed by drive pulleys. The belt assembly is placed in a water bath. The scattering material encompasses the entire Doppler sample volume. The accuracy, linearity, and precision of Doppler velocity measurements can all be assessed over a belt velocity range of 0 to 80 cm/s in both forward and reverse directions. No pulsatile waveforms are possible, however, since the belt velocity cannot be changed rapidly.

Clinical Use

Doppler phantoms cost somewhat more than TM phantoms. Another problem with them, as with normal TM phantoms, is that they eventually fail (i.e., both the latex tubing forming the simulated vessels and the TM material deteriorate). Flow phantoms also require periodic replacement. Their high cost and complex design, plus the lack of a single-phantom comprehensive test method, have restricted their use. None of the current commercially available phantom types has been adopted as the standard for Doppler testing. The most appropriate methods for evaluation of Doppler units are still evolving.

Training

Not only are the Doppler tissue- and blood-mimicking phantoms useful in testing the equipment under simulated clinical conditions, they provide a valuable teaching tool in the training of sonographers. Doppler principles and the effect of operator controls on the Doppler image can be investigated systematically in well-designed laboratory exercises. Pulsed-wave spectral aliasing (Fig. 24-49) and color aliasing are easily demonstrated. When the Doppler sampling line of sight is placed perpendicularly to the direction of flow, the loss of signal content is dramatic (Fig. 24-50). Recovery of signal level occurs if the vessel is interrogated at a proper Doppler angle (Fig. 24-51). Sensitivity to slow flow can be studied. The Doppler imaging artifact of color bleed can be illustrated by increasing the transmit power and color gain (Fig. 24-52).

PURCHASE SPECIFICATIONS

Before the purchase of new equipment, the medical director, lead sonographer, medical physicist, and other staff (as necessary) should determine the functions to be performed and the technical characteristics required to perform these

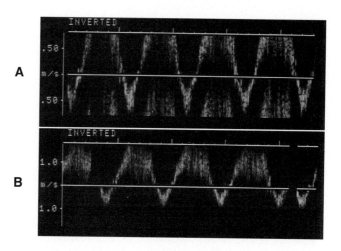

Fig. 24-49 Pulsed-wave spectral waveforms obtained using a Doppler flow phantom. **A,** Aliasing. **B,** Expanding the velocity scale removes the aliasing artifact.

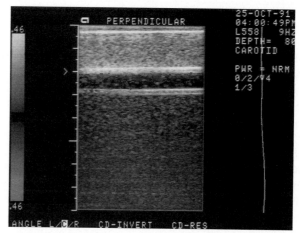

Fig. 24-50 Color Doppler image of the vessel in the flow phantom obtained with a 90-degree Doppler angle. (See Color Plate 21.)

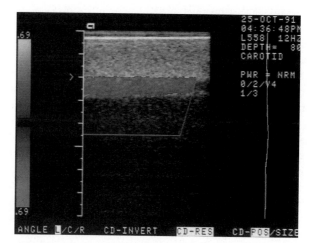

Fig. 24-51 Color Doppler image of the vessel in the flow phantom obtained with a reduced Doppler angle. (See Color Plate 22.)

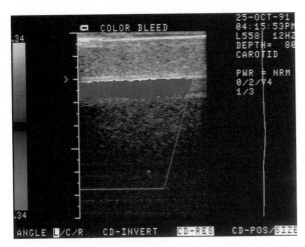

Fig. 24-52 Color bleed artifact generated at high power and color gain with a Doppler flow phantom. (See Color Plate 23.)

functions. Based on these requirements, objective technical specifications should be provided to prospective vendors.

Comparing instruments from different manufacturers is necessary to make rational equipment-purchase decisions. Ascertaining the performance characteristics of various scanners under the same conditions is highly desirable but often difficult. Phantoms offer a unique opportunity to evaluate units with a standard means of comparison.

The final purchase specifications should be in writing and include performance specifications. After the equipment is installed, the medical physicist should conduct appropriate acceptance testing procedures to ensure that the equipment meets the agreed-upon specifications, including federal and state equipment regulations. The equipment should not be accepted until any necessary corrections have been made by the vendor.

SUMMARY

The end product of an ultrasound scan is its image. The quality of the image depends largely on a properly functioning unit. Performance characteristics of the system are evaluated using TM phantoms to measure resolution (axial and lateral), sensitivity, uniformity, dead zone, accuracy of distance markers (vertical and horizontal), and other parameters. Within well-defined limits, these parameters reflect properly functioning equipment.

The display monitor, hard copy camera, and film processing all contribute to the image-recording process. To optimize photographic system performance, the recommendations of manufacturers of the image-recording device, film, and processing chemicals should be followed. The image-recording device should exhibit a full range of gray-scale contrast and an accurate portrayal of size, shape, and relative positions of structures in the displayed image. Matching the response of the display monitor and the hard copy camera is necessary to ensure that what is seen on the monitor is recorded on film.

Flow, string, and belt phantoms are used for checks on Doppler instruments. Velocity (or flow), the Doppler angle

indicator and Doppler sample volume, sensitivity, and the wall filter can be evaluated. An inexpensive, easy-to-use, and accurate Doppler test phantom has not been developed. Standards for testing of Doppler instruments are evolving.

Acceptance testing establishes the baseline performance levels of an ultrasound unit and ensures that the unit meets design specifications.

REVIEW QUESTIONS

1. Name several test parameters that can be evaluated with a general purpose tissue-mimicking (TM) phantom.
2. The attenuation rate of the TM material is normally set at _____ or _____ dB cm^{-1} MHz^{-1}.
3. The maximum depth of visualization of the backscatter in a TM phantom provides an indication of _____.
4. Lateral resolution is affected by scan line density and _____.
5. A urethane phantom has attenuation and scattering properties similar to tissue, except that the _____ is lower than that of tissue.
6. Gray-scale contrast on the display monitor and film is best evaluated using an _____ video/digital test pattern.
7. TM phantoms mimic the acoustic properties of tissue with respect to velocity, _____, and backscatter.
8. What is a hydrophone?
9. What is the dead zone?
10. The accuracy of distance markers and electronic calipers should be assessed along the beam axis and _____.
11. If a multiformat camera introduces distortion in the recorded image, are the internal calipers for distance measurements also in error?
12. The rod groups in the TM phantoms that measure axial resolution are offset horizontally to prevent _____.

BIBLIOGRAPHY

Banjavic RA: Design and maintenance of a quality assurance program for diagnostic ultrasound equipment, *Semin Ultrasound* 4:10-26, 1983.

Boote EJ, Zagzebski JA: Performance tests of Doppler ultrasound equipment with a tissue- and blood-mimicking phantom, *J Ultrasound Med* 7:137-147, 1988.

Browne JE et al: Assessment of the acoustic properties of common tissue-mimicking test phantoms, *Ultrasound Med Biol* 29:1053-1060, 2003.

Goldstein A: Performance tests of Doppler ultrasound equipment with a string phantom, *J Ultrasound Med* 10:125-139, 1991.

Goodsitt MM et al: Real-time B-mode ultrasound quality control test procedures: report of AAPM Ultrasound Task Group No. 1, *Med Phys* 25:1385-1406, 1998.

Gray JE et al: Test pattern for video displays and hard-copy cameras, *Radiology* 154:519-527, 1985.

Hedrick WR, Hykes DL: Image recording devices, *J Diagn Med Sonogr* 7:56-63, 1991.

Hedrick WR, Hykes DL: Image distortion caused by an improperly adjusted hardcopy camera, *J Diagn Med Sonogr* 9:180-183, 1993.

Hedrick WR, Hykes DL: Photographic system quality control, *J Diagn Med Sonogr* 9:62-66, 1993.

Hoskins PR, Loupas T, McDicken WN: A comparison of the Doppler spectra from human blood and artificial blood used in a flow phantom, *Ultrasound Med Biol* 16:141-147, 1990.

Hykes DL et al: Quality assurance for real time ultrasound equipment, *J Diagn Med Sonogr* 2:121-133, 1986.

Phillips DJ et al: Testing ultrasonic pulsed Doppler instruments with a physiologic string phantom, *J Ultrasound Med* 9:429-436, 1990.

Rickey DW, Rankin R, Fenster A: A velocity evaluation phantom for colour and pulsed Doppler instruments, *Ultrasound Med Biol* 18:479-494, 1992.

Walker AR, Phillips DJ, Powers JE: Evaluating Doppler devices using a string target, *J Clin Ultrasound* 10:25-30, 1982.

Zagzebski JA: US quality assurance with phantoms. In Goldman LW, Fowlkes JB, eds: *Categorical course in diagnostic radiology physics: CT and US cross-sectional imaging,* Oak Brook, Ill, 2000, Radiological Society of North America.

CHAPTER 25

Quality Control

KEY TERMS

Baseline values   Quality control
Control limit   Sensitometric strip

An effective **quality control (QC)** program is required to obtain consistent high-quality images and ensure proper equipment performance. It must be simple to implement and easy to maintain. One that is overambitious in terms of complexity or frequency of testing will often cease to be performed at all. At the same time, to be meaningful, the QC tests must be comprehensive and capable of detecting common system problems. Cost efficiency is improved and patient inconvenience is reduced because fewer examinations are repeated. This chapter describes a QC program for real-time ultrasound equipment.

PURPOSE OF QUALITY CONTROL

QC tests provide objective assessment of instrument stability and performance. They have proved to be beneficial in diagnostic imaging facilities when conducted regularly. One of the most important advantages is the documentation of gradual degradation of system performance when compared with clinical impressions of image quality. The value of QC

programs in these areas has extended to other imaging modalities; test objects and tissue-mimicking (TM) phantoms have been designed specifically for diagnostic ultrasound applications.

Long-term performance is evaluated by periodically testing ultrasound equipment under well-defined conditions (e.g., specified instrument settings using appropriate phantoms). The instrument settings must be maintained at the same values, and a phantom that mimics the properties of tissues should be used. The properties of the phantom must remain constant with respect to time.

A good QC program eliminates misdiagnoses because of improperly operating equipment and reduces cost by decreasing the number of repeat examinations. In recognition of the essential relationship between QC and correct diagnosis, the Joint Commission on Accreditation of Health Care Organization (JCAHO) requires periodic QC testing. Recommendations made by other agencies and organizations—the American Institute of Ultrasound in Medicine, the American Association of Physicists in Medicine, and the National Electronic Manufacturers Association—also include routine testing.

RESPONSIBILITY

Responsibility and authority for the overall ultrasound QC program and its monitoring, evaluation, and corrective measures resides with the medical director. Primary responsibility for implementing and maintaining the ultrasound QC program should be delegated to the supervisor of the ultrasound section. The supervisor may designate certain aspects of the program testing to a qualified sonographer but should be responsible for ensuring that the program is executed, corrective actions are monitored, and appropriate people (i.e., service personnel or the medical physicist) are contacted when the need arises.

PERSONNEL

The sonographer who routinely uses the equipment for patient examinations should perform the QC procedures. A more sensitive check on machine malfunction and technical error can thus be made. It requires administrative support to schedule the time necessary for that individual to conduct the QC testing. The time allotment must allow for access to the unit and for the analysis and documentation of results.

Results of the QC procedures should be reviewed periodically by the medical director, the sonographer performing the QC procedures, and if possible, a medical physicist. *The parameters to be tested, the results to be recorded, and the performance limits for each parameter should be specified.*

PHANTOMS

A wide variety of general-purpose TM phantoms have been developed to monitor the performance characteristics of ultrasound scanners. Model 403 from Gammex-RMI, Middleton, Wisconsin, and Model 40 from CIRS Inc., Norfolk, Virginia, are recommended for routine QC testing. New designs with regions of TM material only and that are relatively free of objects would improve testing for sensitivity and image uniformity.

Rubber-based urethane phantoms have also been developed for QC applications. Fig. 25-1 illustrates the rod groups and masses contained within the CIRS Model 42 phantom. The specifications for this phantom are listed in Table 25-1. Three sides of the phantom provide an acoustic window, which allows structures to be interrogated at different depths depending on the side of access. An extended-field-of-view scan of this phantom is presented in Fig. 25-2. The low velocity and frequency dependence of the attenuation coefficient limit the application to monitoring consistency but not accuracy of scanner performance. The physical separation of the vertical rods is 18.6 mm so that the measured axial distance is the stated 20 mm (corrected for the difference in acoustic velocity between urethane and tissue). When the rods are oriented perpendicularly to the direction of propagation, then the measured distance should correspond to actual separation of 18.6 mm.

QUALITY CONTROL TEST SELECTION

While extensive testing is appropriate when the scanner is installed, the purpose of QC is to use tests that are sensitive indicators of overall scanner performance. *The following*

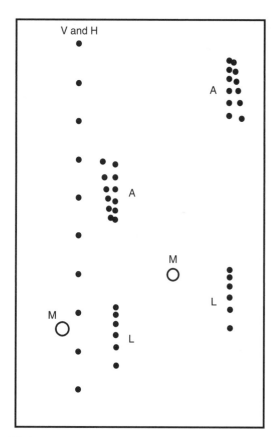

Fig. 25-1 Diagram of the CIRS Model 42 urethane phantom. Vertical and horizontal rod group *(V and H),* axial resolution rod groups *(A),* lateral resolution rod groups *(L),* and simulated anechoic masses *(M)* are indicated.

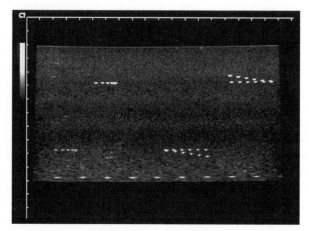

Fig. 25-2 Extended-field-of-view sonogram of the CIRS Model 42 urethane phantom. The scanning surface was oriented parallel to the vertical/horizontal rod group. The width of the field of view was 18 cm, and the scan depth was 10 cm. The center frequency was 6 MHz.

tests are recommended for the quality control program: penetration, distance accuracy, image uniformity, fidelity of image display, and fidelity of image recording. Mechanical inspection of the transducers, power cords, and console should also be included.

Low contrast detectability has not been demonstrated as yet to be a useful monitor of scanner performance. Since a

Table 25-1 Specifications of the CIRS Model 42 Urethane Phantom

Objects	Description	Specification
Vertical group	Number of rods	10
	Depth range	1-19 cm
	Vertical spacing	10 mm and 20 mm
Horizontal group	Number of groups	1
	Depth	3 cm and 10 cm
	Number of rods	10
	Horizontal spacing	18.6 mm
Axial resolution group	Number of groups	2
	Depth	2, 5, 8, 11 cm
	Number of rods	12
	Axial separation between rods	5, 4, 3, 2, 1, 0.5 mm
Lateral resolution group	Number of groups	2
	Depth of each group	2 cm, 5 cm, 8 cm, 11 cm
	Number of rods	6
	Horizontal spacing	5, 4, 3, 2, 1 mm
Anechoic masses	Number of stepped masses	2
	Attenuation coefficient	0.2 dB/cm/MHz
	Diameter	2, 4, 6, 8 mm
	Depth	2, 5, 8, 11, 13, 16 cm

specially designed phantom with hypoechoic spherical objects at various depths is required, this test is not included in the QC program.

The current QC program is a simplified version of those proposed previously. This is attributed to three factors. Scanner reliability has improved. Many instruments have internal diagnostic testing during start-up, which identifies improper electronic operation. The yield from QC tests conducted during the past several years has been evaluated to determine the most sensitive indicators of scanner performance.

BASELINE VALUES

The initiation of a QC program is very important, because the results obtained serve as **baseline values** for future comparisons. The program must be continued even if the patient load becomes high, because a scanner operating under these conditions has an increased probability of failure. The QC program may be able to identify problems before they become major, thus preventing excessive downtime, misdiagnoses, and repeat scans.

PENETRATION

Sensitivity is related to maximum depth of visualization under specified conditions. Factors that influence the penetration include frequency, power, receiver gain, focal zone, attenuation by the medium, and electronic noise.

The transducer is coupled to the phantom, in which a uniform section of the TM material wider than the field of view is scanned. Nylon rod depth markers may be included within the field of view. Many scanners have presets for depth, frame rate, scan lines, persistence, and post processing, which have been optimized for specific applications.

Often, some of these scanning parameters cannot be adjusted individually by the operator. Select an application preset appropriate for the transducer to be evaluated (e.g., liver or breast). Instrument settings are adjusted to maximum output, maximum gain, deepest focal zone, wide dynamic range (>50 dB), reject off or minimum, and time gain compensation (TGC) set at full gain where signal falloff occurs. Mark or record positions of TGC settings so that TGC can be reproduced in future QC checks. The maximum depth at which the tissue texture pattern is visualized is measured (Figs. 25-3 and 25-4).

For a completely stationary transducer, speckle produces a constant spatial pattern of signal levels while noise creates a fluctuating pattern. An alternative method to determine the maximum depth of visualization uses weakly echoic spherical objects distributed throughout the TM material. The depth at which the structures are not perceived is measured. The latter method has the advantage that objects rather than noise denote the limit of detectability. Since monitoring the consistency of performance is the primary goal of quality control, this type of phantom would be a reasonable substitute for testing penetration. However, further expense would be incurred for the purchase of an additional phantom.

The depth of penetration for a particular transducer should not shift by more than 1 cm for identical settings. Variations of output intensity or receiver gain and loss of transducer integrity can cause reduced sensitivity, which decreases the maximum depth of visualization.

DISTANCE ACCURACY

A major application of real-time imaging involves the measurement of length or area. Most ultrasound units employ markers to delineate distance on the monitor and

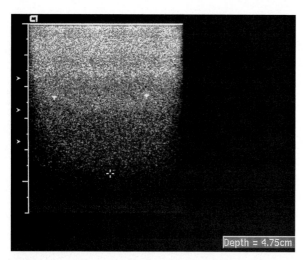

Fig. 25-3 Determination of the maximum depth of penetration using a tissue-mimicking phantom. The fading of parenchymal scatterers indicates that the maximum depth of penetration is 4.8 cm for this linear array transducer operated at a frequency of 14 MHz.

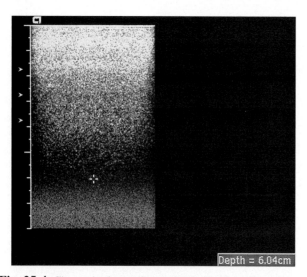

Fig. 25-4 Change in the maximum depth of penetration as frequency is reduced. The fading of parenchymal scatterers in a tissue-mimicking phantom indicates that the maximum depth of penetration is 6 cm for the same linear array transducer as in Fig. 25-3. The center frequency was lowered to 8 MHz.

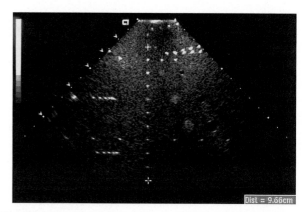

Fig. 25-5 Check of vertical distance accuracy. Measurement when the separation includes several rods in a tissue-mimicking phantom over the extremes of the scanning range. For a known distance of 100 mm, the measured separation is 96.6 mm, which demonstrates poor vertical distance accuracy.

hard copy image. The proper diagnosis depends on the accurate representation of spatial relationships. Accuracy is checked by comparing distance indicators (markers or cursors) in both the vertical (depth) and horizontal (lateral) directions with the known separation between rods in the phantom.

Vertical distance is measured along the axis of the beam. The location of an acoustic interface with respect to the face of the transducer can be determined if the velocity of ultrasound in the medium and the time of flight of the ultrasonic pulse are known. In practice, the velocity of ultrasound in the phantom and patient is assumed to be constant (1540 m/s). The elapsed time between the transmitted pulse and the returning echo is measured, which permits the calculation of the distance to the interface.

The transducer is positioned over the vertical set of rods in the phantom, and scan data are acquired. Instrument settings are adjusted as described previously for the penetration measurement, except gain and TCG are reduced to produce an image with moderate brightness.

Assessment of depth accuracy involves comparing the known distance between rods with the distance indicated by the internal calipers. The image is analyzed by determining the distance between rods located at the extremes of the scanning depth (Fig. 25-5). This measurement is most likely to identify vertical distance miscalibration, because errors are compounded with longer distances. Some sector scanners have distance markers on the outside edge of the sector image with no other indicators available. In this case, handheld calipers in conjunction with the calibration scale must be used for distance measurements on the hard copy image.

The vertical distance indicators should be accurate to within 2% or 2 mm, whichever is less restrictive. Any discrepancy greater than 3% attributed to scanner error should be corrected by the service representative. The performance of the scanner in Fig. 25-5 is poor, since the deviation is greater than 3%. Distance inaccuracy is the result of either machine error or the fact that the velocity of ultrasound in the phantom is not equal to that in soft tissue. Excessive pressure on the acoustic window of the phantom could also cause an error in distance measurement.

Horizontal distance is measured perpendicularly to the beam axis. The ultrasound image is a composite of many lines of sight, each representing the depth information gathered along the axis of the beam. The two-dimensional image, however, also provides spatial relationships perpendicular to the beam axis. Often, information regarding the size of an object in the horizontal direction is desirable. This spatial representation depends on the number of lines of sight, output intensity, resolution of the scan converter (pixel size), resolution of the display, and beam width (lateral

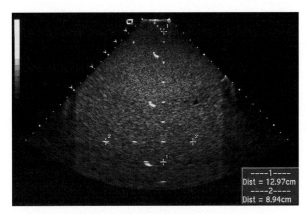

Fig. 25-6 Horizontal and vertical distance measurements on the same image. For a known vertical distance of 130 mm, the measured separation is 130 mm. For a known horizontal distance of 90 mm, the measured separation is 89 mm. Linear phased array transducer operating at 3 MHz.

resolution). Changes in beam formation by a defective transducer and mechanical motor wear associated with annular arrays can degrade horizontal distance accuracy.

A scan of the horizontal rods in the phantom is performed, and the internal calipers are used to measure the separation of rod echo positions in a manner similar to the vertical measurement procedure discussed previously. Often, horizontal and vertical distance measurements are obtained from the same image (Fig. 25-6). The horizontal distance indicators should be accurate to within 3% or 3 mm, whichever is less restrictive. The service representative should correct any discrepancy greater than 5% attributed to scanner error.

UNIFORMITY

Uniformity refers to the ability of the ultrasound system to display echoes of equal magnitude with the same brightness on the monitor throughout the field of view. Because TGC modifies the amplitude of the received signal, the echoes originating at the same depth must be compared across the field of view. Image nonuniformities can conceal subtle variations in tissue texture.

The scanning procedure is the same as the procedure described for maximum depth of visualization. Mechanical sector and curvilinear transducers may not produce a uniform pattern at the edges of the sector, which is caused by poor coupling with the phantom surface. This is a qualitative measurement, which is difficult to assess with any numerical limits. Figs. 25-7 and 25-8 are sonograms obtained with units that demonstrate poor uniformity.

IMAGE DISPLAY

Manufacturers have incorporated various test patterns in ultrasound scanners to aid in the setup and quality control of display monitors and hard copy cameras. These test patterns usually include a gray-scale image in a set of 16 or more bars of varying brightness levels and a grid of equally

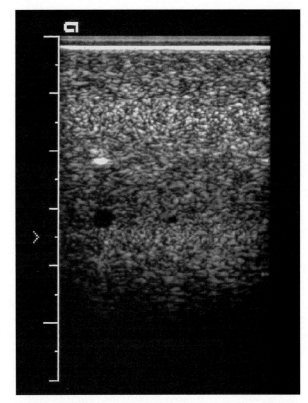

Fig. 25-7 Example of poor uniformity for a linear array transducer. A single-transmit focal zone was set at 3.5 cm. A low-intensity band is present across the image near a depth of 3 cm. This suggests that time gain compensation was not properly applied, but the banding is not constant across the width of the field of view.

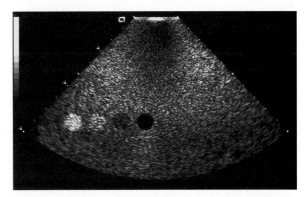

Fig. 25-8 Example of poor uniformity in the central field of view at shallow depths for a linear phased array transducer.

spaced parallel horizontal and vertical lines. The gray scale represents the entire dynamic range of potential signal levels. The grid allows an assessment of spatial distortion.

The brightness and contrast controls were adjusted at the initial setup to achieve the proper gray-scale presentation. The settings should be checked to confirm that they have not been changed. The fidelity of image display on the monitor is assessed by displaying the gray-scale test pattern. Each bar in the test pattern should be distinguished as a separate shade of gray. The gray levels must range from black to white, with midscale bars depicted in gray tones. If tearing or blurring of letters in the text occurs, the brightness adjustment is too high.

A Society of Motion Picture and Television Engineers (SMPTE) test pattern is recommended for quality control of display monitors and hard copy cameras. The ready accessibility of the test pattern as a display option in each scanner facilitates QC monitoring.

IMAGE RECORDING

The end product of an ultrasonic scan is typically a high-quality photographic reproduction of the display—a hard copy visual representation of the interactions of ultrasound with tissue. *The image recorded on film must be a faithful reproduction of the image viewed on the display monitor.* The photographic system should duplicate the structural detail of the displayed image. Additionally, the display monitor and processed film must have the potential to exhibit a full range of shades from black to white. Gray levels must extend from black to white with multiple intermediate shades. Hard copy image quality depends on the matched response between display monitor and image-recording device as well as on proper film processing. Distortion should be minimal. Hard copy images derived from QC testing also provide documentation of properly functioning equipment.

The photographic system may distort the image on the display when the image is recorded on film. The integrity of the hard copy process is evaluated by comparing direct measurements of rod separation on film with those determined from the display.

Film Processing

The assumption by some imaging departments has been that if a film processor does not develop radiographs, a QC program for that film processor is not needed. The implication has been that films from another imaging modality (e.g., ultrasound) are not susceptible to fluctuations in film processing. This is false. Variations in chemistry (replenishment rates, oxidation, and contamination), temperature, agitation, and cleanliness of the film processor all influence image quality. Every ultrasound film processor requires daily monitoring of its performance.

QC checks of the film processor should be conducted at the beginning of the workday, after processor warm-up, and before developing any patient films. This provides the opportunity to identify and correct problems before they impact on clinical practice.

The most important daily QC check is exposure, processing, and evaluation of a **sensitometric strip.** The sensitometer produces a highly stable and controlled light exposure to film that forms density variations in a step-wedge pattern (Fig. 25-9). The optical density of a particular step is measured with a densitometer, which detects the amount of transmitted light and expresses this on a logarithmic scale. The optical densities of various steps of the sensitometric strip shown in Fig. 25-9 are listed in Table 25-2.

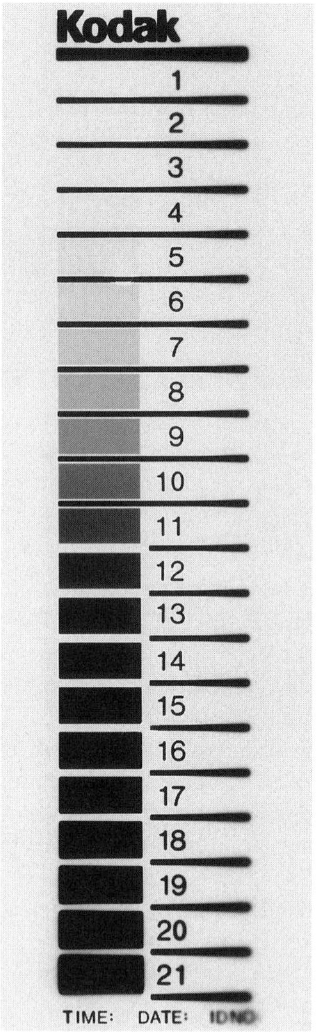

Fig. 25-9 Sensitometer strip.

■ **Table 25-2** Optical Densities of a Sensitometric Strip

Step	Optical Density	Optical Density Minus Base-Plus-Fog
1*	0.16	0
2	0.17	0.01
3	0.17	0.01
4	0.18	0.02
5	0.18	0.02
6	0.2	0.04
7	0.24	0.08
8	0.33	0.17
9	0.52	0.36
10	0.82	0.66
11	1.22	1.06
12	1.72	1.56
13	2.32	2.16
14	2.72	2.56
15	3	2.84
16-21	>3	—

*Denotes base-plus-fog.

A sensitometer with an appropriate light source is not commercially available for laser camera film. An alternate method is used to generate density steps for monitoring film processor performance. Laser cameras are configured with internal test patterns containing various gray scales that can be selected for recording on film. Although this testing procedure does not completely isolate the laser camera from the film processor, the recording of an internal test pattern is very stable.

The three parameters base-plus-fog, speed index, and contrast index have been established for the assessment of film processor performance. Base-plus-fog is the optical density obtained from a clear area on the film where no exposure to light has occurred. Three steps in the sensitometric strip that have optical densities of approximately 0.45, 1, and 2 above the base-plus-fog are identified. The optical density of 1 above base-plus-fog is classified as the speed index. The contrast index is calculated as the difference between the high-density (2) and low-density (0.45) steps.

With the data in Table 25-2 as an example, steps 9, 11, and 13 (with respective optical density of 0.36, 1.06, and 2.16 above base-plus-fog) are selected for quality-control purposes. The optical density of each step is measured whenever the sensitometric strip is processed. For this set of measurements, the speed index is 1.06 and the contrast index, 1.80.

The base-plus-fog, speed index, and contrast index must be determined, and their values recorded daily. Furthermore, each parameter must be compared with the normal operating level to ensure that its current value falls within an acceptable variation (called **control limit**) from the normal operating level. Control limits for the speed index and contrast index are ±0.15. Base-plus-fog should not increase more than 0.05 the normal value.

It is advisable to reserve a box of film (same type as used clinically) exclusively for film processor QC. The sensitometer should produce a light spectrum similar to that of the image-recording device (blue or green light for multi-format cameras), and only the emulsion side of the film should be exposed. Generation of the sensitometric strip must be the same each day (i.e., less-exposed end inserted into the processor first, film edge next to the left [or right] guide, same time delay between exposure and processing, emulsion side oriented up [or down]).

The baseline levels for base-plus-fog, speed index, and contrast index are determined by averaging their respective values for 5 consecutive days. When a new box of processor QC film is opened, five sensitometric strips should be processed to ensure that the speed index and contrast index are unchanged (within 0.02 optical density of the baseline level). Otherwise, new baseline levels must be established. A full sheet of gray-scale test pattern images is recorded in the format and size normally used clinically (i.e., a 6:1 format requires the pattern to be printed six times). Comparisons between the display and the film with these test patterns check for potential loss of contrast.

A quality-control program that faithfully measures and records the sensitometric data will be ineffective if the data are not critically evaluated and corrective action taken when indicated.

Film processors require regular cleaning. A typical cleaning schedule includes crossover racks daily, rack assemblies every 2 to 4 weeks, and tanks whenever chemical solutions are changed. Thorough cleaning of the processor is labor intensive and typically requires at least 1.5 hours.

MECHANICAL INSPECTION

The transducer acoustic surface, housing, and cable should be inspected for cracks and other damage each day of use. If liquids enter the housing, damage to the transducer will result. This also poses an electrical hazard to the operator. The connector should be examined for bent or loose prongs. The power cord should be inspected periodically for wear. Indicator lights and scan parameter displays on the console should function properly.

FREQUENCY OF QUALITY CONTROL PROCEDURES

The most frequently used transducers should be monitored on a semiannual basis, and all other transducers should be tested at least yearly. Mobile scanners are more susceptible to failure and should be tested more frequently, at least quarterly. Film processor checks should be completed each day of use. Image-recording devices should be tested at least on a quarterly basis for gray-scale contrast and at least semiannually for distortion. A scan of the TM phantom should be obtained after the unit is repaired (preferably before the service representative leaves) to confirm proper operation.

Phantom testing, initially on a quarterly basis, allows the sonographer to become proficient in the performance of QC procedures. With experience, this person is more likely to perform QC testing regularly over the long term.

DOCUMENTATION AND RECORD KEEPING

An important aspect of any QC program is documentation. QC test procedures are of little value without an effective means of recording the results for future reference. The primary concern is long-term operating performance of an imaging system, which this information provides. It is essential that all instrument settings (e.g., TGC and power) be specified for all future testing. To facilitate comparisons of results, they should be easily reproducible. Obviously, test results must be recorded. When values exceeding the control limits are obtained, further testing, the results of that testing, any corrective action (including service reports), and the results of that action should be documented.

Documentation provides potential solutions to problems that recur at a later date. Permanent records also aid in identifying problem areas in the system. Documentation of baseline values and abnormal values on a hard copy format is extremely helpful. Film storage is bulky and time

DIAGNOSTIC IMAGING DEPARTMENT
CANTON, OHIO

SCANNER	
Manufacturer	
Model	
ID	

TRANSDUCER	
Model	
Frequency	
S/N	

DATE	IMAGE UNIFORMITY (OK)	PENETRATION (CM)	DISTANCE ACCURACY		IMAGE RECORDING		INITIALS
			Depth	Lateral	Distortion	Gray Levels	

Fig. 25-10 Sample quality control form.

consuming, however; therefore appropriate test results can be recorded on special forms (Fig. 25-10). Hard copy images of results outside of the control limits are useful for proving malfunctions to service personnel, particularly for intermittent problems that disappear when the service representative arrives.

Documentation of machine or sonographer errors for both clinical and QC scans aids in identifying recurrent or systematic problems. Service records, including comments for specific problems, should be maintained.

SUMMARY

The end product of an ultrasound scan is its image. The quality of the image depends largely on a properly functioning unit. Performance characteristics of the system are monitored via a QC program. TM phantoms measure sensitivity, uniformity, and accuracy of distance markers (vertical and horizontal). Within well-defined limits, these parameters reflect properly functioning equipment.

The display monitor, hard copy camera, and film processing all contribute to the image-recording process. To optimize photographic system performance, recommendations of manufacturers of the image-recording device, film, and processing chemicals should be followed. The image-

recording device should exhibit a full range of gray-scale contrast and an accurate portrayal of size, shape, and relative positions of structures in the displayed image. Matching the response of the display monitor and the hard copy camera is necessary to ensure that what is seen on the monitor is recorded on film.

Record keeping is an important aspect of the QC program. Records of routine QC tests provide the means for monitoring performance levels of the unit over long periods. Service records should be included as part of this record-keeping process. The QC program must be structured so that the testing is performed on a consistent basis. Often programs begin with an overambitious schedule that cannot be sustained in practice, and this can result in discontinuation of the entire QC program.

REVIEW QUESTIONS

1. Name five quality control (QC) tests that are considered essential to a QC monitoring program.
2. The Society of Motion Picture and Television Engineers (SMPTE) test pattern provides the best assessment of _____.
3. Why should controls for brightness and contrast for the display monitor not be adjusted during clinical scanning?
4. What are the two major limitations of urethane phantoms?

5. Tests for sensitivity, image uniformity, and distance accuracy are most easily performed with a _____.

6. How often should processor QC be performed when film is used as the recording medium?

7. Measurements for distance accuracy yield 85 mm for a 90-mm separation in the vertical direction and 60 mm for a 60-mm separation in the horizontal direction. Since measurement in the horizontal direction is correct, no corrective action is recommended, because measurements in both directions must be in error to indicate a problem. What is the fallacy in this conclusion?

8. During routine QC testing for penetration, the maximum depth for the visualization of scatterers for a 10-MHz transducer is changed from the baseline value of 6 cm to a current value of 3 cm. What do you do next?

BIBLIOGRAPHY

Hedrick WR, Hykes DL: Image recording devices, *J Diagn Med Sonogr* 7:56-63, 1991.

Hedrick WR, Hykes DL: Photographic system quality control, *J Diagn Med Sonogr* 9:62-66, 1993.

Hedrick WR, Hykes DL: Quality control for real time ultrasound equipment, *J Diagn Med Sonogr* 13:68-75, 1997.

Goodsitt MM et al: Real-time B-mode ultrasound quality control test procedures: report of AAPM Ultrasound Task Group No. 1, *Med Phys* 25:1385-1406, 1998.

Zagzebski JA: US quality assurance with phantoms. In Goldman LW, Fowlkes JB, eds: *Categorical course in diagnostic radiology physics: CT and US cross-sectional imaging,* Oak Brook, Ill, 2000, Radiological Society of North America.

Review Test

1. Acoustic velocity is defined as the _____ .
   A. Speed of the vibrating particles that oscillate back and forth when displaced by the sound wave
   B. Speed at which the ultrasound wave propagates through the medium
   C. Number of cycles per second generated by the transducer
   D. Inverse of the frequency of the ultrasound wave

2. The wavelength of an ultrasonic wave in tissue generated by a 5-MHz transducer is _____ .
   A. 0.31 mm
   B. 0.51 mm
   C. 1.00 mm
   D. 3.22 mm

3. The term *rarefaction* describes a zone of _____ in the medium traversed by the ultrasound wave.
   A. Increased velocity
   B. Decreased molecular density
   C. High pressure
   D. Small molecular particles

4. A longitudinal wave is characterized by _____ .
   A. The ability of the sound wave to penetrate at least 5 cm in tissue

   B. Frequency of vibration greater than 1 MHz
   C. Acoustic velocity equal to 1540 m/s
   D. Particle motion in the same direction as the direction of propagation

5. What is the average acoustic velocity of a 5-MHz ultrasound wave in soft tissue?
   A. 1540 mm/s
   B. 1540 cm/s
   C. 1540 m/s
   D. 1540 ft/s

6. Which engineering prefix equals 10^{-3}?
   A. Micro
   B. Milli
   C. Mega
   D. Centi

7. What is the typical frequency range in ultrasound imaging?
   A. 60 Hz
   B. Less than 1 MHz
   C. 1 to 20 MHz
   D. 1 to 10 GHz

8. Find the period of a wave whose frequency is 2 MHz.
   A. 2 s

B. 2×10^6 s
C. 3.1×10^{-4} s
D. 5×10^{-7} s

9. When an ultrasound wave moves from a medium of low acoustic velocity into a medium with a high acoustic velocity, the wavelength _____ .
   A. Increases
   B. Decreases
   C. Remains constant

10. What are the characteristics of nonspecular reflection (or scattering)?
    A. Provides internal texture of organs in B-mode imaging
    B. Occurs at interfaces with small physical dimensions (less than one wavelength in diameter)
    C. Is strongly frequency dependent
    D. All of the above

11. The piezoelectric effect of a crystal in the transducer allows the conversion of _____ .
    A. Pressure wave to electrical energy
    B. Electrical energy to heat
    C. Ultrasound wave to heat
    D. Radiofrequency wave to video signal

12. Relative sound intensity based on a logarithmic scale is expressed typically in units of the _____ .
    A. Rayl
    B. Decibel
    C. Hertz
    D. Curie

13. If a 2.5-cycle pulse is generated from a 3.5-MHz transducer with a pulse repetition frequency of 1000 pulses per second, what is the spatial pulse length in soft tissue?
    A. 1.1 mm
    B. 1.5 mm
    C. 2.2 mm
    D. 4.4 mm

14. If a 2.5-cycle pulse is generated from a 3.5-MHz transducer with a pulse repetition frequency of 1000 pulses per second, what is the pulse duration?
    A. 1.4 μs
    B. 1 μs
    C. 0.7 μs
    D. 0.2 μs

15. If a 2.5-cycle pulse is generated from a 3.5-MHz transducer with a pulse repetition frequency of 1000 pulses per second, what is the duty factor?
    A. 0.0001
    B. 0.0007
    C. 0.0014
    D. 0.001

16. The signal processing technique of time-gain compensation (TGC) attempts to correct for _____ of the ultrasound beam.
    A. Velocity changes
    B. Attenuation
    C. Reflection
    D. Refraction

17. What is the most commonly used piezoelectric material in real-time imaging transducers?
    A. PZT
    B. Quartz
    C. Lucite
    D. Cesium iodide

18. Electronic focusing in the transmit mode for a linear array transducer is accomplished using _____ for those crystal elements forming the pulsed wave.
    A. Curved crystal elements
    B. Changeable lenses
    C. Time delays to excite crystal elements
    D. All of the above

19. A transmitted pulsed wave is necessary for B-mode imaging, because _____ .
    A. The transducer becomes too hot to handle if continuous sound waves are emitted.
    B. The crystal in the transducer would break under the stress of continuous emission.
    C. The depth of the interface from which the echo originated can be determined.
    D. Lateral resolution is improved by pulsed transmission.

20. In real-time imaging the lateral resolution (along the in-plane direction, which is perpendicular to the direction of wave travel) is influenced by _____ .
    A. Acoustic velocity
    B. Acoustic impedance
    C. Beam width
    D. All of the above

21. Find the maximum pulse repetition frequency if the depth of interest is 15 cm and the velocity is 1540 m/s. Assume the frequency is 3 MHz.
    A. 2565 pulses per second
    B. 5130 pulses per second
    C. 10,260 pulses per second
    D. 3,000,000 pulses per second

22. If each frame is composed of 200 lines of sight and the depth of scanning is 8 cm, what is the maximum frame rate in frames per second?
    A. 10
    B. 24
    C. 48
    D. 75

23. Doppler ultrasound has the potential to determine
_____ .
    A. The depth of the moving reflector
    B. The velocity of the moving reflector
    C. The direction of the moving reflector
    D. All of the above

24. The Doppler shift produced by scanning an interface
moving at a velocity of 80 cm/s is usually
_____ . Assume that the transducer is
operating at 3 MHz.
    A. Above 3 MHz
    B. Variable from 0 to 3 MHz depending on angle
    C. In the audible range
    D. None of the above

25. In continuous-wave Doppler, the reflected wave from
a moving interface is algebraically added with the
reference wave to form the _____
frequency, which is equal to the Doppler shift.
    A. Center
    B. Beat
    C. Offset
    D. Mean

26. Calculate the velocity of the moving reflector if a
Doppler shift of 1600 Hz is observed. The angle of
insonation is 60 degrees. The center frequency of the
transducer is 2 MHz.
    A. 8 cm/s
    B. 33 cm/s
    C. 52 cm/s
    D. 123 cm/s

27. Aliasing is a potential problem in pulsed-wave
Doppler, because _____ .
    A. High-frequency transducers are used
    B. Sampling of the Doppler signal is intermittent,
       not continuous
    C. Dynamic focusing directs the ultrasound beam
       along different paths
    D. Motion of the interface perpendicular to the
       direction of ultrasound wave propagation is not
       detected

28. The bending of an ultrasound wave as the wave
passes from one medium into another is called
_____ .
    A. Reflection
    B. Refraction
    C. Relaxation
    D. Reverberation

29. The placement of the reflector along the beam axis in
real-time imaging (registration of the detected object
in the image) is determined by the _____ .
    A. Amplitude of the detected echo
    B. Wavelength of the detected echo

    C. Shift in frequency between the transmitted pulse
       and detected echo
    D. Elapsed time between the transmitted pulse and
       detected echo

30. Which of the following operator-controlled
acquisition parameters can increase penetration of
the ultrasonic beam in soft tissue?
    A. Frequency of a broadband transducer
    B. Pulse repetition frequency
    C. Edge enhancement
    D. Persistence

31. Which of the following improves axial resolution in
the real-time image?
    A. Increasing transducer frequency
    B. Using a lower Q-value transducer
    C. Shortening the pulse duration
    D. All of the above

32. Which is not a type of real-time transducer?
    A. Linear array
    B. Mechanical sector
    C. Rectilinear scanner
    D. Curvilinear array

33. Which real-time transducer is electronically steered
and focused?
    A. Linear phased array
    B. Mechanical sector
    C. Annular array
    D. All of the above

34. Which real-time transducer is electronically focused
but mechanically swept across the field of view?
    A. Linear phased array
    B. Mechanical sector
    C. Annular array
    D. Linear array

35. If the field of view is expanded while maintaining the
same scanning depth (e.g., increasing the sector
angle for linear phased array), what must accompany
this change so that the lateral resolution is not
degraded?
    A. Increasing the digitization bit depth
    B. Increasing the number of scan lines in a frame
    C. Decreasing the number of pixels in the image
       matrix
    D. Decreasing the acoustic power

36. The matching layer between the crystal and tissue is
designed primarily to _____ .
    A. Insulate the patient from the hot crystal
    B. Reduce the vibration of the transducer
    C. Reduce the acoustic impedance mismatch
       between crystal and tissue
    D. Protect the crystal from mechanical shock

37. Calculate the near-field depth for a 5-mm–diameter crystal operating at 5 MHz.
    A. 20 mm
    B. 10 mm
    C. 5 mm
    D. 2 mm

38. Calculate the angle of the far-field divergence for a 5-mm–diameter crystal operating at 5 MHz.
    A. 4.3 degrees
    B. 2.1 degrees
    C. 1.1 degrees
    D. 0.6 degree

39. If the number of lines per frame in a real-time scanner is kept constant, but the pulse repetition frequency is doubled, what is the effect on the maximum frame rate?
    A. Increases by a factor of 2
    B. Decreases by a factor of 2
    C. Increases by a factor of 4
    D. Unchanged

40. In real-time imaging the transmitted ultrasound beam is not continuously generated but is pulsed. Approximately what fraction of the time is the transducer actively generating ultrasound waves?
    A. 99%
    B. 50%
    C. 10%
    D. 0.1%

41. The rate of attenuation in soft tissue is approximately _____ dB/MHz/cm.
    A. 0.01
    B. 0.7
    C. 15
    D. 40

42. An interface composed of which of the following is most likely to generate the strongest echo?
    A. Fat and soft tissue
    B. Air and soft tissue
    C. Bone and soft tissue
    D. Echo strength does not depend on composition of interface

43. Why is good contact between the transducer and patient's skin important?
    A. It increases the velocity of sound in tissue
    B. It removes air from the transducer/skin interface to enhance transmission of ultrasound waves into tissue
    C. It expands the field of view
    D. It improves axial resolution by reducing the spatial pulse length

44. The signal processing technique to eliminate low-amplitude signals below a certain magnitude is _____ .
    A. Rectification
    B. Enveloping
    C. Integration
    D. Reject

45. Dynamic range refers to _____ .
    A. Variations in signal levels that can be detected, recorded, and/or displayed
    B. Transducer frequency bandwidth that can be transmitted and received by a scanner
    C. The minimum time between successive echoes required for signal processing
    D. The enveloping window in signal processing

46. In the commercial television industry the video signal standard requires that frames are displayed at a rate of _____ frames per second.
    A. 1
    B. 30
    C. 100
    D. 525

47. What is the purpose of subdicing in the construction of a multi-element transducer?
    A. To focus the beam
    B. To reduce grating lobes
    C. To increase transmitted intensity
    D. To alter the transmitted frequency

48. Color flow Doppler imaging depicts moving reflectors with color. Each color-coded pixel displays _____ for the red blood cells in that region.
    A. Maximum velocity
    B. Mean velocity
    C. Spectral distribution of velocities
    D. Signal amplitude (proportional to number of RBCs)

49. Power Doppler imaging depicts moving reflectors with color. Each color-coded pixel displays _____ for the RBCs in that region.
    A. Maximum velocity
    B. Mean velocity
    C. Spectral distribution of velocities
    D. Signal amplitude (proportional to number of RBCs)

50. The Doppler shift produced by flowing arterial blood depends on all the following parameters **except:**
    A. Transducer frequency
    B. Velocity of RBCs
    C. Number of RBCs
    D. Angle between direction of flow and ultrasound beam

51. What is the effect on the maximum frame rate if the center frequency of the transducer is decreased from

5 MHz to 2.5 MHz? The scanning parameters of power, gain, scan range, and TGC are unchanged.
A. Increases
B. Decreases
C. No change

52. Which of the following establishes the velocity limit for detection without aliasing in pulsed-wave Doppler?
A. One half the pulse repetition frequency
B. Twice the pulse repetition frequency
C. One half the center frequency
D. Twice the center frequency

53. What is the maximum velocity limit for a continuous-wave Doppler unit operating at 3 MHz?
A. 1200 cm/s
B. 200 cm/s
C. 100 cm/s
D. No velocity limit for continuous-wave Doppler

54. In the binary system, which of the following represents the decimal number 13?
A. 10101
B. 10000
C. 01000
D. 01100
E. 01101

55. Express the binary number 1010 as a decimal number.
A. 2
B. 4
C. 6
D. 8
E. 10

56. The rate of loss of beam intensity as the pulsed ultrasound wave propagates through tissue depends on _____ .
A. Frequency
B. Pulse repetition frequency
C. Pulse duration
D. Spatial pulse length

57. In pulsed-wave Doppler what is the purpose of the wall filter?
A. Exclude echoes from stationary reflectors
B. Exclude Doppler shifts from slow-moving structures
C. Exclude Doppler shifts from fast-moving structures
D. A wall filter cannot be used in pulsed-wave Doppler

58. What is the effect on maximum frame rate if the number of lines of sight is decreased from 150 to 120 scan lines per frame?

A. Increases
B. Decreases
C. No change

59. The A-mode display depicts _____ .
A. Multiple lines of sight simultaneously
B. Multiple interfaces along a single line of sight
C. Motion of a single interface as a function of time
D. Two-dimensional spatial image of reflectors

60. What is a characteristic of static B-mode scanning?
A. Multiple lines of sight are acquired to compose the image
B. A registration arm is necessary for spatial registration
C. A scan converter (digital memory) is required to store echo data
D. All of the above

61. What is the basis for electronic receive focusing in real-time imaging (beam formation)?
A. Curved crystal elements to focus the beam
B. Time delays to excite crystal elements in an array
C. Variable transmit focal zones
D. Time delays after the echo is detected for different crystal elements

62. Which of the following properties of ultrasound forms the basis for tissue harmonic imaging?
A. Harmonic scattering from microbubbles
B. Nonlinear propagation
C. Tissue-dependent attenuation
D. Stress/strain of tissue

63. Which of the following properties of ultrasound forms the basis for elasticity imaging?
A. Harmonic scattering from microbubbles
B. Nonlinear propagation
C. Tissue-dependent attenuation
D. Stress/strain of tissue

64. Which of the following properties of ultrasound forms the basis for intermittent imaging with contrast agents?
A. Harmonic scattering from microbubbles
B. Nonlinear propagation
C. Tissue-dependent attenuation
D. Stress/strain of tissue

65. All of the following methods are used to eliminate the aliasing artifact in the time-dependent pulse-wave Doppler spectral waveform **except:**
A. Change baseline to include movement toward (or away from) the transducer only
B. Increase pulse repetition frequency to change velocity scale
C. Increase Doppler angle from 30 to 40 degrees
D. Increase power setting by 3 dB

66. How can the frame rate be increased in color Doppler imaging?
    A. Decrease width of the color field of view
    B. Increase color scan line density
    C. Decrease color gain
    D. Increase the packet size

67. The frequency of the ultrasound wave as the wave passes from high velocity medium into low velocity medium _____ .
    A. Increases
    B. Decreases
    C. Remains unchanged

68. Which of the following human tissues demonstrates the highest rate of attenuation of the ultrasound wave?
    A. Liver
    B. Fat
    C. Kidney
    D. Lung

69. The computer parameter that limits the number of brightness levels available for display of the image matrix is the _____ .
    A. Magnetic disk storage capacity in bytes
    B. Number of bits that code for pixel value
    C. Clock speed in megahertz
    D. Number of pixels in the matrix

70. Autoclaving to sterilize transducers is recommended _____ .
    A. Whenever sterilization is required
    B. To remove old coupling gel
    C. On a daily basis
    D. Never

71. Which type of real-time transducer allows electronic focusing in both the in-plane and slice thickness directions?
    A. Linear array
    B. Linear phased array
    C. Curvilinear
    D. Annular phased array

72. Which of the following factors affects the acoustic velocity in a medium?
    A. Density of the medium
    B. Thickness of the medium
    C. Frequency bandwidth
    D. Cross-sectional area of ultrasound beam

73. M-mode is characterized by which of the following?
    A. Presentation of multiple lines of sight simultaneously
    B. Two-dimensional gray-scale image
    C. Movement of a single structure interrogated by multiple lines of sight

    D. Depth of moving reflectors along single line of sight depicted in time

74. Which assumption of ultrasonic imaging is violated when a range ambiguity (depth misregistration) artifact occurs?
    A. Sound waves travel along a straight path
    B. Acoustic velocity is a constant 1540 m/s
    C. Detected echoes originate from the most recent transmitted pulse
    D. Narrow beam width limits the sampling volume

75. A pulsed ultrasound wave is generated by the transducer and transmitted into tissue. The power setting on the scanner is increased. The acoustic pressure in tissue is increased, and the _____ is also increased.
    A. Acoustic velocity
    B. Acoustic impedance
    C. Mechanical index
    D. Wavelength

76. The thermal index indicates _____ .
    A. Maximum temperature rise in tissue
    B. Minutes of exposure time before heating is too great
    C. Seconds of exposure time before heating is too great
    D. Acoustic power in milliwatts

77. The mechanical index gives the likelihood of _____ .
    A. Fetal abnormality
    B. Cavitation
    C. Thermal damage
    D. Rotational motion

78. Comparing the velocity of sound in soft tissue and in blood, the velocity of sound in blood is _____ .
    A. Twice as fast
    B. Slightly faster
    C. Slightly slower
    D. Fifty percent slower

79. Echoes produced by moving red blood cells are _____ in amplitude compared with those created in the surrounding soft tissue.
    A. Weaker
    B. Stronger
    C. Similar

80. The rate of blood flow is directly proportional to the _____ difference along the length of the vessel.
    A. Density
    B. Lumen diameter
    C. Pressure
    D. Viscosity

81. Which pressure source contributes to the overall intravascular pressure within a blood vessel?
    A. Contraction of heart
    B. Static filling pressure
    C. Hydrostatic pressure
    D. All of the above

82. Whose principle describes the conservation of total fluid energy as blood moves through the circulation?
    A. Bernoulli
    B. Charles
    C. Poiseuille
    D. Reynolds

83. If the hematocrit of blood is increased, what is the effect on the viscosity of the blood?
    A. Increased
    B. Decreased
    C. Remains unchanged

84. Energy reduction in the kinetic energy component of the fluid energy is often called _____ loss.
    A. Doppler
    B. Heat
    C. Hydrostatic
    D. Inertia

85. Localized, relatively slow rotation of concentric blood layers is called _____ .
    A. Curls
    B. Eddy flow
    C. Stagnant zone
    D. Whirlpool

86. The ability of arteries to expand and store large quantities of blood is called _____ .
    A. Cardiac output
    B. Compliance
    C. Resistance
    D. Stroke volume

87. Which of the following causes pulsatile flow in the arteries?
    A. Compliance
    B. Heart contraction
    C. Hydrostatic pressure
    D. Peripheral resistance

88. Regulation of volume flow rate is primarily accomplished by changes in _____ .
    A. Aortic valve opening
    B. Blood viscosity
    C. Circulation path length
    D. Peripheral resistance

89. A Reynolds' number above _____ in straight, smooth vessels is an indicator of turbulent flow.
    A. 2
    B. 20
    C. 200
    D. 2000

90. The recording device for a freeze-frame image during Doppler imaging is most often the

    _____ .
    A. Video cassette recorder
    B. Multiformat camera
    C. Color video printer
    D. Laser camera

91. Mechanisms by which biologic effects are induced by ultrasound include all of the following **except:**
    A. Cavitation
    B. Heating
    C. Radiation force
    D. Ionization

92. The temporal-averaged intensity is equal to the product of the pulse-averaged intensity and the

    _____ .
    A. Duty factor
    B. Diameter of transducer
    C. Area of ultrasonic beam
    D. Spatial pulse length

93. Avoiding a local temperature rise above _____ should ensure no thermally induced biologic effects. Choose the highest temperature for which adverse effects have not been demonstrated.
    A. 0.1° C
    B. 1° C
    C. 4° C
    D. None, thermal effects have no threshold

94. Distance error along the direction of propagation is caused by _____ .
    A. Measurements not performed within the transmit focal zone
    B. A pulse repetition frequency below 200 Hz
    C. An incorrect instrument setting for velocity in tissue
    D. Low scan line density

95. What is the purpose of quality control testing of imaging equipment?
    A. Long-term monitoring of scanner performance to ensure high-quality images are obtained consistently
    B. A means to evaluate sonographer competence
    C. Short-term monitoring of image quality during selected time periods (e.g., one quarter per year) for accreditation purposes
    D. Has no relevance to clinical performance

96. Tissue mimicking phantoms are composed of materials designed to exhibit _____ .

A. The same acoustic properties for ultrasound propagation through tissue, including attenuation, velocity, and scattering

B. The same acoustic velocity as ultrasound in tissue without regard to attenuation so that distance accuracy can be evaluated

C. The same attenuation rate without regard to velocity of propagation so that sensitivity can be evaluated

D. The same density and acoustic impedance of tissue

97. Examine the color Doppler image of the fetus in Color Plate 24. The study was interpreted as fetal demise. What is the cause of the color encoding associated with the fetus in this color Doppler image?
    A. Umbilical blood flow
    B. Transducer movement by the operator
    C. Artifact related to the presence of air in the fetal heart
    D. Nonlinear propagation that produces harmonic scattering

98. In pulsed-wave Doppler spectral analysis, the pulsatility index is computed from the time-varying trace of the _____ .
    A. Maximum pressure
    B. Maximum velocity
    C. Velocity variance
    D. All of the above

99. Turbulent flow distal to an 80% stenosis has velocity components characterized by _____ .
    A. Disorder, multiple flow directions
    B. Higher speed than observed at stenosis
    C. Prevalently negative
    D. Uniform flow direction

100. Mild arterial obstruction (50% reduction in lumen area) will cause decreased blood flow in the affected extremity during _____ .
    A. Exercise
    B. Rest
    C. Both rest and exercise
    D. None of the above

101. Body position (e.g., standing or lying down) affects the _____ pressure in the venous system.
    A. Filling
    B. Hydrostatic
    C. Transmural
    D. All of the above

102. Insonation at a large Doppler angle (>60 degrees) is desirable, because _____ .
    A. Doppler signal is increased with higher Doppler angle
    B. Doppler shift is at higher frequency

C. Error in measurement of the Doppler shift is reduced
D. Large Doppler angle is not desirable

103. Which operator control adjusts the dynamic range of the displayed signal amplitudes?
    A. Compression
    B. Receiver gain
    C. Reject
    D. Edge enhancement

104. By placing the transesophageal probe in close proximity to the heart, the scan range is decreased, and thus _____ can be increased.
    A. Frame rate
    B. Transducer frequency
    C. Lines of sight
    D. All of the above

105. Why is a linear phased array with a small footprint desirable for real-time imaging of the heart? The small active area for sound generation allows _____ .
    A. Control of near field sampling volume
    B. High frame rate
    C. High pulse repetition frequency
    D. Reduced attenuation of ultrasound beam

106. Turbulent flow as depicted in color Doppler imaging is characterized by a _____ color pattern.
    A. Linear gradient
    B. Mosaic
    C. Smooth boundary
    D. Uniform

107. Reflectivity of an object interrogated by an ultrasound beam is determined by _____ .
    A. Composition of the interface
    B. Orientation
    C. Physical size
    D. All of the above

108. In M-mode scanning, how is the reflectivity of the reflector presented?
    A. Brightness modulation of trace
    B. Peak height of trace
    C. Line width of trace
    D. Slope of trace

109. What is the image format for a linear phased array transducer?
    A. Rectangular
    B. Sector
    C. Parallelogram
    D. Selectable by the operator

110. Multiple zone transmit focusing with a linear array most likely will cause a reduction in the _____ .

A. Frame rate
B. Pulse duration
C. Axial resolution
D. Transmitted intensity

111. The ability of a real-time scanner to evaluate rapid motion is closely associated with _____ .
    A. Frame rate
    B. Pulse duration
    C. Transmitted intensity
    D. Transducer frequency

112. In color Doppler imaging, increasing the packet size from three to seven pulses per scan line will affect the _____ .
    A. Axial resolution
    B. Strength of the echo signals
    C. Accuracy of velocity estimates
    D. All of the above

113. What effect will increasing the power have on the B-mode image?
    A. Increase the penetration
    B. Improve signal from weak scatterers
    C. Reduce the receiver gain
    D. All of the above

114. Which of the following describes a pixel?
    A. Corresponds to small physical dimensions within the patient
    B. Picture element
    C. Smallest spatial component of a digital image
    D. All of the above

115. Which component controls brightness on a cathode ray tube (CRT) screen?
    A. Deflecting plates
    B. Focusing coils
    C. Electron flow
    D. High voltage from cathode to screen

116. Which component controls position of the electron beam on a CRT screen?
    A. Deflecting plates
    B. Focusing coils
    C. Tube current
    D. High voltage from cathode to screen

117. How many pixels compose an image in which the matrix is described as 400 rows and 400 columns?
    A. 400
    B. 800
    C. 160,000
    D. 64,000,000

118. Main memory has a _____ access time compared with storage devices, such as magnetic disk drives.

A. Shorter
B. Longer
C. Similar

119. The term *capacity* with respect to computer memory refers to _____ .
    A. Speed of information retrieval
    B. Number of storage locations
    C. Address of storage location
    D. Number of communication channels

120. Which of the following describes RAM (random access memory)?
    A. Is assessed in sequence, reading the contents of each location one after another
    B. Can be changed (written to)
    C. Contains the control unit
    D. Is slower than getting information from a magnetic disk

121. Name a method to eliminate the aliasing artifact in the Doppler spectral waveform.
    A. Increase pulse repetition frequency
    B. Increase the transmit power
    C. Decrease the range gate
    D. Decrease the amplifier gain

122. The translation of pixel value to brightness level in the displayed image is called _____ .
    A. Baud transfer
    B. Gray-scale mapping
    C. Interpolation
    D. Smoothing

123. The advantage of a 256×256 image format compared with a 64×64 image format is _____ .
    A. Greater spatial detail is possible
    B. Lower capacity memory is required
    C. Number of shades of gray is increased
    D. Contrast sensitivity is increased

124. What is contrast enhancement as it pertains to digital images?
    A. A change in the digitization of the detector signals to alter pixel brightness
    B. Redistribution of gray scale to emphasize the difference in pixel values over a narrow range
    C. A filtering algorithm
    D. A technique of signal averaging

125. The depth of a reflector is 4 cm from the transducer. How long after the transmitted pulse is the echo from this interface incident on the transducer?
    A. 26 µs
    B. 52 µs
    C. 104 µs
    D. 208 µs

126. Calculate the frequency for the ultrasound wave, which has a wavelength of 0.2 mm in soft tissue.
    - A. 10 MHz
    - B. 7.5 MHz
    - C. 5 MHz
    - D. 2.5 MHz

127. Reflection of the sound beam from a large interface with a rough surface is called _____ .
    - A. Scattering
    - B. Diffraction
    - C. Diffuse reflection
    - D. Nonspecular reflection

128. Which interaction is associated with the divergence of the sound beam after passing through a small aperture?
    - A. Scattering
    - B. Diffraction
    - C. Diffuse reflection
    - D. Nonspecular reflection

129. If the acoustic pressure is increased, the _____ also is increased.
    - A. Acoustic velocity
    - B. Wavelength
    - C. Intensity
    - D. Acoustic impedance

130. What is the design objective to generate an ultrasonic beam for imaging purposes?
    - A. Unidirectional
    - B. Short-duration pulsed wave
    - C. Narrow beam width
    - D. All of the above

131. Which transducer factor characterizes the frequency bandwidth of the transmitted ultrasound wave?
    - A. Acoustic impedance
    - B. Density
    - C. Electromechanical coupling coefficient
    - D. Q-value

132. What component of the transducer is designed to enhance transmission of sound energy into the patient?
    - A. Backing material
    - B. Electrical insulator
    - C. Matching layer
    - D. Radiofrequency shield

133. Transmit focusing by varying the beam aperture is accomplished in a multi-element array by _____ .
    - A. Curved crystal elements
    - B. Changeable acoustic lenses
    - C. Time delays to excite crystal elements
    - D. Variable number of elements to form the pulsed beam

134. Varying the excitation voltage to each crystal in the group used to form the transmitted ultrasound pulse is called _____ .
    - A. Apodization
    - B. Integration
    - C. Interelement isolation
    - D. Subdicing

135. Which operator control affects the maximum frame rate?
    - A. Compression
    - B. Transmit power
    - C. Scan range
    - D. Time gain compensation

136. What detection method is used in color Doppler imaging?
    - A. Autocorrelation
    - B. Fast Fourier transform
    - C. Heterodyne
    - D. Demodulation

137. A color Doppler imaging scanner is described as an asynchronous scanner. The scanner has the following characteristic:
    - A. Gray-scale and flow-scan data are acquired with separate transmitted pulses.
    - B. No velocity limit is imposed for the detection of flowing blood.
    - C. Color and gray scale have the same field of view.
    - D. Design is obsolete and not used clinically.

138. What is the unit for power?
    - A. Pascal
    - B. Watts/cm^2
    - C. Watts
    - D. Megahertz

139. What is the unit for pressure?
    - A. Pascal
    - B. Watts/cm^2
    - C. Watts
    - D. Megahertz

140. Which is a characteristic of transient cavitation?
    - A. Has no threshold
    - B. Is readily observed in tissue at diagnostic intensity levels
    - C. Formation and collapse of microbubbles
    - D. All of the above

141. Small, high-acoustic impedance objects create multiple internal reflections, which when expressed in the image are called _____ artifacts.
    - A. Mirror image
    - B. Comet tail
    - C. Reverberation
    - D. Refraction

142. Which imaging artifact is associated with multiple reflections between two strong reflectors along the ultrasonic path, creating progressively weaker bands in the image?
    A. Mirror image
    B. Comet tail
    C. Reverberation
    D. Refraction

143. The technique of frame averaging (or persistence) during real-time acquisition is designed to _____ .
    A. Increase the signal to noise
    B. Decrease pixel size
    C. Redistribute the gray scale
    D. Enhance spatial resolution

144. Which is a type of study to determine if an association exists between an adverse effect in a population and exposure to a particular agent?
    A. Case report
    B. Epidemiologic
    C. In vitro
    D. In vivo

145. The output display standard (ODS) of mechanical index increases in magnitude as the _____ is decreased.
    A. Acoustic pressure
    B. Acoustic velocity
    C. Frequency
    D. Beam width

146. What parameter as a monitor of film processor performance is obtained by exposure and processing of the sensitometric strip?
    A. Base plus fog
    B. Contrast index
    C. Speed index
    D. All of the above

147. If the frequency of the transducer is changed from 5 MHz to 2 MHz, what is the effect on the observed Doppler shift for a moving reflector?
    A. Increases
    B. Decreases
    C. Remains the same

148. The depth of the focal zone for a single element transducer is established by the _____ .
    A. Excitation pulse voltage
    B. Curvature of the crystal
    C. Pulse repetition frequency
    D. Pulse duration

149. What is the fast Fourier transform?
    A. A mathematic technique that analyzes the frequency components in the echo-induced signal
    B. A means of electronic dynamic focusing according to the anticipated frequency components of the Doppler signal
    C. A specialized piezoelectric crystal whose signal output depends on the frequency of the echo-induced signal
    D. An audible amplifier that drives stereo speakers according to the frequency components in the echo-induced signal

150. Which of the following will affect the acoustic output?
    A. Receiver amplification
    B. Time gain compensation
    C. Frame averaging
    D. Transmit power

151. If the center frequency of a broadband transducer is changed from 2 MHz to 5 MHz, what is the effect on acoustic velocity in soft tissue?
    A. Acoustic velocity is increased
    B. Acoustic velocity is decreased
    C. Acoustic velocity is unchanged

152. The mirror-image artifact in real-time imaging is most likely to occur if _____ .
    A. Refraction by overlying tissues changes the straight-line beam path
    B. A structure is located in front of a strongly reflective interface
    C. An air-filled cavity undergoes resonance
    D. Propagation speed changes along the beam path

153. What are the advantages of color Doppler imaging?
    A. Presents global hemodynamics in real time
    B. Superior gray-scale imaging readily detects plaques
    C. Eliminates the need for Fourier analysis of a vessel segment
    D. All of the above

154. Which of the following does **not** rely on wave interference?
    A. Generation of beat frequency
    B. Beam formation
    C. Huygens' principle
    D. Time gain compensation

155. Rank the following tissues with respect to acoustic velocity (fastest to slowest): soft tissue, bone, air, and fat.
    A. Soft tissue, bone, air, fat
    B. Bone, soft tissue, air, fat
    C. Bone, soft tissue, fat, air
    D. Bone, fat, soft tissue, air

156. What is a potential cause for loss of coherence (reduced net signal) during signal summing in the beam former?

A. High receiver gain

B. Velocity differences along beam paths to crystal elements

C. Low pulse repetition frequency

D. High setting for frame averaging (persistence)

157. Which of the following is **not** associated with nonlinear propagation in soft tissue?

A. High-intensity, transmitted, pulsed wave

B. Generation of harmonic frequencies

C. Distortion of the sinusoidal wave

D. Uniform acoustic velocity throughout the wave cycle

158. At a particular crystal in a multi-element array transducer, the intensity of the echo from a reflector depends on all of the following **except:**

A. Acoustic velocity

B. Composition of the interface

C. Depth of the reflector

D. Transmitted frequency

159. Doppler imaging of a microbubble contrast agent located in the liver shows a color mosaic throughout the parenchyma. What is the source of this color-encoded signal?

A. Broadband transducer

B. Destruction of microbubbles

C. Generation of harmonics in tissue

D. Rapid motion

160. Which interaction between tissue and sound waves is responsible for energy conversion to heat?

A. Scattering

B. Absorption

C. Diffraction

D. Interference

161. Attenuation by a thickness of material equal to one half-value layer corresponds to a loss of intensity of _____ dB.

A. 1/2

B. 1

C. 3

D. 10

162. What component stores scan data during real-time acquisition and then periodically is read line by line for display?

A. Monitor

B. Scan converter

C. Phosphor plate

D. Magnetic disk

163. What is the typical axial resolution for a 5-MHz transducer?

A. 0.1 mm

B. 0.5 mm

C. 3 mm

D. 5 mm

164. Slice thickness for a linear array transducer is _____ throughout the field of view.

A. Constant with depth

B. Variable (minimum slice thickness is within the transmit focal zone)

C. Variable (minimum slice thickness is within the fixed focal zone of the curved elements)

D. Variable (minimum slice thickness depends on beam aperture)

165. Identify the type of scanning system that has B-mode imaging and Doppler (either pulsed-wave or continuous-wave) capabilities.

A. B-mode

B. Duplex

C. Hertz

D. M-mode

166. The region near the transducer/tissue interface in which scan data fails to correlate with objects is called the _____ .

A. Dead zone

B. Insensitivity zone

C. Quiet zone

D. Overlap zone

167. According to the American Institute of Ultrasound in Medicine Statement on Mammalian In Vivo Biological Effects, no independently confirmed significant biologic effects have occurred with spatial peak, temporal average intensities below _____ for mammalian tissues exposed in vivo. Assume unfocused ultrasound.

A. 1 W/cm^2

B. 100 W/cm^2

C. 1 mW/cm^2

D. 100 mW/cm^2

168. Shadowing, an artifact in B-mode imaging, is _____ .

A. Caused by a highly attenuating structure along the beam path

B. Typically observed distal to a cystic structure

C. Caused by noise from radiofrequency wave interference

D. Related to propagation speed errors along the beam path

169. Comparing the spatial pulse length for pulsed-wave Doppler and B-mode imaging, the Doppler technique typically has _____ spatial pulse length.

A. Longer

B. Shorter

C. Equivalent

170. What is the acoustic impedance in Mrayls for muscle whose density is 1080 kg/m^3? Assume the velocity in muscle is 1580 m/s and the frequency of sound is 5 MHz.
    A. 0.86
    B. 1.71
    C. 2.92
    D. 8.55

171. A computer system that allows digitized images from various imaging modalities to be stored electronically for later retrieval, display, manipulation, interpretation, and distribution to remote locations is called _____ .
    A. DICOM
    B. HIS
    C. PACS
    D. RIS

172. What is the advantage of data compression for an image management computer system?
    A. It reduces image storage requirements
    B. It reduces image transmission time
    C. It reduces costs
    D. All of the above

173. What file and communication standard allows devices from multiple manufacturers to be incorporated into an image management network?
    A. DICOM
    B. HIS
    C. PACS
    D. RIS

174. All of the following are essential viewing capabilities/conditions for a workstation used for soft copy interpretation of imaging studies **except:**
    A. Low ambient light level
    B. Indirect lighting
    C. Removal of sources of glare
    D. Flat panel monitor

175. What method is used to isolate the harmonic signal in tissue harmonic imaging?
    A. Autocorrelation
    B. Fast Fourier transform
    C. Pulse inversion
    D. Time domain correlation

176. What is the advantage of multiple beam formers in real-time scanning?
    A. Improve axial resolution
    B. Increase frame rate
    C. Reduce equipment costs
    D. Increase signal-to-noise ratio

177. Which of the following is most likely to affect visualization of a 2-cm–diameter lesion that has

slight differences in scattering properties compared with the surrounding tissue?
    A. Acoustic noise
    B. Center frequency
    C. Scan line density
    D. Spatial pulse length

178. The partial volume artifact such as cyst fill-in is caused by _____ .
    A. Dimensions of the object smaller than the beam width
    B. High acoustic impedance of the cyst
    C. Propagation error for sound transmission across the cyst
    D. Refraction of the beam by the curved surface

179. Which of the following statements describes a multi-element transducer with five rows of crystal elements (1.5D)?
    A. Beam steering in multiple planes for volume acquisitions
    B. Electronic focusing along the slice thickness direction
    C. Scan lines obtained simultaneously from each row of crystals
    D. All of the above

180. How is scan data for the extended-field-of-view image acquired?
    A. With the transducer stationary, the beam is steered over a 120-degree arc
    B. Rocking the transducer back and forth about a single pivot point
    C. As the transducer is moved across the patient surface, a series of B-mode images is obtained
    D. Specially designed 1.5D transducer steers the beam over the wide field of view

181. If the physical size of a cyst is 2 cm in diameter, what is the depicted size in the image? Assume that the acoustic velocity in the cyst is 1000 m/s.
    A. 1.3 cm
    B. 2 cm
    C. 3.1 cm
    D. 6.2 cm

182. Calculate the transmitted angle if an ultrasound beam is directed at a large interface composed of soft tissue and fat. The angle of incidence is 20 degrees. Assume the sound beam to be moving from fat to soft tissue.
    A. 17.7 degrees
    B. 18.9 degrees
    C. 21.2 degrees
    D. 23.4 degrees

183. Which of the following statements is true regarding the Doppler effect?

A. The Doppler shift is the difference between the transmitted frequency and the observed frequency
B. The magnitude of the Doppler shift does not depend on the relative velocity between the source and the receiver
C. The maximum Doppler shift will occur when the direction of ultrasound wave propagation is perpendicular to the motion
D. All of the above

184. Which of the following statements are true regarding analog-to-digital conversion?
    A. Accuracy of the digitization of the echo amplitude is improved by increasing the bit depth
    B. Provides continuously variable output
    C. A bit depth of two is adequate for B-mode imaging
    D. All of the above

185. What is the effect of the postprocessing technique of smoothing applied to image data?
    A. It reduces pixel value variations caused by noise
    B. It decreases pixel size
    C. It redistributes the gray scale
    D. It enhances spatial resolution

186. What does the computer term baud rate describe?
    A. Storage capacity
    B. Clock speed
    C. Data transmission
    D. Program execution time

187. The hard copy recording with a laser camera shows a loss of contrast resolution compared with the image displayed on the monitor. What is the most likely cause of poor film quality?
    A. Persistence (temporal averaging) is set too high
    B. Gain is set too high
    C. Gray-scale response of the monitor and camera is not matched
    D. Data transmission to the laser camera is corrupted

188. What is the major disadvantage of transparency film as an image storage medium?
    A. Limited spatial resolution
    B. Limited contrast scale
    C. Storage space requirements
    D. Poor long-term stability

189. Which of the following is used to evaluate gray-scale contrast on the display monitor and film?
    A. Sensitometer
    B. SMPTE test pattern
    C. Hydrophone
    D. Microbalance

190. Which device measures acoustic pressure in the ultrasonic field?
    A. Sensitometer
    B. SMPTE test pattern
    C. Hydrophone
    D. Microbalance

191. What is the advantage of rectangular array transducers compared with linear array transducers?
    A. Volumetric acquisition without moving the transducer
    B. Reduced channel number
    C. Improved spatial detail
    D. Compact size

192. Which of the following is a source of acoustic noise?
    A. Apodization
    B. Low-power transmitted pulse
    C. Radiofrequency wave interference
    D. Speckle

193. In tissue harmonic imaging, where are harmonics most likely to be formed?
    A. Uniformly within the ultrasonic field
    B. Near the transducer face
    C. Near the beam axis
    D. Distal to the focal point

194. In tissue harmonic imaging, the spatial pulse length is sometimes increased. Why?
    A. To improve axial resolution
    B. To enhance the isolation of harmonic frequency components in the echo signal
    C. To increase harmonic production in tissue
    D. To increase the signal-to-noise ratio

195. A curved nodule is depicted more clearly with spatial compounding. What is the reason for this improvement in image quality?
    A. Autocorrelation detection used in signal processing
    B. Nodule interrogated from multiple angles
    C. Speckle reduced at higher transmitted frequencies
    D. All of the above

196. Image quality is characterized by all the following **except:**
    A. Spatial resolution
    B. Contrast resolution
    C. Mechanical index
    D. Noise

197. Which technique improves spatial resolution by decreasing the B-mode field of view?
    A. Decreased spatial pulse length
    B. Frame averaging
    C. Read zoom
    D. Write zoom

198. As the supervisor, what should you do in response to complaints of poor clinical image quality by a single sonographer?
    A. Ignore them
    B. Call for service
    C. Investigate if the problem is associated with a particular transducer or sonographer
    D. Purchase a new scanner

199. Quality control testing indicates that the distance measurements in the horizontal direction are not accurate. What is the most likely cause?

A. Velocity calibration is not 1540 m/s
B. Problems with beam steering
C. Geometric distortion from nonlinear propagation
D. High-frequency components associated with broadband transducers

200. What adverse effects have been associated with ultrasound exposure in utero?
    A. Cancer
    B. Low birth weight
    C. Congenital malformations
    D. All of the above

Review of Mathematics

VARIABLES

In physics and mathematics, letters are often used to designate variables. They represent numbers and can be treated in the same manner as numbers. Often the value of a variable must be determined based on a given set of conditions (i.e., an algebraic equation must be solved). However, letters are also used to define various legitimate mathematic operations, which are necessary for the establishment of internal consistency. For example, a particular operation may be true for all positive integers. It is certainly more convenient to represent this set of numbers with a letter than to attempt to list all members of the set. In problem solving, as long as we obey the "rules" and perform the mathematic operations in the proper order, the final answer will always be correct. This assumes that the logical interpretation of the problem, particularly a word problem, is correct.

EXPONENTS

The product of identical factors can be represented in exponential notation:

$$3^4 = 3 \bullet 3 \bullet 3 \bullet 3 = 81$$

or as

$$a^4 = a \bullet a \bullet a \bullet a$$

In this example, 3 (or a) is called the base. In the more general form, the variable a represents any real number. The superscript 4 is the power, which indicates how many times the factor 3 (or a) is multiplied times itself. A more inclusive form would be

$$a^n = a \bullet a \bullet a \bullet \ldots a \text{ (n factors)}$$

where n is a positive integer.

The use of exponents makes many operations faster and easier. The power can be extended to include negative integers if the relation between positive and negative exponents is defined:

$$a^{-n} = \frac{1}{a^n}$$

Examples of Negative Exponents

If $a = 2$ and $n = 3$, then

$$2^{-3} = \frac{1}{2^3}$$

$$2^{-3} = \frac{1}{2 \bullet 2 \bullet 2} = \frac{1}{8} = 0.125$$

If $a = 10$ and $n = 2$, then

$$10^{-2} = \frac{1}{10^2}$$

$$10^{-2} = \frac{1}{10 \bullet 10} = \frac{1}{100} = 0.125$$

Note that the final result is a positive number with a value between 0 and 1. Bases raised to negative powers provide a means of expressing small numbers.

Laws for manipulating exponents must be defined. When multiplying variables in exponential form, add the powers together and retain the base:

$$a^m + a^n = a^{m+n}$$

When dividing variables in exponential form, subtract the power of the variable in the denominator from the power of the variable in the numerator and retain the base:

$$\frac{a^m}{a^n} = a^{m-n}$$

In both cases the bases must be the same for the exponents to be combined.

Examples of Multiplication Involving Exponents

$$2^2 \bullet 2^3 = 2^{2+3} = 2^5$$

$$x^4 \bullet x^3 = x^{4+3} = x^7$$

$$y \bullet y^3 \bullet y^5 = y^{(1+3+5)} = y^9$$

$$x^3 \bullet x^{-2} = x^{3-2} = x^1$$

$$(x^2y^3)(xy^2) = (x^2x^1)(y^3y^2) = x^{(2+1)}y^{(3+2)} = x^3y^5$$

$$(4x^2)(3x^3) = (4)(3)x^{(2+3)} = 12x^5$$

Examples of Division Involving Exponents

$$\frac{2^4}{2^2} = 2^{4-2} = 2^2$$

$$\frac{x^5}{x^3} = x^{5-3} = x^2$$

$$\frac{x^2y^4}{y} = x^2y^{4-1} = x^2y^3$$

$$\frac{10^3}{10^6} = 10^{3-6} = 10^{-3} = \frac{1}{10^3}$$

The product of factors in which one of the factors has an exponent equal to zero is given by

$$a^0 \bullet a^n = a^{0+n} = a^n$$

Therefore a^0 must equal 1, because only the product of the number 1 and any other number is the latter number. In general, any base raised to the 0 power is equal to 1. Consider

$$a^n \bullet a^{-n} = a^{n-n} = a^0 = 1$$

Or, substituting numbers

$$2^3 \bullet 2^{-3} = 2^3 \bullet \frac{1}{2^3} = \frac{2^3}{2^3} = 1$$

or

$$= 8 \bullet \frac{1}{8} = \frac{8}{8} = 1$$

or

$$= 2^{(3-3)} = 2^0 = 1$$

Other operations include raising a group of factors to the nth power.

$$(a^m)^n = a^{mn}$$

$$(ab)^n = a^nb^n$$

$$\left(\frac{a}{b}\right)^n = \frac{a^n}{b^n}$$

Examples of Factors Raised to Various Powers

$$(4^2)^3 = 4^6 = 4096$$

$$\text{or } (4^2)^3 = (4^2)(4^2)(4^2) = 4^{(2+2+2)} = 4^6 = 4096$$

$$(x^3)^3 = x^9$$

$$(y^2x^2)^4 = y^8x^8$$

$$\left(\frac{2x^3}{y}\right)^2 = \frac{2^2x^6}{y^2} = \frac{4x^6}{y^2}$$

The allowable values for exponents can be expanded to include exponents expressed in fractional form:

$$a^{1/n} \text{ (nth root of a)}$$

which indicates one of n equal factors of a. That is, a factor multiplied times itself n times equals a. If $n = 2$, then $a^{1/2}$ represents the square root of a; if $n = 3$, then $a^{1/3}$ represents the cube root of a, and so on.

Examples of Roots (Fractional Exponents)

$$4^{1/2} = 2 \text{ or } -2 \text{ because } 2 \bullet 2 = 4 \text{ or } -2 \bullet -2 = 4$$

$$8^{1/3} = 2 \text{ because } 2 \bullet 2 \bullet 2 = 8$$

$$27^{1/3} = 3 \text{ because } 3 \bullet 3 \bullet 3 = 27$$

$$16^{1/4} = 2 \text{ or } -2 \text{ because } 2 \bullet 2 \bullet 2 \bullet 2 = 16$$

$$\text{or } -2 \bullet -2 \bullet -2 \bullet -2 = 16$$

The previously defined rules for multiplication and division also apply to fractional exponents. In addition, operations with fractional exponents include

$$(a^{1/n})^m = a^{m/n} = (a^m)^{1/n}$$

where a is a nonnegative number.

Further Examples of Fractional Exponents

$$(8^{1/3})^2 = 8^{2/3} = (8^2)^{1/3}$$

$$(8^{1/3})^2 = (2)^2 = 4$$

$$(8^2)^{1/3} = (64)^{1/3} = 4$$

$$(x^{1/2})^5 = x^{5/2} = (x^5)^{1/2}$$

SCIENTIFIC NOTATION

In physics we often deal with very large or very small numbers. For example, it is inconvenient to write the frequency of a 5 MHz transducer as 5,000,000 Hz. Fortunately, a method called scientific notation has been developed to represent and manipulate these numbers easily. In scientific notation the number is expressed as the product of a number between 1 and 10 and a power of 10 (base 10 with an integer exponent). If the exponent of the power of 10 is positive, the value of the power of 10 is greater than 1. If the exponent is negative, the value of the power of 10 is between 0 and 1. As with any base raised to the zero power, 10^0 is defined as being equal to 1. Numbers represented in powers of 10 are shown in the following table:

Number	Power of 10 Notation
10,000	10^4
1000	10^3
100	10^2
10	10^1
1	10^0
0.1	10^{-1}
0.01	10^{-2}
0.001	10^{-3}

Note that, for positive exponents, the value of the exponent gives the number of zeros that follow the 1 in the decimal number. For example, 10^4 is equal to 10,000, and there are four zeros after the 1. In the case of negative exponents, the value of the exponent indicates the number of places to the right of the decimal point where the 1 is located. For example, in the case of 10^{-2}, the 1 is located in the second decimal place (0.01).

The numbers 3796 and 0.0214 converted to scientific notation are written as

$$3.796 \times 10^3$$

and

$$2.14 \times 10^{-2}$$

respectively. In each case the representation of the numeric value is identical. The scientific notation form is equal to 3.796×1000, which, in turn, is 3796. Similarly, 2.14×0.01 is 0.0214.

There are a few basic rules for converting a number into scientific notation. The first step is to determine the sign of the exponent. If the number is greater than 1, the exponent is positive. If the number is between 0 and 1, the exponent is negative. The second step is to count the number of decimal places that are moved to have a single digit to the left of the decimal point. This determines the integer value of the exponent. The number 3796 can be pictured with a decimal point after the 6 initially: 3796. The decimal point is moved three places to the left to give a number between 1 and 10 (i.e., 3.796). The final task is to combine this number with a power of 10 so that the product equals the original number. The power of 10 has an exponent of +3, because the original number was greater than 1, and the decimal was moved three places to the left. The final result is 3.796×10^3.

In a similar fashion, a number less than 1 (e.g., 0.0214) is converted to scientific notation. The exponent 10 in this case is equal to –2, because the decimal point must be moved to the right two places to give 2.14. Combining this number with the power of 10 gives the final result 2.14×10^{-2}.

To convert a number expressed in scientific notation back into standard format, the process is essentially reversed; that is, a positive exponent indicates how many places to move the decimal point to the right, and a negative exponent indicates how many places to move the decimal point to the left.

For the number 8.75×10^4 the decimal point must be moved four places to the right (to give 87,500), whereas

6.34×10^{-3} requires the decimal point to be moved to the left three places (to give 0.00634).

When multiplying or dividing numbers expressed in scientific notation, we treat the numeric factors as a group and the powers of 10 as another group. Manipulation of the powers of 10 follows all the laws of exponents. These operations are summarized by

$$(a \times 10^n)(b \times 10^m) = ab \times 10^{n+m}$$

and

$$\frac{(a \times 10^n)}{(b \times 10^m)} = \frac{a}{b} \times 10^{n-m}$$

EXAMPLES USING SCIENTIFIC NOTATION

$$(4 \times 10^2)(1.5 \times 10^3) = (4)(1.5) \times 10^2 \times 10^3$$
$$= 6 \times 10^{2+3}$$
$$= 6 \times 10^5$$
$$(2.2 \times 10^4)(3 \times 10^{-3}) = (2.2)(3) \times 10^4 \times 10^{-3}$$
$$= 6.6 \times 10^{4-3}$$
$$= 6.6 \times 10^1$$
$$\frac{4 \times 10^5}{2 \times 10^1} = 2 \times 10^{5-1} = 2 \times 10^4$$
$$\frac{248,000}{0.0124} = \frac{2.48 \times 10^5}{1.24 \times 10^{-2}}$$
$$\frac{2.48}{1.24} \times 10^{5-(-2)}$$
$$= 2 \times 10^{5+2}$$
$$= 2 \times 10^7$$

ENGINEERING PREFIXES

When a physical parameter is expressed in scientific notation that includes some standard unit (e.g., meter, second, hertz, watt), the prefix replaces the power of 10 and becomes a modifier of the unit.

Examples of Engineering Prefixes

$$3.5 \times 10^6 \text{ Hz} = 3.5 \text{ MHz}$$
$$2 \times 10^{-2} \text{ m} = 2 \text{ cm}$$
$$1.3 \times 10^{-5} \text{ s} = 13 \times 10^{-6} \text{ s} = 13 \text{ μs}$$
$$6.5 \times 10^{-3} \text{ W} = 6.5 \text{ mW}$$

In the previous examples, MHz, cm, μs, and mW are stated as *mega*hertz, *centi*meters, *micro*seconds, and *milli*watts. The prefix may also be replaced by the appropriate power of 10 so the mathematic operations can be performed.

Examples of Numeric Conversions of Engineering Prefixes

$$7 \text{ μm} = 7 \times 10^{-6} \text{ m}$$
$$10 \text{ cm} = 10 \times 10^{-2} \text{ m} = 0.1 \text{ m}$$
$$1 \text{ kHz} = 1000 \text{ Hz}$$

SOLVING EQUATIONS

In algebra, equations are used to express relationships among a collection of variables. Each variable is usually denoted by a letter. When a set of conditions is given, a solution to the equation is sought by manipulating the equation according to well-defined mathematic principles. It is important to realize that the letter corresponding to a variable represents a number and therefore can be treated as a number; that is, the letter can be used in steps of addition, subtraction, multiplication, and division. Consider the equation

A-1
$$2x + 4 = 10$$

The equals sign separates one side of the equation from the other. The left-hand side has two terms (*2x* and *4*) and the right-hand side, one term (*10*). The terms are separated by minus (–) or plus (+) signs of operation. The term *2x* consists of an unknown variable x and the number 2, which is the coefficient. A coefficient is a multiplication factor. In the absence of a coefficient, it is understood to be 1.

Because only one unknown (the variable *x*) is present in Equation A-1, the unknown can be isolated on one side of the equation and its value thus determined. This is the solution to the equation and represents a value that, when substituted for *x,* makes the statement, or equation, true. Two useful techniques are used to obtain the goal of isolating the unknown on one side of the equation:

1. Addition (or subtraction) of the same term to (or from) each side of the equation does not change the value of the unknown.
2. Multiplication or division of each side of the equation by the same factor does not change the value of the unknown. Division must be by a nonzero real number.

Let us apply these techniques to solve for *x* in Equation A-1. All terms that do not contain *x* should be eliminated from the left-hand side. In this case, one term, the *4,* must be removed by subtracting 4 from each side:

$$2x + 4 - 4 = 10 - 4$$
$$2x + 0 = 6$$
$$2x = 6$$

The process of solving the equation is not complete, because the coefficient of *x* is not 1 (*x* is not completely by itself on one side of the equation). If each side is divided by 2, then

$$\frac{2x}{2} = \frac{6}{2}$$
$$x = 3$$

The conditions of the original equation dictate that *x* must equal 3. The solution is tested by replacing *x* with 3 wherever *x* occurs in the original equation. Hence

$$2 \bullet 3 + 4 = 10$$
$$6 + 4 = 10$$
$$10 = 10$$

which is obviously a true condition.

The order in which we apply the manipulation techniques is not fixed. Indeed, both sides of Equation A-1 can initially be divided by 2:

$$\frac{2x + 4}{2} = \frac{10}{2}$$
$$x + 2 = 5$$

Note that each term on each side of the equation must be divided by the same number or variable. To isolate *x*, 2 is now subtracted from each side:

$$x + 2 - 2 = 5 - 2$$
$$x = 3$$

Again, the solution of the equation is found to be *x* is equal to 3, which demonstrates internal consistency.

Another example may be useful. Suppose that

A-2
$$3x + 1 = 4x - 6$$

The variable *x* appears on both sides of the equation. Only like terms can be added or subtracted. Like terms are terms in which the variables, including their respective exponents, are the same. (Terms consisting entirely of numbers are also like terms.) To combine like terms, coefficients are added with coefficients. Begin to isolate *x* by adding 6 to each side:

$$3x + 1 + 6 = 4x - 6 + 6$$

The 6 and *3x* as well as the 6 and *4x* are unlike terms and cannot be combined:

$$3x + 7 = 4x$$

Next, subtract *3x* from each side:

$$3x - 3x + 7 = 4x - 3x$$
$$0x + 7 = 1x$$
$$7 = x$$

This solution is tested by replacing every *x* in the original equation with a 7:

$$3 \bullet 7 + 1 = 4 \bullet 7 - 6$$
$$21 + 1 = 28 - 6$$
$$22 = 22$$

Once more, the operations have been applied properly to determine the unknown *(x)*.

These techniques of manipulating equations can be summarized very concisely by remembering that whatever is done to one side of the equation must also be done to the other side.

Often the relationship among many variables is expressed in one equation. In ultrasound a very useful equation relates the properties of the ultrasound wave:

A-3
$$c = f\lambda$$

where *c* is the velocity, *f* the frequency, and λ the wavelength. It is possible to generate tables listing values for velocity, frequency, and wavelength, but this task would never be complete.

The limitation still exists; only one unknown in a given situation can be determined by solving Equation A-3. This means, however, that if any two of the variables are given, we can solve for the third. Rearranging Equation A-3 by dividing each side by λ yields

$$\frac{f\lambda}{\lambda} = \frac{c}{\lambda}$$ **A-4**

$$f = \frac{c}{\lambda}$$

Similarly, dividing each side by *f* gives

$$\frac{f\lambda}{f} = \frac{c}{f}$$ **A-5**

$$\lambda = \frac{c}{f}$$

Equations A-4 and A-5 express the same relation as Equation A-3 in different forms.

Problem A-1

What is the wavelength of the ultrasound wave in soft tissue with a frequency of 2.5 MHz? (Assume that the velocity is 1540 m/s.)

Answer

$$f = 2.5 \text{ MHz} = 2.5 \times 10^6 \text{ Hz}$$
$$\text{or } 2.5 \times 10^6 \text{ 1/s}$$
$$c = 1540 \text{ m/s} = 1.54 \times 10^3 \text{ m/s}$$

Solution: Using Equation A-5

$$\lambda = \frac{c}{f}$$

$$\lambda = \frac{1.54 \times 10^3 \text{ m/s}}{2.5 \times 10^6 \text{ 1/s}}$$

$$\lambda = 6.16 \times 10^{-4} \text{ m}$$

$$\lambda = 6.16 \times 10^{-1} \text{ mm}$$

Problem A-2

The wavelength of ultrasound in a particular medium is 1 mm and the frequency is 5 MHz. What is the velocity of ultrasound in the medium?

Answer

$$\lambda = 1 \text{ mm} = 1 \times 10^{-3} \text{ m}$$
$$f = 5 \text{ MHz} = 5 \times 10^6 \text{ 1/s}$$

Solution: Using Equation A-3
$$c = f\lambda = (5 \times 10^6 \text{ 1/s}) (1 \times 10^{-3} \text{ m})$$
$$c = 5 \times 10^3 \text{ m/s}$$

Problem A-3

The wavelength in tissue is 0.2 mm. What is the frequency of the transducer?

Answer

$$\lambda = 0.2 \text{ mm} = 2 \times 10^{-4} \text{ m}$$

Solution: The velocity in tissue is assumed to be 1540 m/s. Using Equation A-4

$$f = \frac{1.54 \times 10^3 \text{ m/s}}{2 \times 10^{-4} \text{ m}}$$

$$f = 7.7 \times 10^6 \text{ 1/s}$$

$$f = 7.7 \text{ MHz}$$

It is unnecessary to memorize all the forms of the relationship among velocity, wavelength, and frequency. The equation $c = f\lambda$ is sufficient. By substituting for the known variables and manipulating the equation, we can determine the remaining variable.

Problem A-4

Solve Problem A-3 using Equation A-3.

Answer

$$c = 1.54 \times 10^3 \text{ m/s}$$
$$\lambda = 2 \times 10^{-4} \text{ m}$$

Solution:
$$c = f\lambda$$
$$1.54 \times 10^3 \text{ m/s} = f(2 \times 10^{-4} \text{ m})$$

$$\frac{1.54 \times 10^3 \text{ m/s}}{2 \times 10^{-4} \text{ m}} = f$$

$$7.7 \times 10^6 \text{ 1/s} = f$$

UNIT CONVERSIONS

A description of physical parameter is incomplete unless the units are also specified. If someone were to ask how far Los Angeles is from New York City, the reply would most likely be 3000 miles. The unit "miles" is necessary for the answer to make sense.

Most physical parameters are expressed in units—some combination of length, mass, and time. Wavelength is expressed in terms of length, whereas velocity is in terms of length per time. Both 12 inches and 1 foot represent the same absolute measurement of length. The problem or traditional preference usually dictates which unit is to be used.

Note the importance of retaining units in the problems in the previous section. If this is done correctly, the solution for a particular unknown is always expressed in proper units (e.g., wavelength is found in units of length).

Sometimes unit conversions are necessary to maintain a consistent set of units throughout the problem. Once the relationship between original units and desired units is known, this conversion factor is modified to a fractional form, which is equal to 1. The product of the fractional form of the conversion factor and the original units gives the desired units without changing the absolute value of the physical parameter.

Suppose 10 millimeters (mm) is to be expressed in terms of meters (m). The conversion factor is given by

$$1000 \text{ mm} = 1 \text{ m}$$

The problem can be viewed as

$$10 \text{ mm} \times CF = ? \text{ m}$$

where *CF* is the fractional form of the conversion factor. *CF* must be written so the unit meter is in the numerator and millimeter is in the denominator. Dividing each side of the conversion factor by 1000 mm

$$1 = \frac{1 \text{ m}}{1000 \text{ mm}}$$

$$CF = \frac{1 \text{ m}}{1000 \text{ m}}$$

Substituting for *CF* as the factor times 10 mm

$$10 \text{ mm} \times \frac{1 \text{ m}}{1000 \text{ mm}} = 0.01 \text{ m}$$

Note that millimeters in the numerator and the denominator cancel. We find that 0.01 m is the same as 10 mm. The fractional form of the conversion factor can be inverted to transform meters to millimeters.

To express 0.01 meters in terms of millimeters

$$0.01 \text{ m} \times CF = ? \text{ mm}$$

$$0.01 \text{ m} \times \frac{1000 \text{ mm}}{1 \text{ m}} = 10 \text{ mm}$$

Once again, the original unit cancels with the denominator in the conversion factor, and the desired unit remains.

Problem A-5

A car is moving at a rate of 60 miles per hour. What is the velocity in terms of miles per minute?

Answer

The conversion factor is 60 min = 1 hr

Solution:

$$\frac{60 \text{ miles}}{\text{hr}} \times CF = \frac{? \text{ miles}}{\text{min}}$$

The fractional form *(CF)* must have hours in the numerator. Therefore

$$CF = \frac{1 \text{ hr}}{60 \text{ min}}$$

Substituting for *CF*

$$\frac{60 \text{ miles}}{\text{hr}} \times \frac{1 \text{ hr}}{60 \text{ min}} = \frac{1 \text{ mile}}{\text{min}}$$

Common Conversion Factors	
1000 mm	1 m
10 mm	1 cm
100 cm	1 m
1 MHz	10^6 Hz
1 μs	10^{-6} s
1 ms	10^{-3} s
1 m/s	100 cm/s
1 kg	2.2 lbs
1 Mrayl	10^6 kg/m²/s

TRIGONOMETRY

When two lines cross, they form an angle, which is usually specified in degrees. In Fig. A-1, angle φ is larger than angle θ. A protractor is used to measure the angle. One complete revolution, a straight line, and a right angle correspond to 360 degrees, 180 degrees, and 90 degrees, respectively. The degree is divided into smaller divisions called minutes, and the minute into even smaller divisions called seconds:

$$1 \text{ degree} = 60 \text{ minutes}$$

$$1 \text{ minute} = 60 \text{ seconds}$$

This is similar to the relationship among hours, minutes, and seconds in timekeeping.

Degrees may also be expressed in decimal form, in which case the seconds and minutes must be converted into degrees via the conversion factors. For example

$$30° \; 45' = 30.75°$$

because

$$45 \text{ min} \times \frac{1°}{60 \text{ min}} = 0.75°$$
$$= 0.75°$$

A unit called the radian is also used to describe the size of an angle. A complete revolution is equal to 2π radians, or

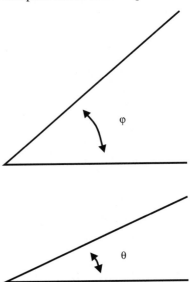

Fig. A-1 Formation of an angle by two lines that cross. Angle φ is greater than angle θ.

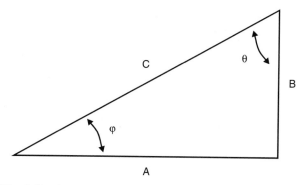

Fig. A-2 Right triangle. The hypotenuse is side C.

identically, one radian is 57.3 degrees. The following table shows various angles expressed in both radians and degrees.

Radians	Degrees
2π	360
π	180
$\dfrac{\pi}{2}$	90
$\dfrac{\pi}{4}$	45

A triangle is a three-sided geometric figure. If one of the angles is 90 degrees, the triangle is a right triangle (Fig. A-2). All the angles of the triangle, when added together, must equal 180 degrees. Therefore angle θ is calculated by subtracting angle φ from 90 degrees and vice versa.

The side opposite the right angle is the hypotenuse (side C in Fig. A-2). The hypotenuse is always the longest side of the right triangle. An opposite side and an adjacent side are designated with respect to the angle of interest. For example, when the angle φ is considered, the adjacent side is side A, and the opposite side is side B.

Early mathematicians noticed some very interesting properties about right triangles. For a particular angle, the ratio of any two sides is constant regardless of the size of the triangle. For example, in Fig. A-3

$$\frac{a}{b} = \frac{A}{B}$$

The ratio was given a name (e.g., sine [sin], cosine [cos], or tangent [tan]) depending on the sides involved:

A-6
$$\sin (\text{angle}) = \frac{\text{Opposite}}{\text{Hypotenuse}}$$

A-7
$$\cos (\text{angle}) = \frac{\text{Adjacent}}{\text{Hypotenuse}}$$

A-8
$$\tan (\text{angle}) = \frac{\text{Opposite}}{\text{Adjacent}}$$

These are the most commonly used trigonometric functions. When problem solving with trigonometric functions,

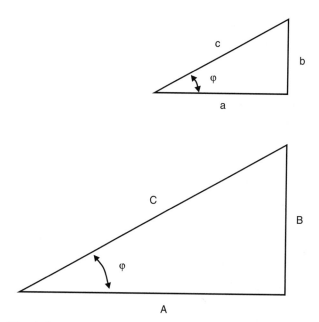

Fig. A-3 Two triangles with equal angles but different lengths of sides.

the angle must be identified, but the numeric value may be unknown. From Fig. A-3, the trigonometric functions are found to equal:

$$\sin \varphi = \frac{b}{c} = \frac{B}{C}$$

$$\cos \varphi = \frac{a}{c} = \frac{A}{C}$$

$$\tan \varphi = \frac{b}{a} = \frac{B}{A}$$

Values of the trigonometric functions have been collected in tables, or they are readily obtainable from scientific calculators. Common trigonometric functions are shown in the following table.

Angle	Sin	Tan	Cos
0 degrees	0	0	1
30 degrees	0.5	0.577	0.866
45 degrees	0.707	1	0.707
60 degrees	0.866	1.732	0.5
90 degrees	1	—	0

Note that this tabulation is used in two ways. Given the ratio of the sides for the particular trigonometric function, read across to determine the angle; this procedure is referred to as taking the arc of the trigonometric function. Likewise, given the angle, read across to find the ratios of the various sides. Think of the trigonometric functions as equations with three variables. If any two of the variables are known, the equation can be solved for the third variable.

Problem A-6

In Fig. A-2 assume that $\varphi = 30$ degrees and that $A = 10$ cm. What is the length of side B?

Answer

$$\tan \varphi = \frac{B}{A}$$

Solution:

$$\tan 30° = \frac{B}{10 \text{ cm}}$$

$$0.577 = \frac{B}{10 \text{ cm}}$$

$$5.77 \text{ cm} = B$$

Problem A-7

In Fig. A-2 assume that side $B = 8$ cm and that side $C = 16$ cm. What is the angle θ?

Answer

$$\cos \theta = \frac{B}{C}$$

Solution:

$$\cos \theta = \frac{8 \text{ cm}}{16 \text{ cm}}$$

$$\cos \theta = 0.5$$

Examine the table for the angle that gives a value of 0.5 for the cosine trigonometric function:

$$\theta = 60°$$

Problem A-8

In Fig. A-2, assume that θ is 60 degrees and that side A is 10 cm. What is the length of side C?

Answer

$$\sin \theta = \frac{A}{C}$$

Solution:

$$\sin 60° = \frac{10 \text{ cm}}{C}$$

$$0.866 = \frac{10 \text{ cm}}{C}$$

$$C = 11.5 \text{ cm}$$

LOGARITHMS

In essence, logarithms are a means to express numbers in terms of a base and an exponent, where the base is understood to be constant. Because the base is known, it does not have to be written explicitly. A number (x) can be represented in the form

$$x = b^y \text{ (x is always greater than zero)}$$

where b is the base and y the exponent. The logarithm to the base b of x is an exponent. Thus

$$\log_b x = y$$

By taking the logarithm of a number, the exponent is found for which the number would be obtained if the base were raised to that exponent. Various types of logarithms exist depending on the base. The two types most frequently used are common logarithms (base 10) and natural logarithms (base e).

In common logarithms, the base is assigned a value of 10. Defining equations are

$$x = 10^y \tag{A-9}$$

and

$$\log_{10} x = y \tag{A-10}$$

A table of logarithms of the powers of 10 follows.

Number (x)	Power of 10	$\text{Log}_{10} x$
1000	10^3	3
100	10^2	2
10	10^1	1
1	10^0	0
0.1	10^{-1}	−1
0.01	10^{-2}	−2
0.001	10^{-3}	−3

Suppose the number x is not a power of 10; then $\log x$ is a decimal number. The number x is written in scientific notation (i.e., the factor times a power of 10). The logarithm is found by adding the characteristic and the mantissa together. The exponent in the power of 10 is the characteristic, and the logarithm of the factor is the mantissa. Because the factor has a value between 1 and 10, the mantissa will have a value between 0 (the log of 1) and 1 (the log of 10). Mathematic tables list the logarithms of numbers between 1 and 10.

Although decimal exponents may be somewhat confusing initially, they can be understood simply as a combination of roots and powers. The square root of 10 can be written as a fractional exponent ($10^{1/2}$), as a decimal exponent ($10^{0.5}$), or as a number (3.16). For example, consider

$$10^{0.25} = (10^{0.5})^{0.5} = (3.16)^{0.5} = 1.78$$

$$10^{0.67} = (10^{2/3}) = (10^2)^{1/3} = 100^{1/3} = 4.63$$

The following examples demonstrate the process of finding the logarithm of a number.

$$\log 42.5 = \log (4.25 \times 10^1)$$

$$= \log (4.25) + \log (10^1)$$

$$= 0.6284 \text{(mantissa)} + 1 \text{(characteristic)}$$

$$= 1.6284$$

$$\log 4250 = \log (4.25 \times 10^3)$$

$$= \log (4.25) + \log (10^3)$$

$$= 0.6284 + 3$$

$$= 3.6284$$

$$\log (0.00302) = \log (3.02 \times 10^{-3})$$

$$= \log(3.02) + \log(10^{-3})$$
$$= 0.48 + (-3)$$
$$= -2.52$$

Numbers greater than 1 that differ only in their powers of 10 have the same mantissa. The logarithm of a number less than 1 but greater than zero is negative. The operation of finding the logarithm of a negative number is not defined.

Scientific calculators make the process of finding the logarithm of a number considerably easier. The number in standard format or scientific notation is entered into the display, and the log key is pressed. The logarithm is calculated and replaces the number in the display.

Suppose that the log x is given; how do we determine the number x? That is, the exponent is known, and x must be calculated. This process is the reverse of finding the logarithm and is called taking the antilogarithm (antilog). The antilog of y is the base 10 with an exponent of y:

$$\text{Antilog } y = 10^y = x \qquad \text{A–11}$$

Examples of Antilogarithms

Given that log $x = 1.6395$, find x.

$$x = \text{Antilog }(1.6395)$$
$$= 10^{1.6395}$$
$$= (10^{0.6395})(10^1)$$
$$= (4.36)(10^1)$$
$$= 43.6$$

Given that log $x = -2.52$, find x.

$$x = \text{Antilog }(-2.52)$$
$$= 10^{-2.52}$$
$$= (10^{0.48})(10^{-3})$$
$$= (3.02)(10^{-3})$$
$$= 0.00302$$

If tables are used, the mantissa must be a positive number between 0 and 1. That is why (–2.52) was rewritten as (0.48 – 3) in this example. If one uses a calculator, this distinction does not have to be made, because the base 10 raised to any power is calculated directly.

Because logarithms are exponents of bases, logarithms have properties similar to the operations defined for exponents. When two numbers are multiplied, we can either take the logarithm of the product or add the logarithms of the individual factors:

$$\text{Log }(x_1 \bullet x_2) = \log(x_1) + \log(x_2) \qquad \text{A-12}$$

For example,

$$\log(2 \bullet 3) = \log(2) + \log(3)$$
$$\log 6 = 0.301 + 0.4771$$
$$0.7781 = 0.7781$$

This property has already been used in obtaining the number of x numbers expressed in scientific notation. In the case of one number divided by another, the logarithm of the divisor is subtracted from the logarithm of the dividend:

$$\log\left(\frac{x_1}{x_2}\right) = \log(x_1) - \log(x_2) \qquad \text{A–13}$$

For example,

$$\log\left(\frac{8}{2}\right) = \log(8) - \log(2)$$
$$\log(4) = 0.903 - 0.301$$
$$0.602 = 0.602$$

The logarithm of a number raised to the mth power is the product of m and the logarithm of the number:

$$\log(x^m) = m \log x \qquad \text{A-14}$$

For example,

$$\log(2)^3 = 3 \log 2$$
$$\log 8 = 3(0.301)$$
$$0.903 = 0.903$$

The second type of logarithm, called natural logarithms, uses the base e, which has a numeric value of approximately 2.7183. The defining equations become

$$\log_e x = y \qquad \text{A-15}$$

or

$$\ln x = y \qquad \text{A-16}$$

and

$$e^y = x \qquad \text{A-17}$$

The latter is called an exponential function and can be pictured as

$$2.7183^y = x$$

where the base (2.7183) is raised to the power of y. The exponent y can be positive or negative or zero, but x is always greater than zero.

The natural logarithms of numbers have been compiled in mathematic tables. They are also readily available via scientific calculators. Natural logarithms do not use characteristics as do common logarithms. The inverse of the natural logarithm is the exponential function, which eliminates the need for the term antilogarithm when referring to natural logarithms. The relationship between e^y and $\ln x$ is shown in the following table.

x or e^y	ln x or y
0.01	−4.6052
0.1	−2.3026
1	0
2.7183	1
10	2.3026
100	4.6052

Scientific calculators provide values for exponential functions. The same properties defined for common logarithms apply to natural logarithms *(ln)*. The relationship between the natural and common logarithms is given by

A-18

$$\ln x = 2.303 \log x$$

A-19

$$e^y = 10^{0.4343y}$$

which permits easy conversion from one type to the other.

For example, the natural logarithm of *x* when *x* equals 100 is solved by using the relationship between natural and common logarithms as follows:

$$x = 100$$

$$\ln 100 = 2.303 \log(100)$$

$$= 2.303(2)$$

$$= 4.606$$

To solve for e^y when $y = 2$

$$e^2 = 10^{(.4343)(2)} = 10^{0.8686}$$

$$= 7.389$$

DECIBELS

In ultrasound the intensity at one point is compared with that at another. Relative rather than absolute values of the intensity are specified. Because many powers of 10 are involved, a logarithmic scale is employed in which the change in intensity is given in decibels (dB). The level in dB is defined by:

A-20

$$\text{level (dB)} = 10 \log \left(\frac{I}{I_0}\right)$$

where I_0 is the intensity at the reference point and *I* the intensity at the point of interest. The ratio of I/I_0 must always be dimensionless; I_0 and *I* must be expressed in the same units.

Problem A-9

Determine the level in decibels if the ultrasound beam enters the material with an intensity of 1×10^5 mW/cm² and exits with an intensity of 2×10^2 mW/cm².

Answer

$$I_0 = 1 \times 10^5 \text{ mW/cm}^2$$

$$I = 2 \times 10^2 \text{ mW/cm}^2$$

Solution: Using Equation A-20

$$\text{level (dB)} = 10 \log \left(\frac{I}{I_0}\right)$$

$$\text{level (dB)} = 10 \log \left(\frac{2 \times 10^2}{1 \times 10^5}\right)$$

$$= 10 \log (2 \times 10^{-3})$$

$$= 10 (-2.699)$$

$$= -26.99$$

The negative sign indicates the intensity decreased from the reference point to the point of interest.

Problem A-10

A 10 dB loss in intensity is observed at a certain depth *(z)* in the medium. If the intensity at the surface is 2.5×10^3 mW/cm², what is the intensity at depth *z?*

Answer

$$I_0 = 2.5 \times 10^3 \text{ mW/cm}^2$$

Level (dB) = −10, because a loss in intensity occurred.

Solution: Using Equation A-20

$$\text{level (dB)} = 10 \log \left(\frac{I}{I_0}\right)$$

$$-10 = 10 \log \left(\frac{I}{I_0}\right)$$

Divide each side by 10:

$$-1 = \log \left(\frac{I}{I_0}\right)$$

Take the antilog of each side:

$$\text{Antilog } (-1) = \left(\frac{I}{I_0}\right)$$

$$0.1 = \left(\frac{I}{I_0}\right)$$

Substitute for I_0:

$$0.1 = \left(\frac{I}{2.5 \times 10^3 \text{ mW/cm}^2}\right)$$

Solve for *I*:

$$I = (2.5 \times 10^3 \text{ mW/cm}^2) (0.1)$$

$$I = 2.5 \times 10^2 \text{ mW/cm}^2$$

Problem A-11

The surface intensity in Problem A-10 is raised to a new value. If the intensity at depth *z* is 8×10^6 mW/cm², what is the intensity at the surface? Assume a 10 dB loss to depth *z*.

Answer

$$I = 8 \times 10^6 \text{ mW/cm}^2$$

$$\text{Level (dB)} = -10$$

Solution: From Problem A-10, the ratio of the intensities is 0.1:

$$0.1 = \left(\frac{I}{I_0}\right)$$

$$0.1 = \left(\frac{8 \times 10^6 \text{ mW/cm}^2}{I_0}\right)$$

$$I_0 = 8 \times 10^7 \text{ mW/cm}^2$$

Problem A-12

Determine the level in decibels if the intensity of interest is half the reference intensity.

Answer

$$I = 0.5 \, I_0$$

Solution: Using Equation A-20

$$\text{level (dB)} = 10 \log \left(\frac{I}{I_0} \right)$$

$$\text{level (dB)} = 10 \log \left(\frac{0.5 \, I_0}{I_0} \right)$$

$$\text{level (dB)} = 10 \log (0.5)$$

$$\text{level (dB)} = 10 \, (-0.301)$$

$$\text{level (dB)} = -3.01$$

If the intensity decreases by a factor of 2, a 3 dB loss results. Each half-value layer (HVL) of material causes a 3 dB reduction in intensity.

Problem A-13

The intensity at the surface is $5 \times 10^6 \text{ mW/cm}^2$. What is the intensity after transmission across a material four HVLs thick?

Answer

Determine the intensity level change caused by the absorbing material:

$$-3 \text{ dB/HVL} \times 4 \text{ HVL} = -12 \text{ dB}$$

$$I_0 = 5 \times 10^6 \text{ mW/cm}^2$$

Solution:

$$\text{level (dB)} = 10 \log \left(\frac{I}{I_0} \right)$$

$$-12 = 10 \log \left(\frac{I}{I_0} \right)$$

$$-1.2 = \log \left(\frac{I}{I_0} \right)$$

$$\text{Antilog} \, (-1.2) = \left(\frac{I}{I_0} \right)$$

$$0.063 = \left(\frac{I}{I_0} \right)$$

$$0.063 = \left(\frac{I}{5 \times 10^6 \text{ mW/cm}^2} \right)$$

$$I = 3.15 \times 10^5 \text{ mW/cm}^2$$

An alternative solution is to recognize that each HVL decreases the intensity by a factor of 2:

A-21

$$I = \left(\frac{I_0}{2^n} \right)$$

where n is the number of HVLs.

$$I = (5 \times 10^6 \text{ mW/cm}^2) \, (1/2)(1/2)(1/2)(1/2)$$

$$I = 3.12 \times 10^5 \text{ mW/cm}^2$$

This does not agree exactly with the previous answer, because the decibel loss per HVL was rounded off to 3.

STATISTICS

Biologic variations occur in populations. Heights of adult human females, birth weights of human fetuses, and mutation rates in mice are three examples of parameters that can be evaluated in the respective populations. Clearly, these parameters are not constant throughout a population. Statistics is the mathematic technique that describes and analyzes numeric data obtained from experimental observations of populations.

Since performing measurements on every member of a large population is not practical, a small representative sample is designated for study. The number of members investigated in this population is the sample size *(N)*. Listing the individual measurements is time consuming and difficult to communicate. Statistical parameters (primarily the mean and the standard deviation) have been developed to characterize a set of measurements.

The mean (x_m) is the arithmetic average, which is calculated by summing the individual measurements (x_i) and dividing by the number of measurements

A-22

$$x_m = \frac{\sum x_i}{N}$$

The standard deviation (σ) indicates the amount of variability and is defined mathematically as

A-23

$$\sigma = \sqrt{\frac{\sum (x_i - x_m)^2}{N - 1}}$$

The standard deviation is expressed in the same units as the mean.

Suppose we have to record the height of women between the ages of 20 and 25 entering a building. The first five observations (in inches) are 64, 60, 64, 63, and 67. These data are presented as a histogram in Fig. A-4. The horizontal axis represents the magnitude of measurement (height in inches), and the vertical axis shows the number of times each height is observed in the population. Graphic formats are useful in presenting large data sets in concise form.

As the sample size is increased, the distribution becomes centrally peaked, with falloff on each side of the peak (Fig. A-5). Irregularities become more smooth. The numeric data are depicted by a bell–shaped curve, called the normal distribution (Fig. A-6). The normal distribution is specified completely by the mean and the standard deviation. The mean corresponds to the horizontal value at the central peak, and the standard deviation indicates the width of the distribution.

Measurements that are fairly uniform yield a low value for the standard deviation and show little spread in the

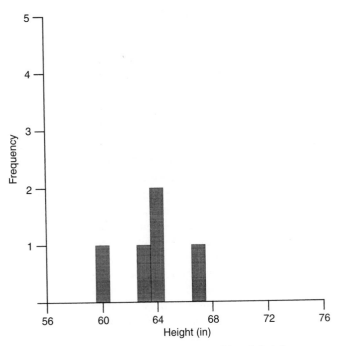

Fig. A-4 Histogram of five observations of female height.

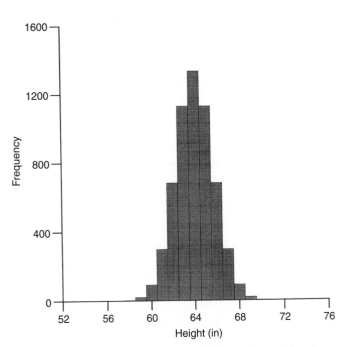

Fig. A-5 Histogram of several thousand observations of female height. The mean is 64 inches, and the standard deviation is calculated to be 3 inches.

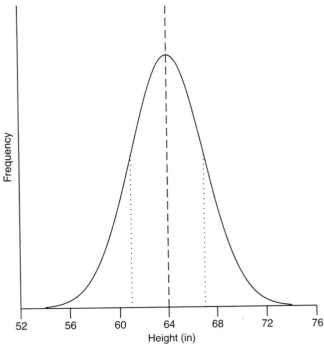

Fig. A-6 Normal distribution of female heights from the data in Fig. A-5. The mean is 64 inches and is shown by the dashed line. The spread of the distribution is denoted by the dotted lines corresponding to one standard deviation on each side of the mean. In this numeric data set the standard deviation is equal to 3 inches.

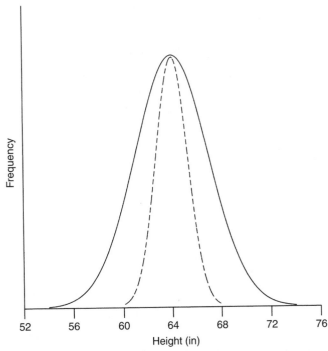

Fig. A-7 Comparison of normal distributions with the same mean but different variability. The standard deviation associated with the distribution represented by the dashed line has a lower numeric value.

normal distribution. Another group of measurements may have the same mean but exhibit more variability (Fig. A–7). An important property of the standard deviation is to denote the fraction of measurements within a range of values. The percentage of all measurements included within $\pm 1\sigma$, $\pm 2\sigma$, and $\pm 3\sigma$ of the mean are 68.3%, 95.4%, and 99.7%. This is true regardless of the absolute value of the standard deviation.

Certainly, the experimental conditions can influence the distribution of the measurements. If we are monitoring the height of female players entering a gymnasium for a basketball game featuring the Russian National Women's Team, the mean height will increase. The standard deviation may actually decrease if the players are similar in height.

Problem A-14

Calculate the mean and standard deviation for the following series of measurements (in inches): 60, 63, 64, 64, and 67. Determine the range for 68.3% and 95% of the measurements.

Answer

Find the mean.

$$x_m = \frac{\sum x_i}{N}$$

$$x_m = \frac{60 + 63 + 64 + 64 + 67}{5}$$

$$x_m = 63.6 \text{ inches}$$

Calculate the standard deviation.

$$\sigma = \sqrt{\frac{\sum (x_i - x_m)^2}{N - 1}}$$

x_i	$x_i - x_m$	$(x_i - x_m)^2$
60	−3.6	12.96
63	−0.6	0.36
64	0.4	0.16
64	0.4	0.16
67	3.4	11.56

The sum of the extreme right column equals $\sum (x_i - x_m)^2$.

$$\sigma = \sqrt{\frac{25.2}{(5 - 1)}}$$

$$\sigma = 2.5 \text{ inches}$$

For the range 61.1 to 66.1 inches, we would expect to find 68.3% of the measurements. For the range 58.6 to 68.6 inches, we expect to find 95.4%.

Two other statistics are often used to describe a collection of measurements. The median is the middle value when data are ranked from lowest to highest. The number of measurements is equally divided above and below the median value. The mode is the prevalent value in the collection of measurements. When presented in graphic format, it corresponds to the highest peak in the curve.

INDICES OF DIAGNOSTIC TEST PERFORMANCE

The growth of ultrasound can, in large part, be attributed to new clinical applications. Researchers must demonstrate that proposed applications selectively identify patients with specific disease. Statistical parameters (typically sensitivity, specificity, and accuracy) have been developed to judge the efficacy of diagnostic tests. The patient may or may not have disease, and the ultrasound examination may or may not have positive findings. Four outcomes are possible:

1. True-positive (TP): The ultrasound findings are positive, and the patient has disease.
2. False-positive (FP): The ultrasound findings are positive, and the patient does not have disease.
3. True-negative (TN): The ultrasound findings are negative, and the patient does not have disease.
4. False-negative (FN): The ultrasound findings are negative, and the patient has disease.

The determination of disease is accomplished independently by using an established procedure (a surgical biopsy). The perfect diagnostic test would identify all diseased persons with positive findings and all nondiseased persons with negative findings. The sensitivity of the diagnostic test is the percentage of all subjects with disease that yield a positive test result. Mathematically

A-24

$$\text{Sensitivity} = \frac{TP}{TP + FN} \times 100$$

Sensitivity describes how well the diagnostic test identifies subjects with disease. Minimizing false-negatives improves the reliability of the diagnostic test. The specificity of a diagnostic test is the percentage of all subjects without disease who yield a negative test result. Mathematically

A-25

$$\text{Specificity} = \frac{TN}{TN + FP} \times 100$$

Specificity describes how well the diagnostic test excludes nondiseased subjects from having a positive test result. Minimizing false-positives also improves the reliability of the diagnostic test. Accuracy of the diagnostic test is the percentage of all subjects tested who are correctly assessed as having or not having disease. The equation for accuracy is

A-26

$$\text{Accuracy} = \frac{TP + TN}{\text{All subject tested}} \times 100$$

Positive predictive value (PPV) indicates the likelihood of disease if the test is positive. Similarly, negative predictive value (NPV) indicates the likelihood of the subject being free of disease if the test is negative. The defining equations are

A-27

$$\text{PPV} = \frac{TP}{TP + FP} \times 100$$

A-28

$$\text{NPV} = \frac{TN}{TN + FN} \times 100$$

Sensitivity, specificity, accuracy, PPV, and NPV are also expressed by fractions between zero and 1 to indicate probability of various outcomes. In this format the factor 100 is eliminated in Equations A-24 through A-28.

Problem A-15

Calculate the sensitivity, specificity, PPV, NPV, and accuracy for an ultrasound examination with the following outcomes when compared with the diagnostic standard.

TP: 53
FP: 18
TN: 70
FN: 4
Total number of subjects tested: 145

Answer

$$\text{Sensitivity} = \frac{53}{57} \times 100 = 93\%$$

$$\text{Specificity} = \frac{70}{88} \times 100 = 80\%$$

$$\text{Accuracy} = \frac{53 + 70}{145} \times 100 = 85\%$$

$$\text{PPV} = \frac{53}{71} \times 100 = 75\%$$

$$\text{NPV} = \frac{70}{74} \times 100 = 95\%$$

Imaging procedures are subject to interpretation by an observer. The observer may or may not correctly analyze the information content of the image. Sensitivity and specificity are dependent on the knowledge and experience of the observer. Consequently, the accuracy of the diagnostic test is expected to vary within a group of observers. A graphic

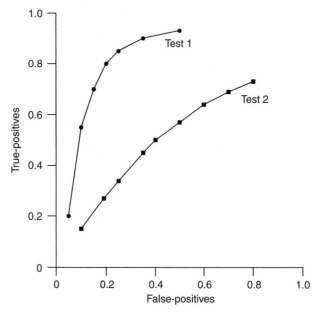

Fig. A-8 Receiver operating characteristic curves for two diagnostic tests. Test 1 is superior to Test 2.

method, called receiver operating characteristics (ROC) curve, summarizes the performance of multiple observers or different test conditions. The fraction of TPs of all subjects with disease (sensitivity) is plotted against the fraction of FPs all subjects without disease (1 − specificity). Data points concentrated in the upper left portion of the graph indicate high sensitivity with a low rate of FPs (the most desirable attributes of a diagnostic test). Example ROC curves are presented in Fig. A-8.

Fourier Analysis

In physics an entity often demonstrates complex behavior that is difficult to describe mathematically. For example, the ultrasound wave produced by a piezoelectric crystal exhibits pressure (or intensity) fluctuations over time and space. Also, the Doppler signal generated by interfaces moving at different velocities has multiple components that are not readily perceived. A simplified description of this complex variation (whether pulsed ultrasound wave or Doppler signal) is essential for understanding and analysis. One method, called **Fourier analysis,** identifies a series of sine wave constituents that, when added together, yield the original waveform. The technique of Fourier analysis has numerous applications in ultrasound physics, but the two most important are the determination of transducer Q-value and Doppler spectral analysis.

A ball suspended from a string exhibits very nearly simple harmonic motion that can be described by a sine wave. The ball, when moved from its equilibrium position, oscillates back and forth. The distance from the center for two different starting positions is plotted with respect to time in Fig. B-1. Shortening the string as demonstrated in Fig. B-2 can increase the rate of oscillatory movement.

Amplitude, frequency, and phase characterize sine waves. **Frequency** is the number of oscillations per unit time. **Amplitude** describes the extent of the vibratory movement, or more generally, the range of values of the physical

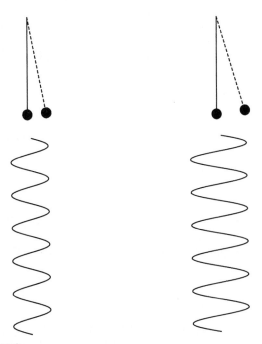

Fig. B-1 A ball suspended from a string oscillates when released from its starting position *(dotted line)*. A sine wave describes the movement of the ball as a function of time. The ball on the right shows greater range of movement.

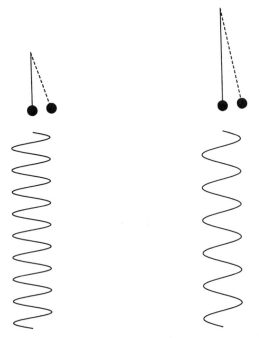

Fig. B-2 The ball on the left, suspended from a shorter string, has a higher rate of oscillatory movement.

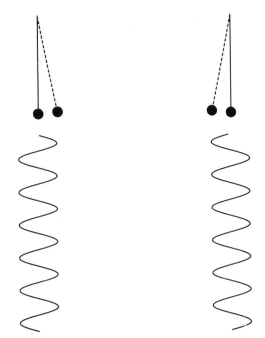

Fig. B-3 Changing the starting position from the right to left side of the center, but equidistant from the center *(dashed lines)*, produces sine waves with equal amplitude and equal frequency but different phase.

entity. **Phase** offsets or shifts the location of maxima and minima.

Fig. B-1 shows sine waves of constant frequency with different amplitudes. In Fig. B-2 the amplitude is kept constant while the frequency is varied. The appearance of the sine wave portraying the movement of the ball suspended from a string is modified by changing the starting position to the left of center, although the frequency and amplitude remain the same (Fig. B-3). This results in a phase shift of 180 degrees. (The maxima of one wave correspond to the minima of the other wave.) In another example a phase shift of 90 degrees moves the two-cycle sine wave one-quarter cycle to the left in Fig. B-4.

The mathematic description of the amplitude of the sine wave (*A*) is given by

B-1

$$A = A_o \sin (2\pi f t + \varphi)$$

where A_o is the maximum amplitude, π is a constant with a value of 3.1416, f is the frequency, t is the variable of time, and φ is the phase. The amplitude at any point in time can be calculated using Equation B-1. Consider the two-cycle wave generated in a time interval of 1 second with a maximum amplitude of 10 mm (Fig. B-5). The phase is zero. The amplitude (*A*) at 0.15 second is determined by substituting the appropriate parameters in Equation B-1 and solving for *A*:

$$A = (10 \text{ mm}) \sin [2 \pi (2 \text{ cycles/sec})(0.15 \text{ sec})]$$

$$A = (10 \text{ mm}) \sin (1.884 \text{ radians})$$

$$A = (10 \text{ mm}) (0.95)$$

$$A = 9.5 \text{ mm}$$

The amplitude at 0.15 second is 9.5 mm. Note that in this application the argument of the sine function is expressed in radians and not in degrees.

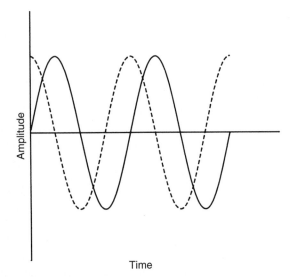

Fig. B-4 Phase shift of 90 degrees. Two-cycle sine waves with a phase angle of 0 degrees *(solid line)* and offset one-quarter cycle to the left *(dashed line)*.

Sine waves can be algebraically added together to depict more complex variation. This superposition of sine waves is also called **interference.** Fig. B-6 shows the result of combining a two-cycle sine wave with a three-cycle sine wave. The addition of sine waves is accomplished by summing the wave amplitudes at each point in time. At 0.15 second the amplitude of the two-cycle wave and three-cycle wave is 9.5 mm and 3.1 mm, respectively. The resultant wave has an amplitude of 12.6 mm at 0.15 second. At a different time (0.22 second) the respective amplitudes

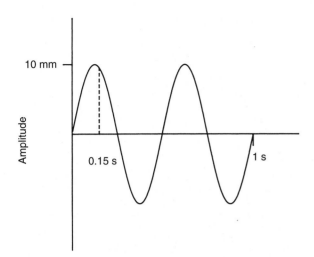

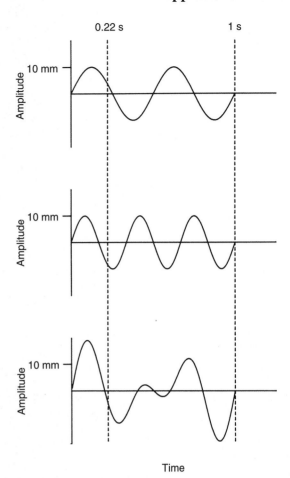

Fig. B-5 The amplitude at 0.15 second is 9.5 mm for a sine wave with a frequency of two cycles per second and a maximum amplitude of 10 mm.

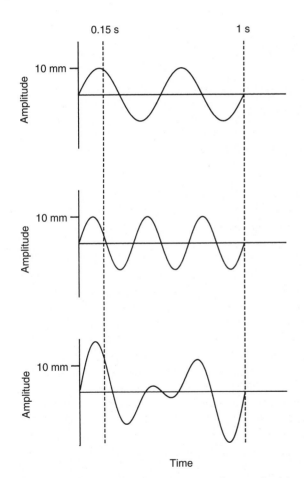

Fig. B-7 Summation of sine waves. A two-cycle wave *(top)* is combined with a three-cycle wave *(middle)* to form the resultant wave *(bottom)*. The vertical dashed line on the left indicates the respective amplitudes at 0.22 second.

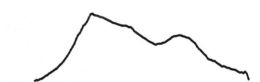

Fig. B-8 Idealized shoreline.

Fig. B-6 Summation of sine waves. A two-cycle wave *(top)* is combined with a three-cycle wave *(middle)* to form the resultant wave *(bottom)*. The vertical dashed line on the left indicates the respective amplitudes at 0.15 second.

(3.7 mm and –8.4 mm) combine to yield a value of –4.7 mm (as demonstrated in Fig. B-7).

Multiple sine waves of varying frequency and amplitude can be combined to form a complex waveform. As an illustrative example, imagine viewing the shoreline from a

distant cliff above the beach. The boundary between the water and sand form an intricate pattern (Figs. B-8 to B-10). This pattern of the idealized shoreline can be analyzed mathematically and then reproduced by combining sine waves; each component in the composite waveform has a well-defined amplitude and frequency based on analysis of the idealized shoreline. The composite waveform more closely represents the idealized shoreline as more sine waves are added together.

The presentation of sine waves in Figs. B-1 to B-7 is in the time domain. (The amplitude is plotted as a function of time.) An alternative method to describe sine waves, however, is to state the maximum amplitude (often in an abbreviated form as amplitude only) and frequency. The basis for comparison is frequency, which is described as the **frequency domain.** The identification of the frequency

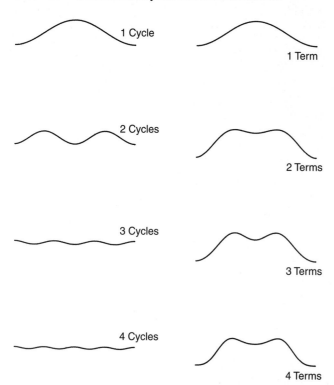

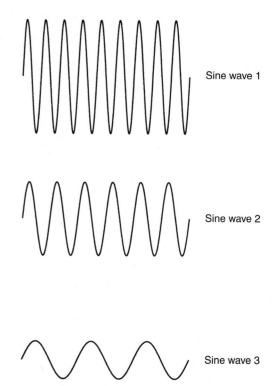

Fig. B-9 A sine wave of single frequency added to other sine waves yields a composite waveform that approximates the idealized shoreline. The first four sine waves are shown individually on the left with their effect on the composite waveform *(right)*.

Fig. B-11 Three separate sine waves. Sine wave 1 has a frequency of nine cycles per second and an amplitude of 0.75. Sine wave 2 has a frequency of six cycles per second and an amplitude of 0.5. Sine wave 3 has a frequency of three cycles per second and an amplitude of 0.25.

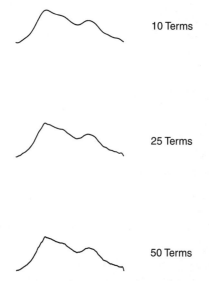

Fig. B-10 As more sine waves with different frequencies and amplitudes are added, the pattern generated more closely represents the idealized shoreline (10 to 50 sine waves).

components is called **spectral analysis.** The frequency domain specification of the sine wave depicted in Fig. B-5 has a maximum amplitude of 10 mm with a frequency of two cycles/sec. This information can be used to generate the sine wave in the time domain via equation B-1. The mathematic term for this process is **transformation.** It is

important to recognize that the frequency domain gives an equivalent representation of the sine wave of interest in a simplified format.

Fig. B-11 shows a time domain presentation of three sine waves; each sine wave has a unique frequency and amplitude. Phase is constant and equal to zero. This same information can be presented concisely in a graphic format in the frequency domain. The amplitude of each wave (labeled as magnitude to indicate the spectral analysis) is plotted as a function of frequency (Fig. B-12).

When the three sine waves in Fig. B-11 are added, the complex pattern in Fig. B-13 is generated. Fourier analysis of this pattern can be performed without previous knowledge of these individualized components and yields the frequency spectrum in Fig. B-14. The magnitude at each frequency describes the relative contribution of that frequency to the original waveform. This recipe calls for a mixture in which we add three parts nine-cycle wave, two parts six-cycle wave, and one part three-cycle wave.

In the previous example the waveform was composed of three sine waves only. Often, many sine waves of varying importance make up the waveform of interest. Upon Fourier analysis, a continuum of sine wave frequencies is obtained (Fig. B-15). The interpretation of this frequency spectrum is that a continuous range of frequency components from 0 to 12 cycles per second are present. The dominant frequency is six cycles per second. The contribution of the sine wave

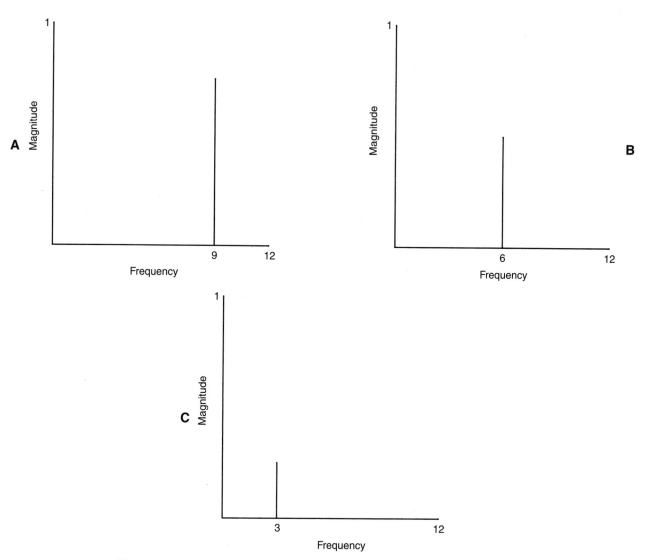

Fig. B-12 Frequency domain representation of the sine waves in Fig. B-11. Each sine wave consists of a single frequency denoted by the position of peak along the horizontal axis. **A,** High frequency. **B,** Middle frequency. **C,** Low frequency.

Sum of 3 sine waves

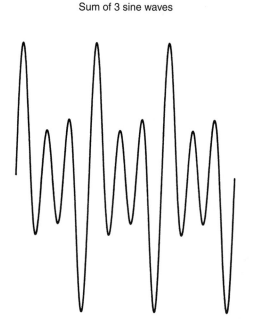

Fig. B-13 A complex pattern that is the sum of the three sine waves in Fig. B-11.

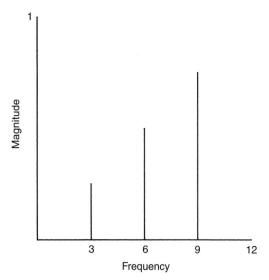

Fig. B-14 Frequency domain representation of the complex pattern in Fig. B-13.

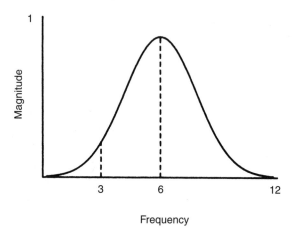

Fig. B-15 Frequency domain representation in which broad range of frequency components contribute to the waveform of interest. The magnitude for three and six cycles per second is 0.22 and 0.88, respectively.

with frequency of three cycles per second is determined by finding the magnitude corresponding to this frequency on the graph. A similar procedure is followed for all other frequencies.

Mathematic algorithms that allow computers to quickly perform Fourier analysis on a data set have been developed. Personal computers can also be programmed to compute the sine wave components of functions.

Answers to Review Questions

CHAPTER 1
BASIC ULTRASOUND PHYSICS

1. Density or compressibility
2. Toward
3. Longitudinal
4. 0.2 μs
5. 2.5 MHz
6. 0.44 mm
7. 1.39 Mrayls
8. 1.1%
9. 99.31%
10. %R = 99.9%, %T = 0.1%
11. $\alpha_R = 0.428$, $\alpha_T = 0.572$
12. 65 degrees
13. 21 degrees
14. 0.7 to 0.8
15. 3 cm
16. 26 μs
17. 20 cm
18. 1500 m/s
19. 1.6 mm
20. 3.33×10^5 Hz
21. 0.5

CHAPTER 2
ATTENUATION IN TISSUE

1. Attenuation
2. 0.7 to 0.8
3. 3.6 dB
4. −29 dB
5. 26.1 dB loss (assuming 0.8 dB/cm/MHz for soft tissue)
6. 39.6 dB loss (assuming 0.6 dB/cm/MHz for fat)
7. 42.8 dB loss (assuming 0.8 dB/cm/MHz for soft tissue)
8. 0.0032
9. 3

CHAPTER 3
COMPUTER FUNDAMENTALS

1. Bit
2. 1110
3. 110
4. 18
5. 134,220,000
6. Address
7. 8
8. Number of bits
9. 31

10. Pixel
11. 65,536 pixels
12. Spatial detail
13. Read-only memory (ROM)
14. Block
15. Low cost, high capacity, stable, compact

CHAPTER 4

SINGLE-ELEMENT TRANSDUCERS: PROPERTIES

1. 3.1 MHz
2. 0.5 mm
3. 0.31 mm
4. Depth of the field of view (scan range)
5. 5133 pulses per second
6. 0.2 ms
7. 0.77 mm
8. 0.5 μs
9. 0.001
10. 8 Mrayls
11. Without the matching layer, the transmission is 15% versus 31% with the matching layer.
12. 50%
13. 0.5 μs

CHAPTER 5

SINGLE-ELEMENT TRANSDUCERS: TRANSMISSION AND ECHO RECEPTION

1. Q-value, frequency, matching layer, and backing material
2. Focusing, crystal size, and frequency
3. Crystal diameter
4. Crystal diameter or frequency
5. 19.5 cm
6. 1.8 degrees
7. To reduce beam width so that lateral resolution is improved
8. Acoustic lens and curved crystal
9. Attenuation
10. TGC, rectification, enveloping, integration, and reject
11. Returning echoes from tissue vary by a factor of 1 million or more. To sort the echo-induced signals on the basis of amplitude requires a wide dynamic range.
12. Weak
13. Secondary lobes of ultrasound energy radiating at an angle to the main beam. Decreasing the Q-value.
14. Decreases dynamic range

CHAPTER 6

STATIC IMAGING PRINCIPLES AND INSTRUMENTATION

1. Signal amplitude
2. 13
3. Equal

4. Brightness
5. Registration arm
6. Scan converter
7. 0.25 mm × 0.5 mm
8. Gate

CHAPTER 7

IMAGE FORMATION IN REAL-TIME IMAGING

1. 42.8 fps
2. 0.013 second
3. Decreases by a factor of 2
4. Lateral
5. 120 to 150 scan lines, but the range can be 50 to 200 scan lines
6. 2000 to 5000 but can be higher
7. 15 to 20 fps but can be higher

CHAPTER 8

REAL-TIME ULTRASOUND TRANSDUCERS

1. Mechanical focusing by acoustic lens or curved crystal
2. Timing delays, aperture, and apodization
3. Selective activation of crystal elements
4. Transmit steering by altering the timing sequence of excitation pulses to the crystal elements
5. Mechanical movement of the transducer
6. Signals from multiple crystals are delayed and then summed to form the net signal (receive beam formation). Receive focal zone is varied with time following transmission (depth) so that a small sampling volume is maintained for all points along the scan line.
7. 0.016 second
8. 1.7

CHAPTER 9

REAL-TIME ULTRASOUND INSTRUMENTATION

1. A communication pathway between a crystal element and the transmitter or summing circuit in the beam former
2. Improved signal by interrogating the reflector from multiple angles
3. Distance from the point of interest to the respective crystal element. A constant acoustic velocity along the path is assumed.
4. If the acoustic velocity is not constant along all paths to the crystal elements, then channel-specific time delays are in error, and beam formation is distorted.
5. Intensity
6. Near the central beam axis
7. Frequency filtering and pulse inversion
8. Multiple scan lines

9. Elasticity imaging
10. Increases signal-to-noise ratio or penetration

CHAPTER 10
DIGITAL SIGNAL AND IMAGE PROCESSING

1. Edge enhancement
2. Write zoom, regional expansion, reduced field of view, zoom
3. 32
4. Contrast enhancement
5. Noise
6. Compression or TGC
7. Spatial smoothing

CHAPTER 11
IMAGE QUALITY

1. Spatial resolution, noise, contrast resolution, lack of geometric distortion, absence of artifacts
2. Image contrast
3. Adding
4. Frequency
5. Physical properties of tissue, acquisition parameters, and preprocessing of scan data
6. Multiple wavefronts from numerous scattering centers are detected simultaneously and produce a net signal by interference. The interference changes with time during the collection of a scan line. A pattern of bright and dark variations is created along each scan line. The two-dimensional presentation of speckle is constant if the spatial relationships of the scattering centers are unchanged. (The signal from interference is the same at each point in the sampling process.)

CHAPTER 12
IMAGE ARTIFACTS

1. The sound wave travels along a straight-line path from the transducer to the object and back to the transducer, attenuation of sound in tissue is uniform along the path, beam dimensions are small in both section thickness and lateral directions, all detected echoes originate from the axis of the main beam only, all received echoes are derived from the most recently transmitted pulse, the ultrasound wave travels at the rate of 1540 m/s, each reflector contributes a single echo when interrogated along a single scan line, and the amplitude of the echo is derived from the object scanned alone and is directly related to the reflective properties of the object.
2. Refraction
3. Reverberation, comet tail, and mirror image
4. PRF
5. Mirror image
6. Acoustic velocity in tissue
7. 15.4 cm
8. Front

CHAPTER 13
HEMODYNAMICS

1. Blood moves in concentric layers. Flow velocities vary across the vessel lumen, the slowest component near the vessel wall, and progressively increase toward the center of the lumen.
2. Pressure difference along the length of the vessel and luminal radius
3. Hydrostatic pressure
4. Bernoulli's equation. Conservation of energy from three sources: work, potential energy, and kinetic energy.
5. Frictional forces. Heat.
6. Inertia
7. Acceleration, curvature of the vessel, branching, obstruction, and diverging cross section
8. Fairly uniform distribution of flow velocities
9. Localized rotation of concentric blood layers
10. Velocity components are not coherent, wide range is present. Cross flow and reversal of flow.
11. 2650. Yes, since Reynolds' number exceeds 2000.
12. High-velocity jet at stenosis, flow reversal and broadening velocity distribution immediately distal, and turbulence more distal

CHAPTER 14
DOPPLER PHYSICS AND INSTRUMENTATION

1. The measured frequency of sound is offset from the true value if there is relative motion between the source of the sound and the receiver of the sound.
2. Velocity
3. Parallel to the sound wave
4. 779 Hz
5. 390 Hz
6. 29 cm/s
7. 1623 Hz
8. It is the algebraic addition of the transmitted and received waveforms and is equal to the difference between the transmitted frequency and received frequency.
9. Remove wall thump
10. False
11. Time the gate is activated
12. Aliasing

CHAPTER 15
DOPPLER SPECTRAL ANALYSIS

1. Scattering from RBCs produces relatively weak echoes compared with soft tissue.
2. Velocity and the relative number of RBCs moving at each velocity
3. Velocity, signal strength of each velocity component, and time
4. Increased velocity and fill-in of the spectral window

5. A time-dependent trace of the maximum velocity obtained in each FFT spectral analysis
6. Spectral broadening becomes greater.
7. The ability to depict rapid temporal changes in the velocity components is improved.
8. It improves signal-to-noise ratio or reduces the velocity range represented by the brightness-modulated dots.
9. Only the slow flow components near the vessel wall would be depicted. The maximum velocity waveform would appear diminished in magnitude.
10. Pulsatility index is independent of Doppler angle.

CHAPTER 16
DOPPLER IMAGING

1. Packet size
2. Autocorrelation
3. Remove signals from stationary reflectors
4. Time domain correlation
5. Lines of sight for gray scale and color flow are collected separately, width of color field of view is adjustable, Doppler angle is adjustable and may be different than gray-scale beam steering.
6. Simultaneous analysis of flow and gray-scale information, high frame rate, and color and gray-scale field of view are the same.
7. Time domain correlation
8. Mean velocity
9. Signal amplitude of moving reflectors
10. Color gate
11. Baseline
12. Increase packet size
13. Decrease line density, decrease packet size, decrease width of color field of view.
14. Aliasing, flash artifact, color bleed, mirror image, color noise

CHAPTER 17
M-MODE SCANNING

1. Reflector depth
2. Straight line
3. B
4. Temporal resolution
5. Echo strength
6. Color Doppler
7. M-mode sampling direction is defined relative to visualized structures.
8. Strip chart recorder, laser camera, videotape, electronic storage (CD-ROM)
9. The distance dimension is unchanged, but the time dimension is elongated to show temporal changes.

CHAPTER 18
CONTRAST AGENTS

1. Particles less than 6 microns can cross the pulmonary capillary bed and are efficient scatterers of ultrasound energy.
2. Controls biodistribution and stability
3. Harmonic
4. Acoustic power
5. Loss of signal following destruction of contrast agent is interpreted as motion and encoded in color.
6. Intermittent sampling
7. Pulse inversion harmonic imaging and power pulse inversion harmonic imaging

CHAPTER 19
IMAGE-RECORDING DEVICES

1. Bulk
2. Silver halide grains
3. Internal CRT
4. The hard copy device must be matched to the monitor. If the monitor settings are changed, then the recorded image will not be the same as shown on the monitor.
5. VCR or CD-ROM
6. Video printers and CD-ROM
7. Sublimation
8. Spatial detail
9. Spatial resolution

CHAPTER 20
PICTURE ARCHIVING AND COMMUNICATION SYSTEM

1. By standardizing file formats and transmission protocols, a PACS network is not limited to one manufacturer. DICOM allows devices from different manufacturers to function on the same network. Purchase decisions can be based on the merits of the desired component, whether ultrasound scanner or laser printer.
2. Data compression reduces the file size for storage and transmission. Smaller file size decreases archival storage costs and network transmission costs.
3. Lossless and lossy
4. Decreased film costs, no lost films, current list of studies for interpretation, prompt access to images from multiple modalities, multiple clinicians can view the same images simultaneously, electronic storage of patient data, image processing, electronic transfer to remote locations
5. Electronic devices fail. If all patient data were stored on one device, which failed, then all information is lost.
6. MODs, magnetic tape, RAID
7. 2.1 seconds
8. Baud rate
9. Low ambient light levels, indirect incandescent lighting, no glare from bright objects or windows, walls with low reflection
10. Gray-scale mapping (changing the window and level)

11. Spatial resolution (number of pixels), lack of distortion, contrast resolution, aspect ratio, maximum luminance, dynamic range, uniformity, persistence, refresh rate

CHAPTER 21
INTENSITY AND POWER

1. SPTP, SATP, SPTA, SATA
2. Megapascal, pascal
3. Pulse averaged intensity, pulse duration, pulse repetition frequency
4. Square
5. I(SPTA), mechanical index
6. Focusing
7. Water

CHAPTER 22
BIOLOGIC EFFECTS

1. Mechanical, thermal, and cavitational
2. Collected works from many researchers combine to form an overall picture of the induced biologic effects. The intensity descriptors, for example, provide a basis for comparison.
3. Biologic effects in human populations exposed to the agent of interest are assessed under actual conditions of use.
4. An increasing number of individuals are exposed to ultrasound examination in utero. Substantial damage can be manifested in large populations even if the probability of the effect is low.
5. 100 mW/cm^2, 1 W/cm^2, SPTA
6. Length of time of the temperature rise

CHAPTER 23
CLINICAL SAFETY

1. Temperature rise
2. Cavitation
3. Square root of the frequency
4. Attenuation coefficient, distance, and frequency
5. Threshold
6. Routine screening for every pregnancy is not recommended by the National Institutes of Health.
7. Measurements in water underestimate the in situ intensity or pressure.
8. There have been no demonstrated harmful effects in patient populations at the intensity levels used in the examination. Numerous studies have been conducted to evaluate potential hazards, and many more continue to be done. Your physician ordered this examination because he or she believes it will provide diagnostic information important for your medical care that outweighs any risk associated with ultrasonic exposure.

CHAPTER 24
PERFORMANCE TESTING

1. Dead zone, distance accuracy, axial resolution, lateral resolution, penetration, image uniformity, focal zone, cyst characteristics
2. 0.5 dB/cm/MHz and 0.7 dB/cm/MHz
3. Penetration (sensitivity or signal to noise)
4. Beam width (focusing)
5. Acoustic velocity
6. SMPTE
7. Attenuation
8. Device to measure ultrasound intensity
9. Region near the transducer in which tissue echoes are not depicted
10. Perpendicular to the beam axis
11. Distance measurements by the scanner would be correct if the hard copy recording device introduces error.
12. Interference from shadowing

CHAPTER 25
QUALITY CONTROL

1. Sensitivity, image uniformity, distance accuracy, fidelity of image display, and fidelity of image recording
2. Fidelity of image display and fidelity of image recording
3. The fidelity of image recording depends on a matched response between the monitor and image recording device. Adjustment of the monitor will cause an erroneous reproduction of the image viewed on the display monitor.
4. Velocity in urethane is less than that in soft tissue and frequency dependence of the attenuation coefficient.
5. Tissue-mimicking phantom
6. Each day of use
7. Spatial mapping of echoes in the image depends on different processes (echo ranging for vertical placement and beam steering for horizontal placement).
8. Check for instrument settings (particularly power) and rescan the phantom. If the problem persists, test the transducer on another unit, if available. Consult with the lead sonographer.

Answers to Review Test Questions

1. B	28. B	55. E	82. A
2. A	29. D	56. A	83. A
3. B	30. A	57. B	84. D
4. D	31. D	58. A	85. B
5. C	32. C	59. B	86. B
6. B	33. A	60. D	87. B
7. C	34. C	61. D	88. D
8. D	35. B	62. B	89. D
9. A	36. C	63. D	90. C
10. D	37. A	64. A	91. D
11. A	38. A	65. D	92. A
12. B	39. A	66. A	93. B
13. A	40. D	67. C	94. C
14. C	41. B	68. D	95. A
15. B	42. B	69. B	96. A
16. B	43. B	70. D	97. C
17. A	44. D	71. D	98. B
18. C	45. A	72. A	99. A
19. C	46. B	73. D	100. A
20. C	47. B	74. C	101. B
21. B	48. B	75. C	102. D
22. C	49. D	76. A	103. A
23. D	50. C	77. B	104. D
24. C	51. C	78. B	105. A
25. B	52. A	79. A	106. B
26. D	53. D	80. C	107. D
27. B	54. E	81. D	108. A

109.	B	132.	C	155.	C	178.	A
110.	A	133.	D	156.	B	179.	B
111.	A	134.	A	157.	D	180.	C
112.	C	135.	C	158.	A	181.	C
113.	D	136.	A	159.	B	182.	C
114.	D	137.	A	160.	B	183.	A
115.	C	138.	C	161.	C	184.	A
116.	A	139.	A	162.	B	185.	A
117.	C	140.	C	163.	B	186.	C
118.	A	141.	B	164.	C	187.	C
119.	B	142.	C	165.	B	188.	C
120.	B	143.	A	166.	A	189.	B
121.	A	144.	B	167.	D	190.	C
122.	B	145.	C	168.	A	191.	A
123.	A	146.	D	169.	A	192.	D
124.	B	147.	B	170.	B	193.	C
125.	B	148.	B	171.	C	194.	B
126.	B	149.	A	172.	D	195.	B
127.	C	150.	D	173.	A	196.	C
128.	B	151.	C	174.	D	197.	D
129.	C	152.	B	175.	C	198.	C
130.	D	153.	A	176.	B	199.	B
131.	D	154.	D	177.	A	200.	B

Glossary

3D imaging An imaging mode in which spatial relationships of structures within a scanned volume are represented in three spatial dimensions. The display of tomographic data is by a surface-rendered image, volume-rendered image, or multiple format planes.

4D ultrasound An imaging mode in which a surface-rendered entity or multiple planes of the sampled volume are displayed in real time.

absorption The process whereby energy is deposited in a medium by transforming ultrasonic energy into other energy forms, primarily heat. It is an exponentially decreasing function and is the major factor in the total attenuation of the beam.

absorption coefficient A parameter that characterizes the rate at which sound energy is absorbed in a medium. Expressed as fractional loss or decibel loss per unit distance. The absorption coefficient increases linearly with the frequency.

acceptance testing The initial testing of equipment at installation that permits one to determine whether the equipment meets the specifications of the manufacturer, as well as the purchaser.

acoustic impedance (Z) A measure of the resistance of a medium to the transmission of sound. The acoustic impedance is expressed as the product of acoustic velocity of the medium and the density of the medium ($Z = \rho c$). The acoustic impedance mismatch at the interface determines the amount of reflection that occurs. See **intensity reflection coefficient.**

acoustic output A measure of the intensity, pressure, or power in the transmitted ultrasound beam generated by a transducer.

acoustic velocity (c) The rate and direction at which sound propagates through a medium. The average velocity of sound in soft tissue is 1540 m/s.

address The designator for a location in computer memory. Random access memory uses the address to write information directly to a specific location or to read information directly from a specific location.

algorithm A prescribed set of well-defined operations for the solution of a problem in a finite number of steps.

aliasing An artifact in pulsed-wave Doppler, in which a high-frequency Doppler shift is incorrectly interpreted as a lower frequency. Aliasing is caused by the intermittent sampling of the Doppler data.

alphanumeric Alphabetic and numeric characters.

A-mode Type of scanning mode in which the amplitude of the signal is plotted versus the depth of the interface. The strength of the reflected echo is represented by the height of a spike.

amplification A technique in signal processing whereby a low-level signal (microvolt or millivolt) is increased to a higher-level signal (volts).

amplitude Normally used to refer to the particle displacement, particle velocity, or acoustic pressure of a sound wave. Amplitude also indicates the strength of the detected echo or the voltage induced in a crystal by a pressure wave.

analog A continuously variable signal, as opposed to discrete values.

analog-to-digital converter (ADC) A device that translates continuously variable signals (analog) into discrete values (digital). The digital form can then be manipulated and stored by computers.

anechoic The area in an image relatively free of echoes. This usually occurs within a fluid-filled structure or behind a very strong reflector.

angle of incidence The angle with respect to a line drawn perpendicular to the surface at which the sound beam strikes the interface.

angle of reflection The angle with respect to a line drawn perpendicular to the surface at which the sound beam is reflected from an interface. The angle of reflection equals the angle of incidence.

annular phased array Type of transducer in which the crystal arrangement is in concentric rings. Electronic focusing is applied for both the in-plane and out-of-plane directions. Sampling along different lines of sight is achieved by mechanical means.

aperture The piezoelectric area of a transducer that is activated to form a transmitted beam.

apodization A transmit and receive technique to reduce grating and side lobes. The transmission process involves varying the excitation voltage for each crystal element across the aperture of a multielement array to be highest at the center and lower in magnitude toward the boundary. The reception process involves varying the gain applied for each crystal element across the aperture of a multielement array to be highest at the center and lower in magnitude toward the boundary.

archival storage Long-term electronic storage of image data and associated patient information.

artifact A structure in the image that does not provide a true representation of the scanned object. Artifacts are created by the inherent nature of sound interactions (e.g., refraction, shadowing, and enhancement) or by the malfunction of equipment or by the improper operation of equipment.

asynchronous scanner In Doppler imaging, flow and gray-scale scan data are acquired independently of each other.

attenuation The decrease in intensity as a sound beam travels through the medium. Attenuation depends on all the interactions of ultrasound with tissues (i.e., macroscopic interactions), which include scattering, divergence, and absorption. Reflection may be included or treated separately as a component of beam intensity reduction.

attenuation coefficient A parameter that characterizes the rate at which sound energy is lost by absorption and scattering in a medium. Expressed as fractional loss or decibel loss per unit distance. The attenuation coefficient increases linearly with the frequency.

attenuation compensated flow volume ratemeter A device to measure volume flow rate that accounts for differences in path-length attenuation.

autocorrelation A processing technique in Doppler imaging whereby a series of echoes from the same reflector (red blood cell group) are examined to assess motion. Very fast data-collection method in which the mean frequency of the Doppler signal is estimated.

axial pressure profile A representation of the acoustic pressure along the axis of the beam. Measurements of acoustic pressure provide an indication of the variation in beam intensity.

axial resolution The ability to resolve, as separate entities, objects located near each other along the axis of propagation. Axial resolution depends on the spatial pulse length.

backing material The material placed behind the crystal in the transducer to dampen ringing of the crystal. Air is used for continuous wave ultrasound where the difference between the acoustic impedances of the crystal and the backing material is large, resulting in maximum ringing and output. The acoustic impedance of the backing material and the acoustic impedance of the crystal are nearly the same for B-mode imaging to prevent ringing.

bandwidth A parameter that describes the distribution of frequency components in a wave (e.g., transmitted ultrasound pulsed wave).

baseline In spectral Doppler flow detection, a control that shifts the center point of the velocity scale to vary the range of velocities displayed in the forward and reverse directions.

baseline values The initial values for performance parameters measured at the start of a quality control program to which future measurements are compared.

BASIC Beginner's All-Purpose Symbolic Instruction Code, a programming language used extensively with personal computers.

baud Data transmission rate of 1 bit per second.

beam aperture The piezoelectric area of a transducer that is activated to form a transmitted beam.

beam cross-sectional area The area on the surface of a plane perpendicular to the beam axis consisting of all points at which the pulse intensity integral is greater than 25% of the maximum pulse intensity integral in that plane.

beam formation (reception) Echo-induced signals from multiple crystal elements are delayed in time and then summed to maximize the net signal associated with the reflector.

beam formation (transmission) Timed sequence of excitation pulses applied to crystal elements across the aperture to enable focusing and/or steering of the ultrasound beam.

beam width The lateral extent of the beam perpendicular to beam propagation. Beam width varies along the beam axis. For an unfocused transducer, beam width is smallest in the near field and increases with depth in the far field. Focusing reduces the beam width and thus improves the lateral resolution within the focal zone.

beat frequency A phenomenon caused by wave interference in which waves of different frequencies, when added together, produce rhythmic cycles or beats. Beat frequencies in Doppler ultrasound obtained by combining the transmitted and received signals indicate the presence of motion.

belt phantom A device to evaluate the accuracy, linearity, and precision of Doppler velocity measurements.

Bernoulli's principle The total energy content of a flowing nonviscous liquid is conserved. Potential energy, kinetic energy, and work contribute to the total energy.

bilinear interpolation A scan conversion method to assign echo amplitude to a pixel, which is not interrogated by a scan line. The interpolation is performed in the axial and angular directions.

binary The number system with a base of 2. Two possible states—either 1 or 0.

bistable scanning Storage of B-mode dots, which results in only a black and white image. The condition of the dot is either "on" or "off" (bright or dark).

bit A binary digit, either 1 or 0. The smallest unit of information in the binary system. Bits are the building blocks of computer bytes and words.

B-mode Brightness mode scanning, which modulates the brightness of a dot to indicate the amplitude of the signal displayed at the location of the interface.

broadband transducer A transducer with a wide frequency distribution. The fractional bandwidth is greater than or equal to 15%.

broker A computer that converts patient data in HL7 to DICOM and vice versa to allow communication between information systems and picture archiving and communication systems.

buffer Electronic storage where information is held temporarily until a device is ready to receive the information.

bulk modulus A physical parameter that quantifies the fractional change in volume when a pressure is applied to material. The bulk modulus is the reciprocal of the compressibility. The velocity of sound in the medium is directly proportional to the square root of the bulk modulus.

byte A group of 8 bits, usually handled together and treated as a unit by a computer.

capture function A Doppler imaging technique in which the highest mean velocity detected at each pixel location during a sampling interval of 1 to several seconds is displayed.

cathode ray tube (CRT) A display device for two-dimensional information that has a cathode (source of electrons) and an anode (phosphor screen) biased with a high potential difference. Electrons are accelerated across the tube to strike the phosphor screen. Focusing cups and magnetic or electronic deflection plates control the size and position of the electron beam on the phosphor screen.

cavitation Dynamic behavior of microbubbles in the medium exposed to an ultrasonic beam. Two types of cavitation are possible: stable and transient. An intensity threshold is associated with transient cavitation.

center frequency The frequency that has the highest magnitude in a graph of the frequency components of the transmitted sound wave.

central processing unit (CPU) Computer hardware that performs mathematic manipulations, interprets logic functions, and coordinates all control operations, including data transfers from one device to another in the system.

channel A communication pathway between a crystal element and the transmitter or summing circuit in the beam former. The total number of channels limit the number of crystal elements that participate in beam formation.

cine loop Multiple frames of a real-time acquisition stored in computer memory for immediate playback.

clutter A type of acoustic noise. Signals induced by echoes created by secondary lobes striking off-axis structures.

C-mode scanning A gated-mode scanning technique that processes data from a specified depth only.

coded excitation Frequency modulation (chirp) or binary encoding of the transmitted pulse to improve signal-to-noise ratio. Upon reception the echo signal must be manipulated mathematically (deconvoluted) to compress the signal waveform.

color aliasing An artifact in Doppler imaging in which high-frequency Doppler shifts above the Nyquist limit are depicted by colors associated with slower flow.

color bleed An extension of color beyond the region of flow in Doppler imaging.

color flash Sudden burst of color associated with tissue movement in Doppler imaging.

color flow imaging or **color Doppler imaging** A real-time acquisition in which flow information encoded in color is superimposed on a gray-scale image depicting stationary structures.

color gain Doppler imaging parameter that adjusts amplification of the Doppler signal.

color gate Doppler imaging parameter that sets the axial length of the Doppler sampling volume.

color map Assignment of various shades or brightness of color to depict different velocities while maintaining directional information.

color M-mode The presentation of the color Doppler image in conjunction with the M-mode trace. The sampling direction for M-mode is shown on the color Doppler image.

color noise Random variations in signal detection cause areas with no flow to be color encoded in Doppler imaging.

color persistence Frame averaging in Doppler imaging.

color reject Doppler imaging parameter that sets an amplitude threshold for the display of Doppler signals.

color threshold Doppler imaging parameter that sets the lower velocity limit for the display of moving reflectors.

color video printer Color image-recording device that receives image data in the form of the video signal. The print medium is paper.

combined Doppler mode The presentation of the color flow image in conjunction with the time display of the pulsed-wave spectral analysis.

comet tail artifact An artifact created from small, highly reflective interfaces. They originate from multiple internal reflections and are seen in normally echo-free areas.

compact disk (CD) Type of optical storage device. Capacity is approximately 650 megabytes.

compiler A computer program that translates high-level language source code into machine language.

compound B-mode scanning A two-dimensional static imaging mode in which brightness-modulated dots indicate the origin and amplitude of the echoes. Special electrical components store the signals, and a registration arm is required to place the induced signals at the appropriate locations.

compound linear array A linear array transducer that steers the beam via electronic phasing to extend the width of the field of view.

compressibility The ease with which a medium can be compressed. The velocity of sound in a medium is inversely proportional to the square root of compressibility of the medium.

compression (computer) A data manipulation technique to reduce the number of bytes needed to represent the data set. Most often applied to digital images to decrease the storage requirements and transmission time of patient studies.

compression (digital processing) A signal processing technique in real-time imaging to reduce the dynamic range of signal values.

compression (wave propagation) A high-pressure region or a region of increased density of particles in a medium created by the action of the sound wave.

computer program A series of coded instructions designed to solve a problem.

constructive interference A process whereby two waves algebraically add together to produce a wave of greater amplitude than either of the original waves.

contrast agent Material introduced to enhance tissue echogenicity.

contrast enhancement An image processing technique that changes the association between signal values and gray levels to display pixels with similar values as different shades of gray.

contrast harmonic imaging An imaging technique to de-emphasize tissue without the presence of contrast agent by detecting the reflected harmonics from microbubbles.

contrast resolution The ability to resolve two objects with similar reflective properties (signal levels) as separate entities.

control limits Range of values for a quality control parameter that are considered acceptable for proper functioning equipment.

converse piezoelectric effect A property of piezoelectric materials whereby an electric stimulus causes the dipolar material to expand and contract, producing a pressure wave (sound wave). This property permits a material to be used as a transmitter of ultrasound. See **piezoelectric effect**.

coprocessing The computer processing of multiple lines of sight simultaneously to maintain high frame rates when multiple fixed transmit focal zones are used in real-time imaging.

Curie temperature The temperature above which dipoles move about freely in a material.

curvilinear array Multiple crystal elements arranged linearly on a curved surface. A curved linear array reduces side lobes and grating lobes, since the lines of sight are always perpendicular to the transducer face. The width of the field of view extends beyond the physical dimension of the row of crystal elements.

cycle A sequence of events recurring at regular intervals in time or space. For example, particle density varies from a maximum in the compression zone to a minimum in the rarefaction zone and back to a maximum in the successive compression zone to complete one cycle. The distance for this cycle is the wavelength.

damping The effect of reducing ringing or shortening the temporal pulse length after the excitation pulse. The damping is affected by the backing material and the Q-value of the transducer.

database A collection of interrelated data that can be accessed and used for one or more applications.

dead zone The distance from the face of the transducer to the closest identifiable echo.

decibel Unit to express relative intensity or power: relative intensity (dB) = $10 \log I/I_0$, where I is the intensity at the point of interest, and I_0 is the original or reference intensity.

deflection plates Magnetic or electronic plates in a cathode ray tube that control the horizontal and vertical position of the electron beam.

degree of focusing A transducer descriptor that indicates location and relative beam width of the focal zone.

delay gain A control of an ultrasound scanner to set the depth at which the time gain compensation is first applied.

demodulation (signal isolation) A signal that has undergone interference with a carrier wave is subsequently isolated from the carrier wave. This procedure is often used in Doppler ultrasound, in which the sum of the reference and received signals produce rapid oscillations that vary in strength at the beat frequency.

demodulation (signal processing) The technique of enveloping the radiofrequency signal by ignoring the rapid oscillations and retaining the maximum amplitude of each cycle.

density (ρ) A physical parameter that describes the mass of a medium per unit volume.

depth of field Length of the focal zone for a focused transducer.

derating factor Fractional reduction in intensity or pressure caused by attenuation.

destructive interference A process whereby waves add together algebraically to give a resultant wave of lower amplitude than either of the original waves.

DICOM (Digital Imaging and Communication in Medicine) Standardized file formats for patient data and images as well as criteria for the transfer, storage, and display of this information.

dielectric constant A transducer parameter that determines the electrical and mechanical matching of the transducer to the rest of the ultrasonic system.

diffraction The spreading out of the beam that results from the beam passing through a small aperture.

diffuse reflection The reflection of an ultrasound beam in multiple directions from a large rough-surfaced object.

digital A numerical representation of discrete values by a series of 1s and 0s.

digital filtering A computer technique designed to modify the value in each pixel throughout the image matrix based on the values in the surrounding pixels.

digital subtraction harmonic imaging A background image acquired immediately following the destruction of the microbubbles is subtracted from the contrast-enhanced image obtained during the destruction of the microbubbles. The resultant image depicts a signal from the contrast agent only.

digitization The process of converting analog signals into digital signals.

dipole Positively and negatively charged regions on a molecule.

dispersion The dependence of the velocity of sound or other physical parameter on the frequency of the sound source.

distortion A parameter of image quality that describes the lack of adherence to the original geometric relationships.

divergence The spreading out of a beam that results from a source of small physical dimensions or diffraction or scattering. Divergence degrades the ultrasonic image by creating a loss of beam intensity.

Doppler angle The angle between the beam axis and the direction of travel for the moving reflector.

Doppler effect Relative motion between the sound source and sound receiver causes a change in the observed frequency.

Doppler imaging Moving reflectors encoded in color and stationary reflectors encoded in shades of gray are depicted throughout the field of view in real time.

Doppler shift The change in frequency between the transmitted frequency (f) and received frequency by reflection from an interface moving with velocity (v) at an angle (φ) to the sound source:

$$\text{Doppler shift} = \frac{2f\, v \cos \varphi}{c}$$

where c is the velocity of sound in the medium.

Doppler spectral waveform The time display of the power spectrum of the Doppler signal.

dry processing The development of transparency film without liquid chemistry.

duplex scanner Instrument that combines real-time imaging with Doppler flow detection.

duty factor The fraction of the time the transducer is actively producing the ultrasound beam. The duty factor is found by dividing the pulse duration by the pulse repetition period. This factor is important when characterizing biologic effects of ultrasound.

dwell time The time required to interrogate one line of sight.

dynamic imaging Echo wavetrains from pulse-inverted transmit pulses along the scan line are manipulated to isolate the harmonic signals from microbubbles and eliminate static tissue signals. Real-time imaging at low power levels is possible.

dynamic range A measure of the span of signal magnitudes that can be represented or processed by the various components of a system.

dynamic receive focusing An electronic focusing method that uses continuously variable delay lines to sweep the receive focal zone through all depths during reception of returning echoes.

ECG-gated scanning A gated-scanning technique that processes information electronically during a specific portion of the heart cycle using the electrocardiographic wave as a trigger.

echocardiography The branch of cardiology that uses ultrasound to study the function of the heart.

echo-ranging A technique to determine the distance of an object from the transducer that relies on reflection. A sound beam is transmitted into a medium and reflected from the object back to the sound source. The elapsed time (t) between the transmitted pulse and the received echo is converted into total distance traveled (z) according to the formula $z = ct$. The velocity of sound in the medium (c) is assumed to be known. The distance from the transducer to the object is equal to half this total distance.

echo wavetrain The succession of echoes detected along a line of sight following the transmitted pulse.

eddy flow A region of swirling motion for a flowing fluid.

edge enhancement A filtering technique to make the boundaries of structures sharper.

elasticity imaging The resistance of tissue to a change in shape when the force is applied is depicted throughout the field of view.

electromagnetic radiation Waves consisting of alternating electrical and magnetic fields perpendicularly to each other. Electromagnetic radiation such as light and x-rays can propagate through a vacuum.

electromechanical coupling coefficient A transducer factor that describes how well the electrical stimulus is converted to acoustic energy and how well the returning echo is converted to an induced electrical signal in the crystal. Mathematically, the electromechanical coupling coefficient is equal to the product of the transmission and reception coefficient. This coefficient can be considered as the total conversion efficiency of the transducer.

electronic focusing Electronic delay lines connected to individual crystals of multi-element transducer are adjusted to cause the ultrasonic beam to reach the point of interest in phase (focus) and to reinforce the induced signals on reception of the echo.

electronic real-time scanner Automated (by electronic means) scanning or steering of the ultrasound beam through the area of interest to collect multiple lines of sight for each image at high frame rates.

endosonography Specialized real-time imaging with small probes that can be inserted into various body cavities (e.g., endovaginal and endorectal).

enhancement An image artifact created behind a low-attenuating object such as a cyst. Reflectors distal to the low-attenuating medium appear with greater amplitude than identical reflectors located in the neighboring region.

ensemble length The number of pulses used to sample a color line of sight in Doppler imaging. Also called packet size.

enveloping The electronic process of surrounding the rectified radiofrequency signal.

epidemiology The study of the factors related to the presence or absence of disease in a population.

extended field of view As a transducer is moved across the patient, successive frames are combined to form a panoramic image. Method to enlarge the field of view of a real-time transducer.

facing material The material applied across the aperture of a transducer to prevent damage to the crystal(s) and to reduce the acoustic impedance mismatch between the crystal and tissue.

far field The region beyond the near field for a nonfocused transducer in which the ultrasound beam diverges rapidly. In this region, lateral resolution becomes increasingly poor with depth.

far gain An instrument setting for time gain compensation that controls maximum amplification in the region far from the transducer. Signals arising from this region decrease exponentially in strength with depth.

fast Fourier transform (FFT) Mathematic algorithm designed to separate a waveform into its various frequency components. Spectral analysis of the complex Doppler signal identifies the Doppler shifts and their relative importance.

feedback microbalance A device that measures the average power over the beam cross-sectional area.

field of view (FOV) The physical region probed by the ultrasound beam that corresponds to the image.

film development The processing of transparency film to produce a gray-scale image. Usually implies that liquid chemistry was used.

firewall A router or computer connection between two networks that controls access to information in one network from the other. A security measure to protect system data.

fixed echo canceller A Doppler signal processing technique in which echoes from stationary reflectors are removed by subtracting identical echoes in consecutive echo wavetrains along the same scan line.

flow phantom A Doppler scanner test device in which volume flow rate is regulated.

f-number Ratio of focal length to the aperture for a focused transducer.

focal length The distance from the front face of the transducer to the focal point.

focal point The point along the beam axis with minimum width and maximum intensity for a focused transducer.

focal zone For a focused transducer, the region defined by the pressure amplitude that is within 3 dB of the maximum pressure amplitude of the transmitted beam. The focal zone corresponds to the region of minimum beam width.

focal zone banding Artifact in which adjacent transmit focal zones are presented with markedly different signal levels.

focusing A process whereby the beam width is reduced by mechanical or electronic means to improve the lateral resolution.

footprint The active piezoelectric area of a transducer that transmits ultrasound waves.

Fourier analysis The mathematic process of converting a complex wave into a series of sine waves of different frequencies (component parts). This process changes the amplitude versus time domain to the amplitude versus frequency domain.

fractional bandwidth The distribution of frequency components in a wave (e.g., transmitted ultrasound pulsed wave) expressed as a fraction of the center frequency.

frame rate The number of images acquired per second.

Fraunhofer zone (far field) The region beyond the near field for a nonfocused transducer in which the ultrasound beam diverges rapidly. In this region, lateral resolution becomes increasingly poor with depth.

free-field measurements Performed in water without reflectors or other disturbances to the ultrasonic field.

freeze frame An image acquired during the real-time scanning is designated for continuous display until this mode is turned off.

frequency (f) The number of wave cycles passing a given point in a given increment of time. The unit is cycles/second or hertz. Frequency is the inverse of the period.

frequency compounding Frequency components in the echo signal are processed separately and then recombined in a single image to improve contrast.

frequency domain processing Combined with quadrature phase detection to generate the spectrum of Doppler shifts.

Fresnel zone (near field) For the nonfocused transducer, the region from the front face extending to the beginning of divergence (corresponds to the last maximum)—the area with the most narrow beam width.

gated-mode scanning A scanning technique that electronically processes selected received signals on command from a specific gated signal (i.e., depth or electrocardiogram cycle).

ghost-image artifact An artifact whereby an object located distal to refractive structures is replicated multiple times in the image.

ghosting A mirror image of the color flow produced when the vessel is located in front of a strong reflector.

grating lobes Secondary intensity lobes created by the regular spacing of crystal elements that are offset from the main intensity lobe. Grating lobes create artifacts in which a detected object is placed at the wrong location in the image.

gray bars The gray-scale test pattern present on most ultrasonic units that can be used to check the photographic system.

gray-scale imaging An alternative name for B-mode scanning. The brightness of the detected signal is displayed in various shades of gray to represent different echo amplitudes.

H and D curve Response of film characterized by a plot of optical density versus exposure or log exposure.

half-value layer (HVL) The amount of material required to reduce the intensity by half of its original value. A half-value layer results in a 3 dB reduction in intensity.

hard copy The recording of the image on printed media (film or paper).

harmonic frequencies Integer multiples of the fundamental frequency.

hertz The unit of frequency that expresses the number of cycles per second. The kilohertz (kHz) is 10^3 Hz, and the megahertz (MHz) is 10^6 Hz.

heterodyne Doppler detection method to identify the direction of motion. An offset signal is combined with the reference signal to place Doppler shifts corresponding to a particular direction within a well-defined frequency range.

high-pass filter A filter that removes the low-frequency components and retains the high-frequency components of the signal.

horizontal distance Measurement of distance in the direction perpendicular to the axis of the beam.

Huygens' principle The division of a large sound source into a collection of small radiating sources. Each small individual source creates its own beam pattern, which interferes with those from the other sources to form a complex beam pattern.

hydrophone A device to measure pressure variations in the ultrasonic field.

hydrostatic pressure Pressure generated by the position of fluid in a gravitational field.

hyperechoic Characterization of relatively strong echoes created in the image compared with nearby regions.

hypoechoic Characterization of relatively weak echoes created in the image compared with nearby regions.

image-recording device A device interfaced to the scanner that produces a hard copy of the image.

inertia loss Slowing the velocity of fluid flow causes a reduction in kinetic energy.

infrasound Low-frequency (<20 Hz) mechanical waves that the human ear cannot detect.

in-line transducer A transducer that does not use an acoustic mirror to reflect the beam. The sound beam follows a direct, straight-line path from the crystal element to the transducer face.

integration An electronic processing technique in which the area under the echo signal is represented as a spike or dot. The area is proportional to the amplitude of the returning echo; thus the height of the spike or brightness of the dot is also proportional to the echo amplitude.

intensity A physical parameter that describes the amount of energy flowing through a unit cross-sectional area of a beam each second. This is the rate at which the wave transmits the energy over a small area. The unit of intensity is the watt per square centimeter or joule per second per square centimeter.

intensity descriptors Parameters used to specify the intensity of the ultrasonic field with respect to space and time.

intensity reflection coefficient The fraction of beam intensity reflected from an acoustic interface, given as

$$\alpha_R = \left(\frac{Z_2 - Z_1}{Z_2 + Z_1} \right)$$

where Z_1 and Z_2 are the acoustic impedances of the media that compose the interface.

interelement coupling The vibration or electrical stimulation of one crystal element in an array affecting adjacent crystal elements.

interelement isolation The process reducing mechanical and electrical coupling between crystal elements in an array.

interface The junction of two media with different acoustic properties.

interference The superposition or algebraic summation of waves. Constructive or destructive interference can occur.

intermittent imaging An image of the distribution of the contrast agent is obtained at a high power level. The process of acquiring the image data destroys the contrast agent present within the field of view. The persistence of the contrast agent is extended by reducing the sampling rate to one frame every one to four cardiac cycles.

kernel A collection of weighting values used in a convolution operation, such as smoothing.

kilobyte Equals 2^{10} (1024) bytes; generally denotes storage capacity.

laminar flow Fluid flow in which neighboring layers are not mixed. The velocity profile incorporates slow-moving components near the vessel wall with faster-moving components toward the center of the lumen.

laser camera Type of image-recording device using transparency film. Optical density is controlled for each pixel by a modulated laser beam.

lateral resolution The ability to resolve, as separate entities, two adjacent objects that lie perpendicular to the beam axis. Lateral resolution depends on the beam width. Focusing the sound beam improves the lateral resolution.

length focusing (in-plane) The focusing of a linear array along the in-plane or length direction of the array to reduce beam width in that direction. This type of focusing is accomplished electronically.

length-mode vibration For a linear array, the expansion and contraction of the rectangular element along the length of the array that can cause interelement coupling, inducing artifacts in the final image.

linear array A multielement transducer in which the crystal elements are positioned one after another in a row. Selective activation of the crystal elements determines the scan line. The image format is rectangular.

linear phased array A multielement transducer in which the beam is electronically steered and focused by time-delayed excitation of the crystals. The image format is sector.

line density The concentration of scan lines within the field of view.

line of sight A line directed along the axis of the beam. Real-time images consist of multiple scan lines collected by mechanically or electronically sweeping the beam through many directions.

liquid crystal display (LCD) Type of solid-state monitor that has smaller overall size compared with cathode ray tubes having the same viewing area.

liquid path A nonattenuating liquid layer (usually water-alcohol mixture) added to the front of the transducer to permit better coupling to the patient. These systems typically use large radii transducers.

longitudinal wave A wave in which the particle motion is along the same direction as the propagation of the wave energy (direction of travel of the wave).

loss of correlation Color Doppler imaging applied to depict the distribution of contrast agent in which the destruction of microbubbles is encoded in color.

low-pass filter A filter that removes high-frequency components and retains the low-frequency components of the signal.

master synchronizer A device that controls the timing sequence of all subsystems in the ultrasonic unit. The master synchronizer provides the "start" pulse to all the subsystem "clocks" at the time of the initial transmitted pulse.

matching layer A layer of material placed next to the radiating surface of the crystal in the transducer to facilitate the transmission of sound energy into the patient.

matrix size The number of rows and columns of pixels composing the image. A 512×512 matrix consists of 262,144 elements.

maximum depth of visualization Limit of the scan range at which parenchyma scatterers are perceived.

maximum frequency The Doppler shift associated with the most rapid motion. An upper cutoff limit between 1% and 5% is applied to the power spectrum in this determination.

maximum velocity waveform The time display of the highest velocity component of the Doppler signal.

mean frequency The average of all Doppler shifts in the power spectrum.

mechanical coefficient (Q) The Q-value of the transducer dictates the pulse length and frequency bandwidth. It is defined as either the energy stored per cycle divided by the energy lost per cycle or as the center frequency divided by the bandwidth.

mechanical focusing The method of narrowing the beam using acoustic lenses or curved crystals.

mechanical index A parameter that describes the acoustic output in terms of the likelihood of cavitation. The cavitation threshold is predicted by the ratio of the peak rarefactional pressure to the square root of the frequency.

mechanical interaction Mechanism by which damage can be induced by movement of objects.

mechanical real-time scanner A real-time imaging device in which a mechanical stepping motor sweeps the beam back and forth to collect the lines of sight.

median frequency The middle frequency when all Doppler shifts in the power spectrum are ranked lowest to highest.

megabyte Equals 2^{20} (1,048,576) bytes or 1024 kilobytes; generally denotes storage capacity.

megarayls Unit of acoustic impedance. Equals 10^6 kg/m²/sec.

microbubbles Encapsulated gas bubbles with a thin outer chemical coating that are strong scatterers of ultrasound. Type of contrast agent.

mirror-image artifact An artifact produced when an object is located in front of a very strong reflector. A second representation of the object is placed at the incorrect location distal to the strong reflector in the image.

misregistration The improper placement of a reflector in the image so that the geometric relationships of the structures are misrepresented.

M-mode scanning A scanning technique that depicts reflector position with respect to time in a two-dimensional display. M-mode scanning was originally called time motion, or TM, scanning.

mode frequency The prevalent Doppler shift in the power spectrum.

modem A device that converts digital signals to analog signals for transmission over telephone lines.

motion discrimination The ability to distinguish moving blood from moving tissue so that color encoding is applied to blood flow only.

multiformat camera Type of image-recording device using transparency film. A light image on a cathode ray tube is recorded on film.

multipath artifact An image artifact that occurs when the beam strikes multiple interfaces before returning to the transducer. The reflector is placed at the incorrect location with improper brightness.

narrowband transducer A transducer with a narrow frequency spectrum. The fractional bandwidth is less than 15%.

near field For the nonfocused transducer, the region from the front face extending to the beginning of divergence (corresponds to the last maximum). This is the area of the most narrow beam width.

near gain Also called the mean gain. An instrument setting for time gain compensation that controls amplification in the region close to the transducer.

neper A unit to describe a logarithmic loss in amplitude (e.g., pressure amplitude) from absorption, scattering processes, or both. The defining equation is

$$\text{loss (neper)} = \ln \frac{p}{p_0}$$

where p_0 is the initial pressure amplitude and p the pressure amplitude at the depth of interest.

One neper equals -8.686 dB.

network System of interconnected computers and devices that exchange data.

noise Random variations in signal amplitude measurements of detected echoes.

nonfocused transducer A transducer with no mechanical or electronic focusing. The beam is normally the width of the crystal in the near field, and it diverges rapidly in the far field.

nonlinear propagation At high intensity the sound wave is distorted from the sinusoidal shape with the introduction of additional frequency components (harmonics).

nonspecular reflector An interface with small physical dimensions (i.e., a wavelength or less in size). Nonspecular reflectors cause speckle in the image.

Nyquist limit The maximum frequency shift that can be measured in pulsed-wave Doppler without aliasing.

offset transducer A real-time transducer that uses a mirror to direct the ultrasound beam from the transducer to the patient and from the patient to the transducer.

optical density The amount of darkening of film, which is expressed as the logarithm of the ratio of incident to transmitted light.

Output Display Standard (ODS) The effect of current operating parameters on acoustic output expressed as the thermal index (TI) and the mechanical index (MI).

packet size The number of pulses used to sample a color line of sight in Doppler imaging. Also called ensemble length.

PACS Picture archiving and communication system—a computer network for the acquisition, display, and storage of images.

panning Translation of the write zoom field of view within the limits of the field of view imposed by the transducer.

parallel filter bank Detector with multiple filters designed to separate the frequency shifts in the Doppler signal.

parallel processing (transducer) The collection and processing of echo information from different scan lines simultaneously to improve frame rate performance.

partial volume The assignment of an intermediate signal level when the ultrasonic beam encompasses objects with different reflectivities.

particle displacement The distance traveled by vibrating particles from their mean positions when acted on by a force.

particle velocity The speed and direction at which the particles vibrate back and forth about their mean positions when acted on by a force. The particle velocity induced by a sound wave is not constant.

pascal A unit of acoustic pressure in the meter-kilogram-second system of measurement 1 N/m^2 (10^5 Pa equals 1 atm).

peak negative pressure The maximum rarefactional pressure produced by the sound wave.

percentage reflection The percentage of the incident beam intensity reflected from an acoustic interface.

percentage transmission The percentage of the incident beam intensity transmitted across an interface. Percentage transmission is calculated by subtracting the percentage reflection from 100.

period The time for one complete wave cycle. The period is the inverse of the wave frequency.

persistence A frame-averaging technique to reduce noise. Temporal resolution is degraded when persistence is activated.

phantom An object that mimics the properties of tissue (velocity, attenuation, and scattering) with respect to sound transmission.

phase aberration Loss of signal coherence during beam formation caused by acoustic velocity differences in tissue.

phased array A multielement transducer (linear phased array, rectangular array, or annular array) in which all the crystal elements are excited at or nearly at the same time. Short time delays (nanoseconds) are used to focus and sweep the beam.

phased linear array Antiquated term to describe the ability of a linear array to electronically focus the beam during transmission.

phosphorescent material A material that emits light when electromagnetic radiation or particles (usually electrons) are incident on the material. The coating on the screen of a cathode ray tube is composed of phosphorescent material.

piezoelectric effect An effect associated with materials having aligned dipolar molecules in which a pressure wave (sound wave) induces an electric signal in the material. This permits the material to be used as a receiver of sound waves. See **converse piezoelectric effect.**

pixel A small square or rectangular picture element in the digital image that represents a portion of the scanned area. The smallest spatial component of an image. Each pixel contains a value indicative of the intensity of the reflected echo.

Poiseuille's equation Volume flow rate in a cylindrical vessel depends on the viscosity of the fluid, the geometry of the vessel, and the pressure.

position generator The component in a static B-mode scanner that determines the displayed position of the interface.

position motion mode An alternate name for M-mode scanning.

position sensor The device in the registration arm that measures the position of the transducer. Signals from the sensor are sent into the position generator, which assigns spatial origin of the detected echo based on transducer position.

power A measure of the total energy transmitted summed over the entire cross-sectional area of the beam per unit time (intensity multiplied by area). The unit of power is the watt (joule per second).

power Doppler Doppler imaging technique in which the signal strength (not velocity) of moving reflectors at each sampling site is encoded by color.

power map Color assignment in Doppler imaging based on the intensity of the Doppler signal.

power pulse inversion harmonic imaging A type of dynamic imaging used in conjunction with contrast agents. Pulse inversion is used to isolate the harmonic components.

power spectrum Graphic representation of the spectral analysis in which the magnitude of each frequency is plotted as a function of frequency.

pressure difference The change in pressure along the vessel. Pressure difference provides a means to regulate flow.

pressure profile Measurements of pressure at various points in the ultrasonic field.

propagation The transmittal of sound energy to regions remote from the sound source.

propagation error The incorrect assignment of reflector size or position caused by acoustic velocity deviation from 1540 m/s along the beam path. Also called velocity error.

pulsatility index (PI) A means of quantifying the maximum velocity waveform with respect to shape. High values of PI indicate pulsatile flow.

pulse average The duration of a single pulse prescribes the time interval over which the intensity is measured.

pulse duration (temporal pulse length) The time interval during which the transmitted pulse is generated. The pulse duration is calculated by multiplying the number of cycles in the pulse times the period.

pulse inversion harmonic imaging A type of dynamic imaging used in conjunction with contrast agents. Pulse inversion is used to isolate the harmonic components.

pulse repetition frequency (PRF) The number of times a transmitted pulsed wave is generated each second. The maximum PRF depends on the scan range (R) and the velocity of ultrasound (c):

$$PRF_{max} = \frac{c}{2R}$$

pulse repetition period (PRP) The time needed to transmit a pulsed wave and detect the returning echoes. It is equal to the inverse of the pulse repetition frequency.

pulser System component that generates electronic signals to stimulate piezoelectric crystal to emit ultrasound waves. Also called the transmitter.

quadrature detection The formation of in-phase and out-of-phase signals by dividing the received signal into two components, mixing with the phase-adjusted reference signal, and demodulating the resulting waveforms.

quadrature phase detection Doppler detection method to identify the direction of motion. The Doppler signal is divided into two components, mixed separately with in-phase and out-of-phase reference signals, and filtered. The relative phase between the two components is examined.

quality control (QC) The routine testing of equipment to ensure proper functioning. An effective QC program is necessary to obtain high-quality images on a consistent basis.

quarter wavelength transducer A transducer that uses a one-quarter wavelength matching layer in front of the crystal to reduce the crystal–tissue impedance mismatch.

Q-value A transducer parameter that characterizes the pulse length and bandwidth of the transducer.

radial mode vibration For a circular or disc-shaped crystal, the expansion and contraction along the face of the crystal, which produces side lobes.

radiation force Acoustic pressure applied over the surface of the object that causes translational or rotational motion.

radiology information system (RIS) A computer system that acts as a dynamic database for patient information associated with imaging procedures.

RAID Redundant array of independent disks—multiple magnetic disks configured in an array for the electronic storage of image data and the associated patient information.

random access memory (RAM) Type of computer memory in which information is written or read by specific location (address).

range ambiguity artifact The misplacement of an interface when the assumption that each echo derived from the most recent transmit pulse is violated.

range gate The selection of a time interval (time delay and time length) after pulsed-wave transmission during which the detected echoes are processed for display. Since distance from the transducer is defined by the elapsed time, analysis is restricted to echoes originating from a specific depth.

rarefaction A low-pressure region or a region of decreased density in a medium created by the action of the sound wave.

raster scan A line-by-line output of information on the display device. The pattern is similar to the way in which we read a book with each line scanned left to right.

rayl The unit of acoustic impedance, which is equal to kilogram per square meter per second.

Rayleigh scattering Scattering from small structures with dimensions less than the wavelength of the sound wave.

read mode The process in the scan converter used to display the image in a continuous fashion. A new scan cannot be obtained while in the read-only mode.

read-only memory (ROM) Type of computer memory that allows access only to read the stored information. The contents of ROM cannot be altered.

read zoom During display, a method to magnify the image size on the monitor.

real-time scanning An automated scanning technique in which a rapid series of images is acquired and displayed one after the other to depict motion or changing field of view.

receiver operating characteristics (ROC) curve A graphic method of summarizing the performance of multiple observers or diagnostic tests to identify patients with and without disease.

reception coefficient A transducer factor that determines how efficiently the returning echo is converted to an electrical signal.

reception zone The region within an ultrasonic field from which echoes can be detected.

rectification The electronic process of changing the negative component of the radiofrequency signal to positive or eliminating the negative components from the signal.

reflection An interaction that results in part of the sound being redirected into the medium from which it came after striking an acoustic interface. The angle of incidence equals the angle of reflection. The intensity of the reflected wave depends on the composition of the interface.

reflectivity The combination of factors—including acoustic impedance mismatch, size, shape, and angle of incidence—that determine the intensity of a reflected echo from an interface.

refraction A process whereby sound enters one medium from another, resulting in a bending or deviation of a sound beam from the expected straight-line path. Refraction obeys Snell's law, which is based on the ratio of the velocity of sound in the respective media. Refraction creates artifacts in the image by the misregistration of structures.

registration arm A mechanical device on which the static B-mode transducer is mounted. The position sensors in the registration arm provide the signals for the position generator.

reject Electronic processing that discards signals that are less than a selected level.

relaxation time A time indicative of the rate in which a molecule returns to its original position after being displaced by a force.

reperfusion imaging An imaging technique to show the temporal changes in the distribution of the contrast agent.

resistive index A means of quantifying the maximum velocity waveform to evaluate downstream resistance to flow.

reverberation An artifact created in B-mode imaging when repeated reflections occur between two strong reflectors.

ring-down artifact An image artifact created when an object vibrates at a characteristic resonance frequency. This artifact resembles a comet tail artifact without the specific banding seen with the comet tail.

ringing The phenomenon of continued expansion and contraction of a crystal after being subjected to a short excitation pulse. A short ring time produces a short temporal pulse length and thus good axial resolution. Ringing depends on the Q-value, matching layer, and the backing material used in the transducer.

risks versus benefits An assessment of the potential harm associated with a particular procedure compared with the expected medical outcome.

scan converter A device that stores scan data as echo signal strengths corresponding to the detected locations of the interfaces. This enables image formation using encoding of echo amplitudes.

scan cross-sectional area For autoscanning systems, the area on the surface through which the beam passes during a scan.

scan line Echoes from reflectors encountered along the path of the directed ultrasound beam are registered linearly with depth. Multiple scan lines compose each real-time image.

scan range The maximum depth from which a returning echo can be detected with the correct assignment of location of origin. The maximum depth of the field of view.

scattering The redirection of sound energy resulting from the sound beam striking an interface whose physical dimension is less than one wavelength. It is also called nonspecular reflection.

scattering coefficient A parameter that characterizes the rate at which sound energy is scattered by a medium. Expressed as fractional loss per unit distance.

sector scanner A real-time mechanical or electronic phased array that produces a pie-shaped field of view.

segmented linear array An array of crystals in which groups of crystals are fired one after the other. The time delay between element group activations is dictated by the depth of interest.

sensitivity (instrument performance) The overall ability of the system to detect weak-reflecting objects at a specific distance from the transducer.

sensitivity (statistic) A statistical index of diagnostic test performance denoting the percentage of all subjects with disease that yields a positive test result.

sensitometer strip A multistep gray-scale pattern used to evaluate film processor performance.

sequential linear array An array of crystals in which each element is fired individually one after the other. The time delay between crystal activations is dictated by the depth of interest.

server A computer that performs specific tasks (data locator, storage, or printing) for other computers within the network.

shadowing The reflectors distal to a highly attenuating object appear lower in signal strength than adjacent reflectors with similar reflectivities.

side lobes Secondary intensity lobes displaced from the main beam, which are created by interference.

signal The voltage variation induced by a pressure wave incident on a piezoelectric crystal. The subsequent manipulation of a time-dependent voltage pattern is called signal processing.

signal processing The manipulation of a received echo signal to enhance the presentation of scan data.

signal-to-noise ratio (SNR) The strength of the echo signal as compared with the noise level. Contrast resolution and sensitivity improve as the SNR is increased.

single-sideband Doppler detection method designed to identify the direction of motion. A filter technique to isolate the forward and reverse motions is employed.

slice thickness The out-of-plane thickness of the body that is scanned for the formation of the ultrasound image.

slope (M-mode) A means to measure velocity of a moving reflector.

slope (TGC) A description of the amount of TGC amplification with depth.

smoothing A spatial filtering technique for reducing noise in the image.

Snell's law A mathematic description of the principle of refraction that relates the bending of the wave with the ratio of the acoustic velocities for the media.

sound Mechanical vibrations or pressure waves that the human ear can detect. The frequency range is between 20 and 20,000 Hz. Sound waves require a medium for propagation. The term *sound* is commonly used in the broad sense to include mechanical vibrations of all frequencies, including ultrasound.

spatial average Average of intensity measurements over the cross-sectional area of the beam.

spatial average intensity The same as spatial average, temporal average intensity (SATA). Generally, this parameter is used when specifying the continuous waveform. National Eclectic Medical Association standard.

spatial average, pulse average intensity (I[SAPA]) The pulse average intensity averaged over the beam cross-sectional area. May be approximated as the ratio of ultrasonic power to the product of duty factor and beam cross-sectional area. National Eclectic Medical Association standard.

spatial average, temporal average intensity (I[SATA]) For autoscanning systems, the temporal average intensity averaged over the scan cross-sectional area on a surface specified. May be approximated as the ratio of ultrasonic power to the scan cross-sectional area or as the mean value of that ratio if it is not the same on each scan. For nonautoscanning systems, SATA is the temporal average intensity averaged over the beam cross-sectional area. May be approximated as the ratio of ultrasonic power to the beam cross-sectional area. National Eclectic Medical Association standard.

spatial average, temporal peak intensity (I[SATP]) The value of the temporal peak intensity averaged over the beam cross-sectional area or scan cross-sectional area for autoscanning systems.

spatial compounding A real-time imaging method in which scan lines for consecutive frames are steered at different angles, and the data collections are summed to form a composite image.

spatial filtering An image-processing technique to reduce noise or enhance boundaries between structures. In Doppler imaging spatial filtering presents areas of flow with more uniform color by allowing pixels to be color encoded only if the adjacent pixels are depicted in color.

spatial peak Location in the ultrasonic field where the measured parameter has the highest value.

spatial peak, pulse-averaged intensity (I[SPPA]) The value of the pulse-averaged intensity at the point in the acoustic field where the pulse-averaged intensity is a maximum or a local maximum within a specified region. National Eclectic Medical Association standard.

spatial peak, temporal average intensity (I[SPTA]) The value of the temporal average intensity at the point in the acoustic field where the temporal average intensity is a maximum or a local maximum within a specified region. National Eclectic Medical Association standard.

spatial peak, temporal peak intensity (I[SPTP]) The value of the temporal peak intensity at the point in the acoustic field where the temporal peak intensity is a maximum or a local maximum within a specified region. National Eclectic Medical Association standard.

spatial pulse length The spatial extent of an ultrasound pulse burst. The spatial pulse length is the product of the number of cycles in the pulse and the wavelength.

specificity A statistical index of diagnostic test performance denoting the percentage of all subjects without disease that yields a negative test result.

speckle Interference pattern incident on a transducer produced by echoes that have undergone multipath scattering. The signal does not exhibit a one-to-one correspondence with the scatters. The speckle pattern is frequency dependent.

speckle tracking A two-dimensional time domain correlation technique for measuring reflector velocity in both axial and lateral directions.

spectral analysis The technique for identifying frequency components in a signal or waveform.

spectral broadening The introduction of additional frequency components in the complex Doppler signal caused by limitations in the detection technique.

spectrum analysis The process of determining the individual Doppler shifts that are present in the complex Doppler signal and the relative importance of each.

spectrum analyzer A device that identifies the frequency components of a signal.

specular reflector An interface larger than the width of the sound beam.

stable cavitation The expansion and contraction of pre-existing microbubbles in response to the applied pressure oscillations.

standard deviation A statistic that indicates the amount of variability in a collection of measurements.

stenosis A narrowing or constriction of a vessel that alters the dynamics of blood flow.

step-down segmental array An electronic array in which a segment of crystals is excited to transmit a pulse and remains silent to listen for echoes before the next pulse is transmitted. The newest segment contains the same number of crystals, but it is offset from the previous segment by one crystal.

string phantom A device to evaluate the flow angle indicators, sample volume, wall filter, and sensitivity of Doppler scanners.

strip chart recorder An output device to record the M-mode tracing.

subdicing The crystal element of an array is divided into several smaller subelements. These subelements are electrically wired together to act conjointly. Subdicing helps reduce the intensity of the grating lobes.

super video home system (VHS) A type of recording format for magnetic tape. Super VHS provides superior spatial resolution compared with VHS.

synchronous scanner A type of scanner for Doppler imaging in which gray-scale and flow data are acquired simultaneously along a line of sight.

thermal mechanism Mechanism by which damage can be induced by the generation of heat.

threshold A value that must be exceeded to cause damage.

temporal average intensity The time average of intensity at a point in space; equal to the mean value of the intensity at the point considered. For nonautoscanning systems, the average is taken over one or more pulse-repetition periods. For autoscanning systems, the intensity is averaged over one or more scan repetition periods for a specific operating mode. National Eclectic Medical Association standard.

temporal peak intensity The peak value of the intensity at the point considered. National Eclectic Medical Association standard.

temporal resolution The ability to depict the movement of structures accurately.

test object A device used to evaluate scanner performance. The material composing the test object usually mimics the velocity of sound in a tissue. Small, strong reflectors are placed in well-defined geometric patterns within the test object to assess axial resolution, dead zone, distance accuracy, and lateral resolution.

thermal index The ratio of the in situ acoustic power to the acoustic power required to raise tissue temperature by 1° C.

thickness mode vibration The normal vibrational mode of the crystal that dictates the center frequency of sound transmitted from the transducer. The expansions and contractions of the crystal occur along the axis of the transducer.

time domain correlation A processing technique in Doppler imaging whereby a series of echoes from the same reflector is examined to assess motion. Reflector velocity is obtained by measuring the time shift of the echoes.

time of flight The time required for an ultrasonic wave to leave the transducer, strike an interface, and return to the transducer.

time gain compensation (TGC) A method of increasing amplification of the signal with depth to compensate for loss caused by attenuation.

time-motion mode An alternate name for M-mode.

tissue characterization The identification of tissue type for a specific pathologic diagnosis by noninvasive means.

tissue harmonic imaging Imaging mode that detects harmonic frequencies created by nonlinear propagation of ultrasound through tissue.

tissue-mimicking (TM) phantom A phantom made of materials that permit it to mimic the ultrasonic properties of tissue with respect to velocity, attenuation, and scattering. Small, strong reflectors are placed in well-defined geometric patterns within the phantom to assess axial resolution, lateral resolution, dead zone, and distance accuracy.

TM-mode scanning The original name of M-mode scanning, because the motion of the interface was plotted with respect to time.

topology Configuration of data communication pathways for components linked together in a computer network.

total reflection A refraction process that prevents sound from entering a second medium from the first medium, because the critical angle is reached or exceeded.

transducer Any device that converts one form of energy into another form. In ultrasound, a piezoelectric crystal converts an electrical stimulus into an ultrasound pulse and the returning echo into an electrical signal.

transient cavitation Short-lived bubbles undergo large variation in size before completely collapsing.

transit time broadening Introduction of frequency components above and below the actual Doppler shift, because sampling is performed with a finite beam size.

transmission coefficient (reflection) A coefficient that describes the fraction of intensity of a beam transmitted through an acoustic interface.

transmission coefficient (transducer factor) The efficiency by which an excitation voltage pulse is converted to ultrasound energy.

transmission-mode scanning An ultrasonic scanning technique that measures the intensity of the ultrasound wave transmitted through a patient. This is the only diagnostic ultrasound imaging technique that does not rely on the echo-ranging principle.

transonography Alternate term for endosonography.

transparency film A hard copy image recording on film in which gray levels are regulated by the amount of transmitted light.

transverse pressure profile A measure of the acoustic pressure perpendicular to the axis of the beam.

transverse wave The motion of the particles in the medium is perpendicular to the direction of wave propagation.

triphasic waveform The maximum velocity waveform exhibits three distinct segments of forward and reverse flow during a cardiac cycle.

turbulence A type of flow in a vessel characterized by cross currents and multiple velocity components.

two-dimensional image The spatial composition of the origins of echoes. The two spatial coordinates for each detected echo are determined by the scan line and the echo-ranging principle.

ultrasonic field The region over which sound energy is transmitted.

ultrasound High-frequency (>20 kHz) mechanical vibrations or pressure waves that the human ear cannot detect.

uniformity Signals obtained for interfaces with similar reflective properties located at the same depth have the same amplitude.

universal serial bus (USB) A serial communication standard for rapid transfer of information between devices connected to the computer.

variance A statistical parameter that indicates the variability in a set of measurements.

variance map Color assignment in Doppler imaging based on the distribution of velocities within the sampling volume.

velocity (c) The rate and direction at which sound propagates through a medium. The average velocity of sound in soft tissue is 1540 m/s.

velocity error The incorrect assignment of reflector size or position caused by acoustic velocity deviation from 1540 m/s along the beam path. Also called propagation error.

velocity map The assignment of various color hues or saturation based on flow velocity in Doppler imaging.

velocity profile The distribution of flow velocities across the vessel. Laminar flow yields a distinctive pattern in which the velocity increases rapidly with distance from the vessel wall.

velocity scale In flow detection, the range of velocities that can be displayed without aliasing.

velocity tag Doppler imaging parameter that allows a selected range of velocities to be depicted in a contrasting color (usually green or white).

vertical distance Measurement of distance in the direction along the axis of the beam.

VHS (video home system) A type of recording format for magnetic tape.

video printer An image-recording device that receives the image data in the form of a video signal. The print medium is paper.

video signal The industry standard television format consisting of 30 frames per second and 525 lines per frame for electronic transmission of images.

videocassette recorder A magnetic tape recorder that records a series of images in real time for subsequent playback. A 1/2-inch magnetic tape in a cassette is used with the videocassette recorder.

viscosity A parameter that describes the ability of molecules in a medium to move past each other.

volume flow rate The quantity of blood per unit time flowing through a vessel.

wall filter A high-pass filter that eliminates low-frequency Doppler shifts associated with slow-moving structures such as the vessel wall.

watt A unit of ultrasonic power. One watt is equivalent to 1 J/sec.

wavefront The compression zone within one wave cycle. Successive wavefronts illustrate the beam pattern generated by an ultrasound source.

wavelength A physical characteristic of a wave that is the distance for one complete wave cycle.

width focusing Focusing of the ultrasound beam in a plane perpendicular to both the beam axis and the direction in which the beam sweeps. Also called slice thickness or out-of-plane focusing.

width-mode vibration For a linear array, the expansion and contraction of the rectangular element along the width (direction of mechanical focusing) of the array. This type of vibration can cause interelement coupling, thereby inducing artifacts in the final image.

word A combination of bits treated as a single entity by the computer. The number of bits in the word dictates the number of different configurations (or values) that can be represented.

word length The number of bits in a computer word.

workstation Computer with specialized graphics for the processing and display of digital images.

write mode Collection of data by the scan converter during the scanning process. As each line of sight is collected, the echoes are mapped in a two-dimensional spatial matrix by the scan converter.

write zoom Magnification technique applied during data collection to improve the spatial detail by mapping the detected echoes in a field of view with reduced physical dimensions.

zero-crossing detector A device that monitors the rate of oscillation of the complex Doppler signal. The rate of zero-crossings is indicative of the frequency shifts present in the Doppler signal.

Index

Page numbers followed by f indicate figures; t, tables; b, boxes.